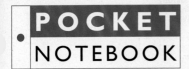

Pocket
INTERVENTIONAL
RADIOLOGY

Edited by

SHIRAZ RAHIM, MD
Vascular and Interventional Radiology Fellow
University Hospitals Case Medical Center
Cleveland, Ohio

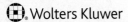

. Wolters Kluwer

Philadelphia • Baltimore • New York • London
Buenos Aires • Hong Kong • Sydney • Tokyo

Senior Acquisitions Editor: Sharon Zinner
Editorial Coordinator: Lindsay Ries
Strategic Marketing Manager: Rachel Mante Leung
Production Project Manager: David Saltzberg
Design Coordinator: Stephen Druding
Manufacturing Coordinator: Beth Welsh
Prepress Vendor: Aptara, Inc.

9 8 7 6 5 4 3 2 1

Printed in China

978-1-4963-8972-5
1-4963-8972-7
Library of Congress Cataloging-in-Publication Data
available upon request

CCS1018

CONTRIBUTORS

John E. Anderson, DO
Radiology Resident
Case Western Reserve University
University Hospitals Cleveland Medical Center
Cleveland, Ohio

Mark W. Anderson, MD
Musculoskeletal Imaging Attending
University of Virginia Health System
Charlottesville, Virginia

Teodora Bochnakova, MD
Vascular and Interventional Radiology Fellow
Harvard Medical School
Massachusetts General Hospital
Boston, Massachusetts

Matthew D. Brocone, MD, MS
Vascular and Interventional Radiology Attending
Case Western Reserve University
Louis Stokes VA Medical Center
Cleveland, Ohio

Ji Buethe, MD
Vascular and Interventional Radiology Attending
Johns Hopkins University
Baltimore, Maryland

Majid Chalian, MD
Musculoskeletal Imaging Attending
University of Texas
Austin, Texas
UT Southwestern Medical Center
Dallas, Texas

Spencer Couturier, MD
Radiology Resident
Stanford University
Stanford, California

Jon C. Davidson, MD, FSIR
Vascular and Interventional Radiology Attending, VIR
Fellowship Director
Case Western Reserve University
University Hospitals Cleveland Medical Center
Cleveland, Ohio

Robert Hunt Dunlap III, MD
Radiology Resident
Johns Hopkins University
Baltimore, Maryland

Jeffrey Farrell, MD
Vascular and Interventional Radiology Fellow
The Ohio State University Wexner Medical Center
Columbus, Ohio

Cree Gaskin, MD
Vice Chair and Chief Medical Information Officer
Musculoskeletal Imaging Attending
University of Virginia Health System
Charlottesville, Virginia

Andrew Gibby, MD
Vascular and Interventional Radiology Fellow
Washington University in St. Louis
St. Louis, Missouri

Karin A. Herrmann, MD, PhD
Abdominal Imaging Attending
Case Western Reserve University
University Hospitals Cleveland Medical Center
Cleveland, Ohio

Paul Hulsberg, MD
Vascular and Interventional Radiology Fellow
University of Florida
Gainesville, Florida

Anouva Kalra-Lall, BA
Medical Student
Case Western Reserve University
University Hospitals Cleveland Medical Center
Cleveland, Ohio

Preet Kang, MD, MSIR
Vascular and Interventional Radiology Attending
Case Western Reserve University
Louis Stokes VA Medical Center
Cleveland, Ohio

Elias Kikano, MD
Radiology Resident
Case Western Reserve University
University Hospitals Cleveland Medical Center
Cleveland, Ohio

Frank Kowalkowski, DO
Radiology Resident
Case Western Reserve University
University Hospitals Cleveland Medical Center
Cleveland, Ohio

Divya Kumari, MD
Radiology Resident
Case Western Reserve University
University Hospitals Cleveland Medical Center
Cleveland, Ohio

Payam Lahiji, MD
Radiology Resident
Case Western Reserve University
University Hospitals Cleveland Medical Center
Cleveland, Ohio

Bahar Mansoori, MD
Abdominal Imaging Clinical Fellow
University of Texas
Austin, Texas
UT Southwestern Medical Center
Dallas, Texas

Janice D. McDaniel, MD
Vascular and Interventional Radiology Attending
Akron Children's Hospital
Akron, Ohio

Eric D. McLoney, MD
Vascular and Interventional Radiology Attending
Case Western Reserve University
University Hospitals Cleveland Medical Center
Cleveland, Ohio

Nathaniel McQuay, Jr., MD
Trauma, Surgical Critical Care and Acute Care Surgery Attending
Case Western Reserve University
University Hospitals Cleveland Medical Center
Cleveland, Ohio

Anna J. Moreland, MD
Radiology Resident
Johns Hopkins Hospital
Baltimore, Maryland

Nicholas C. Nacey, MD
Musculoskeletal Imaging Attending
University of Virginia Health System
Charlottesville, Virginia

Dean Nakamoto, MD
Abdominal Imaging and Intervention Attending
Case Western Reserve University
University Hospitals Cleveland Medical Center
Cleveland, Ohio

Jeffrey T. Nelson, MD
Neurointerventional Fellow
Department of Neurological Surgery
Case Western Reserve University
University Hospitals Cleveland Medical Center
Cleveland, Ohio

Verena Obmann, MD
Radiology Research Fellow
Case Western Reserve University
University Hospitals Cleveland Medical Center
Cleveland, Ohio

Indravadan Patel, MD
Vascular and Interventional Radiology Attending, Section Chief
Case Western Reserve University
University Hospitals Cleveland Medical Center
Cleveland, Ohio

Jennifer Pierce, MD
Musculoskeletal Imaging Attending
University of Virginia Health System
Charlottesville, Virginia

Shiraz Rahim, MD
Vascular and Interventional Radiology Fellow
University Hospitals Case Medical Center
Cleveland, Ohio

Maharshi Rajdev, MD
Radiology Resident
Case Western Reserve University
University Hospitals Cleveland Medical Center
Cleveland, Ohio

Vikram Rajpurohit, MD
Radiology Resident
Johns Hopkins Hospital
Baltimore, Maryland

Jonathan Rischall, MD
Vascular and Interventional Radiology Fellow
George Washington University Hospital
Washington, DC

Daniel J. Scher, MD
Vascular and Interventional Radiology Attending
George Washington University Hospital
Washington, DC

Rishi Sood, MD
Radiology Resident
George Washington University Hospital
Washington, DC

Christopher Sutter, MD
Vascular and Interventional Radiology Attending
Case Western Reserve University
University Hospitals Cleveland Medical Center
Cleveland, Ohio

Sidharta Tavri, MBBS, DABR
Vascular and Interventional Radiology Attending
Case Western Reserve University
University Hospitals Cleveland Medical Center
Cleveland, Ohio

Lisa Walker, MD
Radiology Resident
Case Western Reserve University
University Hospitals Cleveland Medical Center
Cleveland, Ohio

ACKNOWLEDGMENTS

To my mother and father who always believed in me and supported me throughout my journey.

I would like to thank all of the contributors without whom this book would not be possible. This textbook is the culmination of efforts of residents, fellows, and attending physicians at several institutions who are experts in their field and have worked tirelessly to bring their expertise to the pages of this book. I am especially grateful to my mentor, attending physicians, and the interventional radiology staff at Case Western Reserve University, for their guidance throughout my training and the help they provided in evaluating and editing content to ensure it was up-to-date, evidence based, and represented the best and most useful information for the topics included. I would also like to thank my family for their help and support throughout the process of writing this first textbook. Lastly, I would like to thank the publishers and editing team at LWW for accepting my book proposal, for their help throughout the process of creating the final version of this book, and for giving us the ability to bring this text to trainees everywhere.

SHIRAZ RAHIM, MD

PREFACE

Out of all of the specialties in medicine, interventional radiology has probably had one of the most drastic changes in terms of how it is practiced and taught throughout the country. Since its inception with the techniques of Seldinger and the advent of the cardiac catheterization, endovascular and imaging-guided treatments have become a mainstay of patient care. But where interventional radiologists had previously taken the role of technician and only involved themselves as a consultant role in patient care, they have now become a more central part of the interdisciplinary care team and become more and more involved in how care is delivered and how medicine is practiced at most hospitals. This is nowhere more evident than with the creation of the interventional radiology residency, a distinct training pathway that seeks to train physicians to not only become consultants but also primary drivers of medical care and active participants in interdisciplinary management teams. The changes in our field have brought interventionalists back into the spotlight.

With this growing role of interventionalists has come rapid changes in the technologies and tools available to proceduralists. More and more diagnoses can be treated with minimally invasive and imaging-guided techniques. These changes not only make it a great time to be an interventionalist, but also make it essential for new trainees to understand the clinical aspects of the procedures they can now offer in order to continue being an important part of the patient care team. Our patients, referrers, and colleagues expect us to know the research and decision-making process around the types of diseases we can treat.

It is these changes and raised expectations that drove the creation of this text. Although there are several texts already available to teach medical students, residents, and fellows about the techniques in interventional radiology, this text aims to serve the current void in the textbook literature to include clinical aspects of interventional radiology education. It brings together a quick overview of procedures that trainees can use quickly before a procedure and the most current research, tips and tricks, and evidence-based guidelines they should know for making quick management decisions for their patients. Building on the formats of the other books in the Pocket series, it seeks to be a quick reference that offers the reader key updates and important information that can help on a day-to-day basis.

Thank you for turning to this text for your learning needs, and I hope the information contained within will help you achieve the goal that all of us physicians strive daily to perfect: to deliver the best care for our patients.

SHIRAZ RAHIM, MD

CONTENTS

PERI-OPERATIVE WORKUP

Patient Preparation (*JVIR 2016;27:695–9; CIR 2016;39:325–33*)
- **History and Physical:** Guides disease management
  Prior Interventions and Altered Anatomy
  Imaging: Prior imaging (Radiography, US/Echo, CT, MRI, NM) and prior interventions
  Allergies
  Patient Characteristics: Airway management, ability to maintain desired position, refusal of blood products
- **Screening Tests** (*JVIR 2012;23:727–36*)
  Consider complexity/invasiveness and patient risk factors (age, HTN, DM, CHF, ARF/ CRF, coag, medications with common toxicities)
  Hb/Hct, WBC, Platelets, INR, aPTT, LFT

INR/PT	Extrinsic I/II/V/VII/X, Oral AC, Liver dz	0.9–1.1
aPTT	Intrinsic VIII/IX/XI/XII, IV Heparin, von Willebrand, Factor VIII/IX/XI Def, Lupus AC, Liver dz, DIC, Vit K def	25–35 s
Platelet	Thrombocytopenia	150,000–450,000/μL

*Antiplatelet Agents – Consider Platelet Function Assay

- **Informed Consent** (*ACR-SIR Practice Parameter 2016*)
  Capacity: Assessment and proxy algorithm per institutions guidelines (HC POA, next of kin, etc.)
  Obtaining Consent
  1. Basic information (medical condition/need for procedure)
  2. General nature/overview of procedure/analgesia/sedation
  3. Alternatives, benefits, and risks
     - Material risk: Anything a "reasonable person" would consider important
     - Procedure/sedation/radiation risks
  4. Realistic expectations, postprocedure care
  5. Provide time to make decision and option to refuse/seek second opinion
  6. Review consent when significant time has passed or a change in medical status that may affect outcome
  7. Special circumstances
     - Emergencies: Provide treatment only when necessary to save life or prevent significant deterioration
     - Pregnancy: Discuss potential radiation risk
     - Pediatrics: Parents/legal guardian
- **Pre-Procedure Checklist** (*JVIR 2016;27:695–9*): Reduces mortality/morbidity
  Patient identifiers (at least 2), allergies, contrast, premedication, Abx, sedation, lab values, blood products, imaging, specimen collection, radiation, MRI safety, special equipment, consent, pregnancy test
  - **Preprocedure verification**
  - **Site marking**
  - **Time out**

Hemostasis Preparation (*JVIR 2013;24:641–5*)
Risk relates to nature of the procedure

Bleeding risk	Procedure	Management
Low	**V**: Dialysis access, venography, CVC removal, IVC filter/PICC placement **NV**: Drainage cath Ex, Thora/ Para, superficial Asp/Bx/drainage	INR >2.0 for tx (FFP, Vit K) Plt <50,000/μL for transfusion Clopidogrel: Withhold 5 d prior Warfarin: Withhold 3–5 d prior ASA: Do not withhold LMWH: Withhold 1 dose Dabigatran/bivalirudin: Do not withhold Abciximab: Withhold 12–24 h prior Eptifibatide: Withhold immediately prior

Bleeding risk	Procedure	Management
Moderate	**V:** Arterial (size <7F)/venous intervention, chemoembo, UFE, transjugular liver bx, tunneled CVC, port placement **NV:** Intra-abd, chest wall, lung, RP abscess drainage/bx, transabdominal liver bx, perc chole, G-tube placement, RFA simple, spine	INR >1.5 for tx Plt <50,000/μL Clopidogrel: Withhold 5 d prior Warfarin: Withhold 5 d prior ASA: Do not withhold Dabigatran: Defer procedure/if stat withhold 2–5 d dep on CrCl Bivalirudin: Defer procedure/if stat withhold 2–5 h dep on CrCl Abciximab: Withhold 24 h prior Eptifibatide: Withhold 4 h prior
High	**V:** TIPS **NV:** Renal Bx, new biliary interventions, nephrostomy placement, RFA complex	INR >1.5 for tx aPTT: Stop or reverse if >1.5× Plt <50,000/μL Clopidogrel: Withhold 5 d prior Warfarin: Withhold 5 d prior ASA: Withhold for 5 d LMWH: Withhold 24 h/2 doses Dabigatran: Defer procedure/if stat withhold 2–5 d dep on CrCl Bivalirudin: Defer procedure/if stat withhold 2–5 h dep on CrCl Abciximab: Withhold 24 h prior Eptifibatide: Withhold 4 h prior

High-Risk Patients
- **ASA Physical Status Classification:** Common grading of preprocedural physical condition. The score is not a prognostic indicator.

American Society of Anesthesiologists (ASA) Physical Status Classification	
ASA I	Normal healthy patient
ASA II	Mild systemic disease (current smoker, social alcohol drinker, pregnancy, obesity, well-controlled DM/HTN)
ASA III	Moderate to severe systemic disease (functional limitations: Poorly controlled DM, HTN, COPD, morbid obesity, active hepatitis, alcohol dependence, heart failure, ESRD, MI, CVA, CAD)
ASA IV	Severe systemic disease (recent MI, CVA, ongoing cardiac ischemia, severe valve dysfunction, sepsis, etc.)
ASA V	Substantial risk of death within 24 h (ruptured abdominal/thoracic aortic aneurysm, trauma, intracranial bleed, ischemic bowel)
ASA VI	Brain-dead patient whose organs are being removed for donor purposes

- **Non–Insulin-Dependent Diabetes – Metformin** (ACR Manual 2017)
  Category I: No evidence of AKI, eGFR >30; continue metformin, no need to reassess after procedure
  Category II: AKI or severe CKD (stage IV or V), eGFR <30, or undergoing arterial catheter studies that may result in emboli to renal arteries; discontinue at time of procedure and withhold for 48 h subsequently. Reconstitute after renal function re-evaluated.
- **Insulin-Dependent Diabetes**
  Avoid prolonged fasting, schedule early procedures
  Continue long-acting insulin, hold short-acting insulin
  Fluids: D5 to provide basal glucose and avoid hypoglycemia
- **Post-Contrast Acute Kidney Injury/Contrast-Induced Nephropathy**
  (ACR Manual 2017)
  PC-AKI: Deterioration of renal function within 48 h of iodinated contrast administration
  CIN: Specific term to describe renal function deterioration *caused* by iodinated contrast
  Commonly defined as 0.5 mg/dL rise in Cr
  Iso-osmolar iodine contrast may minimize risk
  Minimize use of NSAIDs, ACE-I, loop diuretics

---

*Gadolinium-based contrast media; does not cause CIN/or exceptionally rare

- **Hypertension** (*Radiographics 2015;35:1776–8*)
  Most commonly caused by pre-existing hypertension
  Exacerbated by anxiety/pain. Increased risk of bleeding/hematoma formation
  Control blood pressure to <180/100 mmHg. Avoid drop by more than 25%

Common Periprocedural Antihypertensives	
Hydralazine	2.5–10 mg IV, may cause reflex tachycardia
Labetalol	5–20 mg IV q10
Nitroglycerin	0.4 mg sublingual, paste 0.5–2 in topically
CKD 5 (eGFR <15)	Same as CKD Stage 4 Avoid further contrast for 72 h

Posttreatment Care (*JVIR 2016;27:695–9; CIR 2017;40:481–95*)
- **Documentation:** "Brief OP note," Procedure report
- **Monitoring:** Vital signs, pain, bleeding/hematoma, patient positioning
- **Specific procedure orders:** Catheter/line instructions—drainage/flushing, lung biopsies—chest radiograph for pneumothorax, biopsy—label and submit samples
- **Common overnight admissions:** New drains, angioplasty, TACE, nephrostomy/double J, UAE, lung Bx with pneumothorax → chest tube, tPA infusion, etc.
- **Analgesia**
- **Diet, activity**

CONTRAST, SEDATION, ANALGESIA

CONTRAST

- Anatomic visualizations require sufficient difference in x-ray attenuation between the target and surroundings
- Requires appropriate fluoroscopic parameters and extrinsic contrast agents
- Catheter-specific flow rates, vessels, flow rate, quantity, duration
- Injection considerations: Power injectors vs. manual injection, catheter flow rates, specific vessel imaging
  - Air embolism: Left lateral decubitus, administer 100% O_2, hyperbaric oxygen

General Types of Contrast
- Iodinate contrast material (ICM): Eg, iohexol, iopamidol, iodixanol
  - Iodine load varies (~300 mg/mL) but can be diluted with saline
- Gadolinium contrast material: Eg, gadobutrol, gadobenate, gadopentetate
- Carbon dioxide (CO_2): Negative contrast
  - Subtraction angiography DSA
  - CO_2 rapidly dissolves in blood and is excreted through lungs
  - Used to measure hepatic wedge pressure (TIPSS)
  - Cerebral toxicity: Avoid intra-arterial use above diaphragm or intravenously in pts with left right shunt

Premedication for Contrast Reactions (ACR Manual on Contrast Media 2017)
- Premedication reduces likelihood of mild reactions in average risk pts. Inconclusive evidence for prevention of moderate/severe reactions.
- Premedication risks: Glucocorticoids (transient leukocytosis, hyperglycemia, infection), antihistamines (drowsiness)
- Breakthrough reactions (~2%) similar in severity to index reaction
- Common risks/historic considerations for acute reaction:
  - Prior reaction (5×), atopy/asthma (2–3×)
  - Myasthenia gravis: Conflicting evidence
  - Suspected pheo, thyrotoxicosis (except those in acute thyroid storm), sickle cell disease: No evidence to support specific precautions
  - Beta-blockers: Do not premedicate or discontinue
  - No increased risk if allergic to shellfish or contrast of another class

Premedication is not a substitute for preadministration preparedness

	ACR Premedication Regimens		
Elective	Prednisone 50 mg PO or Hydrocortisone 200 mg IV **13, 7, 1 h** OR Methylprednisolone 32 mg PO **12, 2 h**	Diphenhydramine 50 mg IV/IM/PO 1 h Optional	
Accelerated	Methylprednisolone 40 mg IV or Hydrocortisone 200 mg IV **STAT and every 4 h**	Diphenhydramine 50 mg IV 1 h	At least 4–5 h
	Dexamethasone 7.5 mg IV **STAT and every 4 h**	Diphenhydramine 50 mg IV 1 h	At least 4–5 h 2nd-line if allergy
	Methylprednisolone 40 mg IV or Hydrocortisone 200 mg IV **STAT and every 1 h**		No evidence: Emergent situations only

Contrast Reactions (ACR Manual on Contrast Media 2017)
- Hypersensitive Reactions: Incompletely understood (histamine and other vasoactive mediators) not associated with increased IgE—prior sensitization not required for reaction to occur
- Direct Reactions: Renal (PC-AKI/CIN/NSF/dialysis), cardiac (arrhythmia, pulmonary edema, depressed contractility), vasovagal, hematologic (induce clotting), neurologic (exceedingly rare, requires disrupted blood–brain barrier)
- Reaction rates: Function of complexity and osmolality
  - Nonionic and low osmolar better than ionic and high osmolar

- IV LOCM: Overall rate (0.2–0.7%), serious reaction (0.04%), mortality (~2.1 per million)
- Gadolinium Reactions: Physiologic 0.07–2.4%, allergic rare ~0.004%
  - Dose-dependent deposition in CNS: No current evidence of neurotoxicity
  - Nephrogenic systemic fibrosis: Fibrosing disease, skin thickening, with organ involvement, may be fatal
    - Gadodiamide (Omniscan), Gadopentetate (Magnevist) contraindicated when eGFR <30, on dialysis, or in AKI
    - CKD4 or 5/dialysis can use: Gadobenate(MultiHance), Gadobutrol (Gadavist), Gadoterate (Dotarem), Gadoteridol (ProHance)

CSA 2-2

Review of Acute Contrast Reaction Management

Mild allergic (limited urticaria, edema, congestion, sneezing, itchy throat)	Monitor vitals Diphenhydramine 25/50 mg PO optional
Moderate allergic (diffuse urticaria, erythema, facial edema, wheezing, bronchospasm) + stable vitals	Vitals, IV access, oxygen Diphenhydramine 25/50 mg PO/IV/IM Beta agonist (albuterol) 2 puffs (90 µg/puff)
Severe allergic (moderate + laryngeal edema, hypoxia, hypotension, tachycardia)	Monitor vitals, IV access Diphenhydramine 25/50 mg IV/IM Bolus IV fluids NS if hypotensive Epinephrine 0.3 mL IM(1:1000) q5–15 min t1 mL Call code
Isolated hypotension	Monitor vitals, IV access, oxygen, elevate legs Bolus IV fluids NS
Vasovagal reaction	Vitals, IV, oxygen, fluids Severe: Consider atropine 0.6–1.0 mg Call code
Hypertensive crisis	Vitals, IV access, Oxygen Labetalol 20 mg IV OR Nitroglycerin tablet 0.4 mg q5–10 min Call code
Pulmonary edema	Vitals, IV access, oxygen, elevate HOB Furosemide: 20–40 mg IV slowly
Seizures	Protect, turn to side, suction, vitals, IV access, oxygen Lorazepam 2–4 mg IV Call code
Reaction rebound prevention: May prevent short-term recurrence of severe allergic-like reaction	Hydrocortisone 5 mg/kg IV OR Methylprednisolone 1 mg/kg IV

Sedation and Analgesia (Radiographics 2013;33:E47–60)
Administration of medications which decrease awareness, responsiveness, reduce anxiety, facilitate pain control

Sedation	Response to stimuli	Airway	Spontaneous ventilation	Cardiovascular function
Minimal	Normal response to verbal	Unaffected	Unaffected	Unaffected
Moderate	Purposeful response to verbal/tactile	No intervention required	Adequate	Usually maintained
Deep	Purposeful response after repeated/painful	May require intervention	May be inadequate	Usually maintained
General anesthesia	Unarousable	Intervention required	Frequently inadequate	May be impaired

Preprocedural Assessment: Determine level of sedation needed and safe
- History/physical, documented discussion, risk/benefits/consent, plan of sedation
- Age, BMI, comorbidities, smoking, medications/drug use, allergies
- ASA classification score (see Chapter 1), Mallampati score, Gastrointestinal/fasting status, surgical history
- Confirm availability of resuscitation equipment

- Conservative approach: Can start with local anesthesia and add systemic analgesia and sedatives as needed
- Analgesia: Set expectations prior to procedure

Attempt to use combination of nonsteroid analgesics with opioid analgesics; synergistic effect without increased toxicity

IV acetaminophen 1 g/ibuprofen 800 mg combination may reduce opioid use compared to IV ketorolac 30 mg *(JVIR 2017;28(2):S47–8)*

Local anesthetic	Max patient dose	Onset	Duration
Lidocaine	30 mL of 1%	1–2 min	30–60 min
Lidocaine with epinephrine	50 mL of 1%	1–2 min	60–240 min
Bupivacaine	70 mL of 0.25%	5 min	120–240 min

(From American Society of Anesthesiologists Task Force on Sedation and Analgesia by Non-Anesthesiologists. Practice guidelines for sedation and analgesia by non-anesthesiologists. *Anesthesiology* 2002;96(4):1004–17, with permission.)

Sedative	Patient dose	Onset	Duration
Diazepam	2–10 mg IV	Variable onset	20–100 h
Midazolam	1–2.5 mg IV	Rapid onset	1–4 h
Lorazepam	2 mg IV	Variable onset	15 h

(From American Society of Anesthesiologists Task Force on Sedation and Analgesia by Non-Anesthesiologists. Practice guidelines for sedation and analgesia by non-anesthesiologists. *Anesthesiology* 2002;96(4):1004–17, with permission.)

Analgesic	Patient dose	Potency	
Morphine	2–10 mg IV	1	
Fentanyl	50–100 μg IV	50–100×	Stiff chest syndrome – intubate + succinylcholine
Hydromorphone	1–2 mg IV	4–8×	4–8× potent than morphine Antitussive effects
Meperidine	50–150 mg IM/SQ, less if IV	1/10×	Sepsis-related rigors in recovery
IV Acetaminophen	1 g IV		Postrecovery pain

(From American Society of Anesthesiologists Task Force on Sedation and Analgesia by Non-Anesthesiologists. Practice guidelines for sedation and analgesia by non-anesthesiologists. *Anesthesiology* 2002;96(4):1004–17, with permission.)

Intraprocedural Monitoring
- Monitor respiratory rate and electrocardiogram continuously
- Blood pressure checked every 5 min, before and after each sedative dose
- Moderate sedation: BP, pulse Ox, EKG, capnography
- Deep sedation/anesthesia: BP, pulse Ox, EKG, Temp, capnography, anesthetic gas concentrations, circuit low pressure alarm, ventilator parameters
- Assess for need for reversal agents
  - Naloxone 1.5–3 mg/kg IV: Reverses opioids. Onset 1–2 min, duration 45 min
  - Flumazenil 0.2 mg IV: Reverses benzodiazepines. Onset 1–2 min, duration 30–60 min
    - Caution: Refractory seizures if patient chronically on benzodiazepines

Postprocedural Monitoring
- Monitor for postprocedural complications at least every 15 min for minimum of 30 min after last dosage
- If sedation/analgesia reversal agent used, assess for 2 h
- Predischarge Aldrete score: See Chapter 1
- Discharge instructions: Activity, diet
- Discharge pain medications: Dependent on procedure type
  - Eg, Oxycodone 5 mg PO 3–5 d supply with follow-up

Patient-Controlled Analgesia
- Self-administered small doses of opioids with fixed parameters
- Typical procedures: End-organ embolization, eg, UAE, TACE, etc
- Loading dose, basal dose, patient-administered dose, frequency/lockout period

Drug	Patient dose	Basal dose	Frequency
Hydromorphone	0.2–0.5 mg	0.2–0.5 mg/h	6–10 min
Meperidine	10–15 mg	15–50 mg/h	6–10 min
Morphine	1–2 mg	0.5–1 mg/h	6–10 min
Fentanyl	10–25 μg	25–50 μg/h	2–5 min

(From Kandarpa K, Machan L. *Handbook of Interventional Radiologic Procedures.* 4th ed. Philadelphia, PA: Wolters Kluwer; 2011:731, with permission)

BACKGROUND

- There are multiple drug classes routinely employed in interventional radiology. Knowledge of indications, contraindications, and complications is essential for appropriate patient care.
- This chapter will divide commonly used drugs into these major categories: Anticoagulants, antiplatelets, antihypertensives, antibiotics, vasodilators, thrombolytics, and miscellaneous.

Anticoagulants (Whalen K. *Lippincott Illustrated Reviews: Pharmacology.* 6th ed. Baltimore, MD: Wolters Kluwer Health/Lippincott Williams & Wilkins; 2014; Kandarpa K. *Handbook of Interventional Radiologic Procedures.* Philadelphia, PA: Wolters Kluwer; 2011)

- Heparin
  - Indications: Venous and arterial thrombosis, DVT, pulmonary embolism
  - Contraindications: Active bleeding; history of heparin-induced thrombocytopenia (HIT), recent CNS surgery or bleed
  - Mechanism of action (MOA): Inactivates thrombin and factor Xa
  - Short half-life ~1.5 h
  - Heparin is given SQ or IV drip (gtt). Heparin drip can be stopped 1 h before any procedure.
    - *Tips and Tricks:* Heparin drip is a nice option for anticoagulation because it gives clinicians more control (aka patient starts bleeding, turn off drip)
  - Intraprocedural monitoring can be done with activated clotting time (ACT) with goal of 180–240 s
  - Postprocedural monitoring via PTT with therapeutic goal in 60 s
  - If bleeding occurs, stop drip but keep IV open with saline
  - Reversal agent: Protamine but rarely used
  - If a patient has an allergy to heparin or history of HIT, **ALL** heparin-containing material (eg, heparinized saline) must be exchanged for fondaparinux or bivalirudin
  - HIT develops 5–10 d postexposure to heparin, LMWH, and derivatives
- Low-molecular-weight heparins: Enoxaparin (Lovenox®)
  - Generally used for long-term outpatient anticoagulation and thus have longer half-lives than heparin, eg, enoxaparin: 57 h
  - MOA: Inhibits thrombin and factor Xa after binding antithrombin III
  - Indications: Similar to heparin
  - Contraindications: Bleeding, HIT
- Fondaparinux (Arixtra®)
  - Indications: Similar to heparin, history of HIT
  - MOA: Binds antithrombin III and deactivates factor Xa
  - Half-life up to 21 h
- Bivalirudin (Angiomax®)
  - Indications: Similar to heparin, history of HIT
  - MOA: Reversible, direct thrombin inhibitor
  - Half-life of 30–60 min, GFR dependent
  - Monitor with ACT intraprocedure
- Warfarin (Coumadin®)
  - Indications: Venous and arterial embolism prevention and treatment, atrial fibrillation, and mechanical heart valves
  - Long half-life of 20–60 h
  - Monitor using INR. Preprocedural goal <1.7
  - Reversal agents: Fresh frozen plasma and PCC (prothrombin complex concentrate). Vitamin K takes up to 24 h for effect.
  - Can be difficult for patients as they need routine INR monitoring as outpatients
- New oral anticoagulants: Rivaroxaban (Xarelto®), apixaban (Eliquis®), dabigatran (Pradaxa®)
  - Indications are the same as warfarin
  - MOA: Direct Factor Xa inhibitors
  - No monitoring or reliable reversal agent

Antiplatelets (Whalen K. *Lippincott Illustrated Reviews: Pharmacology.* 6th ed. Baltimore, MD: Wolters Kluwer Health/Lippincott Williams & Wilkins; 2014; Kandarpa K. *Handbook of Interventional Radiologic Procedures.* Philadelphia, PA: Wolters Kluwer; 2011)

- Aspirin (ASA)
  - Indications: Postballoon angioplasty or stenting
  - MOA is similar to NSAIDs: Inhibits COX 1 and 2, preventing platelet aggregation
  - Antiplatelet effects last 10 d
  - Dosages: PO 81 mg baby aspirin or up to 325 mg during acute coronary syndrome
  - Can give platelets for reversal if emergent procedure
  - Monitor via bleeding time
- Clopidogrel (Plavix®); ticlopidine (Ticlid®)
  - Indications: CVA, coronary stents, postvascular stenting
  - Stop 5 d before procedure but consult with ordering M.D. to weigh risk/benefits. Must discuss with cardiologist due to concern for in-stent thrombosis.
  - If emergent procedure needs to be performed, must disregard that patient is on Plavix (eg, obstructed biliary system, septic patient)
  - No consensus on how long to keep patients on Plavix for arterial stenting. However, will often give a loading dose of 300 mg, then 75 mg a d for 3–6 mo
- Cilostazol (Pletal®)
  - Indications: Peripheral arterial disease
  - MOA: Inhibits phosphodiesterase type III, reducing platelet aggregation
  - No need to stop before procedure

Drug	Hold	Resume
Aspirin	5 d	Immediately
NSAIDs	Variable (1–10 d)	Immediately
Clopidogrel	5 d	Immediately
Warfarin	5 d	1 d
Apixaban	3 d	2 d
Rivaroxaban	2 d	2 d
Fondaparinux	2 d	6 h
Lovenox	12 h	6 h
Argatroban	4 h	1 h
Heparin IV	1–4 h	1 h
Heparin sq	4 h	1 h

(JVIR 2012;23:727–36)

Antihypertensives (Whalen K. *Lippincott Illustrated Reviews: Pharmacology.* 6th ed. Baltimore, MD: Wolters Kluwer Health/Lippincott Williams & Wilkins; 2014; Kandarpa K. *Handbook of Interventional Radiologic Procedures.* Philadelphia, PA: Wolters Kluwer, 2011)

- Nitroglycerin
  - Indications: Intraarterial vasospasm during angioplasty embolization procedures such as uterine or prostate artery embolization
  - MOA: Stimulates cGMP production, which causes vasodilation
  - Half-life: 1–3 min
  - Dosages: 100–200 µg direct arterial bolus
  - Side-effects: Tachycardia, headache
  - *Tips and Tricks:* Always keep an eye on blood pressure before administering
- Nifedipine
  - Indications: Intraarterial vasospasm during angioplasty
  - MOA: Prevents calcium reflux into vascular smooth muscle causing relaxation
  - Half-life: 2 h, increases with renal disease
  - Dosages: 10 mg PO
- Hydralazine
  - Indications: Hypertensive crisis
  - MOA: Direct peripheral vasodilator
  - Half-life: 3–7 h
  - Side-effects: Reflex tachycardia
  - Dosages: 10–20 mg IV q2–4h, repeat as tolerated
  - *Tips and Tricks:* Avoid use if heart rate is above 90–100 because of reflex tachycardia. Instead, use a β-blocker

---

*Tips and Tricks: These are not hard and fast rules, but guidelines that the interventional radiologist should know.

- Metoprolol
  - Indications: Tachycardia and hypertension
  - MOA: Selective β-blocker
  - Half-life: 3–4 h IV
  - Dosages: 5–10 mg IV, repeat as tolerated
- Labetalol
  - Indications: Hypertensive crisis
  - MOA: α- and β-blocker
  - Half-life: 7 h
  - Dosages: Start 20 mg IV × 1q10 min (max dose 300 mg)
- Nitroprusside (Nitropress®)
  - Indications: Hypertensive crisis
  - MOA: Direct peripheral vasodilator
  - Half-life: 2 min
  - Dosages: Start 0.3 µg/kg/min IV q10 min
- Furosemide (Lasix®)
  - Indications: Pulmonary edema/volume overload
  - MOA: Loop diuretic
  - Half-life: 30–60 min
  - Dosages: Start 40 mg IV × 1; max: 80 mg IV q1h
  - If sulfa allergy use: Ethacrynic acid (Edecrin®); give 50–100 mg IV × 1 (can repeat once)
- Hypertensive emergency
  - Blood pressure >180/120 with end-organ damage on CNS, cardiac, and renal
  - Treatment: Decrease BP slowly over several hours with IV meds as tolerated
- Volume overload
  - Increased blood volume in the right or left heart
  - Clinically can present as pleural and pulmonary edema
  - Treatment: Stop all unnecessary IV fluids, then diurese with Lasix ® as tolerated

Antibiotics (ABX) (JVIR 2010;21:1611–30)

Interventional procedures can be divided into **four** broad categories per SIR guidelines:
- **Clean:** GI, GU, or respiratory tract is not entered, inflammation is not evident, and no break in aseptic technique
- **Clean-Contaminated:** GI, biliary, or GU tract is entered, inflammation is not evident, and no break in aseptic technique
- **Contaminated:** Entry into an inflamed or colonized GI or GU tract without frank pus, or break in aseptic technique occurs
- **Dirty:** Entering an infected purulent site such as abscess, infected biliary or GU site, or perforated viscus

Per SIR guidelines: "Antibiotic prophylaxis for IR procedures is generally recommended for procedures that are not clean, or for procedures that are considered clean but, as a result of which, a potentially significant volume of necrotic tissue is generated in potentially contaminated areas, eg, embolization with intent to create infarction."

Commonly used Antibiotics:
- Cefazolin (Ancef®)
  - Standard ABX prophylaxis for clean procedures
  - Dosages: 1 g IV 30–60 min preprocedure
  - Half-life: 2 h, rises with renal dysfunction
  - 1st-generation cephalosporin
  - *Tips and Tricks:* If allergic to cephalosporins or penicillin, often times can give clindamycin.
- Clindamycin
  - Dosages: 600 mg IV
  - Half-life: 3 h
- Cefoxitin
  - 2nd-generation cephalosporin
  - Indications: Gram-negative coverage, TIPS, percutaneous biliary drain, nephrostomy tubes
  - Dosages: 1 g IV q6 for 48 h
  - Half-life: 60 min, rises with renal dysfunction
- Ceftriaxone/cefepime
  - 3rd-/4th-generation cephalosporins
  - ABX for GI/GU, intraperitoneal, biliary, renal/splenic embolization
  - Dosages: 1 g ceftriaxone IV 60 min preprocedure; 1–2 g cefepime IV preprocedure
  - Half-lives: 7 h ceftriaxone and 2 h cefepime. Both rise with renal dysfunction.

- Metronidazole
  - Indications: Hepatic chemoembolization (+Ancef®),
  - Dosages: 500 mg IV
  - Half-life: 8 h

Prophylaxis for Common IR Procedures

Procedure	Category	Prophylaxis recommended? Which Abx?
Vascular interventions: Angioplasty, closure devices, stent placement	Clean	No. Will often use *Cefazolin*
Endograft placement	Clean	Yes, *Cefazolin*
IVC filter placement	Clean	No
Central venous access	Clean	No, but will often use *Cefazolin* for Mediports or tunneled venous catheters
Chemo-embolization	Clean-contaminated	Yes, no consensus, but will often use *Cefazolin* or *Cefoxitin*
Uterine artery embolization	Clean-contaminated	Yes, no consensus, but will often be used *Cefazolin*.
TIPS	Clean-contaminated	Yes, no consensus; will always give *Cefoxitin*
G tube	Clean-contaminated	No consensus. Usually will not give antibiotics
Biliary drain	Clean-contaminated, contaminated	Yes, no consensus; will always give *Cefoxitin*
Nephrostomy tube	Clean-contaminated, contaminated	Yes, no consensus; will always give *Cefoxitin*
Tumor ablation	Clean, clean-contaminated	No consensus, but will usually give *Cefazolin*
Abscess drain	Dirty	Yes, no consensus. Very often, patient will already be on an antibiotic regimen.

Vasodilators (Whalen K. *Lippincott Illustrated Reviews: Pharmacology.* 6th ed. Baltimore, MD: Wolters Kluwer Health/Lippincott Williams & Wilkins; 2014; Kandarpa K. *Handbook of Interventional Radiologic Procedures.* Philadelphia, PA: Wolters Kluwer, 2011)

- Nitroglycerin
  - Indications: Intraarterial vasospasm during angioplasty embolization procedures such as uterine or prostate artery embolization
  - MOA: Stimulates cGMP production, which causes vasodilation
  - Half-life: 1–3 min
  - Dosages: 100–200 μg direct arterial bolus
  - Side-effects: Tachycardia, headache
  - *Tips and Tricks:* Always keep an eye on blood pressure before administering
- Nifedipine
  - Indications: Intraarterial vasospasm during angioplasty
  - MOA: Prevents calcium reflux into vascular smooth muscle causing relaxation
  - Half-life: 2 h rises with renal dysfunction
  - Dosages: 10 mg PO (what's the IA dosage??)

Thrombolytics (Whalen K. *Lippincott Illustrated Reviews: Pharmacology.* 6th ed. Baltimore, MD: Wolters Kluwer Health/Lippincott Williams & Wilkins; 2014; Kandarpa K. *Handbook of Interventional Radiologic Procedures.* Philadelphia, PA: Wolters Kluwer, 2011)

- Tissue plasminogen activator (tPA)
  - MOA: Causes fibrin-enhanced conversion of fibrin-bound plasminogen to plasmin
  - Indication: Fibrinolysis of pulmonary embolism, DVT, intraarterial thrombus
    - How to administer – usually drip *1 mg/h*; if 2 catheters (eg, bilateral PE), will drip *0.5 mg/h* through each
      - Make sure to give fluid through sheath—usually give low-dose heparin through sheath
      - Trend fibrinogen levels q6h. If fibrinogen drops below 150, half the dose of tPA. If fibrinogen drops below 100, turn off tPA and run heparinized saline through lysis catheter.
      - How long to run tPA—usually will not go more than a total of 24 mg tPA

- Contraindications: Active bleeding, intracranial neoplasm, recent GI bleed/CVA/intracranial surgery
- Reversal: Turn drip off OR give FFP

Fibrinogen level	tPA dose
>150	1 mg/h
100–150	0.5 mg/h
<100	Turn off tPA: Run saline through catheter

- Other thrombolytics: Streptokinase, urokinase, reteplase—same as tPA

Medications that Reduce Peristalsis (Whalen K. *Lippincott Illustrated Reviews: Pharmacology*. 6th ed. Baltimore, MD: Wolters Kluwer Health/Lippincott Williams & Wilkins; 2014; Kandarpa K. *Handbook of Interventional Radiologic Procedures*. Philadelphia, PA: Wolters Kluwer, 2011)
- Glucagon
  - MOA: Relaxes smooth muscle of stomach and bowel
  - Indication: Used to reduce peristalsis during gastrostomy tube placement (keeps air in stomach)
    - *Tips and Tricks*: Give 1 mg glucagon after patient is prepped for G-tube
  - Contraindications: Avoid in diabetics
  - Half-life: 3–6 min

Antiemetics (Whalen K. *Lippincott Illustrated Reviews: Pharmacology*. 6th ed. Baltimore, MD: Wolters Kluwer Health/Lippincott Williams & Wilkins; 2014; Kandarpa K. *Handbook of Interventional Radiologic Procedures*. Philadelphia, PA: Wolters Kluwer, 2011)
- Ondansetron (Zofran®): Most commonly used
  - MOA: Serotonin receptor antagonists
  - Dosage: 4–24 mg PO, IM, IV 2–4×/d
- Other common antiemetics:
  - Metoclopramide (Reglan®): 5–10 mg PO
  - Prochlorperazine (Compazine®): 2.5–10 g IV, IM, or PO
  - Promethazine (Phenergan®): 12.5–25 mg PO
  - Diphenhydramine (Benadryl®): 25–50 mg PO/IV: While not specifically an antiemetic, can often help with nausea

NONINVASIVE VASCULAR IMAGING MODALITIES

Ultrasound

Background

- Ultrasound (US) imaging is based on sound waves of variable frequencies that are emitted and received by crystals inside a so-called transducer (probe).
- For vascular US of superficial vessels (extremities, neck), high-frequency transducers are used (~5–15 MHz). For vessels in the abdomen or pelvis, low-frequency transducers are preferred (~2–4 MHz). Most endoluminal transducers (endovaginal, endorectal, or endoscopic) have the capacity for flow evaluation.
- Various US techniques are available including gray-scale (B-mode), spectral Doppler, color Doppler, and power Doppler (PW) imaging. These techniques do not require contrast agents.
- Contrast-enhanced ultrasound (CEUS): Relatively new technique since recent FDA approval of US contrast agents; may not be as easily available as standard vascular US techniques due to recent release.
- General limitations for US: Presence of air, bone (skull), and extensive calcifications as well as large body habitus (for abdominal imaging).

Ultrasound Techniques

Gray-Scale (B-Mode)

- Provides information on the anatomy and morphology of the vessels and vessel wall, but not on the blood flow; **Example:** Atherosclerotic soft and hard plaques; thrombus; vessel diameters (aneurysm)

Spectral Doppler US (SD-US)

- SD-US is based on a physical effect called Doppler shift (Doppler effect): A change of the frequency of sound waves when a reflector (ie, moving particles) is moving toward or away from the transducer. Flow toward the transducer is displayed above the baseline, flow away from the transducer below baseline (always refer to scale on each US image).
- SD-US can demonstrate velocity and direction of flow
- Specific waveforms describe the blood flow depending on the cardiac cycle and the effects of respiration: Triphasic, biphasic, or monophasic
- Arterial flow can further be described as high resistance or low resistance; this is indicated by the arterial resistive index (RI)
- RI:
  - Resistance to blood flow within an artery created by the capillary bed of the target organ
  - Defined as peak systolic velocity (PSV) minus the peak diastolic velocity divided by the PSV
  - Values range between 0.0–1.0 (low to high resistance)
  - High resistance (RI >0.7): (Figure 4-1A): Triphasic waveform with high-velocity systolic forward flow—brief, early diastolic retrograde flow—late diastolic forward flow). **Example:** External carotid arteries, extremity arteries, and mesenteric arteries during fasting
  - Low resistance (RI: 0.55–0.7): (Figure 4-1B): High-velocity systolic forward flow – diastolic forward flow. **Example:** Internal carotid arteries, hepatic arteries, renal arteries, and testicular arteries
- Venous flow depends on the proximity to the heart and is respiratory dependent; In general it has a lower velocity compared to the arteries.

Color Doppler (CD; Duplex US)

- Color Doppler (or Duplex) US shows velocity and direction of flow and assigns colors to reflect this
- CD-US depends on the orientation of the transducer; conventionally, red reflects flow toward and blue flow away from the transducer (refer to color scale in each color Doppler US image)
- Yellow/white/green colors usually indicate turbulent flow (see color scale) **Examples:** High-grade stenosis; neck of the pseudoaneurysm
- **Indication:** Evaluation of intravascular flow; atherosclerotic disease and stenosis; vessel occlusion; and vascularity and perfusion of organs

Power Doppler (PW)

- Used when standard Doppler imaging does not demonstrate flow
- More sensitive to flow than standard color Doppler; improves detection of slow flow

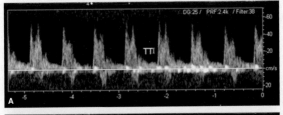

Figure 4-1A. High-resistance waveform (ECA): Sharp and narrow systolic peak, rapid decrease of flow toward baseline and minimal flow in diastole. TT indicates temporal tap which is waveform oscillations during manual tapping of a branch of the superficial temporal artery near the temple. This is a helpful maneuver to distinguish ECA from ICA. **B.** Low-resistance waveform (ICA): Broad systolic peak and continuous decrease of diastolic flow.

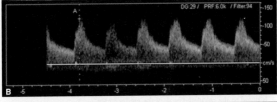

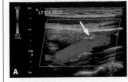 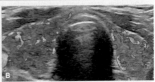

Figure 4-2 (A) Color Doppler US shows small hyperechoic focus in the wall of the proximal ICA (*arrow*) representing a calcified atherosclerotic plaque. **(B)** Color Doppler US shows normal vascularity in the thyroid gland.

- Detects motion (ie, of red blood cells) but is independent and does not indicate the velocity and direction of flow

Ultrasound Contrast Agents for Contrast-Enhanced Ultrasound (CEUS)
- Consist of microbubbles that have a gas core and a lipid shell and typically the size of a red blood cell
- Are strongly echogenic and act as "echo-enhancer"; can show blood flow dynamics, direction, and velocity of blood flow
- Are strictly intravascular and are eliminated by the liver and lung
- Applicable without danger in patients with renal failure
- Are injected intravenously in a superficial venous access and follow typical contrast enhancement phases and timing:
  - Arterial phase: Starts at 10–30 s postinjection; lasts for 35–40 s
  - Portal venous phase lasts for 2 min postinjection
  - No interstitial/equilibrium phase because no extravasation of the contrast agent
- **Indications:** To evaluate vascularity of any tissue, enhancement pattern of focal lesions, and vascular leak and endoleak in stent grafts. To improve the visualization of blood flow in vessels

Computed Tomography Angiography (CTA)

Background
- CTA provides morphologic information of the vessel lumen and vessel wall, specifically calcifications are well visualized

- CTA requires intravenous administration of iodinated contrast agents
- **Advantages:** (1) Widely available, fast, and relatively easy; (2) high spatial resolution (higher than MRA); (3) no vascular artifacts from turbulent or slow flow; and (4) lower cost than MRA
- **Disadvantages:** (1) Ionizing radiation (caution in pediatrics and pregnant women); (2) iodinated contrast; (3) adverse contrast reactions is more common than MRA (require premedication); and (4) less contrast resolution

Imaging Technique

- Images are acquired with thin collimation (typically 0.6–1.0 mm) and reconstructed in thin sections (typically 1–2 mm)
- Postprocessing and 3D reconstruction improves assessment
- Iodinated contrast is injected intravenously. For optimal image quality in CTA, exact timing of the imaging after contrast injection is necessary to obtain maximal arterial enhancement within the target vessel
- Image acquisition should be near the peak of enhancement in the target vessel; this can be obtained by specific techniques (see below)
- Optimal opacification depends on: (1) Anatomic location and diameter of target vessels and organs; (2) difference in cardiac output; (3) and presence of vascular pathology (stenosis or aneurysm)
- Arterial opacification can be increased by: (1) Higher concentration of iodine (contrast agent); (2) higher flow rate (concentrated contrast bolus); and (3) higher volume of contrast (longer bolus)
- Two main techniques to adjust the scan timing for optimal imaging:
  Bolus timing: A single slice low-dose scan is performed in the area near or in the target vessel. A small amount of contrast agent is administered intravenously (~15–20 mL); repeat (dynamic) low-dose scanning is performed until contrast arrives. A region of interest (ROI) is placed in the target vessel to calculate a time–attenuation curve. Subsequent image acquisition of the desired body region is timed to the calculated peak of the enhancement.
  Disadvantages: (1) More contrast; and (2) more time
  Bolus tracking: Similar to bolus timing, an ROI is placed in the target vessel on a low-dose scan. Subsequent automated measurements during contrast injection generates a time–attenuation curve of the arrival of the contrast bolus and image acquisition starts when a set attenuation threshold is reached.
  Disadvantages: (1) Variable scan delay times; and (2) limited troubleshooting

Indications

- *CNS:* Stroke protocol and evaluation for carotid and cerebral artery stenosis
- *Chest:* Acute chest pain protocol to "triple rule out" dissection, acute coronary syndrome, pulmonary embolism
- *Renal arteries:* Renal transplant donor, evaluation of renal vasculature
- *Abdominal aorta:* Aneurysmal disease and surveillance of aortoiliac stents and grafts
- *Peripheral vascular disease:* Aortography with peripheral run-off; evaluation of the vasculature of the extremities in trauma
- *Abdomen and pelvis CTA in trauma and GI bleeding:* Acquired in 3 phases including nonenhanced, arterial, and portal venous phases
  Nonenhanced images: To decrease the false-positive findings from pre-existing hyperattenuating structures (ingested pills, residual contrast in bowel, stool, suture material, surgical clips, foreign body)
  Arterial phase: Key phase to detect extravasation of contrast due to active bleeding.
  Portal venous phase: To confirm active bleeding due to change in appearance and volume of extravasated material with time compared to arterial phase

Magnetic Resonance Angiography (MRA)

Background

- Vascular imaging with Magnetic resonance Angiography (MRA) is performed using contrast-enhanced and noncontrast techniques
- MRA shows vessel morphology, blood flow, flow direction, and static blood products (thrombus). MRA focuses on the vasculature, but often combined with morphologic imaging of the respective body region.
- **Advantages of MRA:** (1) No radiation exposure (preferable for pediatric patients); (2) less nephrotoxicity of contrast agents; (3) unlimited number of acquisitions (phases) after contrast administration; (4) time-resolved angiography (fast repetitive scanning at high temporal resolution); and (5) dynamic contrast-enhanced imaging (DCE) for tissue perfusion and quantification of blood flow, blood volume, permeability, and other parameters.

- **Disadvantages of MRA:** (1) Long image acquisition times (> than CT); (2) Relative contraindications for pacemaker, defibrillator, and certain implanted devices; and (3) Less sensitivity than CT for small calcifications; large calcifications may cause susceptibility artifacts and therefore limit the evaluation.
- **MR safety:**
  - Prior to MR imaging check for:
    - Any type of metallic implant devices within the body (metallic implants, pacemaker, certain surgical clips, cochlear implants, subcutaneous electronic pump devices, etc.)
  - Prior to MR—contrast administration check for:
    - Renal function (serum creatinine <1.3 or glomerulofiltration rate GRF >30 mL/min/1.73 m^2)
    - History of allergic reactions to MR contrast agents

Imaging Techniques

Contrast-Enhanced Magnetic Resonance Angiography (CE-MRA)
- Most frequently used imaging technique for MRA
- Requires the injection of Gadolinium (Gd)-chelate based contrast agents (Gd shortens the T1 relaxation time due to its paramagnetic effect; it appears hyperintense [high signal] on T1-weighted images [T1WI])
- Injection of the contrast agent preferably through peripheral venous access; image acquisition must be synchronized and timed with injection. Imaging occurs at the first passage of contrast bolus through arterial vessel of interest and may be repeated
- **Advantages:** Very high spatial resolution; fast
- **Dosage:** Typical dose: 0.2 mmol/kg/body weight (BW); can be increased up to triple dose. Typical injection volume: 0.1–0.3 mL/kg/BW, between 10–40 mL (higher volumes may provide higher signal-to-noise ratio [SNR] for better delineation of small vessels); typical injection rates: >0.5–4.0 mL/s
- **Contrast agents:**
  - *Extracellular contrast agents:* Most frequently used Gd-based contrast agents; have intravascular (vessel) and interstitial (tissue) components; excreted by the kidney (concern for nephrogenic systemic fibrosis [NSF] if end-stage renal disease [ESRD])
  - *Blood pool agents:* Purely intravascular; remain longer in blood pool; allow longer imaging times; have higher relaxivity for greater vascular detail; no interstitial component; excreted mostly through the kidneys, 9% hepatobiliary (concern for NSF if ESRD) **Indications:** MRA (aortoiliac occlusive disease); MRV (deep vein thrombosis [DVT], May–Thurner syndrome, Nutcracker syndrome, pelvic congestion syndrome, thoracic outlet syndrome)
- **Technical aspects of CE-MRA:**
  CE-MRA is acquired using 3D MR imaging techniques.
  Types of MRA are:
  - *Single timepoint multiphase MRA:* Image acquisition is repeated at multiple fixed time points (phases); emphasis is on high spatial resolution for high morphologic detail; **Example:** MRA for arterial stenosis, vasculitis, small vessel aneurysms
  - *Time-resolved MRA:* Rapid repetitive multi-timepoint image acquisition at fast temporal resolution during contrast bolus passage to demonstrate flow pattern and perfusion pattern; "four-dimensional" evaluation of blood flow. Provides more specific information on hemodynamics in a vessel or tissue including wide range of flow velocities; **Example:** Arteriovenous malformation (AVM), arteriovenous fistula (AVF), shunts
  For optimal quality, CE-MRA requires fast image acquisition (short TR; undersampling acquisition techniques) and exact image timing after injection of the contrast agent. Exact timing is achieved with either fixed time points or bolus tracking:
  - *Bolus timing:*
    - A technique to adjust the time point of optimal imaging to the individual circulation time of a patient by determining the time point of the highest contrast concentration in the target vessel
    - Can be performed using either test bolus or bolus triggering:
      Test bolus: A small amount of contrast agent is injected intravenously; repetitive single slice images are obtained over the target vessel until the contrast agent arrives in the target vessel; a time-signal intensity curve is calculated; subsequent image acquisition is timed to the peak enhancement.
      Bolus triggering: Image acquisition is started automatically or manually when the signal increases within the target vessel with arrival of the contrast bolus on repetitive single slice imaging.

- *Image subtraction:*
  - Digital technique to reduce or remove the anatomic background in an image to focus only on the vessels
  - Images of the same anatomic region obtained before contrast injection are subtracted from images after contrast injection; only contrast-enhanced vessels and structures remain (digital subtraction angiography)
  - **Advantage:** Subtraction improves the visibility of vascular details and small vessels
  - **Disadvantages:** Subtraction reduces the signal-to-noise ratio [SNR]; is susceptible to misregistration artifacts resulting from motion
- **Advantages of CE-MRA over noncontrast MRA:**
  - Less sensitive to artifacts than noncontrast techniques
  - Fast image acquisition in single breath-hold intervals
  - High morphologic detail even in small vessels and with slow flow
- **Disadvantages of CE-MRA:**
  - Need for exact timing and synchronization of image acquisition and contrast material injection (bolus timing).
  - Need for breath hold and completely motion free acquisition period
  - Limitations in pregnancy and in patients with severe renal failure and dialysis (NSF)
- **Vascular territories:**
  - Carotid, vertebral, intracranial arteries
  - Thoracoabdominal arch and its branches including supraaortic, renal, celiac, mesenteric arteries, peripheral arteries of the upper and lower extremities
  - Combined evaluation of arterial and venous vasculature (preferably with blood pool contrast agents (see above)
  - Veins of the upper extremity, pulmonary artery, inferior vena cava (IVC), pelvic veins, portal venous system, lower extremity veins.
- **Indications:**
  - *Atherosclerosis:* Identify and quantify stenosis, vascular occlusion, collateral systems, disease extent and severity
  - *Dilated angiopathy:* Identify aneurysms and pseudoaneurysms
  - *Vasculitis:* Identify and quantify wall thickening, mural edema, late mural enhancement
  - *Dissection:* Evaluate morphology of dissection membrane, flow pattern in true and false lumen, organ perfusion
  - *Vascular malformations:* arteriovenous malformations (AVMs) and vascular neoplasms, AV shunts, arteriovenous fistula (AVF), portosystemic shunts

Noncontrast-Enhanced MRA (NE-MRA)

- No Gd chelates required; can be used in patients with renal failure and/or with known allergy to MR contrast agents
- Superior to CTA for calcified vessels and vessels close to bones
- **Disadvantage:** Long acquisition times; small body coverage; limited to certain anatomic areas of the body
- **Specific techniques:**
  - *Time-of-Flight (TOF):* Flow-related enhancement
    - Background tissue saturated (appears "dark" on imaging)
    - Is used for both arterial and venous angiograms
    - **Advantages:** Relatively robust; low cost
    - **Disadvantages:** Long acquisition times; overestimates stenosis; high-flow artifacts; susceptible to field inhomogeneities
    - **Clinical application:** Cerebral arteries (3D), peripheral vessels (2D), head and neck arteries (2D). Pelvic veins; not standard for extremities
  - *Phase contrast:* Information on flow velocity and flow direction
    - Measures phase shift of spinning protons at two time points; stationary protons have no phase shift
    - **Advantages:** Direction independent
    - **Disadvantage:** Long image acquisition time (3D), signal loss in turbulent flow, sensitive to motion
    - **Clinical applications:** Cerebral veins (3D), cerebrospinal fluid; cardiac valves; hemodynamics, and quantification of flow
  - *Other techniques:*
    - Typically not done routinely, requires supervision by radiologist
    - *Black blood technique:* Evaluates vessel wall morphology in atherosclerosis (carotid arteries, aorta) and arteritis; tumor thrombus; not an angiographic technique
    - *Electrocardiography (ECG)-gated fast spin echo (FSE):* For aorta and branches
    - *Steady state free precession (SSFP):* For coronary arteries, aorta, renal arteries
    - *Arterial spin labeling (ASL) based on SSFP:* For visceral and renal arteries

Thyroid Nodules

Background

- The prevalence of thyroid nodules has been reported in up to 50% in autopsies, however the incidence of malignancy is low (3–7%). With increasing use of imaging studies, the number of incidentally found thyroid nodules continues to increase. The main purpose of dedicated imaging analysis of thyroid nodules is to identify thyroid nodules which require biopsy or continued follow-up due to risk of malignancy.

Imaging Techniques

- Diagnostic imaging tools are US and thyroid scan (I-123).

Benign Thyroid Nodules

- Four patterns of thyroid nodule morphology are described indicating benign nature of thyroid nodules with 100% specificity: (1) Spongiform configuration; (2) Cyst with colloid clot; (3) giraffe pattern; and (4) diffuse hyperechogenicity **(Figure 4-3A, B)**

Figure 4-3A, B. Gray-scale ultrasound of the thyroid shows a cystic lesion with a mural nodule consistent with a cystic colloid nodule/colloid cyst (biopsy proven). **(A).** Predominantly solid colloid nodule is shown in image **B.**

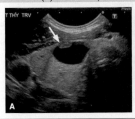
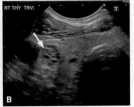

Malignant Thyroid Nodules

- Morphology, size, and growth are important parameters
- Signs of malignancy (depending on size) are:
  - Microcalcifications or coarse calcifications **(Figure 4-4A, B)**
  - Halo appearance
  - Irregular contour
  - Solid or cystic appearance with nodule, singularity

Figure 4-4 Papillary carcinoma: Gray-scale image of the thyroid demonstrates a slightly round ill-defined hypoechoic solid mass with several hyperechoic foci of microcalcifications (*arrow*).

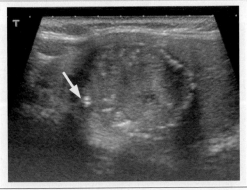

- The Society of Radiologists in Ultrasound (SRS) provides recommendations for the management of thyroid nodules of 1 cm or larger diameter. US-guided fine needle aspiration (FNA) to be strongly considering if:
  - ≥1 cm and presence of microcalcifications
  - ≥1.5 cm and solid or coarse calcifications
  - ≥2 cm and solid, cystic, or entirely cystic with a mural nodule
  - None of the above but substantial growth since prior US examination

  If multiple nodules, consider US-guided FNA of one or more nodules, with selection prioritized on the basis of the above criteria (in order listed) for solitary nodule

LYMPH NODES

Indeterminate Lymph Node

Background
Many cancers spread to locoregional lymph nodes. Distinguishing abnormal suspicious lymph nodes with potential metastatic involvement from reactive nodes is of utmost importance to correctly determine the TNM stage and prognosis. There is no single criterion to distinguish a suspicious lymph node.

Characteristics of Indeterminate Lymph Node
- **Morphology:**
  - Suspicious: Effacement of normal fatty hila; replacement of homogeneous lymphatic tissue with necrosis; cystic change; calcification
  - If nodal calcifications in cervical adenopathy: Indicative of malignant spread of head and neck cancers
  - If calcification in mediastinal nodes: Malignant etiology less likely; Differential diagnosis: Sarcoidosis, silicosis, mycobacteria, granulomatous disease
  - Calcified nodes are seen in treated lymphoma
- **Shape:**
  - Suspicious: loss of the usual reniform configuration from oval to round **(Figure 4-5A, B)**
  - Irregular and indistinct margins
- **Echotexture:** Suspicious: If heterogeneous
- **Distribution:**
  - Asymmetrically prominent nodes or contiguous ≥3 confluent lymph nodes along the lymphatic drainage chain of a primary tumor
- **Size:**
  - Lymph nodes >10 mm in the thorax and abdomen measured in short axis
  - Eccentric cortical thickening >3 mm in axillary adenopathy (important in staging of breast cancer).
- **Vascularity:** Suspicious: Several peripheral blood vessels

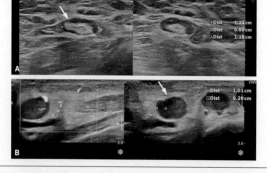

Figure 4-5A. Gray-scale ultrasound of a normal lymph node with reniform configuration, prominent fatty hilum, and no cortical thickening. **B.** Gray-scale and Doppler US of a biopsy-proven metastatic lymph node with rounder configuration, no fatty hilum, and abnormal vascularity.

Pleural Effusion

Background
- **Pleural effusion** is a fluid collection in the pleural space which is a virtual space. Pleural space normally contains up to 15 mL of fluid.
- **Simple pleural effusion** (transudate, usually bilateral); etiology: congestive heart failure (CHF), nephrotic syndrome, volume overload
- **Complex pleural effusion** (exudate, usually unilateral, loculations and septations); etiology: Pneumonia, malignancy, tuberculosis
- **Hemothorax/hematothorax** (blood in the pleural space); etiology: Posttraumatic, malignancy
- **Chylothorax** (lymphatic fluid in the pleural space); etiology: Postsurgical (injury of thoracic duct), congenital

Radiographic Findings
- Small amount on pleural effusion (<50 mL) is only detectable on the lateral radiograph: Blunting of posterior costophrenic angle.
- At least 200 mL is needed to be seen on frontal radiograph: Blunting of the costophrenic angle.
- >500 mL needed to obliterate the hemidiaphragm
- **Meniscus sign** describes the concavity of the fluid level in the pleural space.
- **Hydropneumothorax:** If the pleural space contains air and fluid at the same time, an air–fluid level is seen instead of the meniscus sign.
  Subpulmonic effusion: Presence of fluid between the diaphragm and the lung base. The distance between the gastric bubble and left hemidiaphragm is greater than 2 cm. Lateral decubitus radiograph or US may be needed to confirm the diagnosis.

Radiographic and Sonographic Imaging Findings in Pleural Effusion

Radiography	Ultrasound
- Blunting of costophrenic angle, heart border, hemidiaphragm - Meniscus sign - Diffuse haziness of the hemithorax (supine radiograph) - Fluid within the fissures (associated with fissure sign on Tc-99m perfusion scan) - Lentiform opacity along the pleura (loculated effusion) - White lung +/– mediastinal shift (large pleural effusion)	Simple effusion: Anechoic fluid Complex effusion: Presence of internal echoes and/or septations Nonloculated pleural effusion demonstrates flow on color Doppler; the lung can be seen moving within the pleural effusion

Computed Tomography
- No definitive correlation is seen between CT attenuation values and transudate vs. exudate effusion.
- Additional pleural thickening and nodules are findings in favor of exudative pleural effusion.
- CT allows differentiating pleural thickening from small pleural effusion and diagnosis of complicated pleural effusion and concomitant lung infiltrates. Differentiating lung abscess from empyema is important, given the difference in management. Findings such as consolidation, free air, and septation may be seen with both entities.

Imaging Findings in CT to Distinguish Empyema From Lung Abscess

	Empyema	Lung Abscess
Definition	Infection in pleural cavity	Focal area of infection with destruction of lung parenchyma
Radiologic features	- Split pleural sign: Thickening and enhancement of visceral and parietal pleura - Lenticular shape - Obtuse angle with chest wall	- Thick wall cavity - Round shape - Acute angle with chest wall
Management	Needs percutaneous drainage	Needs IV antibiotics If there is abscess—pleural empyema percutaneous drainage is feasible.

Pneumothorax

Background
Pneumothorax is presence of air in pleural space between the visceral and parietal pleura. There are 2 main subtypes: spontaneous and traumatic subtype

Spontaneous Pneumothorax
- **Primary:** No underlying lung disease; strong association with smoking
- **Secondary:** Known underlying lung disease such as emphysema with bullae, cystic lung disease (Langerhans cell histiocytoma), cavitary lesions, pneumatoceles
- **Catamenial pneumothorax:** Rare entity seen in patients with endometriosis and diaphragmatic implants. Recurrent pneumothorax happens concomitant with menstrual cycles.
- M/F ratio: 1:3.3

Traumatic Pneumothorax
- Blunt or penetrating trauma.
- Iatrogenic pneumothorax: May be caused by mechanical ventilation, interventional, and surgical procedures including venous punctures, biopsies, and surgeries related to the chest wall, lung, esophagus, heart, or mediastinum.

Imaging Techniques

Radiography
- Pneumothorax is best identified on radiographs taken in expiration.
- Visible visceral pleura: Thin radiopaque line paralleling the contours of the chest wall; no lung markings visualized beyond that line. Note that chest wall structures or a skin fold (especially in ICU patients) may mimic a visceral pleural line
- On upright chest radiographs free air is mostly seen in the apical or apicolateral pleural space but may be localized in ventral or diaphragmatic location. On supine radiographs, anteromedial and subpulmonic location are more common.
- **Deep sulcus sign:** A geographic regional lucency overlying the ipsilateral costophrenic angle on supine chest radiograph. It is an indirect sign of a pneumothorax.
- **Tension pneumothorax:** A medical emergency caused by a one-way valve phenomenon in which air accumulates in the pleural space, increases the intrathoracic pressure, causes shift of mediastinal structures, and decreases venous return. Radiographs show a large size pneumothorax, compressive atelectatic lung, mediastinal shift, and variable compression of contralateral lung.

Related IR Procedure: Ultrasound/CT-Guided Thoracentesis
- **Therapeutic/palliative vs. diagnostic thoracentesis:** Specimen sent for protein, LDH, cholesterol, triglycerides, glucose, creatinine, pH, amylase, and cytology, based on the clinical questions.
- **Complications:** Pneumothorax (10%), hemothorax, reexpansion pulmonary edema (drainage of >1 L of effusion), extrapleural bleeding (hematoma).

ABDOMEN AND PELVIS

Ascites

Background
- Ascites is an accumulation of excess fluid in the peritoneal cavity.
- The peritoneal cavity normally contains only a minimal amount of free fluid (<20 mL in females).
- Two main categories of ascites based on total protein content and serum ascites albumin gradient (SAAG): (1) Transudate ascites: common etiology is cirrhosis; and (2) exudate ascites: Common etiology is peritoneal carcinomatosis
- Two main types of intraabdominal fluid collections: Free intraperitoneal fluid and contained (loculated) fluid collections
  - **Free intraperitoneal fluid:** Cirrhosis, heart failure, peritoneal dialysis (Figure 4-6A).
  - **Contained fluid:** Intraabdominal abscess, hematoma, biloma, urinoma, pancreatic pseudocyst

Imaging Techniques

Ultrasound
- Anechoic; freely flowing with patient repositioning
- Easily compressible with probe pressure

Figure 4-6 Ascites and Hemoperitoneum: contrast-enhanced computed tomography (CECT) of the pelvis shows free intraperitoneal fluid (simple ascetic fluid) in image **A**. Layering high-attenuating material as shown with arrow (sedimented red blood cells) is known as the "hematocrit effect" and is consistent with hemoperitoneum **(B)**.

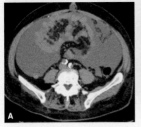 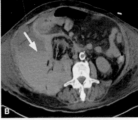

Computed Tomography
- Simple fluid attenuation (<20 Hounsfield unit [HU]) accumulating in dependent areas
- Fluid displaces bowel toward the center of the abdomen **(Figure 4-6A)**

Magnetic Resonance Imaging
- Signal intensity identical to simple fluid (T2-weighted [T2W] high, T1W low-signal intensity); may show artifacts from motion/flow

Hemoperitoneum

Background
- Hemoperitoneum is an important subtype of free intraperitoneal fluid in which the fluid consists of blood or hemorrhagic products.
  Typical causes are:
  - Trauma: Solid organ injury (mostly spleen and liver); mesentery and bowel injury
  - Iatrogenic: Postprocedural
  - Nontraumatic, spontaneous:
    - Complication of anticoagulant therapy
    - Ruptured aneurysm/pseudoaneurysm
    - Ruptured primary or secondary neoplasm
    - Ruptured ectopic pregnancy
    - Ruptured ovarian hemorrhagic cyst

Ultrasound
- Hypoechoic with internal echogenic debris, heterogeneous
- Fluid is not compressible with probe
- No mobility of fluid in repositioning

Computed Tomography
- Intraperitoneal fluid with increased attenuation; the attenuation may vary based on the patient's hemoglobin and age of the hemorrhage. Unclotted blood has an attenuation of 30–45 HU, clotted blood 45–70 HU
- Layering of blood products with fluid–fluid level (sediments) **(Figure 4-6B)**
- **Sentinel clot sign** (high-attenuation clotted blood): Indirect indicator of the source of bleeding in intraperitoneal hemorrhage

Magnetic Resonance Imaging
- Fluid with variable T2W signal intensity: High, intermediate or low depending on the age of the hemorrhage and concentration of blood products; T1W hyperintense compared to muscle; no enhancement

Differential Diagnosis of Contained or Loculated Fluid Collections
- Hematoma
- Intraabdominal abscess **(Figure 4-7A, B)**
- Biloma (injury to liver or bile duct system)
- Urinoma (if injury occurred to the urinary system)
- Postoperative seroma
- Lymphocele (injury to lymph vessel following LN dissection)
- Peritoneal inclusion cysts
- Cystic neoplasms, lymphangioma

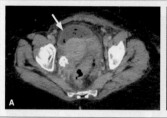
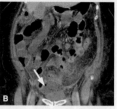

Figure 4-7A, B. Abscess secondary to perforated diverticulitis. Axial and coronal CECT demonstrate a contained, loculated fluid collection with peripheral enhancing wall and air pockets anterior to the uterus consistent with an abscess (Arrow in A and B).

Abscess

Background

- An abscess is a collection of pus and the most common cause for a contained fluid collection.
- An abscess is a complication of an infectious process and a known complication of surgery. CT is the preferred imaging modality in the early postoperative period to evaluate for potential complications.

Common Causes of Intraabdominal Abscess

Organ	Etiology of the Abscess
Liver	Cholecystitis, cholangitis hematogenous (intraabdominal infection such as diverticulitis or septic emboli), contagious spread
Spleen	Hematogenous seeding, trauma, superinfection of hematoma
Pancreas	Necrotizing pancreatitis Pseudocyst superinfection
Kidney	Ascending infection Hematogenous seeding
Psoas	Discitis Contagious spread (intraabdominal or intraosseous infectious process) Hematogenous seeding
Retro-peritoneum	Duodenal ulcer perforation, diverticulitis, Crohn disease
Peritoneum	Postoperative condition of any kind Bowel perforation, penetrating trauma, Crohn phlegmon and fistulizing disease

Imaging Findings

Radiography

- Abscesses are difficult to diagnose on plain radiographs; clues are:
  - Presence of a mass-like soft tissue density
  - Presence of air–fluid levels and/or clustered collection of foci of gas/air in unexpected location
  - Focal ileus (indirect sign)

Ultrasound

- Gray-scale US: Complex fluid collection with:
  - Ill-defined wall
  - Internal echoes or septations
  - Echogenic foci with dirty shadowing (depending on the amount of gas)
- Color Doppler:
  - Hypervascular periphery, avascular center

Computed Tomography

- Heterogeneous fluid collection (HU >50) with variable amount of gas
- Peripheral wall enhancement; adjacent fat stranding
- Mass effect on the adjacent organs (depending on size)

Aorta and Vasculature

Background

- Aortic dissection is one of the most critical acute aortic syndromes; others include intramural hematoma and penetrating ulcer.
- Dissection is a tear in the innermost of the three layers of the aortic wall (intima, media and adventitia). A tear in the intima allows blood to pass between intima and media creating a "false" lumen. Blood flow and velocity is different in "true" and "false" lumen.
- Various classifications exist to describe the location and extent of dissections related to the aorta.

Classifications

Stanford Classification

- Type A (60–70%): Involving the ascending aorta regardless of site of the origin; may extend into the descending aorta **(Figure 4-8A–D)**
- Type B (30–40%): Origin distal to the left subclavian artery and extending distally

Figure 4-8A, D. Aortic dissection Stanford type A. Axial CECT images (**A**, **B**) show an intimal dissection flap within the ascending and descending thoracic aorta extending into the arch branches, specifically right brachiocephalic artery (**A**, *arrow*). What is referred to as "beak sign" is shown (*) on **B**. Mediastinal hemorrhage is tracking in the pericardial recesses and pulmonary artery sheath (**B**, **). **C**: In the abdominal aorta, the dissection flap involves the ostium of the left renal artery; there is no contrast enhancement of the left kidney (*arrow*) and renal artery (*arrowhead*) concerning for ischemia/infarction. **D**: Sagittal 3D reformat demonstrates the full extent of involvement.

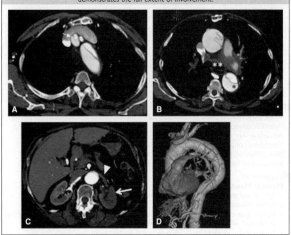

De Bakey Classification

- Type I: Origin in the ascending aorta propagating at least to the aortic arch and often more distally
- Type II: Confined to the ascending aorta
- Type III: Origin in descending aorta propagating distally

Complications

- Complications of aortic dissection vary depending on the type and extent of involvement.

Complications in the Thoracic Aorta and Branches: (Figure 4-8A, B)

- Acute aortic valve regurgitation
- Pericardial tamponade
- Aortic rupture into the left pleural cavity, mediastinum, right ventricle, pulmonary arteries

- Major aortic branch obstruction: Coronary and supraaortic extent such as brachiocephalic dissection with or without limb ischemia, and,
- Neurologic ischemic attack (5–10%)

Complications in the Abdominal Aorta and Branches:
- Occlusion or dissection of the major abdominal aortic branches with organ malperfusion:
  - Splenic or hepatic perfusion abnormalities/infarct (celiac trunk)
  - Kidney infarct or lack of perfusion **(Figure 4-8C)** (renal artery)
  - Mesenteric ischemia/infarct (superior mesenteric artery [SMA]/IMA)
  - Perfusion deficit and ischemia to the lower limbs (common/external iliac arteries and more distally)

Imaging Findings
- On imaging, the false lumen is typically identified as the larger cross-sectional portion of the split lumen with delayed contrast filling. Terms used for its appearance are "cobweb sign," "beak sign," and crescent shape. The false lumen may thrombose.

Ultrasound
- TTE or TEE with Doppler is the modality of choice for unstable patients (good availability; fast performance)
- Ability to identify flap: Transthoracic echocardiogram (TTE): Sensitivity 59–83%, specificity 63–93%; transesophageal echocardiogram (TEE): Sensitivity 94–100%, specificity 77–100%
- Limitation: Operator dependent; small FOV; low sensitivity to identify the complications; no information for surgical planning

Computed Tomography Angiography (CTA)
- CTA is the mainstay for diagnosis of acute aortic syndromes
- High sensitivity (100%), high specificity (98%), high NPV
- CTA Protocol includes non-enhanced computed tomography (NECT) + CECT (use bolus tracking; flow rate of 3–4 mL/s); ECG gating is required (decreases false positives due to motion artifact)
- Role of CECT: To detect the site of tear and origin of dissection; determine extent of involvement, specifically of great vessels; identify the origin of the branch vessels relative to true vs. false lumen
- Role of NECT: Helpful to detect intramural hematoma, blood clots, and acute hemorrhage

3D Contrast-Enhanced MRA
- To be performed if there is contraindication for CT (contrast-related issues or radiation concern)
- Advantage: No radiation
- Limitation: Longer, more complex examination
- Non enhanced-magnetic resonance (NE-MR) may be indicated in patients with limited renal function and concern for contrast nephropathy (GFR <30)

Management
Medical Management:
- Type B uncomplicated dissection; surveillance and blood pressure control

Interventional Management:
- IR management is indicated in Type A dissection and complicated Type B dissection associated with high likelihood of mortality
- Endovascular IR techniques: High technical success rates; low morbidity and mortality; however, no prospective study available comparing open surgery with endovascular techniques
- Widely practiced IR procedures include:
  - Branch vessel stenting
  - Aortic fenestration
  - Aortic endograft placement

THE LIVER

Background

Liver Anatomy
- Dual blood supply by portal vein (75%) and hepatic artery (25%)
- Separate blood supply of the caudate lobe
- Visceral peritoneum covering the liver except at the bare area, the gallbladder bed and the porta hepatis

- Porta hepatis contains the portal triad: Main portal vein, common hepatic artery (CHA) and CBD
- The falciform ligament: A double fold of peritoneum from the anterior abdominal wall to the liver surface; it separates posteriorly to surround the bare area; it carries the remnants of umbilical veins
- The liver is anatomically divided into 8 segments following the Couinaud classification **(Figure 4-9A, B)**. This segmentation is the basis for surgical resections.

Figure 4-9A, B. Couinaud classification of liver segments. **A:** Superior aspect of the liver (above portal vein). **B:** Inferior aspect of the liver (below portal vein). Left (*1*), middle (*2*) and right (*3*) hepatic veins are anatomic landmarks between segments *II*, *IVa*, *VIII*, and *VII* in the superior plane and between segments *III*, *IVb*, *V*, and *VI* in the inferior plane. The caudate lobe (*I*) is located anterior to the IVC.

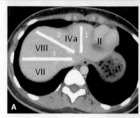 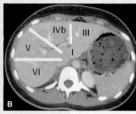

Vascular Variations of the Hepatic Arterial Supply
- Normal, conventional anatomy is seen in 55% of the population; the remainder has replaced the origin of hepatic arteries or accessory origin of hepatic arteries.
- **Normal conventional anatomy:** Celiac artery > CHA > proper hepatic artery (MHA) > right and left branches (RHA, LHA)
- **Replaced origin:** Arterial blood supply from an ectopic location
- **Accessory origin:** Arterial blood supply from typical and ectopic branch. **Most common variations (based on Michel's classification 1955):**
  55%: Trifurcation of CHA into MHA, RHA, and LHA.
  10%: RHA, MHA, and LHA from CHA; replaced LHA from GDA
  11%: RHA and MHA from CHA; replaced RHA from SMA

Vascular Variations of Cystic Artery
- Variations of the cystic artery: 90% from RHA, 7% from LHA, 3% from CHA, and 1% from the GDA
- Coil embolization rarely may cause ischemic cholecystitis; hepatic radioembolization is rarely complicated by radiation cholecystitis.

Imaging Appearance of the Normal Liver

Ultrasound
- Normal liver parenchyma is hyperechoic relative to renal cortex and medulla and less echogenic than spleen and pancreas.
- Hepatic veins and portal veins are anechoic tubular structures with flow; portal vein branches have echogenic walls
- Normal bile ducts and hepatic arteries are only visualized in the porta hepatis.
  Hepatic Artery (Figure 4-10A):
  - Normal RI: 0.5–0.8; normal peak arterial velocity: <200 cm/s. May be artificially elevated if tortuous course of the vessel or kinks
  - Normal arterial waveform: Low resistive flow
  - Normal flow direction: Toward the liver
  Portal Vein (Figure 4-10B):
  - Normal waveform: Monophasic undulating with respiratory cycle
  - Normal flow direction: Toward the liver
  Hepatic Vein (Figure 4-10C):
  - Normal waveform: Triphasic
  - Normal flow direction: Away from the liver toward the IVC

Computed Tomography
  Dedicated Liver CT Protocol (for Focal Lesion Assessment):
  - Late arterial phase: ~30 s postinjection of contrast material
  - Portal venous phase: ~70–80 s

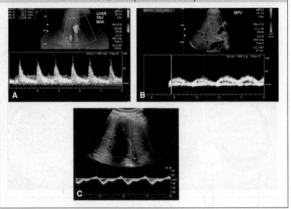

Figure 4-10A: Normal spectral waveform within a hepatic artery in a transplanted liver. Systolic upstroke is sharp and narrow (PSV <200 cm/s, acceleration time <0.08 s). **B:** Normal spectral waveform of a normal portal vein (MVP) in a transplanted liver. Antegrade monophasic flow with undulation (respiratory variation). **C:** Spectral waveform of a normal hepatic vein in a transplanted liver.

- Late venous phase: ~3–5 min
- Optional: 8–10 min delayed acquisition for characterizing hemangioma
- If preoperative workup for resection and arterial vascular supply perform CTA

Normal CT Appearance of the Liver
- Normal liver demonstrates a smooth border and pointed angle of the left liver lobe capsule.
- Liver attenuation: Normal for unenhanced liver: 55–65 HU; exceeds the attenuation of spleen by about 10 HU; if <40 HU: Fatty changes and hepatic steatosis; attenuation >70 HU: Iron deposition (primary or secondary hemochromatosis) and long-term amiodarone therapy

Magnetic Resonance Imaging (MRI)

Contrast Agents Used for Liver MR Imaging
Extracellular agents
- *Prototype:* Gd chelates (macrocyclic or linear)
- *Dosage:* 0.1–0.2 mmol/kg/BW
- *Elimination:* Almost entirely via the kidneys (concern for NSF in ESRD)
- **Indications:** Lesion detection and characterization, vascular anatomy
Hepatobiliary agents
  Gd-based hepatobiliary agents
- *Prototype:* (Agent 1) Gadoxetate/Gadoxetic acid (Gd-EOB); (agent 2) Gadobenate dimeglumine (Gd-BOPTA)
- *Dosage:* (Agent 1) 0.025–0.05 mmol/kg/BW; (agent 2) 0.05–0.1 mmol/kg/BW
- Intravascular and interstitial component; in addition, selective uptake into functional hepatocytes via specific cell-based carrier mechanisms
- *Elimination:* (Agent 1) 50% biliary and 50% renal depending on liver function; (Agent 2) elimination is mostly renal, only 5% through the biliary system
- *Biliary excretion:* First identified at 5 min after injection; optimal hepatobiliary phase depends on agent and is at approximately 20 min (agent 1) with later imaging (>25 min–3 h) preferred if poor hepatic function; for (agent 2) optimal hepatobiliary imaging is at 45–120 min up to 3 h postinjection
- **Indications:** Workup for liver metastasis, characterization of focal nodular hyperplasia (FNH), adenoma, hepatocellular carcinoma (HCC); evaluation of the bile duct system and for biliary leak
Reticuloendothelial agents
- *Prototype:* Superparamagnetic iron oxide nanoparticles (SPIO), (only in few countries; (Ferucarbotran SH U 555), Dosage: <60 kg: 0.45 mmol (0.9 mL): >60 kg: 0.7 mmol (1.4 mL); IV bolus injectable

- *Elimination:* Through intrinsic iron metabolism of the hepatocytes. Storage in reticulo-endothelial system (RES) of the liver
- Imaging is performed 10 min after injection up to 4 h.
- Normal liver parenchyma and benign lesions of hepatocellular origin with functional RES demonstrate signal drop in T2W and T2* imaging
- **Indications:** Detection of HCC in the background of cirrhosis, detection of metastases; does not further characterize lesion as benign or malignant or regarding tissue type

Standard Liver Protocol (Diffuse and Focal Disease)
- Coronal (and axial) T2W SSFSE
- T2W SSFSE or T2W FSE with fat saturation
- Axial In/out of phase GRE T1W for chemical shift
- Axial T1W GRE fat saturated pre contrast administration
- Axial T1W GRE arterial phase (20–25 s postinjection)
- Axial T1W GRE portal venous phase (70–80 s post injection)
- Axial/coronal T1W GRE equilibrium phase (3–5 min post injection)
- Diffusion-weighted imaging (DWI)
- Optional and only in selected cases: 8–10 min delayed acquisition may be helpful to characterize hemangioma and cholangiocarcinoma

Normal MRI Appearance of the Liver
- **Precontrast imaging:** Homogeneous parenchymal signal intensity
  - *T1W sequence:*
    - Types: In phase, opposed or out of phase, fat saturated
    - To depict presence of fat, iron, blood products, hemorrhage
    - Decreased signal intensity on out-of-phase compared to in-phase image: Steatosis
    - Decreased SI on in-phase compared to out-of-phase image: Iron deposition (hemochromatosis; hemosiderosis)
    - Focal increase in SI in all T1W sequence types: Blood products
  - *T2W sequence:*
    - Intermediate signal intensity, homogeneous
    - Markedly low SI indicated iron deposition/hemosiderin, chronic blood products, calcification
    - Intermediate-high SI indicates fatty changes
  - *Diffusion-weighted imaging (DWI)*
    - To detect focal liver lesions (FLL); minor role for characterization of FLL
    - No significant value in diffuse parenchymal disease
- **Postcontrast imaging:**
  - To assess vascular anatomy and patency; evaluation in arterial and (portal-) venous contrast phases
  - To characterize focal lesions due to distinct enhancement patterns over time and compared to liver enhancement
  - To detect perfusion abnormalities; evaluation in all liver phases (including the equilibrium phase)

Cirrhosis

Background
- **Definition of cirrhosis:** End point of fibrosis and scarring of the liver parenchyma following exposure to a toxic agent.
- **Underlying causes** (toxic agents) for liver cirrhosis include: Alcoholic liver disease, infectious (viral) disease, metabolic diseases (diabetes, steatosis, hemochromatosis), autoimmune disease, inflammatory disease (primary sclerosing cholangitis [PSC], primary biliary cholangitis [PBC], nonalcoholic steatohepatitis [NASH], nonalcoholic fatty liver disease [NAFLD], cryptogenic) and toxic drug exposure
- Cirrhosis is associated with an increased **risk** for developing HCC of 1–4% per year.
- **Complications** of liver cirrhosis include portal hypertension (HTN) with ascites, portosystemic collaterals and varices, recanalized umbilical vein, GI bleeding (from varices), splenomegaly, encephalopathy
- **Transjugular intrahepatic portosystemic shunt (TIPS):** Artificially created vascular shunt through the hepatic parenchyma with stent between the hepatic venous system (typically right hepatic vein) and the portal venous system (typically right portal vein branch); created to treat effects of portal HTN.

Imaging Findings in Cirrhosis

Ultrasound
- Nodular contour (best appreciated with a high-resolution [high–frequency] linear or curved array transducer)
- Coarse and heterogeneous parenchyma with nodularity

- Caudate/right lobe ratio >0.65
- Signs of **portal HTN** (hepatic venous pressure gradient >10 mmHg) as evidenced by: Ascites, splenomegaly, increased portal vein diameter (>1.3–1.5 cm), presence of collaterals (recanalized umbilical vein, paraesophageal varices, perisplenic collaterals); reversal of portal vein flow
- Portal HTN is measured by invasive angiographic techniques

Doppler US Evaluation TIPS

Normal TIPS
- Flow within portal venous vessels should be directed toward the TIPS stent (reverse flow in right and left portal branches and antegrade flow in MPV).
- Monophasic pulsatile flow within the stent with velocity of 90–190 cm/s (velocities are measured along the shunt in at least 3 locations proximal at portal vein, middle, and distal near hepatic vein).

TIPS malfunction
- Flow within portal vein branches away from the stent
- Increased velocity >200 cm/s within the stent (indicating stenosis) or <40–60 cm/s (at the stenosis)
- Shunt gradient of >50 cm/s across the stent
- Main portal vein peak velocity drops by <30 cm/s
- New or worsening ascites

Ultrasound Elastography
- Technique to detect and quantify liver fibrosis and cirrhosis by measuring the stiffness of liver tissue
- Increased parenchymal stiffness results in faster propagation of mechanical waves; Supersonic shear-wave elastography provides velocity measurements.
- SRS proposed 3 categories: low risk (elastography normal <5.5–7 kPa; F0 or F1; no follow-up); intermediate risk (F2–3, at risk of progression, follow-up required); and high risk for fibrosis (F3–4; high elastography values [>15 kPa]; need prioritization for therapy).

Computed Tomography
CT in Early Cirrhosis:
- Segmental or lobar hypertrophy of the left liver lobe or caudate lobe (Caudate/right lobe ratio > 0.65)
- Hepatomegaly
- Widening of the porta hepatis, enlargement of the interlobar fissure, expansion of pericholecystic space
- Heterogeneous appearance and enhancement of liver parenchyma

CT in advanced cirrhosis (Figure 4-11A, B):
- Shrinkage of the liver
- Nodular surface and parenchyma
- Lace-like geographic areas or bands of fibrosis

Magnetic Resonance Imaging
- Morphologic MRI findings are similar to CT findings **(Figure 4-11A, B)**
- MRI > CT > US to detect and characterize suspicious focal liver lesions and HCC in the cirrhotic liver

Figure 4-11A. Liver cirrhosis: Axial single-shot (SS) T2-weighted MR shows asymmetric shrinkage of the liver in the right lobe, asymmetric hypertrophy of the left lobe and caudate lobe, enlargement of the interlobar fissure, and nodular surface and parenchyma consistent with advanced cirrhosis. **B.** Axial T1-weighted fat sat postcontrast (70 s) shows lace-like geographic pattern of enhancement of the liver, more pronounced in the right lobe.

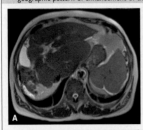
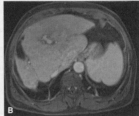

- MRI provides additional information about underlying liver disease such as steatosis or hemochromatosis.
- **MR elastography:** Most accurate noninvasive method to detect and stage liver fibrosis. MR elastographic stiffness (shear modulus in kPa) correlates with the degree and stage of fibrosis (normal <3.0 kPa).

Related IR Procedures
- TIPS
- Diagnostic or therapeutic paracentesis for ascites
- Transjugular hepatic biopsy
- Measurement of portal HTN by hepatic venous pressure gradient
- Portal vein thrombolysis
- Portosystemic collateral embolization

Focal Liver Lesions (FLL)

Background
- FLL are characterized with imaging based on signal intensity (MRI) and attenuation (CT) and enhancement patterns following intravenous contrast administration
- Preferred imaging modality to characterize an indeterminate >1-cm lesion detected on US in a normal liver: CEMR > CECT > NEMR > NECT (American College of Radiology [ACR] Appropriateness Criteria)
- Preferred imaging modality to characterize an indeterminate >1-cm lesion detected on US in the presence of known history of extrahepatic malignancy: CEMR > NEMR > CECT > Biopsy > FDG-PET > NECT (ACR Appropriateness Criteria)

HCC
- **Diagnosis** established based on imaging only without biopsy if characteristic imaging criteria present (size, number, and enhancement pattern)
- Likelihood of diagnosis of HCC in imaging reported based on **LI-RADS** classification system (Liver Imaging Reporting and Data System)
- **Treatment options:** Surgical resection; liver transplant; minimally invasive interventional ablation techniques (if no candidate for surgery or transplant or if multifocal but locally limited disease).

Clinical Classifications and Scoring Systems Related to HCC
- **MELD Score (Model of End-stage Liver Disease):** Classification to score patients with liver failure between 6–40 to indicate liver transplant. Components include serum creatinine (mg/dL), total bilirubin (mg/dL) and INR.
- **Milan Criteria:** Widely used system to evaluate suitability of patients with HCC for liver transplant. Single lesion: ≤5, OR: Up to 3 lesions up to 3 cm in size; no vascular invasion or extrahepatic spread
- **AASLD (American Association for Study of Liver Disease):** Evidence-based guidelines by a committee of experts providing recommendations of preferred approaches to the diagnostic, therapeutic and preventative aspects of care (updated every 5 years)
- **Other classification systems:** Barcelona Criteria, San Francisco Criteria

Radiologic Imaging

Ultrasound
- Imaging modality of choice to screen cirrhotic patients for nodules
- Imaging findings: Nodule of any echogenicity, mostly hypoechoic
- CEUS: Demonstrates hypervascularity with arterial hyperenhancement and washout

Computed Tomography
- Triple-phase imaging with late arterial phase, portal venous phase and delayed-phase imaging is recommended
- **Imaging findings:** Lesion with arterial hyperenhancement, delayed washout (hypodensity relative to liver parenchyma); pseudocapsule (perilesional rim of delayed enhancement)
- **Additional imaging findings:** Intralesional fat, vascular invasion, interval growth of 50% or more on serial imaging 6 mo or less apart

Magnetic Resonance Imaging
- **Imaging findings:** Nodule with isointense or mildly hyperintense signal on T2W imaging; isointensity, hyperintensity, or hypointensity on T1WI, diffusion restriction
  Extracellular contrast agent
  - Arterial hyperenhancement, delayed washout (hypointensity relative to liver parenchyma); pseudocapsule (perilesional rim of delayed hyperenhancement); (similar to CT) **(Figure 4-12A–C)**

Hepatobiliary contrast agent
- **Standard contrast phases:** Arterial hyperenhancement, delayed washout (hypointensity relative to liver parenchyma); pseudocapsule (perilesional rim of delayed hyperenhancement); (similar to CT)
- **Hepatobiliary contrast phase:** Lack of uptake of the hepatobiliary agent within the lesion; note: Well-differentiated HCC may demonstrate uptake in hepatobiliary phase
- **Additional imaging findings:**
  Intralesional fat, vascular invasion, interval growth of 50% or more on serial imaging 6 mo or less apart (as with CT)

Figure 4-12A–C. HCC, LI-RADS 5 lesion: Axial T2WI SSFSE with fat saturation shows mildly hyperintense lesion in liver segment 8 **(A)**. The lesion enhances strongly in arterial phase **(B,** T1WI fat saturated images @25 s) and has washout appearance on portal venous phase **(C;** T1WI fat saturated images @70 s). Note that size >2 cm is an important criterion.

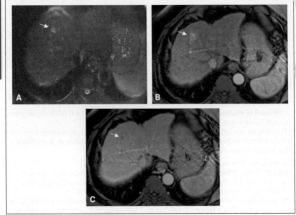

Metastasis
- In general, metastasis shows imaging features similar to the primary neoplasm.
- Metastases may be hypervascular or hypovascular:
  - Hypovascular metastases: Pancreatic and GI adenocarcinoma, cholangiocarcinoma, breast, lung, others
  - Hypervascular metastases: Kidney, thyroid, malignant melanoma, neuroendocrine tumors, sarcoma, breast, others
  - Metastasis containing macroscopic fat are very rare (liposarcoma)

Ultrasound
- Metastasis may demonstrate any echogenicity, central hypoechoic necrosis, target appearance
- Irregular and/or poorly delineated contours

Computed Tomography
- Imaging modality of choice for staging and workup of cancer
- **Imaging findings:**
  - Variable enhancement pattern; mostly heterogeneous enhancement on single portal venous phase
  - *Hypovascular metastasis:* Poor arterial enhancement, peripheral rim enhancement in delayed phases; slow progressive enhancement
  - *Hypervascular metastasis:* Avid enhancement in arterial phase; Note: This type requires multiphase protocol including arterial phase

Magnetic Resonance Imaging
- MRI > CT to detect and characterize a focal liver lesion in the known history of malignancy
- MRI > CT to detect hemorrhage, fat, fibrosis, necrosis
- DWI improves detection of metastasis, specifically if small size

- Hepatobiliary agents improve detection of metastasis, specifically if small size
- **Imaging findings:**
  - In general intermediate to mildly hyperintense on T2WI, except mucinous metastasis which is strongly hyperintense
  - *Hypovascular metastasis:* Hypointense on T1WI, poorly enhancing in arterial phase of dynamic imaging; may exhibit "rim" enhancement; may show gradual enhancement
  - *Hypervascular metastasis:* Best seen in arterial phase; hypointense on T1WI and strongly enhancing in arterial phase
  - Most metastases are heterogeneous (especially when larger) with heterogeneous enhancement. Diffusion restriction is an important feature **(Figure 4-13A–D)**

Figure 4-13A–D. Metastasis. On axial T2W SSFSE **(A)**, a slightly hyperintense lesion is identified in segment 4 which demonstrates diffusion restriction on b-800 DWI **(B).** The lesion enhances peripherally in the arterial phase and (T1WI fs 25 s; **C**) is progressively predominantly heterogeneous on later postcontrast phases (T1WI fs 70 s; **D**).

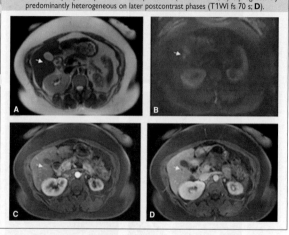

Cholangiocarcinoma
- **Predisposing liver conditions:** PSC, pyogenic cholangitis, hepatitis C, human immunodeficiency virus (HIV), ulcerative colitis, parasitic infections (fluke), chemical carcinogens (Thorotrast, asbestos, nitrosamine).
- **Subtypes:**
  - **Intrahepatic:** 75%, mass-forming type (most common)—periductal infiltrating type—intraductal growing type
  - **Extrahepatic:** Irregular asymmetric wall thickening of the bile duct with abnormally increased enhancement
  - **Extrahepatic subtype** in the hilum (Klatskin tumor) classified based on Bismuth–Corlette classification.
- **Imaging findings:**
- Mass type: Mixed hypoattenuating/hypointense lesion with target appearance; arterial peripheral enhancement and peripheral washout, gradual centripetal progressive enhancement (delayed images may be helpful)
- Capsular retraction, satellite nodules, biliary ductal dilatation
- Shows lack of uptake with hepatobiliary contrast agents

Related IR Procedures
- Biopsy for tissue characterization
  Ablation of FLL
- Percutaneous transhepatic cholangiography (PTHC) for ductal type and Klatskin

Imaging of Post Microinvasive Local Treatment

Background
- **Types of local treatment:** Microwave, cryo and radiofrequency ablation (RFA); chemo- and particle embolization (TACE), radioembolization (Y90).

Figure 4-14A–F. Axial T2-weighted SSFSE, ADC and postcontrast T1-weighted imaging in a patient with HCC treated with radioablation (Y90). The lesion in segment 7 has high signal on T2WI (**A**), no diffusion restriction (**B**) and peripheral rim enhancement which can be seen as postradiation inflammatory change (**C**). On treatment follow-up (T2-weighted SSFSE, DWI, post-contrast T1-weighted: **D, E, F**), lesion enlarges, shows solid components with diffusion restriction in the lateral aspect (**E**, *arrow*) and heterogeneous internal enhancement. These findings are concerning for viable residual or recurrent tumor. Abnormal geographic perfusion in the periphery of the lesion is again radiation-induced change.

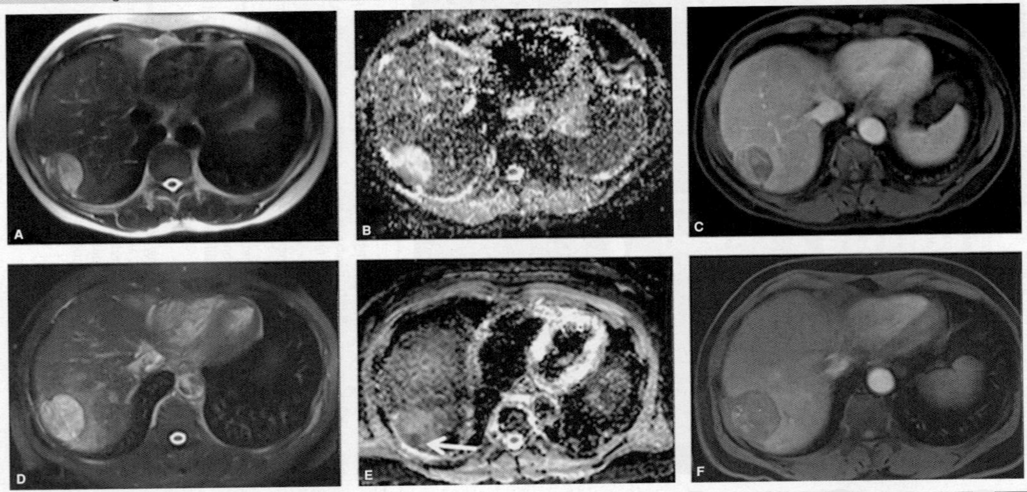

- **Indications:** 1st-line treatment of FLL, bridging and downstaging for subsequent transplant, palliative treatment, limitations to surgery, combined with intraoperative therapy
- Time point for **imaging follow-up** is typically at 6 wk–3 mo postintervention if no suspicion for acute complication

Imaging Findings on Follow-up

Effective treatment
- Area of treatment (ablation): Includes the area of prior lesion in full extent plus safety margin (larger than original lesion); well-demarcated boundaries; CT: Low attenuation; MRI: Hypo-, iso-, or hyperintense on T1WI (hemorrhagic products); hypo- or isointense on T2WI; no or minimal progressive delayed enhancement (preferably assessed on subtraction MR images)
- Decrease in lesional enhancement, peripheral rim enhancement is possible as posttreatment inflammatory reaction
- Decrease in size of the treatment zone on serial follow up imaging
- Stable shape of treatment zone
- No diffusion restriction (subject to artifacts due to susceptibility)

Recurrence
- Revascularization of previously necrotic (nonenhancing) area **(Figure 4-14A–F)**
- New focus of abnormal enhancement at the margin of the treated area
- New focus of diffusion restriction at the margin of treated area
- Change in shape

Pitfalls
- Perfusion changes of the liver parenchyma surrounding the lesion specifically with Y90 (more than with RFA or TACE) due to radiation-induced veno-occlusive changes; may mimic recurrence
- Circumferential faint hyperenhancement in the periphery of the lesion representing inflammatory reaction to treatment, may mimic recurrence; will resolve with time
- DWI: Susceptibility artifacts and pseudorestriction from hemorrhagic changes may mimic true diffusion restriction and recurrence

Complications
- Development of fluid collections (hematoma, abscess, biloma)
  - Pseudoaneurysm, active hemorrhage
  - Vascular dissection or occlusion biliary stricture (at follow-up) and upstream peripheral biliary dilatation

Imaging of Liver Transplant

Background
- Three types of liver transplantation: (1) cadaveric; (2) living donor (left lateral hepatectomy, right and left lobectomy); (3) split liver graft which includes right extended graft (segments I and IV–VIII) and left lateral graft (segments II–IV)
- Three main vascular anastomoses (mostly end-to-end): (1) Portal vein (×1); (2) IVC (×2, unless piggyback technique); (3) hepatic artery (×1)

Nonvascular biliary anastomosis: Three types: (1) choledocho-choledochal (end-to-side, end-to-end); (2) choledocho- to cystic duct; (3) hepaticojejunostomy, preferred in patients with sclerosing cholangitis

Imaging of Posttransplant Liver
- Doppler US is the first imaging modality for the transplanted liver in immediate postoperative period and in follow-up
- If concern for vascular complication on US: Contrast-enhanced US, CTA or MRA are indicated; digital subtraction angiography is used for confirmation and interventional treatment
- If concern for biliary leak: CT or MRI with MRCP; MRI with hepatobiliary agents; ERCP for confirmation and treatment
- If concern for biliary stricture or vascular stricture: MRA, MRI, MRCP

Complications of Liver Transplant

Vascular Complications
  Hepatic artery thrombosis:
  - Most common complication of liver transplant
  - **Doppler US:** Lack of flow (nonvisualization)
  - Be aware of the false-positive findings in the immediate postoperative period due to slow flow or technical factors.
  - **CTA and MRA:** Contrast-filling defect on cross-sectional imaging

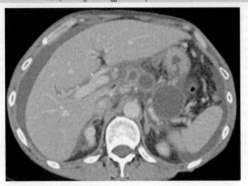

Figure 4-15 Hepatic artery stenosis posttransplant: Tardus-parvus waveform is observed in the proper hepatic artery with decreased systolic upstroke and delayed time to systolic peak resulting in dampening of distal arterial waveform. RI is low (not calculated here). Findings are suggestive of proximal stenosis.

Hepatic artery stenosis: (Figure 4-15)
- **Doppler US:** Low RI (<0.5)
- Prolonged acceleration time (>0.08 s)
- Tardus-parvus waveform distal to stenosis
- Increased PSV at the stenotic site (>200 cm/s) (may be at the anastomosis or anywhere along the vessel)
- High RI within the liver may be seen in 50% in the immediate postoperative period due to edema and decreased diastolic flow
- **CTA and MRA** to confirm US findings and to depict vascular stricture; to guide treatment decision (IR or surgery)

Pseudoaneurysm
- *Extrahepatic:* At the arterial anastomosis site or as complication of angioplasty
- *Intrahepatic:* Complication of percutaneous biopsy, biliary procedures, or infection.
- **Doppler US:** To-fro, turbulent flow, ying-yang patterns
- **CTA and MRA:** Contrast-filled aneurysmal pouch

Arteriovenous Fistula (AVF)
- Usually complication following biopsy
- **Doppler US:** Increased peak velocity with low-resistance waveform (increased diastolic flow, low RI) in the artery; aliasing/ turbulent flow in the fistula; increased velocity and pulsatile flow on the venous end
- **CT and MRI:** Premature enhancement of peripheral portal veins and corresponding wedge-shaped region of liver parenchyma with abnormal perfusion

Portal Vein Stenosis
- **Doppler US:** Peak anastomotic velocity >125/s
- Anastomotic/preanastomotic ratio >3/1
- **CT and MRI:** Anastomotic narrowing on cross-sectional imaging

Portal Vein Thrombosis
- **Doppler US:** Lack of flow within the portal vein; increased heterogeneous echogenicity within the vessel lumen on B-mode US
- Be aware of false positives due to technical factors due to slow flow; use of nondirectional PW technique may be helpful
- **CT and MRI:** Filling defect on contrast-enhanced cross-sectional imaging.

IVC Stenosis
- Caused by anastomotic narrowing or any external compression, for instance by hematoma
- **Doppler US:** A 3–4× increased velocity of the affected IVC, aliasing, distension of hepatic veins with dampening or loss of phasicity of the hepatic waveform (from triphasic to monophasic)

IVC Thrombosis/Hepatic Vein Thrombosis
- Usually caused by surgical factors and hypercoagulability state
- Filling defect and lack of flow in the IVC

Hepatic Vein Stenosis
- **Doppler US:** Venous pulsatility index <0.45; monophasic waveform

Biliary Complications
Biliary Obstruction/Stones
- Obstruction usually secondary to anastomotic stricture, less frequently choledocholithiasis

Bile Duct Stricture
- At the anastomotic site: Secondary to surgical technique or scar formation
- Nonanastomotic site stricture due to posttransplant ischemia or relapse of prior disease (PSC, PBC, etc.)

Bile Leak and Biloma
- Bile leak occurs mostly at the anastomotic site; on **HIDA scan** appears as extravasation of radiotracer and accumulation in abdomen with no morphologic characteristics
- CT and MRI: Loculated fluid collection subhepatic or in porta hepatis. MRI with hepatobiliary contrast agents may be helpful
- Biloma: Contained leak within liver parenchyma or outside

Other Complications
- **Abscess, seroma, and hematoma:** May have similar imaging features. In presence of hematoma, underlying hepatic artery stenosis and biliary necrosis should be excluded.
- **Neoplasm:** recurrence of HCC; posttransplant lymphatic disease (PTLD)

Related IR Procedures
- Biliary percutaneous drain if biliary stenosis
- Arterial angioplasty of transplant artery
- Percutaneous drainage of fluid collections

THE PANCREAS

Acute Pancreatitis and Indications for Intervention

Background
- **Two main clinical presentations of acute pancreatitis:** (1) Interstitial edematous pancreatic; (2) necrotizing pancreatitis. Main difference: Presence of pancreatic necrosis in (2)
- **Atlanta Classification:** Provides standardized nomenclature for acute pancreatitis and its complications; worldwide consensus published and updated in 2016 (revised Atlanta Classification)
- **Pancreatitis-associated fluid collections** are a complication of both forms of acute pancreatitis and are defined as follows:
  - *With interstitial edematous pancreatitis:* <4 wk: Acute peripancreatic fluid collection; >4 wk: Pancreatic pseudocyst
  - *With necrotizing pancreatitis:* <4 wk: Acute necrotic fluid collection, >4 wk: Walled of necrosis
  - *Necrotic collections:* Are further classified as parenchymal, peripancreatic, or combined
- **Pancreatic pseudocyst:**
  - Most common pancreatic cystic mass
  - Develops within 4–6 wk after an episode of acute pancreatitis
  - Fluid collections <6 cm often resolve spontaneously
  - **Complications:** Superinfection, internal hemorrhage, rupture, pseudoaneurysm, mass effect on adjacent organs requiring intervention **(Figure 4-16)**
  - **Other complications:**
  - Splenic vein and superior mesenteric vein thrombosis, splenic artery aneurysm, splenic infarct
  - Colitis

Imaging
- Transabdominal US used as a screening method for collections
- CT and MRI are equally well suited to diagnose acute pancreatitis and associated fluid collections and complications
- MRI > CT to distinguish between necrotic tissue (walled-off necrosis) and pseudocyst
- MRI/MRCP > CT to identify pancreatic ductal injury
- MRI particularly useful to diagnose internal hemorrhage and pseudoaneurysm
- Endosonography used for guidance of endoluminal drainage and cyst-gastrostomy
- **Imaging findings of pseudocyst:**
  US: Well-delineated margin, internal heterogeneity due to debris
  CT: Higher than simple fluid attenuation; heterogeneous, with internal hemorrhagic and/or necrotic products with high SI in T1WI, low to intermediate SI in T2WI, peripheral enhancing rim (pseudocapsule)

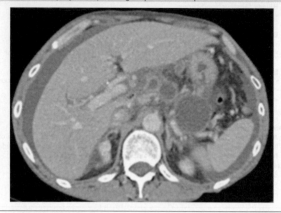

Figure 4-16 Pancreatic pseudocyst. CECT of the abdomen shows several unilocular encapsulated fluid collections with enhancing rim at the expected location of the pancreas (body and tail) following an episode of acute pancreatitis.

Imaging Findings Relevant by Type of Intervention
- **Endoscopic transgastric or transduodenal endoluminal drainage (cystogastrostomy):**
  - Preferably close anatomic vicinity to the stomach, need be of sufficient size; good way of access
  - Interposed prominent vasculature or collaterals is unfavorable
  - Arterialization with formation of pseudoaneurysm and internal hemorrhage may be relative contraindication
- **ERCP and pancreatic ductal stent:**
  - For pancreatic ductal injury, best seen on MRCP imaging
- **US- and CT-guided percutaneous drainage:**
  - Preferred if collection in difficult anatomic location
  - In presence of infection nonresponsive to antibiotic therapy
  - Be aware: Most sterile collections resolve without intervention
- **Intravascular embolization of pancreatic pseudoaneurysm:**
  - Pancreatic pseudoaneurysm: Rare but **life-threatening condition** requiring immediate embolization due to risk of rupture
  - Needs preinterventional contrast-enhanced arterial phase CTA or MRA to show arterial communication between artery and pseudocyst due to chronic erosion
  - **Key imaging finding:** Arterial enhancement of the pseudocyst
  - Most common site of communication: Pancreatic/peripancreatic branches of the splenic artery (splenic artery > hepatic artery).
  - Controversy about the need for a subsequent surgery
- **Surgery**
  - Only if superinfection of pancreatic or extrapancreatic necrosis (gas pockets, strong peripheral enhancement)
  - Should—if possible—be postponed to >4 wk to deal with walled-off necrosis.

THE SPLEEN

Background
- The Spleen is the most frequently injured solid organ during abdominal blunt trauma.
- Main types of injury include: (1) Subcapsular hematoma; (2) laceration (tear, focal lack of perfusion) or intraparenchymal hematoma; (3) splenic rupture and perisplenic hematoma (with or without active hemorrhage); and (4) devascularization
- Treatment: Conservative (1 and 2 with observation), if active bleed embolization may be discussed (3); splenectomy (if unstable; 4)

AAST Spleen Injury Scale (American Association for the Surgery of Trauma) is a widely used grading system

Grade	Description
1	Subcapsular hematoma (SH) ≤10% of surface area (SA), capsular laceration (L) ≤1-cm depth
2	SH = 10–50% of SA; IH = >5 cm or expanding; L = 1–3 cm in depth without involving trabecular vessels
3	SH >50% of SA or expanding; IH >5 cm or expanding; L ≥3 cm or involving trabecular vessels
4	L = involving segmental or hilar vessels with major devascularization >25% of the spleen
5	Shattered spleen, hilar vascular injury with splenic devascularization

SH, subcapsular hematoma; SA, surface area; L, laceration; IH, intraparenchymal hematoma.

Imaging Findings

Ultrasound
- Focused assessment with sonography for trauma (**FAST**) US examination in the emergency room determines presence of free fluid in the abdomen (1st-line diagnosis).
- US is helpful for perisplenic hematoma or subcapsular hematoma; less sensitive for intraparenchymal lesions

Computed Tomography
- CT is the imaging **modality of choice** in a hemodynamically stable patient posttrauma to determine type and degree of injury.
- Multiphase imaging protocol (including arterial + portal venous phases) is strongly recommended to identify active bleed (specifically intraparenchymal);
- Active bleed mostly prompts interventional angiography to confirm the hemorrhage and embolize the relevant vessel(s); requires close postprocedural monitoring for secondary hemorrhage
- Subcapsular hematoma: Elliptoid or crescent shaped, with indentation (mass effect) on the parenchyma;
- Perisplenic fluid with mixed and higher than fluid attenuation; pelvic hemoperitoneum with or without contrast extravasate (active bleed)
- Carefully assess the spleen for the intact capsule
- Carefully assess for arterial dissection or injury to trabecular or hilar vessels (devascularization)

Magnetic Resonance Imaging
- MRI does not play any significant role in the setting of acute trauma

Splenic Abscess

Background
- Splenic abscess may develop as superinfection of a previous hematoma or from infection in the vicinity of the spleen (colitis, pancreatitis, iatrogenic postsurgery); focal abscess can be treated with percutaneous drainage.
- Other etiologies: Septic emboli; systemic infection as in candidiasis, epstein barr virus (EBV), etc.; in these cases often multiple lesions; systemic treatment.

Imaging
- Imaging modality of choice: Computed tomography;
- **Imaging findings:** Fluid collection with expansile, space-occupying character, peripheral enhancement, internal gas
- **US:** Less specific, may identify a perisplenic fluid collection; distinction between an intrasplenic and perisplenic abscess may be challenging
- **MRI:** Limited role due to high cost and less availability

Related IR Procedure
Percutaneous drainage

Splenomegaly

Background
- Normal dimensions of the spleen: 4 cm × 7 cm × 11 cm.
- Enlargement of the spleen: >13 cm largest diameter
- Large spectrum of causes for splenomegaly: Most commonly:
  - *Infection:* EBV, HIV, histoplasmosis, toxoplasmosis, malaria, brucellosis, tuberculosis, leptospirosis, candidiasis (if immunocompromised), echinococcosis, sepsis
  - *Inflammation:* Sarcoidosis, amyloidosis

- *Hematologic disease:* Acute lymphocytic leukemia (ALL), osteomyelosclerosis, AML, CML (acute and chronic myeloid leukemia), non-Hodgkin lymphoma (NHL), hemolytic anemia, malignant lymphoma, polycythemia vera, hemochromatosis
- *Hereditary:* Sickle cell anemia, thalassemia, metabolic
- *Other conditions:* Portal HTN secondary to portal vein thrombosis or liver cirrhosis
- **Treatment:** IR techniques in limited indications: Embolization for thrombocytopenia, splenic parenchymal or vessel injury with active bleed, embolization for varices.
- **Complication** (splenectomy or splenic embolization): Infection; pneumococcal infection

Imaging

- To measure size; US, CT, or MRI are equal, multiple planes
- To evaluate splenic parenchyma for focal lesions
- To assess for abnormal focal or diffuse glucose metabolism (with FDG-PET and PET/CT)

Related IR Procedure

Splenic artery or parenchymal embolization

Splenic Artery Aneurysm

Background

- Third most common site of intraabdominal aneurysms after abdominal aorta and iliac arteries; 4× more common in women; risk of rupture 3× more in male patients
- **Underlying causes:** Spontaneous, portal HTN, pancreatitis, trauma, vasculitis, atherosclerosis, pregnancy
- **Clinical presentation:** Mostly (>95%) asymptomatic; often detected incidentally. Risk of rupture is low if <2 cm, but increases with liver transplantation, portal HTN, and pregnancy. Calcifications are frequent. Presentation of ruptured splenic artery aneurysm: Sudden onset of left upper quadrant abdominal pain; hemodynamic instability, gastrointestinal bleeding.
- **Management:**
  – If asymptomatic, <2 cm, no risk factors: 1-year follow-up
  – If >2 cm in size, rapid increase in size, premenopausal woman, cirrhosis or symptoms: Endovascular treatment (coil embolization)

Figure 4-17A–D. Ruptured splenic artery aneurysm. CT angiogram of the abdomen (**A–C**); portal venous phase in a different patient (**D**). The splenic artery aneurysm enhances in arterial angiographic phase (**A**) and is better appreciated in its full extent on coronal maximum intensity projection (MIP) images (**B**; *arrow*). A large adjacent hematoma (fluid with higher than simple water attenuation) indicates acute hemorrhage (******; **C**), the active extravasation of the contrast is not well seen. **D:** Splenic artery aneurysm in a different patient: Note that the peripheral rim of calcification (*) may be better appreciated on portal venous phase, however can also be seen using CT windowing in arterial phase imaging.

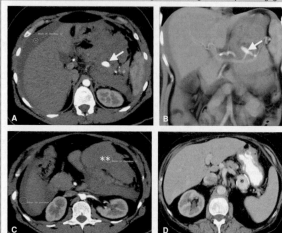

Imaging

- Imaging modality of choice: **CTA** (Figure 4-17)
- **US/Doppler:** Depending on location
- **MRA:** Equal to CTA except for calcifications, limited to selected cases
- **Digital subtraction angiography:** For embolization, not diagnosis
- **Differential diagnosis:** Traumatic injury, pseudoaneurysm, splenic steal

Related IR Procedure
Splenic artery embolization

THE ADRENAL GLANDS

Adrenal Adenoma

Background

- **Clinical presentation:** Adenoma may be secretory or not. Nonsecretory adenomas are asymptomatic. If secretory, clinical presentation depends on the secreted hormone and results in respective endocrinologic syndromes (hypercortisolism—Cushing syndrome; hyperaldosteronism—Conn syndrome; testosterone hypersecretion—hirsutism)
- **Differential diagnosis:**
  Unilateral adrenal mass or asymmetrical enlargement: Benign: Lipid-rich (majority of 70%) or lipid-poor adrenal adenoma, hyperplasia, myelolipoma, hemorrhage, (pseudo)cyst; *Malignant:* Metastasis (most frequent neoplasm), primary adrenocortical carcinoma, pheochromocytoma, paraganglioma
  Bilateral adrenal enlargement: IR may be indicated to perform venous sampling to distinguish between hyperplasia and adenomas. Venous sampling is the standard of reference for the localization of aldosterone-secreting adenomas.
- Venous sampling is performed in the respective renal vein which receives the adrenal veins.

Imaging

- Imaging modality of choice: **CT**

Computed Tomography

- **Dedicated imaging protocol** for adrenal mass including:
  - Noncontrast
  - 60 s postintravenous contrast injection
  - 15 min postcontrast injection
- To determine diagnosis of adrenal adenoma: Calculate the relative and absolute enhancement washout in %:
  Absolute contrast enhancement washout (ACEW) in %:
  $ACEW$ = [(contrast-enhanced HU at 60 s − delayed contrast HU)/(contrast-enhanced HU at 60 s − noncontrast HU)] × 100.
- If ACEW >52%: 100% sensitivity, 98% specificity for adrenal adenoma
- ACEW requires a noncontrast image set for HU measurement
- If noncontrast imaging is not obtained:
  Relative contrast enhancement washout (RCEW) in %:
  $RCEW$ = [(contrast-enhanced HU at 60 s − delayed contrast HU)/(contrast-enhanced HU at 60 s)] × 100.

Magnetic Resonance Imaging

- To identify and distinguish lipid-rich from lipid-poor adenoma and other lesions by chemical shift imaging (T1W in/opposed phase). Ratio between lesion and spleen can be determined as quantitative reference. Lipid-poor adenomas are difficult to discern from other neoplasms
- Contrast-enhanced MRI does not allow for quantification of washout.

Related IR Procedure: Venous sampling

KIDNEYS

Background

- The kidneys are located in the retroperitoneum, usually at the level of the 11th or 12th thoracic to the 2nd or 3rd lumbar vertebral bodies.
- The kidney consists of renal cortex and medulla.
- The renal vasculature and collecting system enter and exit the renal hilum and branch within the renal sinus. The anatomic arrangement within the hilum from anterior to posterior is: Vein—artery—renal pelvis. The renal pelvis is located most posterior in the renal pedicle and nearest the skin of the posterior abdominal wall.
- Due to the embryologic development, a lobulated contour may persist in adolescence/adulthood **(fetal lobulation). Variants:** Pelvic kidney (not in typical orthotopic location), horseshoe kidney (fusion of right and left kidney across the midline), partial or complete duplication of the collecting system (upper/lower moiety)

- The kidneys are surrounded by perirenal fat and the (pre)renal fascia (Gerota fascia). The space surrounding the renal fascia contains the pararenal fat.
- The normal kidney size ranges from 9 to 13 cm in adults.
- **Renal calculi:**
  - Majority of renal stones consist of calcium oxalate (~75%). Other compositions are calcium phosphate (~5–7%), uric acid (5–8%), struvite (with infections), cystine (congenital) ~1%
  - Size and material composition of stones is relevant to determine treatment choice: extracorporeal shock wave lithotripsy (ESWL), extraction, diet
  - Dual energy and spectral detector CT allow, to a certain degree, for material decomposition

Imaging
- Imaging modality of first choice: **US**

Ultrasound
- **Indication for US:** To evaluate size, focal lesions, urinary obstruction, renal calculi, parenchymal abnormality, renal artery stenosis, vascular abnormality. Note that sensitivity is low for renal masses and calculi.
- Renal parenchyma is iso- or hypoechoic relative to liver. Increased echogenicity indicates medical renal disease which is categorized in 4 grades depending on echogenicity and degree of cortical thinning (normal: 8–10 mm measured between papilla and renal capsule).

Computed Tomography
- **Indication for CT:** To detect renal stones (calculi); to characterize cystic and solid renal lesions and renal lesions incidentally detected on prior imaging; to detect urothelial neoplasm, urinary tract infection and abscess; to detect and classify trauma injury; to display vascular anatomy/pathology preop; to detect and quantify renal artery stenosis
- CT is the **method of choice** to stage renal cancer. CT and MRI have similarly high diagnostic accuracy for primary renal lesions.
- **CT protocol:** Imaging evaluation of renal pathology requires multiphase protocol (except renal stones). Imaging phases relevant for renal imaging are (all @ 3-mm slice thickness): (1) NECT; (2) corticomedullary phase: @ 40–70 s postinjection; (3) nephrographic phase: @ 100–120 s; (4) excretory phase: @ 7–10 min postinjection; bolus tracking for contrast injection is recommended
  CT protocols depending on indication:
  (1) *Renal calculi:* NECT only (may be low dose); diaphragm to symphysis pubis
  (2) *indeterminate renal mass* characterization: NECT—nephrographic (@ 100–120 s) diaphragm to iliac crest; optional additional phase: Corticomedullary (@~40–70 s)
  (3) *Known characterized renal mass for pretreatment planning* (partial nephrectomy or preablation): Arterial phase: @ 25–30 s (use bolus tracking)—nephrographic phase (@100–120 s); excretory phase (@ 7–10 min)
  (4) *Workup hematuria incl. urothelial carcinoma:* CT urography: Noncontrast NECT—nephrographic phase (@110–120 s)—excretory phase (@ 7–10 min)
- Excretory (synonym urographic, pyelographic) phase: To differentiate between hydronephrosis, parapelvic cysts and calyceal diverticulum.
- **Renal mass characterization:**
  - Characterization is based on parenchymal enhancement pattern post IV contrast; use of attenuation measurement HU for detection of enhancement
  - Best for detection of enhancing lesions is nephrographic phase
  - Distinction of clear cell vs. papillary or chromophobe renal cell carcinoma (RCC) is supported by corticomedullary phase;
  - Note that there are no imaging features that successfully distinguish RCC from benign oncocytoma or minimal fat angiomyolipoma (AML)
- **Kidney and lesion attenuation:**
  - Normal renal parenchyma has an attenuation of 30–40 HU.
  - Pre/post increase of intralesional attenuation by ≤10 HU indicates no enhancement; increase by 10–20 HU is equivocal or pseudoenhancement, increase by >20 HU indicates enhancement.
  - In lesions with pseudoenhancement (often small (<1 cm, central location) MRI with subtraction may be helpful
  - Lesions with homogeneous density >70 HU and no enhancement are hemorrhagic cysts in >99% of cases
  - Presence of macroscopic fat mostly indicates angiomyolipoma (AML) **(Figure 4-18).** Only 5% of AML have minimal fat. On the other hand, RCC may contain macroscopic fat in rare occasions.

- For detection of urothelial carcinoma, CT urography protocol including excretory phase is imperative.
- CT > MRI: Detection of calcification

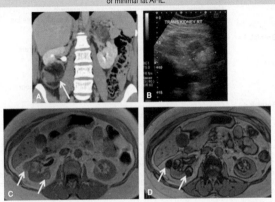

Figure 4-18A–D. Renal angiomyolipoma (AML). Coronal contrast-enhanced CT urogram in excretory phase **(A)** demonstrates a heterogeneous mass with macroscopic fat components arising from the lower pole of the right kidney. On US, macroscopic fat components in AML appear hyperechoic on gray-scale ultrasound and are perceptible if large enough **(B**; different patient). Chemical shift imaging in MRI is particularly helpful to identify fat content. Signal drop on opposed phase GRE images **(D)** compared to in-phase GRE images **(C)** may be seen in the periphery of the lesion facing parenchyma (if macroscopic fat) or within the lesion due to the presence of fat mixed with vascular and soft tissue components within an imaging voxel. This is especially helpful in characterization of minimal fat AML.

Magnetic Resonance Imaging
- CT and MRI are equally effective for renal mass detection and characterization with slight superiority of MRI regarding subtypes
- MRI > CT for tissue contrast; MRI is indicated in equivocal cases of CT and in patients with contraindication for CT or iodinated contrast
- In pregnancy, Gd contrast is discouraged; noncontrast MRI is superior to noncontrast CT for lesion characterization
- Evaluation for urothelial neoplasm requires Gd contrast; due to lack of radiation exposure, theoretically unlimited number of contrast phases are possible (MR urography)
- Timing of postcontrast phases in MRI is identical to CT (see above)
  - **MRI protocol:**
    - Coronal and axial T2W sequence (SSFSE)
    - Precontrast T1W GRE with fat saturation
    - T1W in/out of phase imaging (chemical shift imaging for presence of intravoxel fat)
    - Dynamic postcontrast images
    - Optional, not part of standard imaging: DWI and DCE (perfusion) for characterization of focal lesions/renal cancer subtypes , treatment monitoring and nuclear grade; (https://www.ncbi.nlm.nih.gov/pubmed/22081252)
  - **Lesion enhancement:**
    - Increase in signal intensity between pre- and postcontrast T1W imaging of <15% represents no enhancement, 15–19% equivocal enhancement, ≥20% true enhancement.

Nuclear Medicine
- Functional test for renal excretion

Cystic Kidney Lesions

Background
- Cystic renal lesions are classified according to malignant potential using the Bosniak classification. The Bosniak classification provides recommendations for workup and management. It was established for CT imaging but is also used for other imaging modalities.

Category	Description and Management
Bosniak 1	**Simple:** Cyst with imperceptible wall, rounded, low attenuation (<20 HU) *Work-up:* None
Bosniak 2	**Minimally complex:** A few thin <1-mm septa or thin calcifications (thickness not measurable); nonenhancing high-attenuation (due to proteinaceous or hemorrhagic contents) lesions ≤3 cm; well margined *Work-up:* None
Bosniak 2F	**Minimally complex:** Increased number of septa, minimally thickened with nodular or thick calcifications Perceived (but not measurable) enhancement of hairline—thin smooth septa; Hyperdense cyst >3-cm diameter without enhancement *Workup:* Requires follow-up with no strict rules on the time frame but reasonable at 6 mo
Bosniak 3	**Indeterminate:** Thick, nodular multiple septa or wall with measurable enhancement, hyperdense on CT *Workup:* Requires treatment Preferably partial nephrectomy or ablation techniques including microwave, radio-frequency, and cryo-ablation (in elderly or poor surgical candidates)
Bosniak 4	**Clearly malignant:** Solid mass with a large cystic or a necrotic component *Workup:* Requires treatment Treatment: Partial or total nephrectomy; minimally invasive techniques with cryoablation, microwave, radiofrequency ablation

- **Conditions and syndromes** associated with the presence of **multiple renal cysts**: Autosomal dominant polycystic kidney disease ADPKD (congenital); acquired cystic kidney disease (associated with ESRD and dialysis). Both conditions are associated with increased risk of renal neoplasm.

Imaging
- Imaging modality of choice: **US**

Ultrasound
- **Imaging findings:** *Simple cyst:* Anechoic with through transmission; smooth, thin walled; well delineated, no nodularity, no vascularity *Complex cyst:* Anechoic or hypoechoic with internal echoes (harmonic imaging helps to optimize evaluation), thin walled, well delineated, thin septum or septa without vascularity, thin calcification (hyperechoic with acoustic shadow), no nodularity; *solid lesions:* See Chapter 5

Computed Tomography
- **Indication:** If concern on US or incidental detection on prior imaging
- **Imaging findings:** *Simple cyst:* Attenuation <20 HU; no enhancement; *hemorrhagic/proteinaceous cyst or solid lesion* if attenuation >20 HU (typically 30–70 HU); *hemorrhagic/proteinaceous cyst* is most likely if attenuation is >70–100 HU, no enhancement; *solid lesions:* See Chapter 5
- Note: If diameter less than the double the slice thickness, no confident measurement of HU is possible due to partial averaging effects; lesions are too small to characterize

Magnetic Resonance Imaging
- **Indication:** Contraindication for iodinated contrast or equivocal findings on CT or prior imaging, pregnancy
- **Imaging findings:** *Simple cyst:* Well delineated, thin walled, homogeneous, strongly hyperintense on T2WI; hypointense on T1WI, no enhancement; *hemorrhagic cyst:* Homogeneously hyperintense on T1WI; no enhancement; *solid lesions:* See Chapter 5
- Subtraction imaging is an important tool and of additional benefit

Solid Kidney Lesions

Background
- **Risk factors:** Smoking, HTN, obesity, toxic substances (asbestos, petroleum), drugs (prolonged exposure to analgesics (acetaminophen, aspirin), acquired cystic kidney disease, hereditary syndromes (VHL disease)
- 90% of all solid renal tumors are RCC

- **Histologic subtypes** of RCC include clear cell type (~80%), papillary (~10%), and chromophobe RCC (~5%). Other malignant neoplasms include **oncocytoma** and **metastases**. Differentiating RCC subtypes and other renal neoplasms by imaging may be challenging, particularly differentiating RCC and minimally lipid rich AML and oncocytoma; at times, histologic proof is required.
- **Staging of RCC** depends on: Size (</>7 cm), invasion of perirenal fat within or beyond the Gerota fascia; invasion into adjacent organs (adrenal gland); extent of tumor into venous system (renal vein, IVC below/above diaphragm).
- **Role of imaging:** Detection, characterization, staging, and treatment follow-up for surveillance
- CT imaging should be multiphasic (see imaging protocol); MR imaging should include chemical shift imaging (detection of fat)
- **Criteria relevant for minimally invasive therapy:** Size, location (central vs. peripheral), relationship to pelvicalyceal system (see excretory phase) and arteries (see arterial phase), presence or absence of venous invasion (see nephrographic phase)

Imaging Findings

Ultrasound
- Hyperechoic or hypoechoic solid lesions; lack of through transmission; showing vascularity on Doppler US.

Computed Tomography
- *Clear cell RCC:* **(Figure 4-19)** Heterogeneous, hypervascular; avid enhancement in the arterial phase
- *Papillary and chromophobe RCC:* Mostly homogeneous appearance, hypovascular, poorly enhancing in arterial phase
- 10% may show calcifications
- If *tumor thrombus* within the renal venous system: Tumor thrombus is enhancing, bland thrombus is not; thrombus may be mimicked by inflow of nonopacified blood in early imaging

Magnetic Resonance Imaging
- *Clear cell RCC:* Heterogeneous, mixed hyperintense in T2WI; avid arterial enhancement; may show intravoxel fat content
- *Papillary and chromophobe RCC:* Homogeneous, relatively low SI in T2WI; poorly enhancing in arterial phase.

Figure 4-19A–D. Clear cell RCC with central necrosis. Axial SS T2-weighted MR shows a mass in the lower pole of the left kidney with a rim of intermediate SI and central are with high SI **(A)**. The mass shows slight increased SI on T1WI **(B)**. There is associated avid enhancement of the periphery of the tumor (arrow) on T1-weighted fat sat postcontrast arterial phase **(C)** and continuous enhancement (however lesser degree) on T1-weighted fat sat postcontrast delayed images **(D)**. A right renal cyst is incidentally noted.

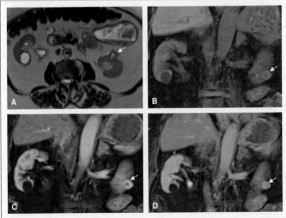

- Differential diagnosis: Hemorrhagic/proteinaceous cyst: Homogeneous hyperintense in T1WI, low to intermediate in T2WI, no enhancement
- MRI is particularly helpful to determine extent of tumor thrombus in the venous system (blood pool imaging)

Oncocytoma

Mostly benign solid neoplasm; malignant behavior has been reported.
- **Imaging findings:** Well defined, sharp borders; heterogeneous, often with central stellate scar: Spoke wheel appearance; may calcify; noninfiltrative pattern
- Radiographically impossible to differentiate from RCC

Renal Angiomyolipoma (AML)
- **Imaging findings:**
  Key finding is intralesional macroscopic fat of variable amount: hyperechoic (US), hypodense (CT), or hyperintense (T1WI) with chemical shift. Fat component may be minimal; careful image analysis for macroscopic fat content is imperative as this can avoid unnecessary surgical excision. **Note:** Unenhanced CT with thin sections and pixel analysis is the most sensitive test to confirm fat: **MRI:** Chemical shift imaging
- **Other imaging findings:** Predominance of tortuous vessels; strong contrast enhancement, flow voids and hyperintensity in T2WI; No calcifications in AML. If calcifications are present, favor RCC
- Increased **risk** of bleeding if size >4 cm.

Related IR Procedures
Biopsy; minimally invasive therapy with ablation

Hydronephrosis

Background
- **Definition:** Dilatation of the urinary pelvicalyceal collecting system of the kidney; hydroureter refers to dilated ureter
- **Most common causes:** Ureteric stones; neoplasms of the ureter, bladder and prostate; extrinsic compression or tumor invasion from other pelvic neoplasms (uterus, ovary, colon, breast, lymphoma); postsurgical ureteral damage, ureteral fistulas, bladder reflux pregnancy (compression by gravid uterus); idiopathic retroperitoneal fibrosis
- **Differential diagnosis:** Renal sinus cysts, extrarenal pelvis, pseudohydronephrosis

Imaging Findings
- Best seen in US (hypoechoic), on CT (hypodense), on MRI (water-isointense very high SI in T2WI, low SI in T1WI)
- Degree of hydronephrosis is graded

Grading	Description
Grade 0	No dilatation, calyceal walls are opposed to each other
Grade 1	**Mild:** Dilatation of the renal pelvis without dilatation of the calyces (can also occur in the extrarenal pelvis)
Grade 2	**Mild:** Dilatation of the renal pelvis (mild) and calyces (pelvicalyceal pattern is retained); no parenchymal atrophy
Grade 3	**Moderate:** Moderate dilatation of the renal pelvis and calyces Flattening of papillae and blunting of the fornices, mild cortical thinning
Grade 4	**Severe:** Gross dilatation of the renal pelvis and calyces, ballooning of the calyces, renal parenchymal atrophy with cortical thinning

Related IR Procedure: Percutaneous nephrostomy

Renal Artery Imaging

Background
- Renal arteries are paired and originate from the abdominal aorta at the level of L1–2, about 1 cm below the origin of the SMA. The left ostium is slightly more cranial than the right.
- Congenital accessory vessels exist in 25% of the population (upper pole and or lower pole arteries) arising mostly from the aorta but also from the lumbar or iliac arteries.

Indications for Imaging
- Arterial HTN secondary to renal artery stenosis (atherosclerosis; fibromuscular dysplasia)
- Traumatic injury: Rupture, dissection, occlusion; hemorrhage
- AVF and malformations
- Aneurysm; arteritis, thromboembolism

- Preoperative or palliative embolization of renal tumors
- Pretransplantation evaluation

Ultrasound
- US including color Doppler/Duplex is screening method for renal artery stenosis (including posttransplant evaluation)
- Advantage: Bedside diagnosis possible
- Main renal arteries are reliably depicted in 95% of patients, but the detection of small accessory renal arteries is less accurate.

Computed Tomography CTA
- Imaging method of choice; very high sensitivity and specificity for detection of vascular pathology and accessory arteries
- Requires optimal arterial contrast bolus
- Good for the detection of calcified plaque; plaques however may limit quantification of stenosis.
- Concomitant evaluation of adrenal glands (pheochromocytoma)

Magnetic Resonance Angiography
- High accuracy for the detection of accessory renal arteries and detection and grading of renal artery stenosis.
- Preferred method in the setting of preorgan donation (noninvasiveness, nonionizing radiation) and pediatric patients (fibromuscular dysplasia)

Imaging Findings: Atherosclerotic Disease

Ultrasound
- **Direct evaluation:** Four main criteria indicating significant renal artery stenosis: (1) PSV within the renal artery at stenosis >200 cm/s; (2) PSV renal/PSV of aorta >3.5; (3) turbulent flow in poststenotic area; (4) indirect criteria; lack of Doppler flow in renal artery suggests occlusion.
- **Indirect evaluation:** Doppler US of intrarenal (parenchymal) arteries: Tardus-parvus waveform indicating upstream stenosis. Quantitative criteria: Acceleration of less than 370–470 cm/s; prolonged time of acceleration >0.05–0.08 s; difference in resistive index of >5% between the right and left renal arteries.
- US findings are used as a predictor for renal revascularization.

MRA (Contrast-Enhanced MR Angiography)
- Excellent visualization of stenosis with sensitivity >95% and specificity >90% and high correlation with conventional angiography
- Allows for quantification of stenosis (source images are essential); provides additional functional information with cine phase-contrast imaging
- Combined evaluation of anatomy, small vessels, stenosis, kidney size, cortical thickness
- Multiplanar reformats improve analysis of renal artery ostia; maximum intensity projection **(MIP)** provides an angiographic overview
- Limitations: Overestimation of moderate stenosis; limited accuracy in small size vessels, branches, and accessory arteries; presence of a metallic stent

ACE Inhibitor Scintigraphy
- Functional nuclear medicine test to evaluate probability of renovascular hypertension (RVH) and/or renal failure
- Normal ACE inhibitor scintigram: Low probability (<10%) of RVH
- Unilateral parenchymal retention of radiotracer after ACE inhibition: High probability (>90%); represents most important criteria for RVH
- A greater than 10% change in the relative uptake of radiotracer after ACE inhibition: High probability of RVH, uncommon

Related IR Procedure
- Renal artery stent angioplasty

Imaging Findings: Fibromuscular Disease

Ultrasound
- Accelerated blood flow in renal arteries at the site of stenosis (may be multiple stenosis)
- Renal size is a marker for disease severity and used for follow-up of disease.

Cross-Sectional Imaging Findings
- Alternating stenosis and dilatations (string of beads) seen in the intimal type (the most common type)
- Focal concentric, long-segment tubular stenosis or diverticular outpouching (less common type)
- Imaging findings in CTA and MRA are similar

Computed Tomography Angiography (CTA)

- 62% sensitivity (inferior to conventional angiography), 84% specificity.
- Advantages: High contrast resolution, fast acquisition time, less pulsation and stair-step artifact (visualization of a greater volume/time)
- Using reformats (MPR, MIP, shaded surface 3D-display) improves the sensitivity and specificity

Magnetic Resonance Angiography (MRA)

- 64% sensitivity (inferior to conventional angiography), 92% specificity
- TOF-MRA in patients unable to undergo CTA or MRA (renal failure, allergy). **Note:** No published studies available to compare TOF-MRA in FMD with conventional angiography or other noninvasive imaging modalities
- Disadvantage: Less spatial resolution compared to CTA

Related IR Procedure

Renal artery balloon angioplasty +/– vascular stent placement

Renal Transplant Evaluation

Background

- Renal transplant may stem from living vs. deceased donor
- Renal transplant is usually placed within the extraperitoneal space in the right or left iliac fossa
- Three anastomoses (usually end-to-end): Typically: Donor renal artery and recipient external (or internal) iliac artery, donor renal vein and recipient external iliac vein and donor ureter to the recipient bladder.

Ultrasound

- **Doppler US of renal transplant artery:**
  - Patency: Presence of flow in color and spectral Doppler
  - Normal RI: 0.6–0.7; high RI (>0.8) may indicate rejection, acute tubular necrosis (ATN), drug toxicity, hydronephrosis, external compression. Low RI: Arterial stenosis, AVF, advanced atherosclerosis
  - Peak arterial velocity: <200 cm/s; PSV in renal artery compared to arterial PSV in adjacent iliac artery gradient <2:1
  - Wave form: Low resistive flow **(Figure 4-20)**
- **Doppler US of renal transplant vein:**
  - Patency: Presence of flow in color and spectral Doppler
  - PSV <3-fold the velocity in adjacent iliac vein **(Figure 4-21)**

Vascular Complications of Renal Transplant

- *Renal artery occlusion/thrombosis:* Absence of flow within the renal transplant artery and within renal parenchyma
- *Renal artery stenosis:* Tardus-parvus waveform; increased PSV in stenosis; if at anastomosis: Comparison to PSV in adjacent iliac artery; gradient PSV renal artery/PSV iliac artery >2:1
- *Renal vein thrombosis:* Lack of flow in renal vein and reverse diastolic flow in renal artery
- *Renal vein stenosis:* Rare; accelerated velocity >3–4 fold compared to iliac vein.
- Pseudoaneurysm (refer to liver transplant section)
- AVF (refer to liver transplant section) **(Figure 4-22)**
- **Note:** Accelerated velocities in transplant vasculature can be observed in tortuous vascular course and temporarily immediately postoperative due to edema

Nonvascular Complications of Renal Transplant

- Hydronephrosis
- Fluid collections: Hematoma/seroma, urinoma (close to the ureteral anastomosis), lymphocele, abscess
- Ischemia/infarction: Segmental or complete lack of flow on Doppler US
- ATN: High RI, low or lack of diastolic flow
- Rejection: High RI (>0.9), low or lack of diastolic flow
- Mass (PTLD, RCC)

Imaging of Kidney Intervention-Related Complications

Background

- Complications after percutaneous nephrostomy and percutaneous kidney biopsy include hemorrhage, AVF, abscess

Hemorrhage

- *Microscopic hematuria:* Very frequent; most often resolves spontaneously
- *Macroscopic hematuria:* Most often resolves spontaneously; may cause clot in the bladder with or without obstruction; occurs with or without acute kidney injury

Figure 4-20A. Spectral waveform of a normal transplant renal artery. Systolic upstroke is sharp and narrow (PSV <200 cm/s, acceleration time <0.08 s). The velocity gradient (PSV in renal artery/iliac artery) should be <2. **B.** Spectral waveform of a normal renal vein in a transplanted kidney. Monophasic continuous flow with minimal phasicity. The velocity gradient (PSV in renal vein/iliac vein) should be <3.

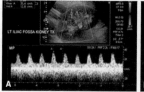 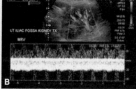

Figure 4-21 Renal pseudoaneurysm in a transplanted kidney. In the center of the renal sinus there is a lobulated anechoic structure **(A)** in which flow is demonstrated using Color Doppler and spectral Doppler imaging. The flow is bidirectional (yin-yang sign) **(B)** indicating turbulent flow. Alternatively, one may see (more typical) to and fro waveforms which were not seen in this case.

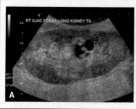 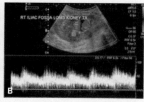

Figure 4-22A, B. Color Doppler **(A)** and spectral Doppler waveform **(B)** of a **postbiopsy AV fistula** in a transplanted kidney. Color flash from high velocity and turbulent flow and from vibration of soft tissue surrounding the AVF is seen in **A**. High velocity is confirmed with the spectral Doppler to be at 187 cm/s within the fistula. Low-resistance flow is demonstrated in the supplying artery. In large AV fistulas pulsatile flow of the main renal vein may be seen (due to arterialization).

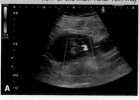 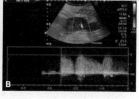

- *Acute anemia* in immediate posttransplant phase
- *Perinephric hematoma:*
  - Mostly self-limiting and resolving if small
  - May become clinically relevant with acute lumbar pain, acute anemia with or without need for blood transfusion.
  - Tendency to self-tamponade; if progressive increase in size or active bleed, intervention may be required (gel foam or coil embolization)
  - CT and US are both well suited to detect hematoma with higher sensitivity for CT (90% vs. 70%).

Arteriovenous Fistula (AVF)
- Resulting from direct injury to a vessel from the biopsy needle
- Mostly asymptomatic; rarely presenting with HTN, high-output heart failure, hematuria, renal failure
- Rarely developing into aneurysm
- Requires confirmation with Doppler US, MRA, or angiography
- On **Doppler US:** High peak velocity, low-resistance flow within the artery supplying the fistula; turbulent flow in the fistula; accelerated pulsatile flow in adjacent vein
- If AVF becomes symptomatic or enlarging on serial Doppler US: Superselective transcatheter arterial embolization or surgery may be indicated

Urinoma
- **US:** Fluid collection next to the transplant or bladder (ureteral insertion)
- **CT:** Urographic/excretory phase is highly specific to show contrast extravasation outside of the collecting system

Imaging of Acute Renal Infection

Background
- Spectrum of acute renal infection includes acute pyelonephritis, renal and perirenal abscess, pyonephrosis, emphysematous pyelonephritis, emphysematous cystitis

Imaging

Ultrasound
- Diffuse or focal hypoechogenicity of the kidney, low specificity

Computed Tomography
- CT is the imaging modality of choice for diagnosis and assessment of severity of acute pyelonephritis and complications
- Preferred CT protocol: CT-urography including noncontrast, nephrographic and excretory phase imaging (assess for obstruction)

Magnetic Resonance Imaging
- Indicated in pregnancy and patients with contraindication to iodinated contrast (including transplant recipients).
- DWI is helpful to differentiate hydronephrosis from pyonephrosis and simple from infected cysts and tumors

Imaging Findings
- **Acute pyelonephritis:**
  - Two possible forms: (1) focal; (2) diffuse pyelonephritis
  - Image appearance **(CT and MRI):** Striated nephrogram = discrete rays of alternating low and high attenuation/SI radiating from the papilla to the cortex; **(Figure 4-23)** (1) focal: Wedge-shaped area of edema and decreased enhancement; (2) diffuse: Global organ enlargement, poor enhancement of the parenchyma, absent excretion if obstruction
- **Early abscess:**
  - Poorly marginated, nonenhancing focal area with decreased attenuation in **CT** and near-fluid characteristics in **MRI**
- **Mature abscess:**
  - Sharply marginated, complex cystic mass with central necrosis and a peripheral enhancing rim (abscess pseudocapsule)
  - **US:** Hypoechoic with internal echoes, septations, loculations; **CT:** enhancing peripheral rim, central hypodensity, enhancing septations **(Figure 4-24)**; **MRI-DWI:** diffusion restriction within abscess
- **Pyonephrosis:**
  - Dilated pelvicalyceal system with or without obstruction
  - **US:** Hypoechoic with internal echoes indicating debris; fluid–fluid levels. **CT:** Increased attenuation of urine with contrast layering.
  - **CT/MRI:** Renal pelvic wall thickening and enhancement. MRI-DWI helpful to differentiate hydronephrosis from pyonephrosis (pyonephrosis tends to show restricted diffusion).
- **Emphysematous pyelonephritis:**
  - Life-threatening condition, necrotizing infection with gas formation; associated with diabetes mellitus or immunocompromised state
  - **US:** Nondependent echoes with dirty shadowing (gas) within the parenchyma and collecting system. **CT:** To evaluate severity, extent of disease, parenchymal destruction, fluid collections, and abscess formation

Figure 4-23A–D. (A) Pyelonephritis with mild hydronephrosis (*arrowhead*) of the left kidney due to mid ureteral obstructing stone (not shown). Note the diffuse swelling of the left kidney compared to right and several areas of linear and wedge-shaped hypoattenuation (*arrows*) in the anterior renal cortex indicating pyelonephritis. **(B)** Placement of double-J-stent catheter, improvement of the hydronephrosis, and interval development of subcapsular hematoma (*). Presence of air is most likely postprocedural. **(C)** Interval removal of double-J-stent catheter; interval evolution and liquefaction of the perinephric hematoma. However the collection is more discrete with an enhancing wall. **(D)** Interval placement of percutaneous nephrostomy catheter and interval decrease in size of the fluid collection.

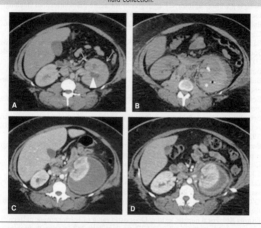

Figure 4-24A–D. Intraparenchymal renal abscess. Ultrasound of the kidney **(A, B)** reveals a hypoechoic well-delineated complex renal cystic lesion in the superior pole of the right kidney with internal echoes and absent central vascularity **(A, B).** CECT (Axial and Coronal) in the same patient on nephrographic phase shows the right kidney is enlarged, edematous with mild perinephric stranding; the cystic lesion has a thick-walled enhancing rim (pseudocapsule) as well as internal septations **(C, D).**

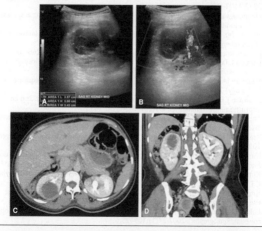

REFERENCES

1. Abramowitz Y. Pleural effusion: characterization with CT attenuation values and CT appearance. *AJR Am J Roentgenol* 2009;192(3):618–23.
2. Agrawal GA, Johnson PT, Fishman EK. Splenic artery aneurysms and pseudoaneurysms: clinical distinctions and CT appearances. *AJR Am J Roentgenol* 2007; 188(4):992–9.
3. Akbar SA. Complications of renal transplantation. *Radiographics* 2005;25(5): 1335–56.
4. Albiin N. MRI of focal liver lesions. *Curr Med Imaging Rev* 2012;8(2):107–16.
5. Artigas JM. Multidetector CT angiography for acute gastrointestinal bleeding: technique and findings. *Radiographics* 2013;33(5):1453–70.
6. Baliga RR. The role of imaging in aortic dissection and related syndromes. *JACC Cardiovasc Imaging*. 2014;7(4):406–24.
7. Barr RG, Ferraioli G, Palmeri ML, et al. Elastography Assessment of liver fibrosis: Society of Radiologists in Ultrasound Consensus Conference Statement. *Radiology* 2015;276(3):845–61.
8. Bintcliffe O. Spontaneous pneumothorax. *BMJ* 2014;348:g 2928.
9. Bobbio A. Epidemiology of spontaneous pneumothorax: gender- related differences. *Thorax* 2015;70(7):653–8.
10. Boll. DT. Diffuse liver disease: strategies for hepatic CT and MR imaging. *Radiographics* 2009;29(6):1591–14.
11. Bonavita JA, Mayo J, Babb J, et al. Pattern recognition of benign nodules at ultrasound of the thyroid: which nodules can be left alone? *AJR Am J Roentgenol* 2009; 193(1):207–13.
12. Bosniak MA. Angiomyolipoma (hamartoma) of the kidney: a preoperative diagnosis is possible in virtually every case. *Urol Radiol* 1981;3:135–42.
13. Daseler E. The cystic artery and constituents of the hepatic pedicle; a study of 500 specimens. *Surg Gynecol Obstet* 1947;85(1):47–63.
14. Das CJ, Ahmad Z, Sharma S, et al. Multimodality imaging of renal inflammatory lesions. *World J Radiol* 2014;6(11):865–73.
15. D'Onofrio M, Crosara S, De Robertis R, et al. Contrast-enhanced ultrasound of focal liver lesions. *AJR Am J Roentgenol* 2015;205(1):W56–W66.
16. Elsayes KM. Focal hepatic lesions: Diagnostic value of enhancement pattern approach with contrast enhanced 3D gradient-echo MR imaging. *Radiographics* 2005;25(5):1299–300.
17. Frates MC, Benson CB, Charboneau JW, et al. Management of thyroid nodules detected at US: Society of Radiologists in Ultrasound consensus conference statement. *Radiology* 2005;237(3):794–00.
18. Gandhi SN. MR contrast agents for liver imaging: what, when, how. *Radiographics* 2006;26(6):1621–36.
19. Hamm B, Ros PR, eds. *Abdominal Imaging*. Berlin Heidelberg: Springer-Verlag; 2013:1601–21.
20. Hennedigea T. Imaging of hepatocellular carcinoma: diagnosis, staging and treatment monitoring. *Cancer Imaging* 2012;12(3):530–47.
21. Hernandez Muñiz S, Olmedilla Arregui P, García de Vicente A, et al. *Imaging review of pleural effusion: diagnosis and intervention*. Presented at ESTI 2014.
22. Jang HJ. Imaging of focal liver lesions. *Semin Roentgenol* 2009;44(4):266–82.
23. Jinzaki M, Tanimoto A, Narimatsu Y, et al. Angiomyolipoma: imaging findings in lesions with minimal fat. *Radiology* 1997;205:497–502.
24. Kaufman JA. *Vascular and Interventional Radiology: The Requisites*, (Requisites in Radiology) 2nd Ed. Elsevier Saunders; 2014;57–60.
25. Kaufman J, Lee M. *Vascular and Interventional Radiology: The Requisites*. 2nd Ed, Imprint: Saunders, Published Date: 19th August 2013.
26. Kapoor A, Morris T, Rebello R. Guidelines for the management of the incidentally discovered adrenal mass. *Can Urol Assoc J* 2011;5(4):241–47.
27. Kielar AZ. Imaging after local tumor therapies: kidney and liver. *Semin Roentgenol* 2013;48(3):273–84.
28. Kim JK, Park SY, Shon JH, et al. Angiomyolipoma with minimal fat: differentiation from renal cell carcinoma at biphasic helical CT. *Radiology* 2004;230:677–84.
29. Kim S, Kim TU, Lee JW, et al. The perihepatic space: comprehensive anatomy and CT features of pathologic conditions. *Radiographic* 2007;27(1):129–43.
30. Kim YH, Saini S, Sahani D, et al. Imaging diagnosis of cystic pancreatic lesions: Pseudocyst versus nonpseudocyst. *Radiographics* 2005;23:671–85.
31. Lubner M, Menias C, Rucker C, et al. Blood in the belly: CT findings of hemoperitoneum. *Radiographics* 2007;27(1):109–25.

32. McMahon MA. Multidetector CT of Aortic Dissection: A Pictorial Review. *Radiographics* 2010;30(2):445–60.

33. McNaughton DA. Doppler US of the liver made simple. *Radiographics* 2011; 31(1):161–88.

34. Michel NA. Blood supply and anatomy of the upper abdominal organs, with a descriptive atlas. Philadelphia, PA: Lippincott; 1955. Observations on the blood supply of the liver and gallbladder (200 dissections) pp. 64–9.

35. Miyazaki M, Lee VS. Nonenhanced MR angiography. *Radiology* 2008;248:20–43.

36. Patel PJ. Endovascular management of acute aortic syndromes. *Semin Intervent Radiol.* 2011;28(1):10–23.

37. Seo N. Cross-sectional imaging of intrahepatic cholangiocarcinoma: development, growth, spread, and prognosis. *AJR Am J Roentgenol* 2017;209(2):W64–W75.

38. Singh AK. Postoperative imaging in liver transplantation: What the Radiologist should know *Radiographics* 2010;30(2):339–51.

39. Singh AK, Cronin CG, Verma HA, et al. Imaging of preoperative liver transplantation in adults: what radiologists should know. *Radiographics* 2011;31(4):1017–30.

40. Soni NJ, Franco R, Velez MI, et al. Ultrasound in the diagnosis and management of pleural effusions *J Hosp Med.* 2015;10(12):811–6.

41. Stark DD, Federle MP, Goodman PC, et al. Differentiating lung abscess and empyema: radiography and computed tomography. *AJR* 1983;141(1).

42. Sureka B. Variations of celiac axis, common hepatic artery and its branches in 600 patients. *Indian J Radiol Imaging* 2013;23(3):223–33.

43. Hassan R, Abd Aziz A, Md Ralib AR, et al. Computed tomography of Blunt splenic injury: a pictorial review. *Malays J Med Sci* 2011;18(1):60–7.

44. Kahn SL, Angle JF. Adrenal vein sampling. *Tech Vasc Interv Radiol* 2010;13(2): 110–25.

45. Farrugia FA, Martikos G, Surgeon C, et al. Radiology of the adrenal incidentalomas. Review of the literature, 10.1515/enr-2017-0005.

46. Lopes Vendrami C, Parada Villavicencio C, DeJulio TJ, et al. Differentiation of Solid Renal Tumors with Multiparametric MR Imaging, *Radiographics* 2017;37(7): 2026–42.

47. Motzer RJ, Agarwal N, Beard C, et al. Kidney cancer. *J Natl Compr Canc Netw* 2011; 9(9):960–77.

48. Silverman SG, Mortele KJ, Tuncali K, et al. Hyperattenuating renal masses: etiologies, pathogenesis, and imaging evaluation. *Radiographics* 2007;27:1131–43.

49. Varennes L. Fibromuscular dysplasia: what the radiologist should know: a pictorial review. *Insights Imaging* 2015;6(3):295–307.

50. Whittier WL. Complications of the percutaneous kidney biopsy. *Adv Chronic Kidney Dis* 2012;19(3):179–87.

DEVICES (WIRES AND CATHETERS)

Units of Measurement		
Access and biopsy needles	Gauge	Outer diameter of needle
Catheter and dilators	French	Outer diameter of catheter
	Inches	Inner diameter of catheter
	Cm	Length
Sheath	French	Inner lumen size
	Cm	Length
Guidewires	Inches	Outer diameter
	Cm	Length

Measurement Conversions	
Access and biopsy needles	**Small needle (larger gauge) vs. large needle (smaller gauge)** • 19G fits a 0.035-inch guidewire • 21G fits a 0.018-inch guidewire
Catheters and dilators	**Smaller catheter (smaller French) vs. larger catheter (larger French)** *Remember that the French size denotes the external diameter* • 1F = 0.3 mm (eg, 3F = 1 mm, 6F = 2 mm, 9F = 3 mm) **Inner diameter of catheter (inches) will match the wire that it fits** (eg, standard 0.035 wire will go through a 4F catheter and larger)
Sheath	**The French size of the catheter tells you which sheath the catheter will fit through.** *Remember that French size denotes inner diameter of the sheath and are sized by the largest catheter they will accommodate.* • Add 1.5–2F (~0.6 mm) to get the outer diameter (eg, 6F sheath + 2F = 8F skin incision)
Guidewires	0.035-inch is ~1 mm **Diameter** • Standard diameter = 0.035-inch thick • Microwire diameter = 0.014–0.018-inch thick **Length** • Typical wire length = 145–180 cm • Shorter wires = 50–100 cm • Longer wires = 260–300 cm

VASCULAR IR DEVICES

Access Needles
• Initial step in all vascular cases, providing access into the vasculature for the guidewire
• **Sizes:** Commonly range from 18–21G
• **Types**
  • Single-wall needle: Sharp hollow beveled needle. The notch on the hub indicates where the bevel is pointing.
  • Trocar needle: Outer blunt hollow cannula + Inner sharp solid stylet
    • The sharp inner stylet allows for initial puncture. Afterward, the inner stylet is removed leaving an atraumatic hollow blunt stylet.

Coaxial Micropuncture Set
• Allows for minimally invasive initial access
• **Components**
  • **21G needle** for initial puncture
  • **0.018 micropuncture guidewire** (made of stainless steel or nitinol) for insertion through needle after puncture
  • **Locking sheath and dilator** (4F or 5F sizes) exchanged for a needle. Subsequently, the inner dilator and microwire are removed. This leaves the 4–5F microsheath, which will accept a standard 0.035-in guidewire.

Peel-away Sheath
• Allows for easy insertion of catheter or instruments through the sheath by decreased friction and improved angles
• Make sure that the catheter intended for insertion can pass through the sheath

- **Components**
  - **Dual knob and plastic sheath bonded at midline:** Allows for the sheath to be peeled away and removed
  - **Valved or nonvalved:** The valve prevents the inadvertent introduction of air into the vasculature

---

Figure 5-1 Peel-away sheath before and after the "peel-away." Note that the inner dilator is removed which allows for insertion of a catheter.

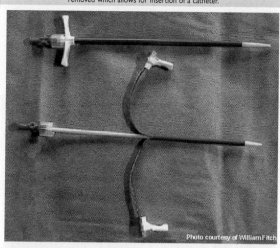

Photo courtesy of William Fitch

Central Venous Lines
- **Background**
  - The specific type of central line placed is determined by the indication, duration, and frequency of therapy and patient factors.
- **Properties:**
  - Catheters are usually made of silicone elastomer or thin polyurethane and come in various sizes and lengths
  - The lumens are variable and range from a single, double, triple, or quadruple lumen
  - Various tips of the catheter also exist. For example, end hole, valved-tip (Groshong), dual lumen with a staggered tip
  - Central lines are also power injectable vs. nonpower injectable. The maximum power injectable amount is labeled on the catheter.
- **Types of central venous catheters**
  - **Peripherally inserted central catheters (PICC lines)**
    - **Types:** Power PICC, Navilyst Power injectable PICC, Spectrum PICC. Can be open-ended vs. close-ended (Groshong). Can be nontunneled or tunneled with a Dacron or Velour cuff.
    - **Access sites:** Basilic, brachial, or cephalic vein
    - **Components:**
      - Catheter tubing with single or multiple lumens
      - Hub which allows for sutures or sutureless attachment
      - Clamps and extension tubing with a Luer lock hub
  - **Temporary (nontunneled) central venous catheters**
    - **Types:** Quinton, Groshong, dialysis, trialysis, apheresis catheter
    - **Access sites:** Internal jugular, subclavian, or femoral vein. Less commonly, the external jugular vein if the IJ is occluded without central venous obstruction.
    - **Components:**
      - Catheter tubing with single or multiple lumens
      - Hub which allows for sutures or sutureless attachment
      - Clamps and extension tubing with a Luer lock hub

- **Permanent (tunneled) central venous catheters**
  - **Types:** Hickman, Broviac, Permcath, Groshong
  - **Access sites:** Internal jugular, subclavian, or femoral vein. Less commonly, the external jugular vein if the IJ is occluded without central venous obstruction.
  - **External portion:** Subcutaneous tissues of the upper chest
  - **Components:**
    - Catheter tubing with single or multiple lumens
    - Velour or Dacron cuff positioned in the subcutaneous tissues near the external portion of the catheter to promote tissue ingrowth
    - Clamps and extension tubing with a Luer lock hub
- **Implantable ports**
  - **Types:** Port-a-Cath, BardPort, Mediport, PowerPort
  - **Access sites:** Internal jugular
  - **Components:**
    - Catheter tubing
    - Single or double lumen port which can be made of plastic, titanium, or stainless steel

Figure 5-2 Different types of central venous catheters (left to right): Temporary apheresis catheter, tunneled central venous catheter, mediport (single and double lumen), PICC line.

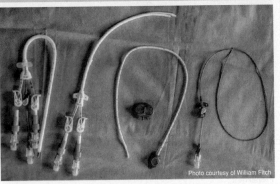

Photo courtesy of William Fitch

Guidewires

- **Background**
  - Guidewires provide catheter support and allow catheter steering. Two broad categories exist: steerable and nonsteerable. These categories will be discussed in further detail below.
  - Most wires are constructed of steel or nitinol with a stiff inner core wire which has a fine wire coiled around the outside.
    - The "floppy tip" of some wires is the point where the inner core ends, and the wire is only constructed of the outer wire coil. This end is designed to be atraumatic relative to the stiff back end of the wire. Some wires have a movable core, which allows you to vary the flexibility of the tip of the guidewire.
    - The length of the floppy portion of a wire is variable between different types of wires. Keep in mind that the longer the floppy end, the lesser the chance of vessel dissection.
    - Take great care if advancing a catheter, dilator, or sheath over the floppy portion of the wire. Since there is no inner core "backbone" in the tip, severe damage to the vessel could occur.
- **Properties**
  - **Diameter**
    - Measured in inches
    - Standard diameter is 0.035 in, which will fit through a 4F or larger catheter
    - Typical microwire diameter is 0.014–0.018 in, which are used with microcatheter systems
  - **Length**
    - Typical wire length is 145–180 cm, which works well for most procedures

- Shorter wires (50–100 cm) may be suitable for procedures such as drain placements
- Longer wires (typically 260–300 cm) are considered "exchange length" wires since they allow enough length on the external end so that a new catheter may be introduced without losing internal wire purchase. Used when working with long catheters (90 cm and above), when working on the upper limb via groin access (or vice versa), and when using through-and-through wires "body flossing."
- **Hydrophilic guidewires** have a special coating, which makes the wire "slippery" when wet, aiding in crossing narrow vessels or stenosis. These wires should be kept wet in a bowl of saline when not in use.
  - Guidewires should be wiped with either saline soaked gauze or a lint-free pad to clean the wire of any clot, fibrin, or dried contrast
- **Steerability**
  - **Steerable guidewires** have variable shapes and angulations of their tips and are designed to be easily turned or torqued
    - The most commonly used steerable wire is an angled glidewire. Many microwires have tips that can be shaped manually.
  - **Nonsteerable guidewires** function predominantly for support or catheter/sheath introduction. Many of these wires can be used as steerable wires if used with an angled catheter.
    - Commonly used wires include the following:
      - **Bentson wire:** Soft catheter with a floppy "atraumatic" 5 cm distal tip. Often used in combination with steerable catheters to traverse stenosis and occlusions. Helps with negotiating tortuous iliac vessels, and the floppy tip helps to select visceral arteries without causing a dissection.
      - **J-guidewire:** Commonly used during vascular access to pass through the micropuncture dilator. The J tip is designed to avoid plaque and branch vessels. The wire has an associated curve radius measurement.
        - Number associated refers to the radius of the curve (eg, 3 mm, 5 mm, 10 mm). Larger curves are better for selecting smaller branch vessels.
      - **Rosen:** Straight or J tipped. Provides support for catheter advancement, and can be used when placing drainage catheters. Good choice for an exchange length wire.
      - **Amplatz:** Stiff wire with a flexible tip. Used if additional support is needed during catheter/sheath advancement over tortuous or calcified arteries, or if there is significant soft tissue scarring. Comes in super stiff, if needed. Useful with angioplasty or stenting.
      - **Meier wire/Lunderquist wire:** Heavy duty guidewires used with large caliber and stiff devices, such as EVAR devices.
      - **Platinum plus:** 0.018-in stiff microwire with a short flexible tip. Useful with stenting or angioplasty of smaller vessels (renal arteries, tibial arteries).
- **Stiffness**
  - There is a large variance between different wires. The key is to know the intended purpose of the wire and choose appropriately.
  - Some wires (such as a Glidewire) come in both regular and stiff shafts
  - Figure 5-3 sums up the stiffness of the commonly used wires in IR

Dilators
- **Background**
  - Short-tapered catheters which go over a guidewire to dilate the soft tissues and vessel. Sequential dilation allows for safer upsizing of a catheter.
  - Dilators are referred to by French (outer diameter of the catheter)

Catheters
- **Background**
  - Like wires, catheters come in a variety of shapes, sizes, and lengths. Different catheters can be used for the same purpose, and many times which catheter is used comes down to operator preference.
  - Three key characteristics to review prior to selecting a catheter: Length, inner diameter, and outer diameter
    - **Length:** Measured in cm, from tip to hub. For visceral work from the groin, 65 cm is usually sufficient. For pulmonary, upper-extremity, or contralateral lower-extremity work, 90 cm catheters or longer may be needed.
    - **Inner diameter:** Refers to the lumen, measured in inches. This tells you how large of a microcatheter or guidewire can be passed through.

Figure 5-3 Example of different types of guidewires.

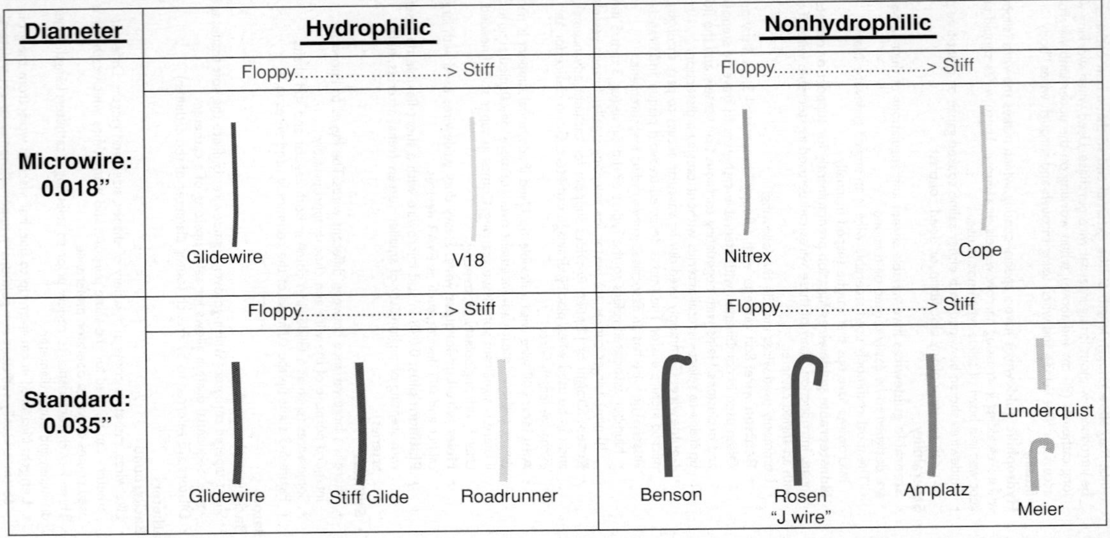

Diameter	Hydrophilic			Nonhydrophilic		
Microwire: 0.018"	Floppy..........> Stiff			Floppy..........> Stiff		
	Glidewire	V18		Nitrex		Cope
Standard: 0.035"	Floppy..........> Stiff			Floppy..........> Stiff		
	Glidewire	Stiff Glide	Roadrunner	Benson	Rosen "J wire"	Amplatz / Lunderquist / Meier

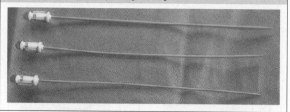

Figure 5-4 Example of different types of dilators from 5–7F (bottom to top). Note that they are larger the larger the French size.

- **Outer diameter:** Measured in French size. 3F = 1 mm. For most angiographic work, 4–5F catheters are sufficient. The French size of the catheter tells you which sheath the catheter will fit through.
- Catheters are typically referred to by their trackability, their pushability, and their torquability
  - **Trackability:** How the catheter follows over the guidewire without losing wire access
  - **Pushability:** How the catheter translates a forward force applied to the hub to the tip
  - **Torquability:** How the catheter tips steers when the hub of the catheter is spun
- Catheters may be end-hole catheters or side-hole catheters
  - **End-hole catheters:** Have only one hole at the end of the catheter. Care must be taken when selecting flow rates, as the jet coming from the end hole can displace the catheter, dislodge plaque, or result in dissection. Care must also be taken when aspirating, which will not be possible if the end of the catheter is against a vessel wall.
  - **Side-hole catheters:** Have additional holes near the tip of the catheter. This allows for the safe and rapid bolus of contrast. These catheters should never be used during embolotherapy, as particles can escape into nontargeted vessels.
- **Flow rates** during angiography
  - Vary by catheter depending on its length, internal diameter, and the number of side holes
  - The maximum flow rate and injection pressure (psi) are specified on the packaging
- **How to flush a catheter**
  - Catheters should be flushed before, during, and after use to assure patency.
  - **"Single flush" technique:** Commonly used outside the cerebrovascular circulation. This is simply aspirating the catheter until a drop of blood is seen in the syringe, then carefully injecting saline. This is best done at a 45-degree angle to allow any air to rise.
  - **"Double flush" technique:** Used in the arch or above to make sure there is no inadvertent injection of small thrombi. Attach a syringe, then aspirate until blood flows freely into the syringe. Discard this first syringe, attach a second saline filled syringe, then flush per the single flush technique.
  - If you are unable to aspirate blood, many problems may be present:
    - The catheter tip may be up against a wall → rotate and pull the catheter back, then try again
    - The catheter may be occluded → in which case it will need to be replaced
    - The catheter may be wedged in a small vessel → slowly pull back until you are able to aspirate
    - The catheter may be kinked → check with fluoroscopy; if it is kinked, it will need to be replaced
- **Types**
  - Many different types of catheters exist, which are too numerous to go into detail, and only the more commonly used catheters will be discussed. Note that the same shape of the catheter may have a different name, depending on the vendor.
  - There are two broad categories of catheters: Selective and nonselective
    - **Selective catheters:** These have tips which are shaped for optimal access to the target vessel
      - **Cobra:** As the name suggests, the tip of the catheter is shaped like the head of a cobra. Commonly used for visceral angiography, especially in downgoing

Figure 5-5 Commonly used catheters in interventional radiology.

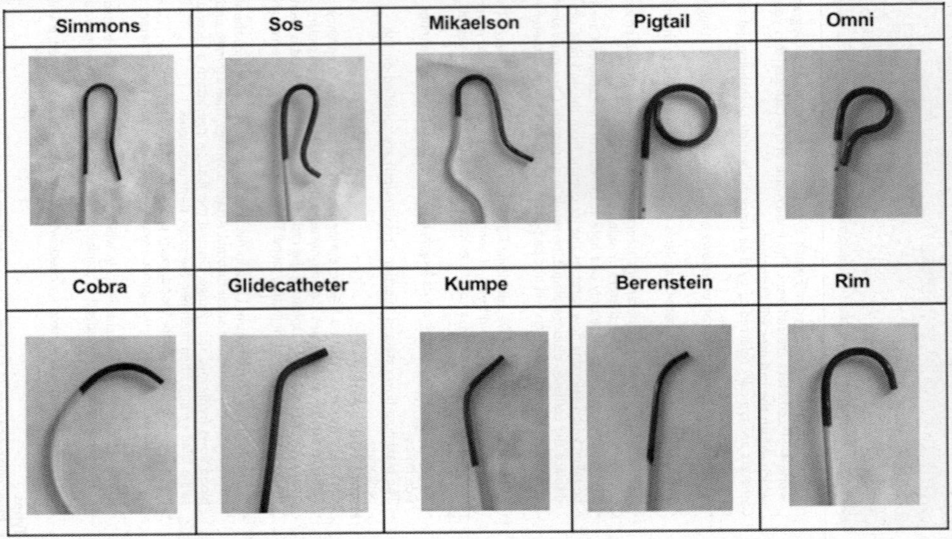

vessels. Advanced by pushing, and removed by pulling. Three variants, C1–C3, exist, with a progressively widening curve. Also comes in a "glide"-type catheter with a hydrophobic coating.
- **Visceral selective/Sos:** Reverse curve catheter with a shorter reverse curve than a Simmons. Commonly used for visceral and renal angiography. Pulled down to engage a vessel, and pushed forward to subselect. Also comes in three variants, with a progressively widening curve.
- **Simmons/Sidewinder:** Catheter with a large reverse curve, and needs to formed either in the aortic arch or over the iliac bifurcation. Useful for the great vessels, visceral work, and can be used for easy selection of the left adrenal vein. Similar to the visceral selective catheter, it is pulled down to engage and pushed forward to subselect.
- **Rosch inferior mesenteric:** Catheter with a short U-shaped reverse curve. Good for selecting the IMA, and can be useful to select the contralateral inferior epigastric artery.
- **Mikaelson:** Looks similar to a VS catheter, only with a "bump" on the back end to stabilize the catheter. Useful for bronchial arteries.
- **Chung:** Catheter with an elongated U-shaped reverse curve. Useful for bronchial arteries, or for visceral arteries with a tight inferior origin.
- **Renal double curve:** Catheter with a downward pointing curve, designed for renal work.
- **Headhunter:** Forward facing primary curve catheter. As the name suggests, primarily used for head and neck vessels.
- **Van Aman/Grollman:** Similarly shaped catheters used for pulmonary arterial work. Shaped like a pigtail catheter with an angle down the shaft of the catheter.
- **Roberts uterine catheter:** Catheter with a very large and tight reverse curve, which is shaped like a pre-formed Waltman's loop. Must be formed over the iliac bifurcation.
- **Angled catheters:** A variety of catheters exist with a simple angle at the end which is variable in length. Examples include Kumpe, Berenstein, MPA, and hockey stick.
- **Nonselective (flush) catheters:** These have tips with multiple side holes, primarily used for aortography and vena cavography.
  - **Pigtail:** Catheter with a "pigtail" shaped loop at the end. The loop measures approximately 15 mm and contains numerous side holes to allow greater flow.
  - **Straight flush:** Straight shaped catheter with numerous side holes. Used in vessels too small to accommodate a pigtail or Omni.
  - **Omni flush:** Catheter with a tight reverse curve and numerous side holes. Although not a selective catheter, it is a good "up-and-over" catheter.
- **Other types of catheters**
  - **Guide-catheters**
    - Large catheters which provide a safe pathway for a conventional catheter to target a vessel
    - Come in a variety of shapes and usually come in 6F, 7F, or 8F sizes
    - These catheters have a much stiffer shaft and larger internal diameter to provide support for guidewires, macrocoils, balloons, and stents. The catheter is positioned in the target vessel ostium. After that, a conventional catheter is used for distal catheterization.
    - Although long introducer sheaths can serve the same function as a guide catheter, the shape variety of guide catheters is a distinct advantage over a long sheath
    - Must be introduced through an appropriate sheath, as guidewires are too small for this large caliber catheter. A disadvantage is the larger sheath size required for the guide catheter.

Guide catheter	Introducer guides (long sheaths)
Sized by outer diameter	Sized by inner lumen size (as other sheaths)
Eg, 6F guide catheter will not fit a 6F catheter or stent through it	Eg, A 6F introducer guide will fit a 6F catheter or stent

  - **Microcatheters**
    - Small catheters, usually 2–3F
    - Flexible, and optimized for catheterization of small, tortuous vessels. Examples include subselection of visceral, hepatic, and peripheral vessels. Used by passing it through the selective catheter after initial catheterization of the targeted proximal vessel.

- **How to select the proper catheter**
  - Choose a catheter that points in the direction you want to go. For example, if a celiac artery is pointing down, a cobra or visceral selective catheter is usually adequate. But if the celiac artery is pointing up, you may need a catheter such as MPA.
  - Assess the other characteristics of the target vessel and parent vessel, and choose accordingly
    - A: Tip length: A longer length gives you more stability in the target vessel. However, you lose some torquability.
    - B: Primary curve: Assess the angle of the target vessel from the parent vessel
    - C: Secondary curve: Assess the width of the parent vessel
    - D: Tertiary curve: Assess the curvature of the parent vessel
    - E: Overall catheter length depending on the target

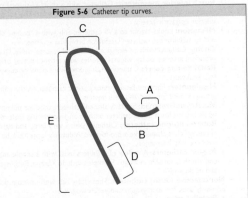

Figure 5-6 Catheter tip curves.

Sheaths
- Hollow plastic tube with a hemostatic valve and a clear side-port for flushing
- Used to provide atraumatic passage of catheters and wires into the vasculature. Maintains access especially in cases where multiple catheters and wires are used.
- Like catheters, they need to be flushed regularly. Some operators prefer to attach a pressurized saline flush to the side-port throughout a case.
  - If a sheath will not aspirate, use fluoroscopy to check for a kink.
    - Kinks usually result from a steep angle of entry into the artery. If a sheath is kinked, try to straighten it by flattening it against the patient's body. If this fails, advance a wire until resistance is felt. Carefully readvance the dilator to this point, and apply gentle traction to attempt to straighten it. If this fails, exchange the sheath.
  - Try to aspirate with a larger caliber syringe (20 cc or larger). If aspiration fails to return flow, exchange the sheath.
- Sheath size corresponds to the size of the catheter that passes through the sheath. Therefore, the outer diameter of the sheath is 1–2F larger than the size of the sheath. For example, if a 4F sheath is used, the outer diameter (and therefore the hole in the vessel) is 5.5–6F.

Embolization
- **Background**
  - Defined as reducing or obstructing blood flow by injecting an occluding material
  - Occlusion may be proximal at the level of a main artery or arteriole or may be distal at the level of the capillary bed, depending on the type of embolic material used
  - The goal is to selectively block target vessels while minimizing embolization to nontarget vessels
    - When injecting particles, stop when there is slow flow. If the vessel is embolized to complete occlusion, there is a high risk of nontarget embolization due to reflux. The goal is a "tree-in-winter" appearance of the vasculature, or for the contrast to take 3–5 heartbeats to clear after injection.
  - Occlusion may be either temporary or permanent, based on the clinical indication and materials used

Figure 5-7 Introducer sheath and dilator.

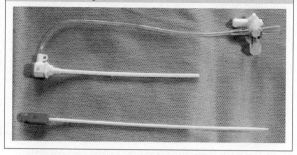

- Temporary occlusion may be used due to trauma, as it allows an otherwise healthy vessel to heal before flow is re-established
  - Options for temporary occlusion include gelfoam and autologous blood clot
- Permanent occlusion may be used in an abnormal vessel (AVF, aneurysm), or for tumor
  - Options for permanent occlusion include coils, particles, and glue
- **Types of embolic material**
  - **Mechanical**
    - **Coils**
      - Permanent, and made of stainless steel or platinum
      - Coils are sized based on the diameter of the coil (0.014–0.018-inch), the unconstrained length, and the diameter of the formed coil
        - When choosing coil size, oversizing slightly helps to minimize coil dislodgement
      - Work by damaging vascular intima, causing the release of thrombogenic agents and activating platelets
      - Designed with thrombogenic fibers to increase the surface area, increasing the speed of thrombosis
      - May be deployed by pushing through an end-hole catheter (either with a wire or a coil pusher), or they may be "shot" into the artery with a saline syringe
      - Detachable coils remain attached to the wire until a specific action is performed. This allows you to test the stability of the coil prior to detachment.
      - Note that when proximal embolization is performed, collateral arteries will rapidly form in the distal vascular bed
        - Take care if choosing proximal embolization, as the coil is permanent, and future access to the artery will not be possible
    - **Vascular plugs (Amplatzer)**
      - Permanent self-expandable nitinol mesh plugs
      - Mounted on a wire, but will expand into a 3D disc upon deployment
        - Similar to detachable coils, they will remain attached to the wire until the lock is unscrewed on the back of the wire
      - Similar to coils, they should be oversized to the target vessel diameter by 30–50%
      - Useful when a larger vessel (such as an internal iliac artery or splenic artery) needs to be embolized
      - May be deployed first as a scaffold for additional embolization with coils or gelfoam
  - **Particulates**
    - **Gelfoam**
      - Temporary hemostatic agent made from purified skin gelatin
        - Since it is temporary, it is useful to stop bleeding during trauma, acute bleeding in an otherwise normal vessel, or for preoperative devascularization of a targeted area to decrease surgical bleeding
      - Works by slowing flow and giving structural support for thrombus
      - Resorbed completely, with vessel recanalization in a few weeks
      - Gelfoam pledgets/sheets → occlude to the level of the arterioles and do not cause tissue infarct

- Gelfoam powder → occlude to the level of the capillaries and can cause tissue necrosis
- There are several methods for embolization
  - "Torpedoes" which are small, rolled strips which are injected. While this may be performed intravascularly, it is particularly useful for embolizing the needle tract after biopsy.
  - "Gelfoam slurry" method, where gelfoam is loaded into a syringe, then attached via 3-way stopcock to a second syringe filled with contrast. After vigorous pumping back and forth between the syringes, a suspension of smaller particles is made, which can then be injected. The density of the slurry is determined by the initial amounts of gelfoam and contrast.
- **Autologous blood clot**
  - A sample of the patient's blood is collected and allowed to clot; this is then injected. This causes only temporary occlusion and only rarely used.
- **PVA**
  - Permanent agent made of irregularly shaped shavings from a block of polyvinyl alcohol
  - Uses include: Uterine fibroid embolization, bronchial artery embolization
  - Available in sizes ranging from 50–1200 μm
    - Choose the size based on the level of occlusion desired. At the capillary bed, use smaller particles; at the arteriole level, use larger particles. Take care when choosing particle size, as the particles tend to clump.
  - Embolize by both occlusion of the vessel as well as activation of thrombin
  - Supplied either dry (PVA particles in a vial), or as part of a solution in a syringe
- **Microspheres**
  - Permanent agent made of spherical embolic material
  - Compared to PVA particles, these have less clumping and clogging of catheters, leading to easier injection and a more predictable level of occlusion
  - Available in sizes from 40–1200 μm
  - Supplied as part of a solution in a syringe
- **Drug-eluting particles**
  - Allow not only for mechanical embolization but also sustained controlled drug release
  - PVA particles loaded with doxorubicin, used for TACE procedures
- **Liquid embolic agents**
  - **Nonsclerosants**
    - **Onyx (Ethylene-Vinyl Alcohol Copolymer)**
      - Liquid embolic which dries at a slow rate from the outside in for more controlled delivery
      - Uses include neuro procedures such as hypervascular spinal tumors, AVMs, and aneurysms
    - **Glue**
      - Permanent agent made of cyanoacrylate
      - Immediately solidifies once it contacts any anionic substance. This not only includes blood but saline as well.
        - Must be mixed with D5W. The catheter must be thoroughly flushed with D5W prior to glue injection, or it will solidify in the catheter.
        - Ethiodol can be used to prolong the time the glue takes to solidify. The ratio of ethiodol to glue can be tailored to the length of time needed for solidification. If the time to solidification is made too long, the glue can pass into the venous circulation and result in pulmonary emboli.
        - All mixtures should be made on a separate side table to prevent cross-contamination
        - The catheter should be changed after each injection. The catheter should not be left in place for long, as it may become glued in place.
      - Causes an intense fibrotic response and vessel necrosis
      - Commonly used to treat AVMs, but can be used anywhere (particularly for portal vein embolization)
  - **Sclerosant**
    - **Alcohol**
      - Damages all tissue it contacts, causing dehydration related cell death and eventual fibrosis
      - Can be used intravascularly, but with great care
        - Only use in vascular beds without significant collaterals. The catheter should be placed as subselectively as possible. Only inject small volumes.

- Can also be used to sclerose cysts or lymphoceles. Regardless of the volume of the cyst/lymphocele, never inject more than 60 mL due to the risk of systemic toxicity. Never let any extravasate, as this can cause damage to the skin or any surrounding nerves.
- **Sodium tetradecyl sulfate (SDS)**
  - Generally a safe, easy-to-use sclerosant
  - Detergent made into a foam after agitating with air which causes red blood cell sludging and thrombosis
  - Good for low flow malformations

Balloons

- **Background**
  - Most balloons are over-the-wire, with a balloon mounted on the end of a catheter, which has a central lumen used to pass over a guidewire
  - The force applied by a balloon is dependent on the inflation pressure, balloon length, material, and the degree of stenosis
  - Balloons may be standard (0.035-inch guidewire compatible), or small vessel (0.014–0.018-inch guidewire compatible)
  - Venous balloons tend to be of larger diameter. Angioplasty of venous structures tends to be less successful due to the large compliance of veins.
  - Arterial angioplasty is indicated for shorter noncalcified stenosis
  - Balloons can be used to tamponade any bleeding caused during procedures
- **Balloon selection**: Choose balloon based on the length and diameter of the vessel being treated. Keep in mind that there is balloon material proximal and distal to the radiopaque markers.
  - Balloon diameter: Ideal size is 10–20% over the normal adjacent artery diameter
  - Balloon length: Long enough to span the lesion but no longer than 1 cm on either side of the lesion
  - Occasionally, a longer balloon may be required to treat a focal lesion, as a small balloon may "watermelon seed" and move either proximal or distal to the stenosis during inflation
- **Types**
  - Constructed of either compliant/semicompliant material or noncompliant material. The balloon is selected by anatomic location and type of lesion.
    - **Compliant/semicompliant balloons:** Will stretch beyond the predetermined diameter with an increase in inflation pressure. These are good for tight lesions and tortuous anatomy, as well as predilation prior to stent deployment.
      - Before opening a larger stent, you can overinflate the smaller stent to achieve a larger vessel diameter (ie, overinflation of a 5-mm balloon may produce a diameter of 5.3 mm), which may fix the stenosis without having to open a larger balloon
    - **Noncompliant balloons:** Will not stretch beyond the predetermined diameter. These are good for resistant or heavily calcified lesions, ostial lesions, and postdilation of stents.

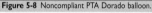

Figure 5-8 Noncompliant PTA Dorado balloon.

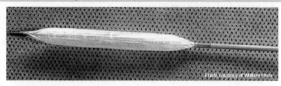

Photo courtesy of Wilken Tech.

- **Specialty balloons**
  - **Fogarty**
    - Compliant balloon used to "sweep" clot during dialysis work
  - **Cutting/scoring balloons**
    - Noncompliant balloons with metal "blades" along the length of the balloon. The balloon should never be advanced by itself, it should be placed through a sheath, then "unsheathed" before use.
    - Rarely used in the vasculature, but can be used for postoperative biliary or urinary strictures that have failed regular angioplasty
  - **Drug-eluting balloons**
    - Angioplasty balloons coated with drugs meant to prevent restenosis

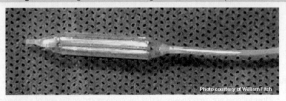

Figure 5-9 Cutting balloon with microsurgical blades and noncompliant balloon.

Photo courtesy of William Fitch

- **Balloon Angioplasty Technique**
  - First "prime" the inflator lumen with contrast by attaching a contrast syringe and aspirating forcefully several times
  - If using an inflator, never use more than 50% contrast, as it will make it difficult to deflate the balloon
  - Always watch when moving a balloon through a stent. The balloon could get stuck in the stent (especially after deflation), or the wire may have found its way through a strut in the stent.
  - Slowly inflate the balloon using an inflator, keeping an eye on the pressure. Also, watch the "waist" in the balloon during inflation.
  - Successful angioplasty when there is <30% residual stenosis

Vascular Stents

- **Background**
  - Stenting may be performed in the arterial or venous systems. Less commonly, stenting can also be performed in the GI tract, tracheobronchial tree, or biliary tree.
- **Stent selection:**
  - While the brand of the stent placed is dependent on operator preference or availability, several factors determine which stent to place
    - **Vessel diameter:** Generally size 1–2 cm longer than the stenosis and 1–2 mm wider than the unstenosed vessel lumen. This is due to the reduction in luminal diameter after stent deployment and poststenting neointimal hyperplasia.
    - **Location:** As above, due to their superiority with placement precision, BE stents are best for ostial lesions and bifurcations. Areas experiencing any external compression should be treated with SE stents.
    - **Length:** Shorter focal lesions are well treated with BE stents, while longer lesions tend to be treated with SE stents
    - **Vessel calcification:** Densely calcified arteries may require the additional radial force supplied by BE stents
- **Types:** There are two broad categories of stents: Balloon expandable (BE) and self-expandable (SE). Type is selected by location.
  - **Balloon expandable stents**
    - Premounted on a balloon, which must be inflated to deploy the stent
    - Made of stainless steel or cobalt/chromium
    - Have higher radial force compared to SE, and can be placed more precisely than SE stents (eg, renal ostium)
    - Are less flexible than SE stents, and are usually unsuitable for tortuous vessels, or vessels that may experience external compression (eg, SFA)
    - Examples: Palmaz, Palmaz Genesis, Omnilink Elite, Assurant Cobalt
  - **Self-expandable stents**
    - Compressed in a delivery catheter, which must be unsheathed to deploy the stent
    - They differ from balloon-expandable stents in that the stent diameter cannot be increased by increased balloon dilatation.
    - Made of nitinol or elgiloy
    - Have "shape memory" and are very flexible. They also retake their shape after compression, making them good candidates for areas experiencing external compression (eg, SFA or carotid)
    - Have lower radial force than BE stents, and placement is not as precise making them poor candidates for ostial lesions or bifurcations
    - Examples: Zilver, SMART stent, Wallstent, and Absolute

- **Other stents**
  - **Stent-grafts**
    - Metal stent (nitinol or stainless steel) which has an outer sleeve (PTFE, polycarbonate, Dacron) lining the stent
    - May be balloon expandable or self-expandable
    - Have different functions depending on the indication. For example: To divert blood flow in vessel rupture, to exclude an aneurysm (ie, endovascular aortic aneurysm repair) or pseudoaneurysm, or for benign or malignant strictures.
    - Examples: Viabahn, Fluency, and Wallgraft
- Some modern stents have additional functionality due to different finishes or coatings (eg, drug-eluting and radioactivity)

NONVASCULAR IR DEVICES

Biopsy Needles
- **Background**
  - Soft tissue biopsy devices should be chosen with the intended target site, and pertinent patient data in mind as a wide variety of biopsy devices exist. Needle selection is typically subject to operator familiarity, target location, biopsy technique, and patient-specific factors.
  - Biopsy needle size is typically measured in gauge (larger gauge = smaller needle)
- **Size of Needle**
  - Fine-gauge biopsy needles (20–25G)
    - Thin-walled hollow needles in which a gentle to and fro motion is used to obtain cells for cytology or used for aspiration
    - Subtypes:
      - Sharp bevel-tipped needles
        - Eg, spinal needle or chiba needle
      - Cutting tip needles
        - Eg, Tuner, Franseen, Westcott, Green, Madayag
  - Large-gauge biopsy needles (14–19G)
    - Has inner stylet with a partially hollow core and an outer stylet with a spring-loaded handle which closes to cut the sample
    - Automated devices are needles which are equipped with a firing mechanism which is "loaded" before use. Automated devices tend to reduce procedure time and yield more uniform/higher quality tissue samples compared to manually acquired tissue samples.
    - Can be used with a coaxial system. The coaxial needle is 1G larger (eg, an 18G biopsy needle has a 17G coaxial needle) and is used to maintain needle position. This allows access to lesions without having to puncture the capsule more than once or allows repeat biopsy access to difficult lesions. Also allows for deployment of gelfoam pledgets or other hemostatic devices to aid in hemostasis if there is bleeding after the biopsy.
    - Eg, Tenmo or Bard
    - Subtypes:
      - Side-cutting needles generally work best in soft tissue masses
      - End-cutting needles generally work best in solid masses
- **Technique**
  - **Fine-needle aspiration**
    - Obtains cells for cytology
    - Performed with fine-gauge needles
    - In general, aspiration needles are safer than cutting needles
  - **Cutting/core needle biopsy**
    - Obtains tissue for biopsy diagnosis
    - Performed with a large-gauge automatic cutting needle such as a Tenmo or Bard coaxial system. May be used with or without a coaxial system.

Other Biopsy
- **Musculoskeletal Biopsy Needles**
  - Most procedures performed under CT or fluoroscopy. Needle choice depends on biopsy site (soft tissue or bone) and lesion type (osteoblastic vs. osteolytic)
  - In general, needles are large caliber with a serrated edge
  - Examples include the Turkel needle (Turkel Instruments), Franseen Needle (Cook Medical), and Ackermann needle (Becton–Dickinson)
  - Generally, a cannula is inserted into the targeted tissue, through which a biopsy needle is placed to harvest tissue

- For lytic lesions with an intact cortex, tools such as the Bonopty Coaxial Biopsy System are utilized. The Bonopty system uses a blunt cannula with a stylet and an eccentric drill to obtain samples
- **Breast Biopsy Equipment**
  - Percutaneous image-guided breast biopsy has become standard of care in many locations compared to standard surgical biopsy. Percutaneous biopsy is faster, cheaper, and less invasive.
  - Wide range of needles is available for use under ultrasound or stereotactic guidance
  - Fine-needle aspirations have largely been replaced by core biopsies utilizing vacuum-assisted devices
  - Commonly utilized vacuum systems include Mammotome system (Ethicon Endo-Surgery) and ATEC (automated tissue excision and collection) system (Suros Surgical Systems)
  - Mammotome system draws tissue into one end via a vacuum which is then excised via a rotating cutter. Suction draws the sample into the device without having to remove the needle. Can be used with ultrasound, stereotactic, and MRI guidance.

Nonvascular Catheters
- **Abscess drainage catheters**
  - **Types:**
    - Single lumen (nonsump) vs. double lumen (sump)
      - Sump catheters are especially good for intra-abdominal abscesses since the outer lumen helps to prevent blockage of side holes when the catheter is adjacent to an abscess cavity wall
    - Locking tip (Cope) vs. nonlocking tip
      - Locking tip catheters are especially useful for deep pelvic abscesses, as well as transrectal or transvaginal drainage
    - Straight-tipped, J tipped, or pigtail tipped
  - **Sizes:** Commonly available in 6–14F sizes, for thicker/more viscous fluid collections, use larger French
- **Internal/external biliary catheters**
  - Has a pigtail tip, which will have multiple side holes. Side holes will extend along the length of the catheter, and end at a radiopaque marker.
    - Side holes should be placed both above and below the site of an occlusion. If extra side holes are needed, these can be cut manually.
  - **Sizes:** Available in 8.5, 10.2, 12, and 14F sizes, ranging from 30–40 cm in length
- **Percutaneous cholecystostomy catheters**
  - **Sizes:** Pigtail tip catheter available in 6–14F in size, ranging from 25–35 cm
- **Nephrostomy catheters**
  - Locking pigtail tip to secure the catheter in the renal pelvis
  - **Sizes:** Typically, an 8F or 10F catheter is placed, though additional sizes are available. Ranges from 25–35 cm in length.
- **Nephroureteral catheters**
  - Has a distal locking pigtail in the bladder, and a proximal locking pigtail in the renal pelvis
  - Allows for both internal and external drainage
  - When placing, the length between the bladder and renal pelvis should be measured to determine the length between pigtails that will need to be placed. Catheters come in 22–28 cm. Typically sized 8F and 10F.
  - A solely internal "double-J" nephroureteral catheter is also available

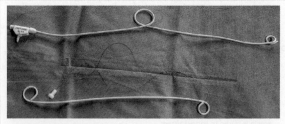

Figure 5-10 Top: Nephroureteral stent. **Bottom:** Double J stent.

ADDITIONAL RESOURCES

1. Funaki B. Central venous access: A primer for the diagnostic radiologist. *Am J Roentgenol* 2002;179:309–18.
2. Kandarpa K, Lindsay M. *Handbook of Interventional Radiologic Procedures*. Lippincott Williams & Wilkins; 2011.
3. Matthew M. *Image-Guided Interventions E-Book: Expert Radiology Series*. Elsevier Health Sciences; 2013.
4. LaBerge J. *Interventional Radiology Essentials*. Lippincott Williams & Wilkins; 2000.
5. *Interventional Radiology Procedures in Biopsy and Drainage*. Springer London; 2011. doi:10.1007/978-1-84800-899-1
6. Kessel D, Robertson I. *Interventional Radiology: A Survival Guide*. Elsevier Health Sciences; 2016.
7. Kaufman J, Lee M. *Vascular and Interventional Radiology: The Requisites. 2nd ed*. Elsevier Health Sciences; 2013.
8. Northcutt BG, Shah AA, Sheu YR, et al. Wires, catheters, and more: A primer for residents and fellows entering interventional radiology: Resident and fellow education feature. *RadioGraphics* 2015;35:1621–22.

PREPROCEDURE MANAGEMENT

- Check the patient's allergies, including allergies to contrast agents
- Check labs
  - Platelet count should be >50,000
  - INR should be <1.5, although exceptions can be made for venous procedures or lower-risk procedures
  - GFR >30. Exceptions can be made if the GFR is lower, but this may require the use of CO_2 for contrast
- Check current medications
  - Heparin should be stopped 2 hours prior to arterial or venous puncture
  - Warfarin, aspirin, and plavix should be stopped for several days prior to an arterial puncture, if possible
    - As this may not always be possible, exceptions can be made. If the procedure carries a high bleeding risk and the patient cannot stop anticoagulation, they may need to be admitted and transitioned to a heparin drip.
- Obtain a full history and perform a physical exam
  - Include pulse checks, both at the site of access and distally. Doppler may be needed for distal pulses.
  - Check the patient's blood pressure. Many times, patients forget to take their blood pressure medications when NPO, even when told to take them with sips of water.
  - If crossing the heart, include an ECG to check for a left bundle branch block, as a wire in the right ventricle can cause a temporary right block
- Make sure the patient is NPO
  - 2–4 h for clear liquids, and 6 h for solids
- Consent the patient after explaining the procedure and common risks of vascular access, including bleeding, infection, and damage to surrounding tissues

ARTERIAL ACCESS

Background

- A micropuncture kit is typically used for vascular access. This kit includes:
  - 21G access needle
  - 0.018-in microwire
  - 4F or 5F dilator sets with stiffened cannula may be used for scarred or calcified arteries. Starting with a stiff cannula may be a good idea if accessing near prior surgical sites.

Access Points

- **Retrograde Femoral Artery Access**
  - The most common site of access. Allows for easy access to the visceral arteries, renal arteries, the bilateral iliac arterial system, and the contralateral femoral artery.
- **Antegrade Femoral Artery Access**
  - Used for interventions on the ipsilateral superficial femoral artery (SFA), popliteal, or tibial arteries
  - May be used if contralateral retrograde access is difficult (scarring, EVAR, ABF), or the required length of balloon/stent is too long for contralateral access
  - More prone to dissection, as the access angle is in the same direction as the blood flow
  - Consider development of dissection if the patient begins to complain of severe or "tearing" pain near the site of intervention
- **Brachial Artery Access**
- Used for interventions on the visceral arteries, renal arteries, aorta, or iliac arterial system
- May be used if femoral artery access is not able to be obtained (scarring, occluded iliac artery, occluded aorta)
- The left brachial artery is preferred. Accessing the right brachial artery requires crossing the arch vessels, which has a risk of dislodging plaque or causing emboli into the CNS circulation.
- Even though the risk of stroke is small, this should be explained to the patient during consent
- **Radial artery access**
  - Used for interventions on the coronary arteries, visceral arteries, renal arteries, and occasionally for ease of access to both internal iliac arteries (ie, for uterine fibroid embolization).

- Not optimal for stenting/angioplasty of the aorta or iliac arteries due to the sheath size required for these procedures
- May be used based on operator or patient preference
- **Other less common arterial puncture sites include:**
  - Tibiopedal: For tibial or popliteal artery interventions, such as limb salvage procedures or infrapopliteal occlusions
  - Popliteal: Used for limb salvage or arterial occlusions when access via femoral artery is not possible
  - Translumbar: Used to puncture the excluded aortic aneurysm sac, typically for evaluation of endoleak after EVAR

Creating Arterial Access
- **Retrograde Femoral Artery Access**
  - Anatomy is defined, lateral to medial, by:
    - Nerve, artery, vein, lymphatics (Fig. 6-1). Remember the mnemonic, NAVL.
  - The artery is best accessed in the inferior 1/2 of the femoral head (Fig. 6-1)
    - This assures you are above the femoral artery bifurcation, but are below the inferior epigastric artery
    - This allows proper compression for hemostasis after the procedure, as you can compress the vessel against the femoral head
      - If the artery is accessed too high, there is a risk of retroperitoneal hematoma
      - If the artery is accessed too low, there is a risk of pseudoaneurysm
      - These complications are due to inability to properly compress the artery for hemostasis

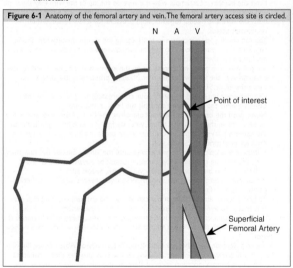

Figure 6-1 Anatomy of the femoral artery and vein. The femoral artery access site is circled.

N   A   V

Point of interest

Superficial Femoral Artery

- Start by first palpating the artery, then placing a hemostat over the palpable pulse.
  - Do a spot fluoro check to make sure the hemostat tip is over the inferior femoral head
  - Never just use the inguinal crease as a guide without checking fluoroscopy. Based on body weight, a patient may have a high or low inguinal crease compared to the femoral head
- Numb the skin with 1% lidocaine. Try not to have your fingers on the patient when you numb them, as they may flinch and cause an accidental needle stick.
  - Leave the hemostat where it was and numb at the tip, mark the spot with a skin marker, or simply use a cutaneous landmark
- Make a small skin nick with a scalpel appropriate for the anticipated sheath size. This can be made after the needle puncture depending on operator preference.

- Advance the access needle toward the artery at a 45° angle. Steeper angles may be needed in cases of severe atherosclerotic disease.
- Feel the pulsation as the needle approaches the vessel. Pulsation will decrease and you may feel resistance as you enter the vessel.
- Check for pulsatile backflow. This will not be present in venous punctures and may not be present in highly calcified or stenotic femoral arteries.
  - Lack of backflow may also indicate you have gone through-and-through the back wall of the vessel. Slowly pull the needle back, checking for backflow. A syringe with saline can be attached to the needle, with negative pressure applied while removing the needle. Blood will be drawn into the syringe when you have re-entered the vessel.
- At this point, do not lift your ultrasound hand (if accessing with ultrasound), or palpating fingers (if accessing by feel), especially in obese patients. The rebounding soft tissue may pull the needle out of the artery.
- Slowly advance the microwire through the needle. Advance the microwire so that the stiff section of the wire is within the vessel. Wires should be advanced under fluoroscopic guidance.
  - Never force the wire, as this may dissect the vessel, or the wire may have found its way up a branch of the femoral artery (typically the circumflex iliac). Stop if you feel any tension or resistance, and check your wire with fluoroscopy.
  - If there is resistance, slowly readjust the angle of the needle to flatten it, then gently try the wire again. Spinning the wire as it is advanced can help it navigate through plaques and tortuosity.
  - Limit the number of attempts with the wire, as the tip of the wire may shear off and embolize. Whenever there is concern that the wire won't advance, remove both the wire and needle together, hold pressure for a few minutes, then re-attempt access.
  - You can check your puncture site by assessing the transition between needle and wire. If the puncture is too high or too low, pull the needle and wire out, hold pressure, then re-access.
- Once the wire is in place, hold pressure on the artery with one hand, and remove the needle over the wire with the other. Maintain pressure on the artery, and advance the 4F or 5F dilator over the wire.
  - Use the index finger and thumb of your compressing hand to advance the catheter, while the other hand controls the back of the wire
  - Never push the catheter in without controlling the back of the wire, as this may cause a kink in the wire (with a kink, you may feel the wire being pushed in by the catheter). Trying to push a catheter when there is a kink may result in the catheter puncturing the vessel wall.
    - If there is a kink, pull back on the wire until the kink is outside the skin, then re-advance the catheter. If the catheter cannot be advanced, the wire will likely need to be replaced, possibly with a new needle stick.
  - Movements should always feel smooth. Whenever there is any doubt, check positioning with fluoroscopy.
  - To help prevent any buckling of the catheter in the soft tissues, compress the soft tissues to minimize the distance between the vessel and the skin nick.
- After the micropuncture dilator is in place over the wire, unscrew and remove the inner stiffener with the wire. You should see brisk pulsatile flow through the outer dilator.
- Advance a Bentson wire through the micropuncture dilator. Watch under fluoroscopy as you advance the wire, establishing wire access into the abdominal aorta.
- At this point, femoral access is secured. Remove the micropuncture dilator over the wire, and advance the desired catheter or sheath over the wire.
- Note that the artery may be accessed "blind" (by palpation), or with ultrasound
  - For blind access, follow the initial steps as above
    - After the skin nick is made, place one finger above the nick and one below. This lets you delineate the course of the artery
    - If the patient experiences pain in the anterior leg, or shooting pain down the leg, the puncture is too lateral and hitting the nerve
    - If blood return is a slow flow and darker red, the puncture is too medial and in the femoral vein
    - Make sure you feel the pulsation pushing directly against you, indicating you are on top of the vessel. If you feel pulsations pushing the needle medially or laterally, you are on the side of the vessel.
  - For ultrasound access, always scan toward the feet to find the femoral artery bifurcation to make sure the patient doesn't have a high SFA origin

- To make your puncture at a 45° angle, check your artery depth with ultrasound. Make your skin entry site the same distance away from the center of the probe (ie, if the artery is 2 cm deep, make your skin entry 2 cm away from the center of the probe).
- **Antegrade Femoral Artery Access**
  - Aim to access the artery in the same place, at the inferior 1/2 of the femoral head
  - Start similarly to retrograde access by first placing a hemostat over the pulse and checking with fluoroscopy
  - Place an ultrasound over the tip of the hemostat, then remove the hemostat. Sweep inferiorly with ultrasound to assess the femoral bifurcation, then move the ultrasound back to its original position.
  - Numb the skin with 1% lidocaine
  - Access the artery at a steep >60° angle. A shallower 45° angle will require a large amount of soft tissue to be crossed, especially in overweight/obese patients.
  - After access is gained, advance the wire as discussed previously
    - Antegrade access is usually obtained for ipsilateral femoral or popliteal intervention, so flow down the profunda is typically brisker compared to the SFA. Therefore, the wire will frequently find its way down the profunda branch of the artery instead of the SFA.
    - Accessing the artery toward the SFA in a slight lateral-to-medial direction facilitates wire access into the SFA
- **Brachial Artery Access**
  - Brachial artery access as a higher risk of complications compared to both femoral artery and radial artery access
  - Must understand the artery's relation to the median nerve and biceps tendon to avoid injury to these structures
  - Access around 1 cm above to the antecubital fossa, as this will be above the biceps tendon, and will allow for hemostasis with compression against the distal humerus
  - Always check radial and ulnar pulses both before and after the procedure
  - This should be performed under ultrasound guidance
  - Heparin should be given after access is obtained, although ACT does not routinely need to be checked
  - Proper hemostasis after the procedure is imperative, as a hematoma can compress the median nerve in the medial brachial fascial compartment
  - The patient will likely need to be carefully watched after the procedure, as most patients have difficulty keeping their arm still
- **Radial Artery Access**
  - You must ensure good collateral flow from ulnar artery using the Barbeau test
    - Place Pulse Ox on the 1st or 2nd finger
    - Look at the waveform and ensure that it is normal
    - Occlude the radial artery with compression
    - The waveform should go back to normal by 2 min if there is good ulnar collateral flow (Fig. 6-2)
    - If it does not (Waveform D), the vessel is occluded or variant anatomy is present and radial access is contraindicated
  - As the smaller arteries are prone to spasm, a combination of Verapamil 2.5 mg, nitroglycerine 0.25 mg, and heparin 2500 IU is administered to reduce spasm and thrombosis
  - The artery may be accessed blind or with ultrasound

Postprocedure Management
- In general, catheters should be removed over a wire. This is especially true if a reverse curve catheter or pigtail catheter is used as these catheters can catch on plaques and stents and dislodge them.
  - If a reverse curve catheter is used for visceral or renal interventions, push the catheter up to de-select the artery
  - Next, advance the wire until you feel resistance. At this point, the wire is likely in the reverse portion of the catheter. Push an additional 2–3 cm of wire to straighten the catheter tip. Remove the wire/catheter combo as a unit.
- Compress the vessel as you remove the sheath or catheter (if not using a sheath). A good pulse should be felt proximal and distal to the site of vascular entry prior to removing devices.
- Remember that the arterial puncture site is not the same as the skin entry site. The arterial puncture site must be compressed.

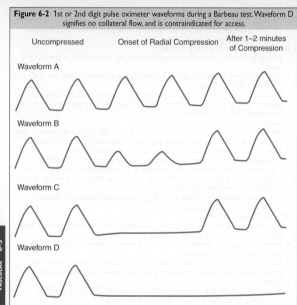

Figure 6-2 1st or 2nd digit pulse oximeter waveforms during a Barbeau test. Waveform D signifies no collateral flow, and is contraindicated for access.

Uncompressed   Onset of Radial Compression   After 1–2 minutes of Compression

Waveform A

Waveform B

Waveform C

Waveform D

- For retrograde femoral artery access, if compressing with the left hand, use your ring finger to compress the arterial puncture above the skin nick. Use your middle finger to compress the skin nick site, and use gentle pressure with your index finger below the skin nick to make sure you feel a pulse below where you're holding pressure (ie, you are not occluding the vessel).
  - If no closure device is used, hold pressure for 3 min × French size catheter used (ie, if a 4F catheter is used, hold for 12 min)
  - Remember to add additional time to this calculation if using a sheath (since a 4F sheath makes a larger hole in the vessel than a 4F catheter)
- Do not use sponges or gauze while holding pressure, as any bleeding should be visible
- Bed rest for 4–6 h. This may be shorter if a closure device is used.
- Check vitals q15 min × 4, then q30 min × 6
- If a hematoma forms, hold additional pressure. Mark the area and monitor for increasing size.

Venous Access

- Complete the previously discussed preprocedural steps
- In general, sedation is not used for temporary central venous catheter placement or PICC line placement. Sedation should be used for tunneled catheters and mediports.
- Prior to prepping and draping, evaluate the vein under ultrasound
  - Ensure that the vein is compressible
  - Check for thrombus both proximal and distal to your planned site of entry
  - If the vein is small, or you see a large number of surrounding collaterals, check the central veins with ultrasound to assess for possible central venous stenosis/ occlusion
- Prep and drape the patient as per hospital guidelines
- Place the ultrasound over the planned entry site
- Numb the skin with 1% lidocaine
  - Aspirate prior to injection to avoid injecting lidocaine intravascularly
- Make a skin nick appropriate for the catheter size
- A micropuncture kit is used for vascular access. An 18G access needle can be used instead, if doing direct 0.035-in system access.

- Advance the needle through your skin nick toward the vessel
- Once at the vessel, advance the needle into the lumen with a quick motion to prevent compression of the pliable walls of the vein
  - If the vessel is tenting, a quick spin of the needle may facilitate entry
  - As with arterial access, if the vessel is traversed through-and-through, slowly pull the needle back until you see it in the vessel with ultrasound, or have blood backflow
    - Attaching a syringe and pulling back with suction may also be performed until you see blood pulled into the syringe
- After the needle is in the vessel, advance the 0.018-in wire through the needle
  - Take the same precautions with the wire as you would with arterial access. Always check your wire position with fluoroscopy before advancing the catheter.
  - Occasionally with IJ access, the wire may course cephalad after deflecting off the IJ valve. If the wire is unable to be manipulated into the SVC, you may have to re-access below the valve.
- After checking your wire position, remove the needle over the wire, and advance the micropuncture dilator
- Remove the inner stiffener and wire together, then advance a Bentson or J tip wire through the outer dilator to secure access
- If getting access from the IJ/EJ, ideally the wire should be advanced into the IVC
  - If there is difficulty getting the wire into the IVC, asking the patient to inhale may facilitate wire advancement
- Any time there is difficulty advancing any catheter or wire, contrast may then be injected through the micropuncture dilator to check anatomy and positioning

Common Sites of Venous Access
- Always be aware of normal anatomy as well as common variants. Check the patient's prior cross-sectional imaging, if available. When assessing prior imaging, identify sites of stenosis, thrombosis, occlusion, altered anatomy, or other vascular findings that might change the planned course and difficulty of the procedure.
- **Internal Jugular Vein**
  - The right jugular vein allows straight access to the SVC, and is preferred over the left
  - The left jugular vein may be used if there is stenosis/occlusion of the right, or if the patient has a dialysis graft/fistula on the right
    - Access through the left jugular vein is more challenging as it first drains into the brachiocephalic vein, which may be tortuous. From left IJ access, the wire tends to enter the azygos arch. Due to these factors, a directional catheter may be needed to advance a wire from the left IJ into the IVC.
- **Femoral Vein**
  - The vein is medial to the artery and is best accessed at the inferior half of the femoral head
  - The right femoral vein has a straighter course to the IVC
- **Subclavian Vein**
  - Not routinely used as access is challenging and is associated with higher risk of pneumothorax
  - Puncture is made inferior to the clavicle, approximately 1/3 distance from the distal end
- **Upper-Extremity Veins**
  - Used for PICC line placement, arm ports, or intervention for central venous stenosis/occlusion
  - Choices include the basilic, cephalic, and brachial veins
  - The basilic vein is usually the vein of choice, as it is away from the artery
  - The cephalic vein is prone to spasm and thrombosis
  - The brachial vein has close proximity to the artery, and is associated with increased risk of complications
  - Many times, however, the choice of vein is made simply by which vein is largest on ultrasound
- **Less Common Puncture Sites**
  - Axillary vein
  - Median cubital vein
  - External jugular vein
    - Used if the IJ is occluded without central occlusion

Postprocedural Management
- Achieve hemostasis with gentle compression
- In cases of jugular/subclavian vein procedures, raising the patient's head above the heart can help reduce bleeding

- Have the patient rest in bed for 1–2 h
- Check vitals, and monitor for bleeding or hematoma every 30 min

Types of Central Venous Access
- **Nontunneled Central Venous Catheter**
  - These catheters can be placed with local anesthesia at bedside, but may be done in IR suite for difficult cases
  - Advantages include ease of access and removal
  - Only suitable for short-term use (<2 w)
  - May be used for hemodialysis, plasmapheresis, IV fluids, medications, etc.
  - For placement
    - Access the desired vein, as above
    - For IJ access, if the line is temporary (ie, for trauma patients), it may be placed in the mid or low IJ
    - If there is a possibility that the patient may need a tunneled catheter, it is best to access the low IJ vein so the same access point may be used to convert the catheter
    - After the flexible 0.035-in wire is placed, remove the micropuncture dilator, and predilate the vein with the dilator supplied in the kit
      - Always watch dilator placement under fluoroscopy! If there is a kink in the wire, or the wire is inadvertently pulled back prior to dilation, the SVC can be ruptured.
    - After predilation, simply advance the catheter over the wire to the appropriate location
      - Catheters placed cranial to the heart should be placed with the tip at the SVC/RA junction
      - Catheters placed caudal to the heart should be placed with the tip at the IVC/RA junction
      - If the catheter tip is placed within the right atrium, it may be kept there as long as there is no evidence of arrhythmia
      - Keep in mind that the catheter tip position will change once the patient sits/stands upright
    - Remove the wire after catheter positioning is confirmed
    - Flush and dwell all catheter's lumens with the appropriate volume of heparin
    - Secure the catheter to the skin with a nonabsorbable suture, and place a sterile dressing
- **PICC lines**
  - With ultrasound, choose the desired vein for access
    - A tourniquet may be placed in the upper arm to distend the veins, if required
  - After numbing the skin, advance a 21G needle into the vein as discussed in the venous access section
  - Once in the vein, advance a 0.018-in wire through the needle, checking its position with fluoroscopy
  - Advance the wire centrally
    - If the wire will not advance, there may be spasm. Injection of saline can help to distend the venous system. Contrast may also be injected.
  - Make a small skin nick
  - Exchange the needle over the wire with the supplied peel-a-way sheath
  - To measure the proper catheter length, place the wire at the SVC/RA junction, then place a clamp on the wire as it exits the peel-a-way. Remove the wire, and cut the PICC line to the appropriate length. Remember to subtract the external hub of the peel-a-way in your measurement.
  - Advance the PICC line through the peel-a-way using the stiffening stylet to the appropriate location
  - Remove the stiffening stylet and peel-a-way sheath
  - Check PICC function by aspirating and flushing the PICC line
  - Secure the PICC to the skin with the supplied catheter lock or nonabsorbable suture and apply a sterile dressing
  - Save a spot fluoroscopic image at the end of the procedure to confirm final positioning
- **Tunneled Central Venous Catheters**
  - Placed for chronic access for patients requiring dialysis, plasmapheresis, TPN, antibiotics
  - The main contraindication is cellulitis at the site of access. Tunneled lines should also be avoided in patients who are septic or bacteremic.
  - The procedure should be performed under conscious sedation. As such, the patient should be NPO for 4–6 h.

- There is no consensus regarding antibiotics prophylaxis
  - May give 1 g cefazolin for prophylaxis
- Access the internal jugular vein, as above. The femoral vein may also be used, but is highly prone to infection.
- After micropuncture dilator placement, choose the exit site for the subcutaneous exit site
- Thoroughly anesthetize the subcutaneous tract using lidocaine
- Make an appropriate skin nick to allow the catheter (ie, larger for dialysis catheters, and smaller for tunneled PICC lines)
- A hemostat can be used to dilate the tract (from both the superior and inferior skin nicks) prior to advancing the tunneler for ease of access
- Attach the catheter to the tunneling device. For ease of placement, a small curve can be placed on the tunneler.
- Advance the tunneler and catheter through the inferior skin nick, and out the venous access site. A gentle curve should be made in the tract. Remove the tunneler from the catheter tip.
- Pull the catheter through the tract enough so that the cuff is 1–2 cm deep to the skin nick on the chest wall
- At this point, attention is again turned to the IJ access. Remove the micropuncture dilator over the wire, and predilate the vein using the supplied dilators.
- After predilation, place the supplied peel-a-way sheath over the wire
  - As with dilators, it is extremely important to watch advancement of the peel-a-way under fluoroscopy. This is especially true for left IJ access, which has a greater number of angles.
- Remove the wire, and advance the catheter tip through the peel-a-way
  - Although most kits now come with a valved peel-a-way to prevent air embolus, ask the patient to maintain positive intrathoracic pressure by humming during catheter insertion
  - Should an air embolus occur, place the patient in the left lateral decubitus position to attempt to contain the air within the right atrium. Try to then aspirate the air from the atrium.
- Position the catheter at the cavoatrial junction. Aspirate and flush the catheter.
- Dwell the lumen with the appropriate volume of heparin
- Secure the catheter to the skin with a nonabsorbable purse-string suture. Place a sterile dressing over the catheter exit site. Remember that the patient's chest will pull down after sitting up, which can pull on the catheter if it is sutured to a mobile area of the chest.
- Many times, the neck entry site does not require a suture, and may simply be closed with Dermabond or steri-strips

- **Implanted Ports**
  - Implanted ports are used for more permanent access, generally for patients requiring chemotherapy or chronic transfusions
    - They are less conspicuous, and have lower rates of infection compared to tunneled catheters
  - The main contraindication is cellulitis at the site of access. Again, if the patient is bacteremic or septic, a port should not be placed.
  - As with tunneled catheters, conscious sedation as well as local anesthesia is usually used
  - There is moderate risk of bleeding, therefore labs should be checked
    - 81 mg aspirin may be continued, but the patient should hold 325 mg aspirin for 5 d
  - Access the internal jugular vein, as above
    - If the jugular veins are occluded, or if the patient prefers, a port may be placed in the patient's nondominant arm
  - After micropuncture dilator placement, choose site for port placement
  - Administer copious lidocaine to numb the area where port will be placed
    - Make sure to anesthetize the incision site, below the incision site where the port will be placed, as well as the route of the tunnel tract
  - Using a #15 blade scalpel, make an incision just wide enough to accommodate the port. The incision should be parallel to the dermatome.
  - Using Metzenbaum scissors and blunt dissection with your fingers, create an appropriate sized pocket for the chosen port
    - If the pocket is too deep, the port will be difficult to access
    - If the pocket is too shallow, the port can erode through the skin
    - If the pocket is too wide, the port can flip over
    - If the pocket is too narrow, excessive tension can lead to wound dehiscence

- Flush the pocket with sterile saline. Some providers will use antibiotics to flush the pocket, but this has not been shown to decrease port infections.
- Attach the catheter to the tunneling device, and tunnel the catheter from the pocket to the neck entry site, with a gentle curve made along the tract
- Attach and secure the catheter to the port reservoir. Place the port securely within the pocket.
- Measure the appropriate catheter length with a wire, and trim the catheter
- At this point, attention is again turned to the IJ access. Remove the micropuncture dilator over the wire, and place the supplied peel-a-way sheath.
  - Always watch peel-a-way placement under fluoroscopy

Figure 6-3 Implanted port placement. The catheter is placed through the chest pocket and into the peel-away. The tip of the catheter lies at the cavoatrial junction.

Cavoatrial junction

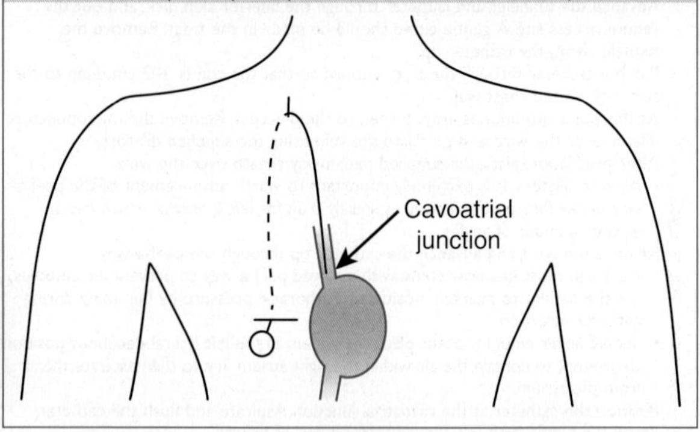

- Remove the wire, and place the catheter tip through the peel-a-way sheath. The catheter tip should be at the cavoatrial junction (Fig. 6-3)
- Prior to closure, assure that the catheter is functional. Access the port with the supplied non-coring Huber needle and verify that the catheter aspirates and flushes easily. Dwell the port and catheter with the specified heparinized solution.
- Close the pocket with a two-layer closure. The deep layer should be closed with 3-0 absorbable sutures, which the superficial layer should be closed with a running subcuticular 4-0 absorbable suture.
- Note that based on operator preference some of these steps may be rearranged. i.e. the catheter tip may be placed through the peel away prior to trimming the catheter, and positioned at the cavoatrial junction. The catheter may then be trimmed at the port side, attached to the port, and then placed within the pocket

Complications during Central Venous Catheter Placement
- Malposition
  - Rare with the use of image guidance
  - Take care when placing catheters in women with large or pendulous breasts, as soft tissue tension may cause dislodgment immediately after placement
  - If the catheter is too long, it can be pulled back. If the catheter is too short, it likely will need to be replaced
  - If a PICC line cannot be aspirated immediately after placement, its tip may be lying against a vessel wall, or the catheter may be kinked. Aspirate while slowly withdrawing the catheter until you aspirate blood freely. If the catheter is kinked, straighten the kink out with a wire.
- Pneumothorax
  - Risk of pneumothorax is low with image guidance; however, post-procedural XR is recommended
  - There is a higher risk with subclavian access as compared to IJ access
  - The size of pneumothorax is typically small, without any symptoms. Follow-up CXR for stability is usually acquired.
  - If the patient is symptomatic, a chest tube may need to be placed

- Vascular or cardiac perforation
  - Although rare, can be fatal. Other symptoms include hemodynamic instability, cardiac tamponade, or hemothorax.
  - This may occur if a dilator or peel-a-way sheath is advanced over a guidewire that is kinked, or if the wire had been inadvertently pulled back prior to placement of the dilator.
  - Always watch placement of dilators or sheaths under fluoroscopy
  - Left IJ lines are more prone to this due to the numerous sharp angles along the course of the central veins from the left IJ
  - The catheter may need to be removed in the OR. If the patient is acutely decompensating, balloon tamponade or a stent graft should be placed.
- Air embolus
  - The risk of air embolus is low, especially as most new sheaths contain a valve
  - This complication is caused by low intrathoracic pressure during instrumentation. Although patients are at higher risk with large sheaths (such as a peel-a-way), it may also occur with small sheaths or dilators.
  - Cap all catheters with a syringe when the catheter is not actively being used
  - When placing a catheter through a peel-a-way, have the patient hum to increase intrathoracic pressure
  - As stated above, place the patient in left lateral decubitus position to contain the air within the right atrium. Administer 100% oxygen, and attempt to aspirate the air.

Complications After Central Venous Catheter Placement
- Infection
  - Infection is the most common complication
  - While cellulitis or pus at the access site are obvious signs of infection, occasionally the patient may only be febrile with an elevated WBC. In these cases, the line is assumed to be the source of infection.
  - The line should be removed, as above, and the tip cultured
  - If a new line is indicated, blood cultures should be negative and the patient should be afebrile for 48 h prior to new line placement
  - In patients with limited options for future access, there are two possible options
    - The line may simply be replaced over a wire, the tip cultured, and the patient put on appropriate antibiotics
    - The line may be left in place, but dwelled with antibiotics. This has a low success rate, and there should be a low threshold to remove the infected catheter.
- Malposition
  - Although the catheter position is confirmed prior to the patient leaving IR, over time, the catheter tip may migrate to an unwanted location
  - Clues that the catheter may be incorrectly positioned include pain during injection/aspiration, or the loss of the ability to aspirate a catheter that can still be flushed
  - In most cases, if the catheter tip has migrated, the catheter will need to be replaced
    - Usually, this is easily performed using an over-the-wire exchange
    - For mediports the indwelling catheter may occasionally be salvaged by obtaining femoral access, snaring the tip of the catheter, and pulling it back to the proper location
- Catheter-related venous thrombosis
  - Patients with pre-existing venous stenosis are at higher risk
  - The patient may develop symptoms similar to SVC syndrome, such as face or arm swelling
  - Generally treated with anticoagulation without removing the catheter, as removing the catheter can dislodge the clot and cause an embolus. Occasionally, however, the catheter may need removed/replaced.
  - If the patient has a pre-existing stenosis that caused the thrombosis, they may need angioplasty or stenting
- Fibrin sheath formation
  - Fibrin sheath is the most common cause of catheter malfunction
  - This is caused by a proteinaceous coat of inflammatory cells that envelop the catheter
  - The catheter may be able to be flushed, but cannot be aspirated
  - Evaluate the catheter positioning with fluoroscopy. Inject contrast, which will typically show pooling at the catheter tip, or retrograde flow of contrast along the catheter along the fibrin sheath.

- First, try to treat with tPA. Administer 2 mg tPA through the catheter, and allow it to dwell. Wait approximately 30 min, then attempt to aspirate the catheter. If function is not regained, a second dwell time of 90 min should be performed.
- If the catheter will not function after tPA infusion, it should be exchanged.
  - Many times, the fibrin sheath will need to be broken up with angioplasty, otherwise the new catheter will be placed in the formed fibrin sheath, and will be nonfunctional as well
  - Advance a guidewire through the sheath, then use a balloon to angioplasty along the length of the fibrin sheath
  - Remove the balloon, and place the new catheter over the wire
  - Inject contrast to assure proper function and to assure that there is no longer a fibrin sheath
- For mediport catheters with fibrin sheaths, occasionally sheath stripping may be needed. A loop snare should be placed via femoral vein access and used to strip the fibrin sheath from the catheter.
- **Device Removal**
- **Tunneled Central Venous Catheter Removal**
  - These catheters can be removed at bedside with local anesthesia
  - After proper cleansing of the skin and catheter, place sterile towels around the catheter and exit site
  - Anesthetize the skin exit site and around the cuff
  - Using blunt dissection with a hemostat and manual traction, free the cuff. Sharp dissection may occasionally be needed, but this must be perform with great care.
- Once the cuff is free the catheter may be removed
- Hold pressure over the venotomy site for hemostasis
  - Raising the head of the bed will assist with hemostasis. Be careful when raising the head, as vessel spasm after catheter removal may lead to lightheadedness.
- Place a sterile dressing over the catheter exit site, which should be allowed to heal by secondary intention
- If removing the catheter due to infection, always send the catheter tip for culture
- Be aware that tunneled catheters may break during removal. This typically occurs at the junction of the catheter and cuff. Should this occur, clamp or compress the catheter within the tunnel using your hand along the catheter tract. Make a small incision proximal to the cuff, and remove the catheter.
- **Port removal**
  - Performed in the angiography suite under sterile conditions
  - Use copious lidocaine over the prior incision site and port pocket
  - Make an incision over the prior incision site
  - Find the hub of the port. Typically, there will be scarring over the port hub, requiring blunt dissection to free the hub.
  - Remove the catheter, hub, and port as a unit
  - If the pocket is not infected, close the pocket as you would
  - If the pocket is infected, clean it with copious irrigation. Pack the pocket with iodoform packing strips, and allow the incision to heal by secondary intention.
  - As always, send the tip for culture if there is concern for infection

Lymphangiograms
- These are generally performed due to extensive chyle leak (usually postsurgical and iatrogenic versus malformation of lymphatics)
- Review MRI or CT imaging
- Consent patient for procedural risks:
  - Infection, bleeding, damage to adjacent structures
  - Lymphedema
  - Very rare possibility of embolization if using glue
- There are two methods of performing lymphangiograms:
  - Pedal lymphangiogram
    - Mix 3 mL lidocaine with 2 mL methylene blue and inject into the tissues between the 1st and 2nd toes
    - Identify the lymphatic duct after it has been filled with dye
    - Make a small vertical incision over the duct and insert a microcatheter into the lymphatic vessel
    - Lipophilic contrast (typically Ethiodol) is inject at a rate of 6 mL/h, not to exceed a total of 20 mL to avoid fat pneumonitis
    - Once the thoracic duct is opacified, it can be cannulated percutaneously in the upper abdomen

- Although this has a high success rate, the procedure requires substantial time for contrast to travel from the foot to the thoracic duct (several hours to up to 24 h)
- Intranodal lymphangiogram
  - Used to bypass the lower-extremity lymphatics and shorten the procedure length
  - Ultrasound is used to locate bilateral groin lymph nodes
  - After anesthetizing, a needle is advanced to the hilum of the lymph nodes
  - Small amount of lipophilic contrast is injected
  - Reposition the needle if contrast extravasates and does not enter the lymphatics
  - Once in position, 3–6 mL of lipophilic contrast is injected bilaterally
  - Saline may help to advance the contrast further within the lymphatics

Normal Hemostasis
- **Virchow's Triad:** Intrinsic coagulability of blood (coagulation cascades), loss of laminar flow (slow or turbid flow), and endothelial response to injury. Endothelial injury results in vasoconstriction and/or spasm.
- **Clot/Thrombus:** Ball of fibrin, platelets, and intrinsic proteins (clotting factors). Clot is stabilized by balance of fibrinolysis and coagulation.

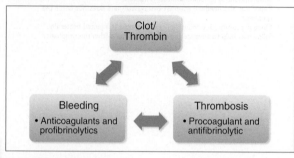

Lab tests (JVIR 2012;23(6):727–36)
- **INR/PT:** Normal 0.9–1.1. Measures the extrinsic pathway. Altered by oral anticoagulants and liver disease.
- **aPTT:** Normal is 25–35 s. Measures the intrinsic pathway. Altered by Heparin, vWB disease, factor VIII, IX, or XI deficiency.
- **Platelet Count:** Normal is 150–450 K/μL. Altered by thrombocytopenia, HIT, thrombocytosis. Transfusion typically recommended for PLT below 50K.
- **Hgb and HCT:** Hgb is the protein, measured in g/dL. HCT is the percent volume of RBC/whole blood.
- **Bleeding Time:** Not used

Consensus Guidelines for Image-Guided Procedures

	Procedure (Vascular)	Procedure (Non-Vasc.)	Lab Testing	MGMT	Meds
Class 1 (Low bleeding risk)	Dialysis int., venography, central line removal, IVC filter, PICC	Drain exchange, thora, para, superficial aspiration/ biopsy, superficial abscess drain	INR: Only pts with liver dz or on warfarin aPTT: Pts on IV heparin PLT: Not recommended HCT: Not recommended.	INR: >2 PTT: N/a HCT: N/a PLT: >50,000	Clopidogrel: Hold for 5 d. Aspirin: Do not hold. LMWH: Hold 1 dose prior.
Class 2 (Moderate bleeding risk)	Angio, venous int., chemoembo, UFE, TJLB, tunneled CVC, Port	Retroperitoneal and chest drain/ bx, lung bx, TALB, Perc chole, G-tube, simple RFA Spine int.	INR: Check aPTT: Pts on IV heparin PLT: Not recommended HCT: Not recommended.	INR: <1.5 PTT: N/a HCT: N/a PLT: >50,000	Clopidogrel: Hold for 5 d. Aspirin: Do not hold. LMWH: Hold 1 dose prior.
Class 3 (Significant bleeding risk)	TIPS	Renal bx, new biliary int, neph tube, complex RFA	INR: Check aPTT: Pts on IV heparin PLT: Check HCT: Check	INR: <1.5 PTT: Reverse hep. HCT: N/a PLT: >50,000	Clopidogrel: Hold for 5 d. Aspirin: Hold for 5 d. LMWH: Hold 24 h prior.

Bleeding disorders (Haemophilia 2017)

- **von Willebrand disease:** Most common bleeding disorder. 1% of population and 1% of those are symptomatic. **Type 1** – decreased amount of vW factor, treat with desmopressin (DDAVP). **Type II and Type III** improper configuration/function of vWF, treat with cryoprecipitate or factor VIII.
- **Hemophilia A:** 1 in 5000 males. Deficiency in factor VIII. 2/3 have severe disease. Prolonged aPTT. Treat with recombinant factor or plasma derived factors. Acute bleeding, treat with Factor VIII 50 μ/kg.
- **Hemophilia B:** 1 in 30,000 males. Deficiency in factor IX. ½ have severe disease. Prolonged aPTT. Acute bleeding, treat with Factor IX 100–120 μ/kg.
- **Acquired Bleeding Disorders:** Liver disease, uremia, cardiac bypass, multiple myeloma/macroglobulinemia, trauma (esp after massive transfusion), antiphospholipid syndrome
- **Platelet Disorders:** Bernard–Soulier, Wiskott–Aldrich, Glanzmann thrombasthenia

Recognizing Hemorrhage (Injury 2014;S35–8)
- **Hemorrhagic Shock:**
  - A severe imbalance between oxygen supply and demand resulting from a lack of red blood cells to carry oxygen to tissues
  - A significant amount of blood (30%) may be lost prior to exhibiting the 1st signs or symptoms due to compensatory mechanisms
  - These compensatory mechanisms are the reason not all hemorrhage results in shock
  - Young patients typically have more "reserve" than elderly patients and may lose a significant amount of blood before symptoms become apparent

ATLS® Shock Classifications

	Class 1	Class 2	Class 3	Class 4
% Blood loss	<15	15–30	30–40	>40
HR (bpm)	<100	>100	120	>140
BP	Normal	Normal	Decreased	Decreased
RR (bpm)	14–20	20–30	30–40	>35
Mental status	Anxious	Anxious	Anxious/conf	Conf/lethargic

- **Compensation:**
  1. Increased cardiac output
  2. Increased extraction of oxygen
  - Anaerobic metabolism, leading to lactic acid formation
  - Lactic acidosis can cause coagulation cascade activation and systemic inflammatory response
  - Check a lactate level!
- **Imaging** (American College of Radiology Appropriateness Criteria www.acr.org):
  - Must be **actively** bleeding to be detected on imaging
  - **CT Imaging:** Often the 1st step after trauma, suspected vascular injury, or GI bleeding in patients who are stable enough to go to the scanner.
    - Helpful for localization and management planning
    - Need 2 phases—usually arterial and venous
    - If you miss the arterial phase, get venous and delayed phases
    - If you can only have 1, choose **venous** (may miss the bleed on arterial phase)
    - If drains are present, rapid filling of drainage tubing with contrast may obscure detection on CT
    - CTA can detect bleeding rates of 0.3–0.5 mL/min
  - **Angiography:** Alternate to CT, especially if intervention is planned and is 1st line in unstable patients with lower GI bleed, pelvic trauma
    - Pseudoaneurysm, blush, abrupt cutoff of vessel, contrast where it shouldn't be, early venous filling which indicates an arteriovenous fistula
    - Can detect bleeding rates of 0.5–1.0 mL/min
  - **Tagged RBC Scan:** Used for lower GI bleed, though time consuming
    - Can detect bleeding rates at 0.1–0.5 mL/min
  - With upper or lower GI bleeding, call GI! 1st step in upper GI bleed is endoscopy and is the 1st step in a stable patient with lower GI bleed

Intraoperative Management of Hemorrhage
- **Massive Transfusion Protocol** (JAMA Surg 2013;127–36):
  - Classically defined as receiving greater than 10 units of RBCs in 24 h
  - Actual protocols vary from center to center

- Typical resuscitation protocols call for 2 L of warmed lactated ringers; then, if BP is not responsive, blood products starting with 2 U PRBCs
- Plasma and platelets are administered in a 1:1 or 1:2 ratio to prevent coagulopathy
- Fibrinogen target is usually >1 g/L
- Cryoprecipitate is given for deficits
- Check blood parameters at least every 30–60 min during massive transfusion
- **Inotropes and Vasopressors** (*JAMA* 2006;509–18):
  - Used sparingly in hemorrhagic shock and used only if all other options are not able to maintain adequate perfusion, with a goal MAP of ≥65
  - Norepinephrine is 1st line, titrated up to 12 units/min
  - Vasopressin added at 0.03 units/min to increase MAP
  - Epinephrine can be added as an additional agent. Titrate up to 10 μg/min
  - Dopamine as an inotrope can be added if cardiac output is insufficient despite adequate MAP. Titrated up to 20 μg/kg/min

Managing Coagulopathy (*JVIR* 2012;23(6):727–36)
- **Whole Blood:**
  - No longer used
  - Separated into transfusable components
- **Packed RBC:**
  - In a hemodynamically stable patient, transfusion is indicated for HGB <6, likely indicated at levels of 6–7, and may be appropriate for levels of 7–8
  - 1 U raises HGB ~1 g/dL and 1–3% HCT
- **FFP:**
  - Contains coagulation proteins
  - Reverses coagulopathy secondary to clotting factor deficiencies
  - 2 U can correct INR in 2.5 range
  - May be given in concert with Vit K
  - FFP has INR of ~1.6 and therefore cannot lower INR below 1.6
- **Cryoprecipitate:**
  - Contains fibrinogen, factor VIII, vWF
  - Indicated for acquired or hereditary deficiencies
  - 10 U increase fibrinogen level by 75 mg/dL
- **Platelets:**
  - Dosed as 6-pack
  - Each unit (6-pack) increases platelets ~50K
- Be prepared to handle refusal of blood components on the basis of religion, eg, Jehovah's Witness, history of transfusion reaction, not willing to take on risks
- Risks: Allergic reaction, Infection (HIV 1 in 2000000, Hep B 1 in 205000, Hep C 1 in 1000000), TRALI, Immune reactions (*NIH* 2012)
- After transfusion wait 15 min before rechecking labs in stable patients

Postoperative Management
- **Bed rest** (*Heart* 2003;447–8):
  - Historically, 6–8 h of bed rest prior to sitting or mobilization has been the standard after arterial puncture
  - Currently, postangiography bed rest recommendations for femoral approach: Sit up at 1 h and mobilize at 2.5 h if using standard compression and a 6F sheath. Take it easy for 1–2 d, no lifting for 5–7 d, no sports for 5–7 d. Shower and remove bandage next day.
  - For radial approach: Early mobilization. Wear a radial compression device for 30–120 min depending on procedure. Little if any local complications. Pressure dressings ease postop care and comfort. No lifting for 24 h, no sports for 1–2 d. Shower and remove bandage next day.
  - Approximately 1 in 14 conversion to groin approach rate secondary to technical challenges
  - Closure devices can lead to early mobilization
- **Hematoma Formation:**
  - One of the most common complications after arterial or venous puncture
  - Manual pressure for 5–10 min often stops any ongoing oozing or bleeding
  - With continued expansion, get ultrasound probe to localize the bleeding to ensure focused pressure and continue holding pressure
  - Hematomas can be very painful; ensure adequate analgesia!
  - Mark the margins of the hematoma with a skin marker to track evolution
  - With continued expansion or inability to stop bleeding, check vitals, get IV fluids, and consider contrast CT with call to vascular surgery

- Last ditch effort and temporizing measure is angioplasty balloon tamponade via alternate access site

Local Hemostasis (Puncture Site) (*JVIR* 2012;73–84)
- **Manual Compression:**
  - Most common and is **Gold Standard**
  - Manual pressure over artery puncture site
  - Start with occlusive pressure, then gradually reduce over 15–20 min
  - If continued bleeding, keep pressure and repeat the process
- **Vascular Closure Devices (VCD):**
  - Can significantly decrease time to hemostasis by up to 17 min
  - Consider reprepping and draping/regloving to minimize complications and infections
  - No data to support prophylactic antibiotic use prior to closure device deployment
  - Types include:

	Name	Function and Specs
Passive/ Compression	Axera	*Low angle vascular access channel. 5–6F. Create low angle access to self-seal. Requires manual compression.*
	Catalyst III	*Nitinol disc 5–7F. Nitinol disc provides hemostasis to allow arteriotomy recoil to 18g wire.*
		Rigid plastic frame with stiff balloon inflated over arteriotomy for approx. 15 mins.
Arterotomy Closure	Femstop	*Collagen Plug. 6, 8F. Intraluminal anchor attaches to extraminal plug with suture. Resorbed in 60–90 d.*
	Angio-Seal	*Polyethylene glycol Plug. 5–7F. Extravascular plug while intraluminal balloon tamponades. Resorbed in 30 d.*
	MynxGrip	
	Exoseal	*Polyglycolic acid plug. 5–7F. Extravascular plug. Resorbed in 60–90 d. Suture device. 5–21F. Delivers pre-tied suture to physically close the arteriotomy. No resorption.*
	Perclose	
	Proglide	
	Starclose	*Nitinol Clip. 5–6F. Permanent clip outside vessel.*
	Vascade	*Collagen plug. 5–7F. Intraluminal anchor and extraluminal collagen plug. 60–90 d.*
External Hemostasis	Syvek Patch, Clo-Sur, Chito-Seal, D-Stat Dry	*Topical procoagulant pads, used with manual compression.*

- Closure device failure reported at 4%, usually secondary to calcific atherosclerosis
- **Complications:**
  - Reported incidence of 2–6% and include, arterial thrombosis, hematoma, AV fistula, and pseudoaneurysm
  - Increased risk in patients older than 65, females, peripheral atherosclerosis, diabetes, hypertension, and patients receiving anticoagulation
- **Contraindications**:
  - Malpositioned arteriotomies such as proximal to inferior epigastric arteries, superficial/profunda femoral arteries, multiple arteriotomies
  - Some devices are contraindicated if the patient has had an ipsilateral arteriotomy in the previous 30 d
  - Be sure to familiarize yourself with the specific device and contraindications prior to use
  - No data for or against VCD use through vascular stents or grafts
  - **Local Hemostasis After Venotomy/Central Venous Catheter Removal**
  - Preremoval labs are not warranted
  - Ask patient to Valsava or hold their breath and remove in steady, swift motion
  - May require multiple attempts
  - Check catheter tip to ensure no fracture!
  - Manual compression for 5 min is often sufficient
  - If still bleeding, hold for 5 min longer

DRAINAGES

Background
- Percutaneous image-guided drainage is defined as the use of image guidance for catheter placement in order to provide continuous drainage of a fluid collection. Placement is via a transorificial or transcutaneous route.
- One of the most commonly performed interventional radiology procedures
- It is the mainstay treatment for a wide range of abdominal and pelvic fluid collections

Indications
- Suspicion that the collection is causing patients symptoms (eg, septic patient)
- Suspicion that collection arises from abnormal fistulous pathway
- To characterize fluid (eg, to determine if collection is sterile or infected)

Contraindications
- Absolute
  - No safe pathway
- Relative
  - Coagulopathy
  - Hemodynamic instability
  - Poor patient cooperativity
- Complex situation
  - Tumor abscess: Often will not completely resolve and catheter will often need to stay in place for the rest of patients lifetime
    - *Tips and Tricks:* Very rarely will drain a tumor abscess

Image Guidance Options
- Ultrasound
  - Real-time imaging: This allows imager the ability to monitor needles and catheters while they are being placed
  - No ionizing radiation
- Fluoroscopy
  - Usually used in combination with either ultrasound or CT
- Computerized tomography
  - Improved spatial resolution
  - Most accurate assessment of structures around catheter placement route (eg, allows visualization of loops of bowel)

Catheter Routes for Pelvic Collections
- Transversal of organs

Safe to transverse as a transcavity route	Vagina, rectum
Safe to transverse in needle aspiration and catheter placement	Liver, kidney, stomach
Safe to transverse for needle aspiration; Unsafe to transverse for catheter placement	Small bowel, bladder
Avoid in needle aspiration and catheter placement	Large bowel, spleen, ovaries, uterus, pancreas, large vascular structures

- Alternative routes to transabdominal percutaneous approach
  - Transgluteal:
    - CT guidance is used
    - Care should be made to avoid sciatic nerve. Needle placement should be placed at the level of the sacrospinous ligament as ***medial*** as possible near the sacrum.
    - Route should be inferior to the piriformis muscle, because traversing the piriformis muscle has been associated with higher rate of postprocedural pain
  - Transvaginal:
    - Should be considered in deep pelvic abscess located adjacent to the vagina
    - Major issue is patient discomfort during and after procedure
  - Transrectal:
    - Usually ultrasound guidance used
    - Especially helpful for prostate abscess in males and presacral abscess in females that are difficult to access
    - Major issue is that it is difficult to maintain/fix catheter in place

Techniques

Trocar Technique
- One-stick procedure
- Guiding wire and catheter placed in tandem
- Major advantage: Speed as it is quick to deploy
- Disadvantage: Difficult to redirect if the first pass is not optimally positioned

Seldinger Technique
- First a hollow needle is placed for access. Subsequently, a guiding wire is placed and used for serial dilation and placement of the catheter.
- Allows for more precise placement of the catheter
- Disadvantage: Increased risk of guidewire kinking which can result in loss of access

Catheter Size
- 12F–14F catheters are preferred for larger collections
- Can use smaller diameter catheter (as low as 7F) for smaller collections

Considerations for Hepatic or Renal Abscess Drainage
- Most small abscess (<3 cm) can effectively be managed by medical therapy alone
- Drainage should be considered for larger collections or those who fail medical management
- In the case of abscess rupture, surgical drainage is required

Treatment Considerations for Ascites
- Paracentesis: Procedure in which a needle is placed within the peritoneal cavity in order to remove fluid either for diagnostic or therapeutic purposes
  - While the procedure can be preformed without image guidance, ultrasound guidance improves the safety. Use imaging to find the largest pocket and avoid large vascular structures such as the **inferior epigastric artery.**
    - *Tips and Tricks:* Always try and stay lateral to inferior epigastric artery
  - Complications include: Leakage at paracentesis site, bleeding, damage to adjacent organs such as bowel
- Tunneled Peritoneal catheter: Allows drainage directed by patient or caregiver at home. Palliative option for patients with recurrent ascites.
  - Inability of patient or caregiver to care for catheter
  - Relative contraindications: Inability of patient of caregiver to care for catheter, loculated collections, **active infections.**
  - Technique: Following access of the peritoneal cavity, a subcutaneous tract is made with exit medial and cranial to the access site. Following serial dilation, 15.5F peritoneal catheter is placed and access site is closed.
  - Major complications include bleeding, infection, development of loculated collections, and catheter malfunction
- Peritoneovenous shunt (*Denver Shunt*): Single direction iatrogenic connection is made from the peritoneal space to the venous circulation in order for continuous paracentesis. A subcutaneous tract is made between the catheter's venous and peritoneal components.
  - Used in treatment of malignant, chylous, and cirrhotic ascites
  - Role in the treatment of refractory ascites (ascites not controlled by dietary modifications or medical therapy): Consider a third-line therapy following large volume paracentesis and portosystemic shunts/TIPS. Limited applications due to the high complication rate (including increased risk of bacterial peritonitis).

Postprocedure Care of Drainage Catheters
- Occlusion prophylaxis: Catheter should be flushed with 10 cc of normal saline three times a day. Flush **toward** the collection.
- When to reimage the collection:
  - Less output than expected or sudden decrease in output, (<10 cc over a 24-h period)
  - Failure of symptom resolution
  - If there is higher output than expected, consider the presence of a fistula. Fistulagram can be obtained for confirmation. If fistula is present, leave catheter for 4–6 w and then reassess.
- Tissue plasminogen activator (tPA):
  - Can be instilled when the collection remains on reimaging and there is poor output in order to facilitate better drainage.
- Catheter Removal: When drainage is less than 10–20 mL/d and there is improvement of patient's clinical symptoms

1. Wallace MJ, Chin KW, Fletcher TB, et al. Quality improvement guidelines for percutaneous drainage/aspiration of abscess and fluid collections. *J Vasc Interv Radiol* 2010;21:431–35.
2. Maher, MM, Gervais DA, Kalra MK, et al. The inaccessible or undrainable abscess: How to drain it. *Radiographics* 2004;24:717–35.
3. Gervais DA, Brown SD, Connolly SA, et al. Percutaneous imaging-guided abdominal and pelvic abscess drainage in children. *Radiographics* 2004;24:737–54.
4. Mavilia MG, Molina M, Wu GY. The evolving nature of hepatic abscess: A review. *J Clin Transl Hepatol* 2016;4:158–68.
5. Kandarpa K, Machan L, & Durham JD. *Handbook of interventional radiologic procedures.* 2016.
6. Martin, LG. Percutaneous placement and management of the Denver shunt for portal hypertensive ascites. *Am J Roentgenol* 2012;199(4):W449–53.

BIOPSIES

Thyroid Biopsies

Background

- Up to 4–7% of US have palpable thyroid nodule
  - Thyroid cancer accounts for 1% of all cancers and 0.5% of all cancer deaths (*N Eng J Med* 2004;351:1764–71)
- Overall thyroid cancer incidence of 7.98 per 100000, with an incidence-based mortality of 0.44 per 100000 person-years
- Women (75%) and white patients (82%) comprise the majority of the cases (*JAMA* 2017;317(13):1338–48)

Indications

- FNA can be considered for nodules >1 cm if there are suspicious features; suspicious features are more important for identifying malignancy than size
- See TI-RADS chart at end of section for further details regarding scoring system
- US features associated with malignancy: Solid component, hypoechogenicity, microlobulated or irregular margins, microcalcifications, and taller-than-wide shape. Two or more features is an indication for tissue sampling (TIRADS 4b and higher) (*Radiology* 2011;260(3):892–9)
- Malignancy risk in nodules with one malignant feature or less can be followed by Ultrasound (TIRADS 3 or 4a) is 0.8% and can be followed (*Radiology* 2015;274(1):287–5)

Procedure

- Informed consent outlying risk of hematoma and infection
- Coagulation panel is not routinely needed but anticoagulation therapy should be stopped 5–7 d before the procedure
- Patient is placed supine with neck extended. The most suspicious nodule is identified by ultrasound using grayscale and color Doppler and the overlying skin is cleaned with iodine or chlorhexidine-based solution
- High-resolution linear probe (7.5–15 MHz) is used with a sterile cover
- Local 1% lidocaine can be used in skin/subcutaneous tissue
- FNA (*RadioGraphics* 2008;28:169–89)
  - 22G–27G needles with or without an attached syringe is advanced into the nodule under ultrasound
  - The needle is moved back and forth and side to side within the nodule with or without applying suction on the syringe. At least two aspirations should be taken.
  - Collected aspirate is smeared on glass slides and fixed in 95% EtOH if using Pap smear or air-dried if Diff-Quick or Giemsa stain is used. Consult with local pathology department about preference.
- Core needle Biopsy CNB (*Radiology* 2003;226:827–32):
  - 16G–18G spring-loaded core biopsy needle is advanced to optimal position taking into account the throw-length of the needle with notch of side-cut needles within the lesion. At least two cores is optimal.
  - Specimens are placed in 10% buffered formalin

Results

- 10–20% of fine-needle aspirations yield nondiagnostic results *(Eur Radiol 2017;27:431–36; Radiology 2015;274(1):287–5)*
- Rapid onsite evaluation by pathology was shown in a recent meta-analysis to increase average adequacy rate from 83–92% *(Am J Clin Pathol 2013;139:300–08)*
- 81–84% of nodules with nondiagnostic results that underwent repeat Fine Needle Aspiration or surgery were finally proved to be benign *(Radiology 2015;274(1):287–5)*
- Core needle biopsies are almost 4× more effective in cases of repeat biopsy after nondiagnostic FNA *(Eur Radiol 2017;27:431–36)*

Complications
Complications include parathyroid hematomas which are usually self-limited

Post Procedure Care
Cover with sterile bandage

ACR Thyroid Imaging Reporting and Data System (ACR TI-RADS)

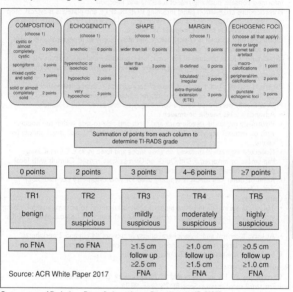

Source: ACR White Paper 2017

ADDITIONAL RESOURCE

1. Tessler FN, Middleton WD, Grant EG, et al. ACR Thyroid Imaging, Reporting and Data System (TI-RADS): White Paper of the ACR TI-RADS Committee. *J Am Coll Radiol* 2017;14:587–95.

RENAL BIOPSIES

Focal Renal Biopsy

Background
- Small renal masses (≤4 cm) make up to 66% of new kidney cancers *(BJUI 2011;10(9): 867–72)*
- Small renal masses benign in 20–30%, role of surveillance and ablation expanding *(Urology 2012;79:372–78)*

- Need for better patient selection for surgery in large or metastatic renal masses
  (Urol Oncol 2017;35:87–91)

INDICATIONS (BJUI 2011;10(9):867–72; Urology 2012;79:372–78; Urol Oncol 2017;35:87–91)
- For small masses:
  - Rule out malignancy in atypical renal masses, differentiate from infection, suspected lymphoma, grading tumor, diagnosis before ablation and recurrence after ablation, and aid in management of small renal masses
- For large masses (>4 cm):
  - Traditionally for renal mass and extrarenal tumor, suspected lymphoma or infection
  - Newer indications include: Pathologic diagnosis for pts not treated surgically, improve informed consent and patient selection for cytoreductive nephrectomy, and improve patient selection for node dissection

Procedure
- Informed consent outlining risk of bleeding and infection
- Preprocedure coagulation panel including PT/INR, aPTT, and platelets is typical. Stop anticoagulation: Aspirin 5–7 d before, Warfarin 5 d before, LMWH 1 dose, Heparin 4 h before. NSAIDs may be stopped 3 d before.
- Blood pressure control is critical before and after biopsy as hypertension is a risk factor for bleeding after native kidney biopsy (140/90 suggested)
- Ultrasound is ideal because of low cost, high availability, and high success rate in skilled hands. CT may be also used if there is overlying gas or poor sonographic visibility from body habitus.
- Patient is usually placed prone, subcostal approach to reduce pneumothorax
- Local 1% lidocaine can be used in skin/subcutaneous tissue
- FNA is usually performed before core biopsy to decrease blood in sample
  - Advance a 21G needle or smaller
  - Vigorously move the needle back and forth and side to side within the nodule with or without applying suction on the syringe. At least 2 aspirations should be taken.
  - Collected aspirate is smeared on glass slides and fixed in 95% EtOH if using Pap smear or air-dried if Diff-Quick or Giemsa stain is used. Consult with local pathology department about preference.
  - RPMI or other cell media is typically used for flow cytometry per Pathology department
- Core Biopsy
  - 16G–18G spring-loaded core biopsy needle is advanced to optimal position taking into account the throw-length of the needle with notch of side-cut needles within the lesion
  - At least 1 central and 1 peripheral biopsy in tumors ≤4 cm and 2 peripheral biopsies in larger tumors. No need to cross normal parenchyma.
  - Specimens are placed in 10% buffered formalin

Results (Eur Urol 2016;69:660–73)
- Core biopsy 99.1% sensitivity and 99.7% specificity for malignancy overall
  – For small renal masses: Sens. 99.7% Spec. 98.2%
  – For cystic renal masses: Sens 83.6% Spec. 98%
- FNA: Sensitivity 93.2% Specificity 89.8%
- Tumor Grade for core biopsy: Mean concordance with surgery 62.5%. In simplified evaluation of high vs. low grade, concordance is 86.5%

Complications (Eur Urol 2016;69:660–73)

Perinephric Hematomas 4.3%, 0.7% Requiring Trusion
- Self-limiting hematuria 3.15%
- Lumbar pain 3%
- Rare (<1%) complications: Pneumothorax, admission for urinary clot retention, pseudoaneurysm formation, tract seeding

---

NONFOCAL RENAL BIOPSY

Background
Imaging evaluation of renal failure in native kidneys and rejection or failure in transplant kidneys is currently nonspecific and most cases need histopathologic evaluation to make a diagnosis. Final diagnosis differs from the main hypothesis in up to one third of cases (World J Nephrol 2014;3(4):287–94)

Indications

Bleeding

- Native Kidneys: Further evaluation of proteinuria, microscopic hematuria, renal manifestations of systemic disease, and unexplained renal failure
- Transplant Kidneys: Evaluate for rejection in the setting of elevated Creatinine, decreased urine output, fever, hypertension, edema, or proteinuria *(Semin Intervent Radiol 2004;21(4):275–81)*
- Transjugular biopsy can be considered in chronic renal failure patients with bleeding diathesis, solitary kidney, high BMI, or uncooperative patients *(Cardiovasc Intervent Radiol 2008;31:906–18)*

Contraindications

- Absolute (Percutaneous biopsy): Bleeding diathesis, uncontrolled severe hypertension, an uncooperative patient, and a solitary native kidney
- Relative: Severe azotemia, anatomic abnormalities of the kidney which may increase risk (ie, arterial aneurysm, skin infection over the biopsy site), drugs which alter hemostasis, pregnancy, and urinary tract infection

Procedure (Percutaneous)

- Preprocedural workup is the same as for focal renal biopsy except a linear transducer can often be used in transplant kidneys as they are closer to the surface
- Core biopsy
  - Local 1% lidocaine can be used in skin/subcutaneous tissue
  - 16G–18G spring-loaded core biopsy needle is advanced to optimal position taking into account the throw-length of the needle with notch of side-cut needles within the lesion
  - On-site pathology or nephrology is usually required to ensure samples have at least 15 or more intact glomeruli
  - Specimens are placed in 10% buffered formalin

Procedure (Transjugular) *(Cardiovasc Intervent Radiol 2008;31:906–18)*

- Preprocedural workup is similar to the percutaneous workup but stopping anticoagulation may be contraindicated
- Often done under conscious sedation and a history and physical including ASA assessment should be performed
- Local 1% lidocaine can be used in skin/subcutaneous tissue
- Supine position and right IJV access preferred.
- IJV access can be obtained with a micropuncture set under ultrasound or an 18G needle with eventual insertion of a 7F sheath
- 5F Cobra catheter is introduced and engaged with the main renal vein (right preferred for favorable angle and shorter course from IVC)
- Guidewire advanced as distal as possible into subcortical vein followed by the catheter and then the 7F sheath after which guidewire and catheter are removed
- Venogram performed to assess venous anatomy via sheath and to ensure peripheral wedging (cortical enhancement distal to sheath) which will increased change of true cortical sampling
- 60 cm 19G Quick-core biopsy needle with beveled end and 2 cm notch inserted into a 70 cm 5F straight catheter which is shortened by 15 cm to accommodate length of biopsy needle. This system is advanced until it reaches the tip of the 7F sheath.
- Sheath and catheter withdrawn to expose needle tip and samples taken with spring-loaded gun
- On-site pathology or nephrology is usually required to ensure samples have at least 15 or more intact glomeruli
- Specimens are placed in 10% buffered formalin
  - Catheter injected with small volume contrast to exclude capsular perforation
    - Embolization can be performed for significant extravasation accompanied by hemodynamic compromise
  - 24-h observation with monitoring of vitals every 15 min for 2 h then 30 min for 4 h, then hourly

Results

In one study *(J Comput Assist Tomogr 2013;37:176–82)*, three passes were adequate for histological diagnosis in 84% of all kidney biopsies, with 4 passes adequate in 94% with statistically significantly lower number of passes for transplant (2.78) vs. native (3.1) kidneys. Transplant kidneys had a significantly higher number of glomeruli per pass (7.2 vs. 6.1) Transjugular biopsies were diagnostic in 95% of patients in one study *(Cardiovasc Intervent Radiol 2008;31:906–18)* with mean glomeruli 10.3 on light microscopy and 2.6 on electron microscopy.

Complications (Am J Kidney Dis 2012;60(1):62–73)

Percutaneous
- Perinephric hematoma 11.6% biopsies (5% when only evaluated for when symptomatic)
  - Require angiographic intervention 0.6% of biopsies
  - Urinary tract obstruction 0.3% of biopsies
- Macroscopic hematuria 3.5%
  - Require transfusion in 0.9% of cases.
- Major bleeding requiring surgery or AV Fistula 0.1–0.5%
- Death <0.1%
- Risk factors for transfusion requirement include lower gauge needle (14 vs. 16/18), Cr ≥2 mg/dL, AKI

Transjugular (Cardiovasc Intervent Radiol 2008;31:906–18)
- Complications more common because of indications for transjugular approach
- Major Complications: 7/59 patients (12.5%), 5 needing transfusion, 2 needing invasive intervention
- Minor Complications: 6/59 (10.2%) including hematuria, pain
- Capsular Perforation seen in 59% of successful biopsies. 24/34 of capsular perforation patients had no clinical sequelae.

LIVER BIOPSIES

Focal Hepatic biopsy

Background
- Primary liver malignancies account for approximately 7% of all cancers and 90% of those are HCC (World J Hepatol 2015;7(9):1157–167)
- Overall year survival rate of Liver cancer is 18%; 31% if local at diagnosis, 11% if regional metastasis, and 3% if distant metastasis (Cancer Facts & Figures 2017. Atlanta, Ga: American Cancer Society; 2017)
- Overall, MRI is more sensitive (76–82%) than CT (60–66%) but both have equivocal specificity (85–91% and 81–92%) for diagnosis of HCC. Lesions <1 cm have lower MRI sensitivity (69%) and specificity (46%) (Radiology 2015;275:97–109). Lesions >1 cm can usually be diagnosed by imaging alone.

Indications (Radiol Clin N Am 2015;53:1049–59)
- Troubleshooting lesions in cirrhotic patients which do not fulfill imaging criteria for HCC or if there is history of malignancy which could alter the treatment algorithm if metastatic. If lesion meets imaging criteria for HCC, no biopsy is indicated.
- Strongly recommended for transplant workup for small nodules to determine malignancy; if benign, transplant may be obviated (J Clin Exp Hepatol 2014;4(Suppl 3):S67–73)

Contraindications
- Absolute: Bleeding diathesis, not a candidate for any treatment
- Relative: Decompensated cirrhosis, Ascites

Procedure (Radiol Clin N Am 2015;53:1049–59; J Vasc Interv Radiol 2010;21:1539–47)
- Informed consent outlining risk of bleeding and infection
- Preprocedure coagulation panel: INR <1.5, PT <15 s, aPTT <40 s, Plts >50K
- Stop anticoagulation: Aspirin/Antiplatelet Tx 5–7 d before, Warfarin 5–7 d before, LMWH 1 dose, Heparin 4 h before. NSAIDs may be stopped 3 d before.
- Ultrasound is ideal because of low cost, high availability, and high success rate in skilled hands. CT may be also used if not sonographically visible.
- Patient is usually placed supine or left lateral decubitus depending on lesion location. Masses close to the dome or anterior may need careful patient coaching of deep breathing.
- Local 1% lidocaine can be used in skin/subcutaneous tissue
- Coaxial technique is generally preferred
- US-guidance: Grayscale is used to localize the lesion and Color Doppler is used to avoid major vessels including the epigastric arteries
- CT-guidance: Noncontrast CT performed for localization. Contrast can be used if the lesion is not visualized on noncontrast scan. Needle is advanced to the optimal location with periodic limited CT scans to confirm proper trajectory and needle position.
- 15G or 17G introducer needle is advanced to the optimal position with inner stylet present ideally with a needle trajectory which passes through about 3–4 cm normal parenchyma before the lesion.

- FNA is usually performed before core biopsy to decrease blood in sample
  - Advance a 21G needle or smaller through the introducer needle
  - Vigorously move the needle back and forth and side to side within the nodule with or without applying suction on the syringe. 3–5 aspirations should be taken.
  - Collected aspirate is smeared on glass slides and fixed in 95% EtOH if using Pap smear or air-dried if Diff-Quick or Giemsa stain is used. Consult with local pathology department about preference.
  - RPMI or other cell media is typically used for flow cytometry per Pathology department
- Core Biopsy
  - 16G–18G spring-loaded core biopsy needle is advanced through the introducer needle
  - At least 3 core biopsies are obtained
  - Specimens are placed in 10% buffered formalin or 0.9% Saline

Results *(J Vasc Interv Radiol 2010;21:1539–47)*
- Diagnostic yields for core needle biopsy and FNA range from 83–100%
- Overall success rate for FNA is 72.5% and 93.3% for core needle biopsy, 95.5% when combined. Combined FNA/Core negative predictive value 98.8%
- No significant difference between CT or US guidance
- Success rate in cirrhotics less (93.7%) if lesion >1.5 cm

Complications

Perinephric Hematomas 4.3%, 0.7% Requiring Trusion
- Hemorrhage requiring transfusion ranges from 0–3.4% *(Radiol Clin N Am 2015;53:1049–59)*
- Seeding is more common with liver biopsies than other types of biopsies with an incidence of 2.7% in HCC *(Radiol Clin N Am 2015;53:1049–59)* and up to 17% in colorectal metastasis *(Br J Surg 2005;92:1165–68)*

NONFOCAL HEPATIC BIOPSY

Background
Cirrhosis and chronic liver disease represent the 12th leading cause of death overall and fifth leading cause of death for patients 45–54 in 2009. Cirrhosis prevalence in the United States is 0.27% with Hepatitis C, alcohol, and diabetes (nonalcoholic steatohepatitis) accounting for 53.5% of cases *(J Clin Gastroenterol 2015;49:690–96)*.

Noninvasive tests based on serology or imaging for the detection of cirrhosis are becoming more accurate; highest noninvasive accuracy for fibrosis found in shear wave elastography, with sensitivity 76–90% and specificity 81–92% *(J Gastrointestin Liver Dis 2016;25(4):525–32)*. Tissue diagnosis, however, remains the gold standard for many forms of liver and biliary disease as well as fibrosis staging.

Indications
- Common indications for nonfocal liver biopsy include diagnosis of cirrhosis, hepatitis, nonalcoholic fatty liver disease, primary biliary cirrhosis, autoimmune hepatitis and post-transplant for diagnosis of rejection
- Less common indications include direction of treatment for hemochromatosis, primary biliary cirrhosis, and Wilson's disease
- Transjugular biopsy may be more appropriate for patients with severe coagulation disorder or ascites

Contraindications
- Absolute: Bleeding diathesis
- Relative: Decompensated cirrhosis, Ascites. For transjugular biopsy thrombosis of the right IJ vein, thrombosis of hepatic veins, cholangitis, or lack of patient cooperation.

Procedure (Percutaneous)
- Preprocedural workup is the same as for focal liver biopsy
- Core Biopsy
  - Local 1% lidocaine can be used in skin/subcutaneous tissue using a 22G needle. A longer 22G needle is advanced to the edge of the liver capsule and lidocaine is injected forming a small pocket over the surface of the capsule
  - 16G–18G spring-loaded core biopsy needle is advanced to optimal position taking into account the throw-length of the needle, avoiding large vascular structures. Coaxial technique can be used. Left lobe is often most accessible via a subxiphoid

- approach, right lobe subcostal, or low intercostal (along the top of the rib) to avoid pleural transgression
- Ideal sample length is >3 cm which is often smaller in cirrhotic patients (*Hepatology* 2009;49(3):1017–44). Specimens are placed in 10% buffered formalin
- Patients are observed for 2 h and then can be discharged if there are no complications

Procedure (Transjugular) (*Diagn Interv Imaging* 2014;95:11–5)
- Preprocedural workup is similar to the percutaneous workup but stopping anticoagulation may be contraindicated
- Often done under conscious sedation and a history and physical including ASA assessment should be performed
- Local 1% lidocaine can be used in skin/subcutaneous tissue
- Supine position and right IJV access preferred
- IJV access can be obtained with a micropuncture set under ultrasound or an 18G needle with eventual insertion of a 9F sheath
- 5F end-hole catheter is introduced under fluoroscopy with a 0.035" J-tipped flexible hydrophilic wire and advanced into the right hepatic vein, position confirmed by 10 mL contrast injection under fluoroscopy. Right hepatic vein is preferred to control distance to capsule.
- Stiff 0.035" guidewire advanced through 5F catheter and catheter is exchanged for a 7F curved-end long sheath. Deep inspiration and hold is helpful for this step.
- FlexCore or Quick-Core semi-automatic needle systems are commonly used and advanced to the end of the catheter. These systems advance by at least 24 mm and care should be taken to avoid the capsule especially with ascites. US or CT confirmation may be helpful.
- Two to three samples are taken. Each sample should be 10 mm long.
- Samples fixed in 10% formalin
- Injection of contrast under fluoro is performed to check for capsular transgression
- Hepatic venous pressure gradient is usually taken as it is an important prognostic factor in patients with portal hypertension
- Patient should remain recumbent and monitored for 4 h

Results
Insufficient samples are obtained in about 2.04% of cases for percutaneous liver biopsy (*Radiology* 2012;265:819–31)

Diagnostic samples were obtained in 96.1% of transjugular biopsies, technical failure in 3.2% usually from failure to catheterize the hepatic vein (*Diagn Interv Imaging* 2014;95:11–15).

Complications
Percutaneous (*Hepatology* 2009;49(3):1017–44)
- Pain 84% (usually mild)
- Bleeding 18–20% of patients have bleeding on US with only 0.75% needing transfusion or intervention
- Death 1 in 10000 biopsies
- Other less common complications include pneumothorax, perforation of adjacent organs, bile peritonitis, infection, hemobilia

Transjugular (*J Hepatol* 2007;47:284–94)
- Minor complication in 7% of cases including abdominal pain (1.6%), Subclinical capsular perforation (1.4%), pyrexia (1%), and neck hematoma (0.8%)
- Major complications in 0.6% of cases including intraperitoneal hemorrhage (0.2%), hematoma (0.05%), arrhythmia (0.05%), and pneumothorax (0.05%). Death in 0.1% of cases, most commonly from intraperitoneal hemorrhage (0.06%).

LUNG BIOPSIES

Background (*Radiol Clin N Am* 2017;55:1163–81)
- Lung cancer is the second most common malignancy in men and women with about 222500 new cases expected in 2017 and is responsible for more deaths than any other cancer
- Lung cancer is curable in early stages without spread. 5-y survival rate for regional spread is 28% and 4% for distant spread making early diagnosis crucial

Indications (*Insights Imaging* 2017;8:419–28; *Radiology* 2017;284:228–43)
- New or enlarging pulmonary nodule >8 mm
  - Use of PET-CT can decrease the need for biopsy although false positives are possible with inflammation (TB, histoplasmosis, rheumatoid nodules), and false negatives are possible with low-grade adenocarcinoma and carcinoid tumor

- Diagnosis of hilar mass after negative bronchoscopy
- Undiagnosed mediastinal mass
- Biopsy or re-biopsy of known malignancy for targeted therapy

Contraindications *(Insights Imaging 2017;8:419–28)*
- Absolute contraindications: Bleeding diathesis, inability of the patient to cooperate, suspected AVM or hydatid cyst
- Relative contraindications: Severe chronic obstructive pulmonary disease, pulmonary artery hypertension, cardiac insufficiencies, poor respiratory reserve, lesion adjacent to large vessel

Procedure *(Insights Imaging 2017;8:419–28; 4)*
- Informed consent outlining risk of bleeding and infection, pneumothorax
- Preprocedure coagulation panel: INR <1.5, PT <15 s, aPTT <40 s, Plts >50K
- Stop anticoagulation: Aspirin/Antiplatelet Tx 5–7 d before, Warfarin 5–7 d before, LMWH 1 dose, Heparin 4 h before. NSAIDs may be stopped 3 d before.
- Ultrasound is ideal for superficial pleural-based or mediastinal lesions but CT is the mainstay for the majority of cases
- US-guidance: Grayscale is used to localize the lesion and Color Doppler is used to avoid major vessels including the epigastric arteries. Hydrodissection can be used to displace adjacent lung and increase the biopsy window
- CT-fluoroscopy allows reduction of needle passes and procedure time but increases the radiation dose
- CT is performed with or without contrast for planning. Ideal pathway is the shortest without traversing pleural fissures and avoiding bone, bullae, or large vessels including internal mammary vessels. A metallic grid can be used to localize the site of entry in slice of interest by measuring the distance needed on the scanner and marking the area on the patient.
- Patient is positioned so the previously planned access is superior. A metallic grid can be used to localize the site of entry in slice of interest by measuring the transverse distance from the desired site on the scanner and marking the area on the patient.
- Local 1% lidocaine can be used in skin/subcutaneous tissue and the small needle can be left in place for another scan to estimate the angle of trajectory.
- Coaxial technique is generally preferred to decrease number of passes through the pleura
- 17G or larger introducer needle is advanced to the optimal position with inner stylet to the optimal location with periodic limited CT scans to confirm proper trajectory and needle position.
- FNA is usually performed before core biopsy to decrease blood in sample
  - Advance a 21G needle or smaller attached to a syringe through the introducer needle
  - Vigorously move the needle back and forth and side to side within the nodule with or without applying suction on the syringe. 3–5 aspirations should be taken.
  - Collected aspirate is smeared on glass slides and fixed in 95% EtOH if using Pap smear or air-dried if Diff-Quick or Giemsa stain is used. Consult with local pathology department about preference.
  - RPMI or other cell media is typically used for flow cytometry per Pathology department. A sterile container can be used for culture.
- Core Biopsy
  - 18G or larger spring-loaded core biopsy needle is advanced through the introducer needle
  - At least 3 core biopsies are obtained
  - Specimens are placed in 10% buffered formalin or 0.9% Saline
- Rapid on-site evaluation (ROSE) by pathology at the time of biopsy is ideal and can essentially guarantee specimen adequacy

Post Biopsy Care *(Handbook of Interventional Radiologic Procedures. 5th ed. Philadelphia, PA: Wolters Kluwer; 2016)*
- Patient is placed biopsy-side down
- Blood Patch can be performed to reduce the risk of pneumothoraces, need for chest tube, and hospital admission *(J VascIntervRadiol 2017;28:608–13)*. A small amount of the patient's blood is injected into the peripheral 2 cm of the needle tract through the 17G coaxial needle. Bullae will reduce efficacy of blood patch. Alternatively, gelfoam slurry may be used to embolize the tract *(Cardiovasc Intervent Radiol 2014;37: 1546–53)*.
- Immediate post-biopsy CT or CXR is obtained. If there is no pneumothorax and the patient is asymptomatic, patient is observed for 2 h with puncture side down. At 2 h,

a CXR is performed and if negative the patient can be discharged with instructions to return if symptomatic.
- A pneumothorax must be treated if the patient has dyspnea or chest pain, the pneumothorax is greater than 30% of lung volume, or if the pneumothorax continues to increase in size. An immediate pneumothorax can be aspirated with an 18G angiocath on a 3-way stopcock and observed for 2 h. If it increases in size or the patient's symptoms persist, a chest drain can be placed and the patient can be admitted for observation.

Results
- Diagnostic accuracy >90%, sensitivity and specificity >95%, adequate samples obtained in 87.2% *(Clin Radiol 2017;72:1038–46)*
- Core needle biopsy can increase the rate of definite benign diagnosis compared to FNA from 52% to 91% *(Semin Intervent Radiol 2013;30:121–27)* and increase the rate of correct diagnosis (90% vs. 82%) as well as providing a cancer type/subtype (97% vs. 64%) *(J VascIntervRadiol 2016;27:674–81)*
- Overall sensitivity/specificity for ground-glass lesions 94% and 92% *(Br J Radiol 2014;87: 20140276)*

Complications

Perinephric Hematomas 4.3%, 0.7% Requiring Trusion
- Minor complications include small pneumothorax, pulmonary hemorrhage, and transient hemoptysis. A recent meta-analysis showed significant decreases in rate of pulmonary hemorrhage (18% CNB, 6.4% FNA) and transient hemoptysis (4.1% CNB, 1.7% FNA) *(Eur Radiol 2017;27:138–48)*
- Major complications include large pneumothorax requiring intervention, hemothorax, air embolism, needle tract seeding, and death which were not significantly different between CNB and FNA *(Eur Radiol 2017;27:138–48)*
- Pneumothorax incidence between 8–64% *(Clin Radiol 2017;72:1038–46)*
- Increased risk of chest tube placement with smaller lesions, use of FNA, COPD, and Core Needle Biopsy

---

MESENTERIC LYMPH NODE AND OMENTAL BIOPSIES

Background
- Peritoneal metastasis often originates directly from masses in the ovary, stomach, pancreas, colon (including carcinoid), uterus, and bladder or from hematogenous spread of melanoma, breast, and lung cancer. Lymphoma is the most common cancer found at biopsy in patients with no known primary *(J Vasc Interv Radiol 2017;28:1569–76)*. Primary peritoneal cancer includes mesothelioma, and pseudomyxoma.
- In some areas of the world, tuberculosis the most common source of peritoneal implants *(Eur J Radiol 2009;70:331–5)*
- Nonneoplastic tissue diagnosis is seen in up to 21.5% of biopsies *(J Vasc Interv Radiol 2017;28:1569–76)*

Indications *(J Vasc Interv Radiol 2017;28:1569–76; Eur J Radiol 2009; 70:331–35; World J Surg Oncol 2013;11:251; Radiology 2011;261(1):311–7; Ultrasound Q 2011;27:255–68)*
- Diagnosis of occult malignancy in the setting of peritoneal carcinomatosis, ascites of unknown origin, lymphadenopathy, or mesenteric reticular infiltration without mass
- Staging in the setting of known cancer
- Concomitant malignancies where diagnosis may alter treatment regimen
- Mass/mesenteric infiltration with possible tuberculosis infection or history of sarcoidosis

Procedure *(J Vasc Interv Radiol 2017;28:1569–76; Ultrasound Q 2011;27:255–68)*
- Informed consent outlining risk of bleeding and infection
- Preprocedure coagulation panel: INR <1.5, PT <15 s, aPTT <40 s, Plts >50K
- Stop anticoagulation: Aspirin/Antiplatelet Tx 5–7 d before, Warfarin 5–7 d before, LMWH 1 dose, Heparin 4 h before. NSAIDs may be stopped 3 d before.
- Ultrasound-guidance is ideal because of low cost, high availability, and high success rate in skilled hands but mesenteric/omental lesions may not be visualized sonographically and CT-guidance may be needed.
- Traversing bowel or other solid organs can be performed but increase the risk of complication. Small bowel contents are sterile and complications of traversal are low but large bowel should be avoided if possible.
- Patient is usually placed supine depending on lesion location. Posterior approach in the prone position is possible but may need CT-guidance.

- Local 1% lidocaine can be used in skin/subcutaneous tissue
- Coaxial technique is generally preferred and may lower the risk of tract seeding
- US-guidance: Grayscale is used to localize the lesion and Color Doppler is used to avoid major vessels including the epigastric arteries
- CT-guidance: Noncontrast CT performed for localization. Contrast can be used if the lesion is not visualized on noncontrast scan. Needle is advanced to the optimal location with periodic limited CT scans to confirm proper trajectory and needle position
- Transgluteal approach should be below the level of the piriform muscle to avoid sacral plexus and gluteal vessels (RadioGraphics 2004;24:175–89)
- 17G introducer needle is advanced to the optimal position with inner stylet present
- FNA:
  - Advance a 21G needle or smaller through the introducer needle
  - Vigorously move the needle back and forth and side to side within the lesion with or without applying suction on the syringe. 3–5 aspirations should be taken.
  - Collected aspirate is smeared on glass slides and fixed in 95% EtOH if using Pap smear or air-dried if Diff-Quick or Giemsa stain is used. Consult with local pathology department about preference.
  - RPMI or other cell media is typically used for flow cytometry per Pathology department
- Core Biopsy
  - 18G spring-loaded core biopsy needle is advanced through the introducer needle
  - 2–4 core biopsies are obtained
  - Specimens are placed in 10% buffered formalin or 0.9% Saline

Results

Omental and Mesenteric Masses (J Vasc Interv Radiol 2017;28:1569–76; AJR Am J Roentgenol 2009;192:131–6)
- Technical success rate 99.5%
- Nondiagnostic in 0.5–11% of technically-successful samples
- Sensitivity 93–95%, Specificity 86–100%, NPV 50–78.3%, more accuracy with addition of core needle biopsy
- In one study for patients with known cancer, metastatic disease confirmed in 44.1%, second primary found in 5.9%, and nonneoplastic diagnosis in 21.5% (J Vasc Interv Radiol 2017;28:1569–76)

Reticular Infiltration without Mass (Radiology 2011;261(1):311–7)
- Accuracy US-guided biopsy is 84%, for malignancy sensitivity was 89% and specificity was 100% in one study
- In reticular infiltration without mass, malignancy was found in 43%, TB in 36%, and nonspecific inflammation in 20%

Peritoneal or Retroperitoneal Lymphadenopathy
- US-guided biopsies successful 86% of the time with 91% of successful biopsies adequate for cytologic or histologic analysis (AJR Am J Roentgenol 1996;167:957–62)
- CT-guided biopsy accuracy 82–98% in abdomen, pelvis, and retroperitoneum (Radiology 1989;171:493–6)

Complications (J Vasc Interv Radiol 2017;28:1569–76; AJR Am J Roentgenol 2009;192:131–6)
- Major complications include bowel perforation with abscess formation (0.5%) and large mesenteric hematoma requiring transfusion (0.5%)
- Minor complications include pain, local bleeding at puncture site (1.6–2.7%)

ARTHROGRAPHY—GENERAL PRINCIPLES

Background

The earliest arthrography dates back to 1933 when air was injected into the shoulder joint to evaluate capsular integrity after shoulder dislocation (*Röentgen praxis* 1933;5:589–90; *AJR Am J Roentgenol* 2004;182(2):329–32). Severin described the utility of the first hip arthrography in children with congenital dislocation of the hip in 1939 (*JBJS* 1939;21(2):304–13). Iodinated contrast media was utilized soon thereafter to evaluate for rotator cuff defects. The introduction of computed tomography (CT) and then magnetic resonance imaging (MRI) then revolutionized the evaluation of the soft tissues of the joints. Better equipment, optimized techniques, and use of newer contrast media have resulted in better image quality, allowing for continued improvements in arthrography. MR and CT arthrography have almost completely replaced conventional arthrography, by revealing subtle pathologies, which contribute significantly to patient care and management.

Indications

The indications for arthrography have been redefined over the past several years, with the introduction of state-of-the-art MR scanners and dedicated joint coils that provide high-quality images. However, there is still an important role for combining these with arthrography to evaluate fine articular soft tissues such as labrum, cartilage, and intracapsular ligaments. The following are the most common indications for an MR arthrography:

1. Improved evaluation of intra-articular structures such as labrum, biceps tendon, and rotator cuff tears
2. Improved evaluation of ligamentous structures
3. More precise evaluation of the cartilage than noncontrast MRI

MR arthrography is the gold standard for the majority of internal derangements. However, there are times when a CT arthrogram is preferred. The main advantages of CT arthrography over MR are its sub-millimeter resolution, better delineation between bone and cartilage, and fast image acquisition. The following are the most common indications for CT arthrogram:

1. Patients with contraindications to MR scanning (eg, pacemaker)
2. Claustrophobia
3. Lack of patient cooperation such as motion
4. Significant susceptibility artifacts related to metal making MR scanning nondiagnostic
5. More precise evaluation of cartilage defects

Contraindications

- Hypersensitivity to any of the injection components. In these cases, apply appropriate premedication in a timely fashion before the procedure.
- Overlying skin infection is a relative contraindication so as to avoid the introduction of bacteria into the underlying noninfected joint. Try a different approach or entry site that appears clear of obvious infection.
- Bacteremia and sepsis are relative contraindications.
- Coagulopathies and anticoagulation are relative contraindications, although little data exists regarding the actual risk. Anticoagulation may need to be stopped before certain procedures depending on the medication, but the risk of stopping the anticoagulation must be weighed against the potential risk of a hemorrhagic complication.

Equipment

- C-arm fluoroscopy table can obtain imaging in oblique planes for small joints, spine injections, and when it is difficult for patients to achieve optimal positioning
- Standard fluoroscopy table can be used for many simple joint procedures
- Skin marker and radio-opaque marker
- Almost all joints can alternatively be injected under ultrasound with appropriate technique

Supplies

- Skin sterilization (1 × gauze for alcohol and 3 × gauze for iodine disinfectant like Betadine antiseptic solution OR a scrub with a chlorhexidine prep kit)
- Self-adhesive fenestrated drape
- 16G–18G drawing needle
- 25G needle for lidocaine injection

- 22G spinal needle for deep joints, short 25G needle may reach smaller, superficial joints such as elbow, wrist, and ankle
- 5-cc syringe for lidocaine
- 3-cc syringe for CT contrast medium (eg, Omnipaque 300)
- 30-cc syringe (knee), 20-cc (for other large joints) or 10-cc (for medium- and small-sized joints) syringe for gadolinium mixture
- 1-cc syringe for gadolinium chelate
- Topical cold spray (ethyl chloride spray) for hand, foot, and ankle injections
- Connection tubing
- Extra gauze pads
- Adhesive bandage

Medications

For diagnostic injections, a variety of injectates have been utilized in varying arthrogram cocktails. There is no global consensus on the ingredients of these cocktails. Having said that, a dilution of 1:200 to 1:250 of gadolinium chelate (reaching a concentration of 0.0020–0.0025 mmol/mL) and iodinated contrast medium (at a concentration of 240 mg/mL or less) are the essentials for MR and CT arthrography, respectively (*Insights Imaging* 2015;6(6):601–10).

Following injectates (Table 9-1) are based on University of Virginia, Department of Radiology and Medical Imaging institutional protocol for MR arthrography

Table 9-1 Recommended injectate for MR arthrography in mL (following clinical protocols at the University of Virginia, Department of Radiology and Medical Imaging)

	Shoulder	Elbow	Wrist	Hip	Knee	Ankle
Gadolinium	0.1	0.05	0.05	0.1	0.15	0.05
Sodium chloride 0.9%	15	8	8	15	25	8
Bupivacaine 0.25%	5	2	2	5	5	2
Total volume	20	10	10	20	30	10
Injected volume	12	3–6	1–4*	20	30	2–5

Should there be concern that MRI may not be successful due to artifact or claustrophobia, some institutes substitute iodinated contrast for some or all of the saline in the aforementioned formulas. This modification enables switch to CT arthrography if needed.

*Injected volume depends on which compartments are opacified: DRUJ, 1 mL; midcarpal, 1–2 mL; radiocarpal, 2–3 mL.

- To prepare injectate for **CT arthrography** simply substitute sodium chloride 0.9% with Omnipaque 300 in the same volumes mentioned in Table 9-1. Obviously, there is no need to add gadolinium to the cocktail.
- When there is metal and you are not sure if MRI will work well, or when you are in doubt that patient would tolerate MR scanner, inject 12 cc of a mixture of 0.04 cc of gadolinium and 20 cc of Omnipaque 300 (for joints like hip and shoulder) or 30 cc of 0.06 cc of gadolinium and 30 cc of Omnipaque for knee. Adding iodinated contrast decreases maximum achievable gadolinium signal. Iodinated contrast shifts the curve of gadolinium signal versus dilution. Therefore, lower concentration of gadolinium should be used when adding iodinated contrast (*Radiology* 2014;272(2):475–83).
- Local anesthetics are divided into two main groups based on their chemical structure. Generally, allergy or hypersensitivity to an amide local anesthetic does not "cross react" with ester local anesthetics, and vice versa. Therefore, if allergic to lidocaine, substitute for lidocaine and bupivacaine with any of the anesthetics in the esters group (Table 9-2).

Table 9-2 Local anesthetics—main structural subgroups

Amides	Esters
Lidocaine (Xylocaine®)	Procaine (Novocaine®)
Bupivacaine (Marcaine®)	Chloroprocaine (Nesacaine®)
Levobupivacaine	Tetracaine
Mepivacaine	Benzocaine
Prilocaine	Tetracaine
Ropivacaine	Risocaine
Etidocaine	Proparacaine
Carticaine	Amylocaine
Cinchocaine	Cocaine
Articaine	Piperocaine

Complications
- Bleeding
- Infection (cellulitis, septic arthritis, osteomyelitis)

- Transient aseptic synovitis
- Drug-induced allergic reactions
- Transient weakness/paresthesia from local anesthetic injection near nerves
- Vascular injury

Useful Hints
- Always make sure that MRI is safe for the patient based on MRI Safety Screening Questionnaire before injection occurs
- Be aware of patients' allergies and address them accordingly (do a pre-procedure "time-out" including allergy review)
- Iodinated contrast used in CT arthrography is FDA approved for joint injection, whereas gadolinium is still off-label (although commonly utilized)
- Wet-to-wet connections must be made at the junctions of the needle hub and tubing as well as the end of the tubing and the injectate syringe, to ensure lack of air bubbles within the joint, which could result in subsequent MRI misinterpretation
- Record pre- and postprocedure pain levels if intra-articular anesthetic is administered. This can be of diagnostic significance to confirm an intra-articular origin of pain.

Postprocedure Care
- Observe patient for 15 min after procedure
- Ask patient to try to hold the injected joint relatively still until imaging is performed. Extensive movement may cause extra-articular leakage of contrast.
- Inform patient about possibility of soreness at the needle puncture site, transient feeling of fullness and stiffness, signs and symptoms of more serious problems such as infection or motor dysfunction
- Provide patient with the name and contact information of a physician who can help if any problem were to arise

---

PAIN MANAGEMENT—GENERAL PRINCIPLES

Background
Intra-articular steroid injection frequently used by clinicians for treating inflammatory conditions of the joints. Janet Travell, MD (1901–97), first introduced muscle injections as a safe and effective adjunct to other pharmacologic and physical therapies. While technically more challenging, intra-articular injections also can be of great value in the patient's recovery (*Clin Radiol* 2015;70(11):1276–80). There is huge pool of data regarding the effectiveness and risks of joint injections, which may even be contradictory and confusing. However, there appears to be a decent overall consensus on short-term effectiveness of these injections for pain management.

Indications
- Ameliorate pain, swelling, and stiffness due to osteoarthritis, rheumatoid arthritis, acute gout, bursitis, epicondylitis, tenosynovitis, or other internal derangements
- Defer or avoid joint replacement surgeries
- Diagnostic injection to confirm intra-articular origin of pain (sensitivity of 91% and specificity of up to 100%) (*J Arthroplasty* 2010;25(Suppl.):129e33)

Contraindications
Following are the most common contraindications for intra-articular steroid injection.
- Hypersensitivity to any of the ingredients
- Active infection in or near the joint
- Systemic infections unless appropriate therapy is employed
- Uncontrolled diabetes mellitus as relative contraindication
- Coagulopathies and anticoagulation are relative contraindications, although little data exists regarding the actual risk. Anticoagulation may need to be stopped before certain procedures depending on the medication, but the risk of stopping the anticoagulation must be weighed against the potential risk of a hemorrhagic complication.
- Impending joint replacement surgery as relative contraindication
- Kenalog® (triamcinolone) is ONLY for intra-articular/intramuscular administration. The safety and efficacy of administration by other routes has yet to be established. Therefore, administration by other routes (IV, intrathecal, epidural, or intraocular) is contraindicated.

Equipment
- C-arm fluoroscopy table can obtain imaging in oblique planes for small joints, spine procedures, and when it is difficult for patients to get optimal positioning
- Standard fluoroscopy table can be used for many simple joint procedures
- Skin marker and radio-opaque marker
- Almost all joints can be injected under ultrasound with appropriate technique

Supplies
- Same as "Arthrography-Supplies," just substitute 3-cc syringe for injection of steroids ± anesthetics for syringe for gadolinium mixture injection

Medications
Different injectates are being utilized for pain management. There is no global consensus on the ingredients of these cocktails. Following injectates (Table 9-3) are based on University of Virginia, Department of Radiology and Medical Imaging institutional protocol for pain management.

Table 9-3 Recommended injectate for pain management in mL (following clinical protocols at the University of Virginia, Department of Radiology and Medical Imaging)			
	Small	**Medium**	**Large**
Kenalog® 40 mg/mL*	0.25	0.5	0.5
Bupivacaine 0.25%	0.25	1.5	2.5

*Kenalog®: Triamcinolone Acetonide

Small joint/bursa/space such as foot/hand joints, acromioclavicular or sternoclavicular joints, tarsal tunnel injection

Medium joint/bursa/space such as ankle and elbow

Large joint/bursa/space such as shoulder, hip, knee, trochanteric, or ischial bursa

Viscosupplementation
In 1997, the FDA approved viscosupplementation with hyaluronate (HA) derivatives for knee osteoarthritis. In 2007, the European Medicines Agency (EMEA) extended approval of HA to treatment of patients with ankle and shoulder OA. Based on FDA criteria, hyaluronic acid derivatives are indicated for the treatment of pain in osteoarthritis (OA) of the knee in patients who have failed to respond adequately to conservative nonpharmacologic therapy, simple analgesics (eg, acetaminophen), NSAIDs, tramadol, or intra-articular steroid injections. Table 9-4 presents the list of HA derivatives available for viscosupplementation:

Table 9-4 Common hyaluronate acid (HA) derivatives available for viscosupplementation with required numbers of injections		
Product	**No. of injections**	**Frequency of Injection**
Synvisc	3	1 w apart
Synvisc-One	1	1 time
Euflexxa	3	1 w apart
Durolane	1	1 time
Gel-One	1	1 time
Gelsyn-3	3	1 w apart
GenVisc 850	5	1 w apart
Hyalgan	5	1 w apart
Hymovis	2	1 w apart
Monovisc	1	1 time
Orthovisc	3–4	1 w apart
Supartz/Supartz FX	5	1 w apart

Data for single knee injection. Synvisc, Synvisc-One, and Euflexxa are the preferred HA derivatives.

Complications
- Infection (cellulitis, septic arthritis), the most common complication mentioned in some reports (Tech Reg Anesth Pain Manag 2007;11(3):141–7)
- Bleeding
- Transient aseptic synovitis
- Drug-induced allergic reactions
- Transient weakness/paresthesia
- Vascular injury
- Systemic side effects of steroids do not typically occur with intra-articular injection when recommended dosage regimens are administered via proper techniques
- Localized skin discoloration and subcutaneous fatty atrophy (Irrigate the injection needle and tubing with small amount of normal saline after steroid injection before taking the needle out to prevent this complication)
- Osteonecrosis with joint destruction if repeated intra-articular injections are given over a long period of time
- Tendon rupture if repeated injections along the tendon sheath are given over a long period of time

- Facial flushing can be experienced by many patients for a day or 2 after injection, but is self-limited
- Potential worsening of arthritis due to chondrotoxicity of steroid and/or anesthetic
- Worsening of blood glucose levels temporarily in diabetics
- Synovitis (after viscosupplementation)

Useful Hints
- Since the duration of effect is variable (approximate half-life of 26 d), repeat injections should be given when symptoms recur and not at set intervals
- Avoid injection into the tendon substance while trying to inject into a tendon sheath. Repeated injection into inflamed tendon has been shown to cause tendon rupture. Therefore, peritendinous injection around the Achilles tendon should be minimized due to absence of true tendon sheath.
- Record pre- and postprocedure pain levels. This can be of diagnostic significance to confirm an intra-articular origin of the pain.

Postprocedure Care
- Observe patient for 15 min after procedure
- Patients should be advised to avoid overuse of joints/tendons after symptomatic relief, particularly tendons, given the potential increased risk of tendon rupture
- Intra-articular anesthetic agent will be effective for a few hours (Bupivacaine duration of action 2–8 h) while steroid onset of action is usually more delayed (24–48 h). Therefore, instruct patients on possibility of transient return or even exacerbation of pain after procedure.
- Inform patient about possibility of soreness at the needle puncture site, transient feeling of stiffness, signs and symptoms of more serious problems such as infection and motor dysfunction
- Provide patient with the name and contact information of the physician who can help if any problem were to arise

ARTHROCENTESIS—GENERAL PRINCIPLES

Background
Arthrocentesis refers to aspirating fluid from a joint for therapeutic or diagnostic purposes. The *Corpus Hippocraticum* provides the first mention of the existence of fluid inside the joints (Tratados quirúrgicos. Introduction, translation and notes by Lara D, Torres H, Cabellos B, Madrid: Editorial Gredos; 1993). At that time, the removal of body fluids to maintain balance among the four humors (earth, fire, air, and water) was the basis of many therapeutic procedures. Centuries later, Fabricius Hildanus (1560–1634), a surgeon, seems to have been the first to puncture an infected fluid that resulted from a previous open wound in the knee (Newer tractat von der Glidwassersucht welche Ichor, Meliceria, Hydrarthros oder Hydrops Articulorum genant wird. In: Wund-Artzeny. Translated by Greiffen FJ. Frankfurt am Main: Beyers, 1652). It was in 1792 when Jean Gay in France reported major advance in therapeutic arthrocentesis (*Rheumatology (Oxford)* 2003;42(1):180–3). Joint aspiration can provide significant pain relief and improve mobility and range of motion.

Indications
- Acute monoarticular arthritis may be caused by septic arthritis, crystalline arthropathy, rheumatoid arthritis, osteoarthritis, lupus, and trauma. In patients where there is concern for septic arthritis in a native joint, aspiration should be performed emergently as extensive cartilage destruction can occur within 24 h. Patients with a joint replacement can typically be aspirated the next day unless they are septic and acute surgical intervention is being considered.
- Evaluate indolent monoarticular arthritis
- Evaluate prosthetic complications such as infection (a more indolent process) or metallosis (although controversial; *BMC Musculoskelet Disord* 2015;16:393)
- Pain relief for tense joint effusion
- Identify cause of unexplained joint effusion

Contraindications
There is no absolute contraindication for arthrocentesis especially in emergent circumstances. Following are the most commonly mentioned relative contraindications for arthrocentesis in the literature:
- Overlying skin infection is a relative contraindication so as to not introduce infection into an underlying noninfected joint. Try to identify a different approach that avoids obvious infection.
- Coagulopathies and anticoagulation are relative contraindications, although little data exists regarding the actual risk. Anticoagulation may need to be stopped before

certain procedures depending on the medication, but the risk of stopping the anticoagulation must be weighed against the potential risk of a hemorrhagic complication.

Equipment
- C-arm fluoroscopy or standard fluoroscopy table
- Skin marker and radio-opaque marker
- Almost all joints can be aspirated under ultrasound with appropriate technique

Supplies
- Same as "Arthrography-Supplies," just substitute 16G–18G needle (larger gauge needle is needed in aspiration cases in the event complex fluid is encountered, spinal needle in needed for deep joints) and 10–20-cc syringe for aspiration for the syringe for gadolinium mixture injection

Medications
No medication is needed other than lidocaine for local anesthesia unless there is specific request for pain management
- There is growing concern that the bacteriostatic nature of lidocaine and/or other local anesthetic agents may compromise culture results (*Ann Emerg Med* 2016;68:324–34; *Rheumatol Int* 2009;29:721–23). Therefore, it is recommended to use preservative-free anesthetics for joint aspiration, especially when there is concern for underlying infection. Anesthetic should be injected around the joint cavity, but not within the joint itself
- Preservative-free, sterile normal saline may be used to lavage the joint space in the case of a dry tap, if the referring service is in agreement. Lavage material can be sent for culture, but the fluid WBC counts will be inaccurate due to dilution effect.

Complications
- Bleeding
- Cellulitis
- Introduction of infection from an overlying soft tissue infection
- Transient aseptic synovitis
- Drug-induced allergic reactions to lidocaine
- Transient weakness/paresthesia
- Vascular injury

Useful Hints
- Aspirate should be split between bacterial culture and synovial fluid profile (to assess WBC count, crystals, etc.). Synovial fluid WBC counts >50000/mm^3 are typically associated with septic arthritis.
- Use your aspirate wisely when small volume (usually less than 1 cc) is aspirated, as splitting the aspirate between synovial fluid profile and culture may result in an adequate volume for both. Decision should be made based on the clinical concern and discussion with the referring provider.
- Preservative-free vials of anesthetics should be penetrated only once and then discarded
- In prosthetic joints, the joint pseudocapsule can be heavily thickened, generating resistance to the needle creating a relatively firm endpoint. Be sure to feel metal.
- If dry tap after passing into the joint, you can confirm intra-articular location of the needle with small amount of Omnipaque 300 followed by injection of small volume of preservative-free sterile normal saline to lavage the joint space if in agreement with referring service. Our adult reconstruction surgeons ask that we not lavage in the setting of a prosthesis.
- Bedside ultrasound can be used prior to intervention to identify the presence of clinically significant joint effusions and/or to identify overlying soft tissue abscess to help avoid unnecessary procedures or complications. If there is doubt regarding the significance of the effusion, comparison views of the contralateral joint can be helpful.
- Joint fluid can have different appearances on ultrasound depending on the nature of the fluid. Simple noninflammatory fluid will appear anechoic. Infected or traumatic effusion may also appear anechoic but could also be heterogeneous with septations and/or debris.
- The needle should be rotated once in the joint if no aspirate is obtained, as this can move the bevel off of thickened synovium and allow for free aspiration of fluid

Postprocedure Care
- Observe patient for 15 min after procedure
- Patients should be advised to avoid overuse of joints after procedure
- Inform patient about the possibility of soreness at the needle puncture site, transient feeling of stiffness; signs and symptoms of infection if not already exists; and signs and

symptoms of more serious problems such as decreased range of motion, motor dysfunction, and increasing pain
- Provide patient with the name and contact information of a physician who can help if any problem were to arise

COMMON JOINTS—TECHNIQUE

Hip

Hip Injection (Arthrography or Pain Management)
Hip arthrography is usually performed in younger patients when there is concern for labral tear
- Prepare the injectate (arthrography or pain management per protocol)
- Patient in supine position on fluoroscopy table
- Position lower extremity in mild internal rotation (use sand bag or tape feet together)
- Always palpate for femoral artery, although it is typically medial to typical approaches unless a bypass procedure has been done previously

1) Anterior Approach
  - Mark lateral femoral head–neck junction (Figure 9-1A)
  - Skin preparation with antiseptic solution and sterile drape
  - Anesthetize the planned needle tract with lidocaine
  - Advance 22G spinal needle perpendicular to table with bulls-eye technique (ie, needle hub superimposed over the needle tip) under intermittent fluoroscopy until needle tip hits the bone
  - Remove the stylet, attach connection tubing to syringe and inject small volume of Omnipaque to confirm intracapsular location (Figure 9-1B)
  - Attach connection tubing to injectate syringe and inject slowly to the desired volume
  - Take the needle out, clean the skin, and apply a small adhesive bandage

2) Oblique Approach
Advantageous in larger patients as it may help to avoid pannus of abdominal wall
  - Mark over greater trochanter
  - Advance 22G spinal needle transversely at a roughly 45° angle to the body under intermittent AP fluoroscopy to hit the femoral head–neck junction. Alternatively, C-arm fluoroscopy can be rotated to the same oblique angle and the needle can be bulls-eyed on the femoral head–neck junction or other intracapsular location along the femoral neck.
  - If needle is superimposed along the medial femoral neck, stop, pull back, and re-advance more steeply
  - Other technical details are the same as in "Hip Injection Anterior Approach"

Useful Hints
- Consider joint aspiration if there is suspected effusion to avoid overdilution of contrast for arthrography
- Air bubbles may look like small filling defects within the joint and be misinterpreted as intra-articular bodies on CT or MR images. Avoid introducing air for arthrography by filling the connection tubing with and dripping Omnipaque and MR contrast into the needle hub to create wet-to-wet connection as well as holding the syringe vertically while injecting.
- Contrast should flow freely away from the needle tip outlining the capsular boundaries, moving from lateral to medial across the femoral neck. If contrast is extra-articular, slightly adjust needle position and re-contact bone before re-checking with additional contrast injection.
- Abdominal wall pannus must be avoided in larger patients by either taping out of the way or utilizing oblique approach in order to avoid risk of intestinal injury

Hip Arthrocentesis
- Mark lateral femoral head–neck junction
- Skin preparation with antiseptic solution and sterile drape
- Anesthetize the planned needle tract with preservative-free lidocaine
- Advance the needle (16G–18G) perpendicular to the table using bulls-eye technique for a native hip and from a slightly lateral approach for hip prosthesis to be able to see the needle while advancing under intermittent fluoroscopy until needle tip hits the bone/prosthesis
- Remove the stylet and try to aspirate with a 20-cc syringe
- If dry tap, advance the needle laterally past the femoral neck/prosthesis and aspirate as you pull back

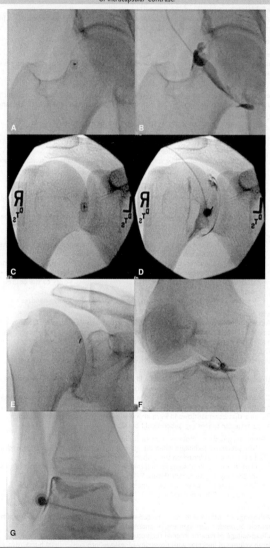

Figure 9-1 Fluoroscopic images demonstrating injections of different joints via bull's-eye needle placements. Needle hub bull's-eye at superolateral femoral head–neck junction **(A)** and normal hip joint distribution of contrast **(B).** Glenohumeral joint before **(C)** and after **(D)** injection for arthrography via Schneider technique, as well as the needle placement for the rotator interval approach **(E)** for pain management. Anterior approach **(F)** for knee joint injection. Lateral clear space approach **(G)** for ankle injection and normal distribution of intracapsular contrast.

- If still dry tap after passing the femoral neck/prosthesis, you can confirm intra-articular location of the needle with small amount of Omnipaque 300 followed by injection of 10-cc preservative-free sterile normal saline to lavage the joint space if the referring service is in agreement. Our adult reconstruction surgeons do not want us to lavage prosthetic joints.
- Inject the fluid into the collecting tubes as instructed in "Arthrocentesis—General Principals."

Useful Hints
- In a prosthetic hip, the joint pseudocapsule can be heavily thickened simulating a firm endpoint like metal or bone. Be sure to feel metal.

Shoulder

Glenohumeral (GH) Joint Injection (Arthrography or Pain Management)
This can be performed in different positions based on patient and operator preference. In addition, shoulder injection can be performed using ultrasound as well.

1) Anterior Approach—Schneider Technique
There are varying opinions between individuals and institutes regarding the best technique for shoulder arthrography. This is the preferred technique for GH arthrography based on the authors' experience.
- Prepare the injectate (arthrography or pain management)
- Patient in supine position on fluoroscopy table
- Position upper extremity in supination/external rotation (palm up), use sand bag on palm to ensure that shoulder stays in external rotation
- Mark the junction of middle and inferior thirds of the humeral articular surface, over the medial cortex (Figure 9-1C)
- Skin preparation with antiseptic solution and sterile drape
- Anesthetize the planned needle tract with lidocaine
- Advance 22G spinal needle perpendicular to table with bulls-eye technique (ie, needle hub superimposed over the needle tip) under intermittent fluoroscopy until needle tip hits the bone. This can alternatively be performed by the same needle used for superficial anesthesia if the patient is thin and the injection volume is low (eg, steroid injection, but not for arthrogram)
- Pull back 1 mm and turn the bevel laterally toward humeral head directing the needle tip medially, advance few mms, and fell the needle drop into the joint
- Remove the stylet, attach connection tubing to contrast syringe and inject small volume of Omnipaque to confirm intracapsular location (Figure 9-1D)
- Attach connection tubing to injectate syringe and inject slowly to the desired volume
- Take the needle out, clean the skin, and put on a small adhesive bandage

Useful Hints
- Advantage of Schneider technique—To be able to inject into a more capacious portion of the intracapsular space. This is especially important in arthrography while adding large volume.
- Disadvantage of Schneider technique—Injection into subscapularis muscle or tendon, GH ligament, or anterior-inferior labrum with contrast *(Insights Imaging 2015;6(6):601–10)*
- Use same technique described in "Hip Injection" to avoid introducing air bubbles into the joint space (ie, use wet-to-wet connections)
- Contraction of subscapularis tendon due to pain while advancing needle may medially deviate the needle tip. Advance under intermittent fluoroscopy.
- Be sure that contrast flows in intra-articular pattern to avoid injection into extra-articular spaces (eg, subcoracoid bursa)

2) Anterior Approach—Rotator Interval Technique
This is the preferred technique when the volume of injectate is small (making it ideal for GH pain injection) based on the authors' experience
- Mark the junction of superior and middle thirds of the humeral head, along the medial edge of the cortex (Figure 9-1E)
- Other technical details are the same as in "GH Joint Injection; Anterior Approach—Schneider Technique"

Useful Hints
- Advantage of rotator interval technique—Less chance of injection into subscapularis muscle or tendon, GH ligament, or anterior-inferior labrum
- Disadvantage of rotator interval technique—Suboptimal for arthrography due to large volume of injectate with possibility of leakage into subacromial bursa. Also, can be problematic in patients with adhesive capsulitis due to rotator interval scarring.

3) Posterior Approach

The posterior approach is the favored approach when injecting under ultrasound guidance (AJR Am J Roentgenol 2016;207(3):484–94). This approach may also be used when there is concern about anterior shoulder instability. An additional advantage is the lack of extracapsular contrast within the anterior soft tissues and thus no interference with the evaluation of subscapularis tendon and anterior labro-ligamentous complex (AJR 2002;178:433–34).

- Patient in prone position on fluoroscopy table
- Elevate shoulder with a triangular foam pad placed under patient's torso to place the GH articulation in profile
- Position upper extremity in neutral or slight internal rotation
- Other technical details are the same as in "GH Joint Injection; Anterior Approach—Schneider Technique"

Posterior Approach GH Injection Under Ultrasound

- Same position as Posterior Approach under fluoroscopy
- Find scapular spine and then align transducer in an oblique axial orientation along the long axis of infraspinatus muscle
- Identify humeral head, glenoid rim, posterior labrum, and infraspinatus myotendinous junction
- Advance needle to penetrate infraspinatus tendon from a lateral to medial approach, contacting the posterior aspect of the humeral head just lateral to the posterior labrum

Useful Hints

- The required needle trajectory is often steeper than most operators realize. Be sure that the patient and ultrasound probe are positioned so that the posterior humeral head can be successfully reached.
- Complications of posterior approach injection are possible neurovascular bundle injury (suprascapular nerve) and injury to circumflex scapular vessels if needle is placed too far medially (Skeletal Radiol 2010;39:575–79), but this is unlikely if one is sure of the anatomical landmarks by ultrasound.

GH Joint Arthrocentesis

- GH joint aspiration is similar to injection in terms of approach and majority of technique
- Utilize a 16G–18G needle in case complex or thick fluid is encountered
- Advance under intermittent fluoroscopy until needle tip hits the bone/prosthesis
- If dry tap, attempt could be made to reposition the needle within the joint
- If still dry tap after passing into the joint, you can confirm intra-articular location of the needle with small amount of Omnipaque 300 followed by injection of 10-cc preservative-free sterile normal saline to lavage the joint space, if in agreement with referring service
- Inject the fluid into the collecting tubes as instructed in "Arthrocentesis—General Principals"

Useful Hints

- In the case of a prosthetic joint, the joint pseudocapsule can be heavily thickened simulating bone or metal. Be sure to sense a very firm endpoint from metal.
- GH joint aspiration can be performed under ultrasound guidance via posterior approach with high rate of success if there is enough fluid.

Knee

Knee injection and aspiration can be performed under ultrasound or fluoroscopy via different approaches.

Knee Injection (Arthrography/Pain Management)

Knee arthrography is usually combined with CT or MR imaging for the postoperative evaluation of the meniscus. Therapeutic injection for pain management or injection of viscosupplementation is common.

1) Anterior Approach

The anterior approach is the least technically challenging method in patients with morbid obesity (typical patients referred for injection under fluoroscopic guidance) and/or in patients with severe patellofemoral compartment osteoarthritis (Clin Sports Med 2005;24:83–91)

- Prepare the injectate (arthrography or pain management)
- Patient in supine position on fluoroscopy table
- Position knee in extension with minimal flexion
- Angle the image intensifier slightly toward feet to have mild inferior-superior needle trajectory
- Mark over anteroinferior aspect of the femoral condyle. Medial side is preferred to avoid traversing patellar tendon (Figure 9-1F).

- Skin preparation with antiseptic solution and sterile drape
- Anesthetize the planned needle tract with lidocaine
- Advance 22G spinal needle perpendicular to table with bulls-eye technique (needle hub superimposed over the needle tip) under intermittent fluoroscopy to reach the femoral condyle
- Remove the stylet, attach connection tubing to contrast syringe and inject small volume of Omnipaque to confirm intracapsular location. Contrast should flow freely from the needle tip, generally into the suprapatellar recess.
- Attach connection tubing to injectate syringe and inject slowly to the desired volume
- Take the needle out, clean the skin, and put on a small adhesive bandage
- Ask patient to flex and extend knee (or ambulate to the scanner) in order to distribute about the knee and into potential meniscal tears

2) Medial Patellofemoral Approach
- Mark the mid-portion of the patellofemoral articulation
- Advance a 22G spinal needle (can be performed by the same needle used for anesthesia if patient is thin) under intermittent fluoroscopy until needle tip comes to rest against the patellar cartilage near the center of the patella
- Other technical details the same as in "Knee Injection: Anterior Approach"

Useful Hints
- Medial approach injection is technically less challenging due to wider joint space compared to lateral side. However, injection can be performed via lateral patellofemoral approach as well. Some experts recommend lateral approach because soft tissues are thinner laterally and also the medial approach requires traversing the vastus medialis obliquus (VMO) (AJR Am J Roentgenol 2016;207(3):484–94).
- Connect a syringe of local anesthetic to the needle and apply gentle pressure to the plunger while inserting the needle. Sudden loss of resistance indicates an intra-articular position.

Knee Arthrocentesis
Ultrasound is generally preferred to use for knee joint aspiration because one can see the fluid and target it directly

1) Ultrasound Technique
- Patient in supine position on fluoroscopy table
- Position knee in extension with minimal flexion
- Initially place the probe parallel to the long axis of the distal quadriceps tendon, revealing distal femur and looking for underlying suprapatellar effusion
- Position the probe transversely to optimize needle visualization as the needle passes into the suprapatellar recess
- Scan in a plane to see the patellar shadow, lateral femoral condyle, and the patellofemoral recess, then mark the skin and advance the needle from a lateral-to-medial approach after prep and drape
- Other technical details the same as in "Knee Injection: Lateral Patellofemoral Approach"
- Inject the fluid into the collecting tubes as instructed in "Arthrocentesis—General Principals"

2) Fluoroscopic Technique
- Knee joint aspiration is similar to injection in terms of approach and majority of technique
- Don't forget to use a 16G–18G needle for aspiration in case the fluid is thick
- Advance under intermittent fluoroscopy until needle tip hits the bone/prosthesis
- If dry tap, attempt could be made to reposition the needle
- If still dry tap after passing into the joint, you can confirm intra-articular location of the needle with small amount of Omnipaque 300 followed by injection of 10–20-cc preservative free sterile normal saline to lavage the joint space if in agreement with referring service
- Inject the fluid into the collecting tubes as instructed in "Arthrocentesis—General Principals"

LESS COMMON JOINT—TECHNIQUE

Ankle
Ankle arthrography is usually combined with CT or MR imaging to evaluate for articular cartilage lesions, intra-articular bodies, and anterolateral and anteromedial impingement (AJR Am J Roentgenol 2016;207(3):484–94). Other indications include therapeutic steroid injection and diagnostic anesthetic injection.

Fluoroscopic-Guided Ankle Injection (Arthrography/Pain Management)

Multiple approaches have been described to access ankle joint space
- Prepare the injectate (arthrography or pain management)
- Patient in supine position on fluoroscopy table
- Position knee in flexion and ankle in mid plantar flexion

Lateral Clear Space Approach
- Profile ankle in mortise view to see the clear space
- Mark between the articulating surfaces of the upper three-quarters of the talofibular articulation (lateral clear space, Figure 9-1G) *(Skeletal Radiol 2014;43(1):27–33)*

Anterior Approach
- Always palpate for dorsalis pedis artery and avoid it
- Mark anteromedial talar dome in between the extensor hallucis longus and tibialis anterior tendons. The anterior ankle capsule inserts on the talar neck making the talar dome an intra-articular structure *(Radiol Clin North Am 2008;46:973–94)*.
- Use topical cold spray (ethyl chloride spray) and anesthetize the planned needle tract with lidocaine (if needed)
- Anesthetize the planned needle tract with lidocaine
- Advance same needle used for anesthesia under intermittent fluoroscopy until needle tip passes the joint capsule
- Attach connection tubing, inject small volume of Omnipaque and confirm ntracapsular location. Contrast should flow away from the needle and across the talar dome.
- Attach connection tubing to injectate syringe and inject slowly to the desired volume
- Take the needle out, clean the skin, and put on a small adhesive bandage

Ultrasound-Guided Ankle Injection

Anterior long-axis approach is the simplest way to access ankle under ultrasound
- Positioning the same as above (fluoroscopic guided)
- Mark the dorsalis pedis artery and extensor tendons
- Obtain a long-axis view of the tibialis anterior tendon
- Translate the transducer just medial to the tibialis anterior tendon and localize the anterior recess
- Advanced the needle under ultrasound guidance into the anterior ankle joint recess to contact the talar dome
- Other technical details same as in "Fluoroscopic Guided Ankle Injection"

Ankle Arthrocentesis

Ankle joint aspiration can be performed under ultrasound or fluoroscopic guidance using aforementioned approaches

Useful Hints
- Please refer to "Arthrocentesis—General Principals" for more details and useful hints

Elbow

Elbow Injection (Arthrography/Pain Management)

Elbow joint arthrography is generally combined with CT or MR imaging to evaluate the collateral ligament tears, articular chondral defects, or the existence of intra-articular bodies *(AJR Am J Roentgenol 2016;207(3):484–94)*. Injection is also requested for pain management. This can be done via posterior *(Skeletal Radiol 2009;38(5):513–6)* or lateral approaches:

1) Posterior (Trans-triceps) Approach
   - Prepare the injectate (arthrography or pain management)
   - Patient in either prone position on fluoroscopy table with the arm over the head and elbow flexed 90° or seated beside the table with the arm abducted and elbow flexed 90°
   - Mark just above and lateral to the olecranon process (Figure 9-2A)
   - Skin preparation with antiseptic solution and sterile drape
   - Anesthetize the planned needle tract with lidocaine
   - Advance the same needle parallel to table under intermittent fluoroscopy until you hit the bone in posterior olecranon fossa
   - Attach connection tubing to contrast syringe and inject small volume of Omnipaque to confirm intracapsular location. Make sure you see contrast flowing to the anterior recess of the joint to ensure that it is not pooling in the posterior fat pad (Figure 9-2B)
   - Inject slowly to the desired volume
   - Take the needle out, clean the skin, and put on a small adhesive bandage

Useful Hints
- Oblique trajectory of needle (Figure 9-2A) could be obtained in posterior approach by marking the skin 1 cm above the olecranon fossa and advancing needle distally

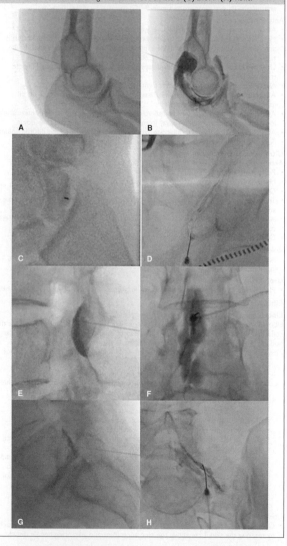

Figure 9-2 Fluoroscopic images demonstrating puncture sites for different joint injections, epidural steroid injection (ESI), and nerve block. Posterior approach for elbow injection **(A)** with normal distribution of contrast into anterior joint recess **(B)**. Puncture site for radiocarpal joint injection **(C)**. Sacroiliac joint injection with small amount of contrast delineating the joint space **(D)**. Normal distribution of contrast during ESI on lateral **(E)** and AP **(F)** views. Attention to normal meniscoid distribution of contrast in epidural space on lateral view. Ideal needle tip position for nerve root block at posterior superior aspect of the neural foramen. Contrast delineates right L5 nerve root on lateral **(G)** and AP **(H)** views.

until hitting bone. This will help to enter a more patulous space of the olecranon recess.
- The posterior approach decreases the likelihood of iatrogenic contrast leakage in the lateral elbow structures, which could create a diagnostic dilemma in arthrography cases, particularly when an injury to the lateral elbow structures is suspected (Skeletal Radiol 2009;38(5):513–6)

2) Lateral Approach
  - Patient in either prone position on fluoroscopy table with the arm over the head and elbow flexed 90° or seated beside the table with the arm abducted and elbow flexed 90° with the medial aspect of the elbow flat on the table. Hand in supination with thumb up to maximally open the joint space.
  - Mark the ventral portion of the radiocapitellar joint
  - Advance the needle into the joint
  - Other technical details the same as in "Elbow Injection: Posterior Approach"

Elbow Arthrocentesis
Elbow joint aspiration can be performed under ultrasound or fluoroscopic guidance using aforementioned approaches

Useful Hints
- Please refer to "Arthrocentesis—General Principals" for more details and useful hints

Wrist
The wrist is composed of three joint compartments, which normally should not communicate with each other—the radiocarpal (RC) joint, midcarpal (MC) joint, and distal radio-ulnar joint (DRUJ). Wrist arthrogram could be single compartmental (RC), double compartmental (RC with either DRUJ or MC), or triple compartmental (RC, MC, and DRUJ) based on the clinical concern for full-thickness vs. partial-thickness tear and the location of the pain. Typically, only the RC compartment is injected while looking for contrast flow into other compartments.

Wrist Injection (Arthrography or Pain Management)
- Prepare the injectate (arthrography or pain management)
- A dorsal approach is used to inject all wrist compartments
- Patient in either prone position on fluoroscopy table with the arm over the head and wrist in pronation flat on the table or seated beside the table with the arm abducted, elbow flexed 90°, and wrist in pronation flat on the table
- Mild passive flexion (supported by small sponge or towel) or ulnar deviation can help open up the RC joint space

RC Injection
Routine approach: Mark the proximal radial cortex of the mid scaphoid (Figure 9-2C). The needle should have a slightly distal to proximal course to avoid the dorsal lip of the radius.
Alternative approach (in patients with radial sided pain, to avoid masking pathologies): Mark the proximal cortex of triquetrum adjacent to pisiform (in patient with radial sided pain, to avoid masking pathologies) (Radiol Clin North Am 2005;43:709–31).

MC Injection
Routine approach (4-corner approach): Mark the confluence of the triquetrum, lunate, capitate, and hamate
Alternative (3-corner approach): Mark the confluence of the lunate, capitate, and trapezoid

DRUJ Injection
Mark the radial cortex of the distal ulna just proximal to its physeal scar
- Skin preparation with antiseptic solution and sterile drape
- Use topical cold spray (ethyl chloride spray) and anesthetize the planned needle tract with lidocaine (if needed)
- Advance the same needle perpendicular to table under intermittent fluoroscopy until you hit the bone
- Attach connection tubing to contrast syringe and inject small volume of Omnipaque to confirm intracapsular location
- Inject slowly to the desired volume
- Take the needle out, clean the skin, and put on a small adhesive bandage

Useful Hints
- Leakage of contrast after RC injection into MC or DRUJ indicates a full thickness tear of the scapholunate (SL) or lunotriquetral (LT) ligaments or triangular

fibrocartilage complex (TFCC), respectively. Injection into other compartments may rarely be requested to attempt to delineate partial thickness tear of these structures.
- MC joint may normally communicate with the common carpometacarpal joint. However, communication with the RC joint is not normal and indicates a full-thickness tear of the one of the interosseous ligaments (SL or LT).
- For arthrography injections, attempt to avoid extensive subcutaneous lidocaine infiltration as this can obscure pathology in the extensor tendons on MR imaging. If MR or CT arthrography is planned, use wet-to-wet tubing connections to avoid injecting air bubbles into the joint.

Wrist Arthrocentesis

Wrist joint aspiration can be performed under ultrasound or fluoroscopic guidance using aforementioned approaches

Useful Hints
- Please refer to "Arthrocentesis—General Principals" for more details and useful hints

Foot

Foot Injection (Pain Management)

Foot injections are almost always for pain management. Different joints can be accessed and injected based on imaging findings and location of the pain. Joints such as the talonavicular and MTPs are concave/convex joints so the technique of advancing onto the convex edge or surface applies.
- Prepare the injectate (pain management)
- Patient in supine position on fluoroscopy table. Generally, the ipsilateral knee is flexed and the foot of interest is flat on the table. However, different positions with various tube angulations can be obtained to place the desired joint space in profile. The image intensifier should be obliqued until the joint space is well seen such that it can be targeted by a "bulls-eye" needle approach. Table 9-5 enlists the common foot joints and injection approaches.
- Skin preparation with antiseptic solution and sterile drape
- Use topical cold spray (ethyl chloride spray) and anesthetize the planned needle tract with lidocaine (if needed)
- Advance the same 25G needle under intermittent fluoroscopy until you pass the joint capsule
- Attach connection tubing to contrast syringe and inject small volume of Omnipaque to confirm intracapsular location
- Attach injectate syringe directly to needle hub and inject slowly to the desired volume given the small joint volume
- Take the needle out, clean the skin, and put on a small adhesive bandage

Table 9-5 Recommended position and approach to inject foot joints	
Joint	**Position and Approach**
Posterior subtalar	Lateral approach just posterior to the fibula, image intensifier typically moved cranially to demonstrate posterior subtalar joint
Middle subtalar	Medial approach along the superior aspect of the sustentaculum tali if posterior subtalar approach not possible
Sinus tarsi	Lateral approach
Talonavicular (TN)	AP approach, with lateral confirmation as needed
Naviculocuneiform (NC)	AP approach
Calcaneocuboid (CC)	Lateral oblique approach, with image similar to an oblique foot radiograph
1st TMT	AP approach
2nd and 3rd TMT	AP approach (usually communicate)
4th and 5th TMT	AP approach (usually communicate)
MTPs, PIPs, and DIPs	AP approach

TMT, tarsometatarsal; MTP, metatarsophalangeal; PIP, proximal interphalangeal; DIP, distal interphalangeal.

Useful Hints
- Rarely, arthrography of a metacarpophalangeal, metatarsophalangeal, or interphalangeal joints is requested and can be performed by targeting the dorsal joint recess under fluoroscopic or ultrasound guidance. Approximately 1 cc of diluted contrast can be injected.
- Ultrasound has been increasingly utilized for foot and ankle intra-articular injections and aspiration (*Foot Ankle Int* 2009;30(9):886–90)

- Shorter 25G needles can be used for MTP, PIP, and DIP joints to ensure that one doesn't pass the needle through or along the joint space to the plantar aspect of the foot with subsequent contamination

Foot Arthrocentesis

Both ultrasound and fluoroscopy could be used for this purpose. However, ultrasound could be a better choice for foot aspirations allowing for direct visualization of the often small volume of effusions.

Useful Hints
- Please refer to "Arthrocentesis—General Principals" for more details and useful hints

Sacroiliac (SI) Joint Injection

SI joint, a true diarthrodial joint, permits only minimal movement. The upper third is a syndesmosis, connected by powerful anterior, interosseous, and posterior ligaments, and lacks synovium. The lower two-thirds are lined by articular cartilage, although the middle third is a purely cartilaginous joint while the lower third is the only part lined with synovium. Therefore, the lower one-third of the SI joint should be targeted for a therapeutic injection.

- Prepare the injectate (pain management)
- Patient in prone position on fluoroscopy table
- With the tube straight, mark the inferior margin of the SI joint
- Angle the image intensifier toward the head (25–35°), which will better profile the posterior position of the inferior SI joint
- Skin preparation with antiseptic solution and sterile drape
- Anesthetize the planned needle tract with lidocaine
- Advance a 22G spinal needle **perpendicular to table** under intermittent fluoroscopy until the inferior margin of the SI joint is encountered (Figure 9-2D)
- Walk the needle toward the joint until you feel the needle slips into the joint
- Remove the stylet, attach connection tubing to syringe and inject a small volume of Omnipaque to confirm intracapsular location
- Attach injectate syringe directly to the needle hub and inject slowly. Relative resistance may be expected due to small size of the joint space.
- Take the needle out, clean the skin, and put on a small adhesive bandage

Useful Hints
- Angling the tube toward the patient's head will profile the posterior inferior aspect of the joint. The needle needs to be advanced perpendicular to the table even though the image intensifier is oblique in the craniocaudal direction.
- If intra-articular access cannot be achieved after a few attempts, medication may be injected in a periarticular location, which typically results in a similar degree of pain relief as an intra-articular injection *(AJR Am J Roentgenol 2016;207(5):1055–61)*.
- Avoid injecting too much contrast when attempting to access the joint. This can obscure the landmarks and make it difficult to visualize the joint.

Acromioclavicular (AC) Joint

Injection and aspiration of the AC joint can be performed under either fluoroscopic or ultrasound guidance. We describe the fluoroscopic technique hoping ultrasound technique is self-explanatory with the provided information.

AC Joint Injection
- Prepare the injectate (pain management)
- Patient in supine position on fluoroscopy table
- Angle tube to see AC joint in profile (usually image intensifier toward feet)
- Mark the middle or central portion of the joint space
- Skin preparation with antiseptic solution and sterile drape
- Anesthetize the planned needle tract with lidocaine
- Advance the same needle (a longer spinal needle may be needed depending on body habitus) perpendicular to the table with bulls-eye technique (ie, needle hub superimposed over the needle tip) under intermittent fluoroscopy until you touch a bony margin or feel you have penetrated the joint capsule. Avoid advancing the needle too deeply.
- Attach connection tubing to the contrast syringe and inject a small volume of Omnipaque to confirm intracapsular location by seeing linear contrast parallel to joint line
- Inject slowly to the desired volume. High resistance may be encountered due to small size of the joint.
- Take the needle out, clean the skin, and apply a small adhesive bandage

Sternoclavicular (SC) Joint

Injection and aspiration of the SC joint can be performed under either fluoroscopic or ultrasound guidance. However, given close proximity to the lungs and potential for pneumothorax, ultrasound is preferred in most institutes due to its superficial position and better ability to access depth. We describe the fluoroscopic technique hoping ultrasound technique is self-explanatory with provided information.

SC Joint Injection
- The same technique as AC joint injection
- Target bone on either side of the joint to avoid overpenetration beyond the posterior joint margin

SC Joint Arthrocentesis
- SC joint aspiration is similar to injection in terms of approach and majority of technique
- Don't forget to use a 16G–18G needle to aspirate in case of thick fluid
- Target bone on either side of the joint to avoid advancing too deeply
- If dry tap, attempt could be made to reposition the needle within the joint
- If still dry tap after passing into the joint, you can confirm intra-articular location of the needle with small amount of Omnipaque 300 followed by injection of 1-cc preservative free sterile normal saline to lavage the joint space
- Inject the fluid into the collecting tubes as instructed in "Arthrocentesis—General Principals"

SPINE INJECTIONS

See Interventional Pain Management Chapter for More Details

Useful Hints
- Make sure the needle is properly positioned over the interlaminar space before connecting contrast tubing so that the needle can be smoothly passed into the epidural space without contacting bone
- Advance the needle slowly while injecting contrast somewhat firmly once posterior epidural space. Mixed epidural/intrathecal injections are possible if the needle is advanced too quickly.
- In large patients, causing photon starvation, it may be difficult to see the flash of epidural contrast. Relying more on the loss of resistance in this situation may be necessary.
- If the needle tip is intrathecal, contrast will move anteriorly and flow with gravity if the table is tilted with contrast outlining nerve roots. If this pattern is seen, the needle should be removed. Injection can be re-attempted at a different level or the patient can come back on another day.
- Ensure that the epidural space is filling. Interlaminar approach injections can inadvertently fill facet joints, the subligamentous space superficial to the ligamentum flavum, or the subdural space all of which can potentially mimic epidural filling.
- If the needle is approaching the spinolaminar line on the lateral view and epidural contrast is not yet seen, check the AP view and make sure the needle has not yet crossed midline. If the needle is across midline, this suggests the obliquity of approach is too shallow such that the needle is skirting the ligamentum flavum but not entering the epidural space. The needle should be pulled back and re-advanced at a steeper angle. The opposite is true if the needle tip is not yet to the middle on the AP view.

Postprocedure Care
- Observe patient for at least 15 min after procedure
- Patient must have a driver in case delayed leg numbness and/or weakness occurs
- Patients should be advised to avoid overuse for the day after the procedure
- Epidural anesthetic agent will be effective for a few hours (Bupivacaine duration of action 2–8 h) while steroids onset of action is usually more delayed (24–48 h). Therefore, instruct patients on possibility of transient return or even exacerbation of pain occurring hours after the procedure.
- Inform patient about the possibility of soreness at the needle puncture site, transient feeling of stiffness, signs and symptoms of more serious problems such as infection, motor dysfunction, and increasing pain
- Provide patient with the name and contact information of a physician who can help if any problem were to arise

Nerve Root Block

See Interventional Pain Management Chapter for More Details on Stellage Ganglion Blocks

Indications
- Clinical and/or MRI evidence of single or potentially two site lumbar nerve impingement. Medication placement in a nerve block is more localized to a specific nerve compared with an epidural injection.
- Nerve blocks can also provide diagnostic information; if a patient's pain resolves after injection of a certain nerve then that is likely the patient's pain generator

Contraindications
- Diffuse lumbar spinal disease is better treated by ESI as the medication is spread more diffusely
- Same as ESI

Equipment
- C arm fluoroscopy is preferred for obtaining multiplanar imaging to accurately determine needle position
- Skin marker and radio-opaque marker

Supplies
- No flush is necessary as the desire is for the medication to stay near the targeted nerve root
- Otherwise same as ESI

Medications
- Local anesthetic must be free of preservatives, particularly methylparaben, as these compounds may be neurotoxic
- Dexamethasone is currently recommended for any transforaminal procedure, as it is the only currently available nonparticulate steroid. Rare cases of cord infarction have been reported when using a particulate steroid for transforaminal injection as low as S1. At the author's institution, 1 cc of 10 mg/mL dexamethasone is mixed with 1 cc of 0.5% Bupivacaine. Dosage may need to be decreased in patients receiving multiple nerve blocks, as dexamethasone since patients may be particularly prone to causing facial flushing reactions at larger doses.

Technique
- Preprocedure imaging reviewed to evaluate degree of stenosis at exiting nerve root, amount of perineural fat, and presence of any foraminal/far lateral disk herniation
- Curved needle technique
  - Manually place a 20–30° curve on the distal-most 2 cm of the spinal needle with the curve going away from the bevel, opposite the raised marker on the needle hub. The needle intrinsically courses away from the bevel; so placing the above curve on the needle exacerbates this tendency.
  - Mark the skin approximately 1 cm lateral to the vertebral body, just under the level of the pedicle on an AP scout
  - After anesthetizing the skin, place the curved spinal needle through the skin, keeping the needle tip perpendicular to the skin surface
  - Alternate between AP and lateral fluoroscopy until the needle tip approaches the posterior superior aspect of the neural foramen (Figure 9-2G)
- Oblique approach technique
  - Obtain 30–45° oblique images such that the vertebrae have a "Scottie dog" appearance
  - Mark along the inferior aspect of the "Scottie dog" head, just anterior to the facet
  - After anesthetizing the skin, a straight (noncurved) spinal needle should be placed in a Bulls-eye position over the target
  - Alternate between oblique and lateral fluoroscopy until the needle tip approaches the posterior superior aspect of the neural foramen
- On the lateral view, slowly advance needle to the mid superior portion of the neural foramen. If the patient experiences radicular pain, the nerve was likely contacted, and the needle should be pulled back 1–2 mm. Avoid the anterior superior portion of the neural foramen as radiculomedullary arterial branches may lie in that quadrant. An inferior location in the neural foramen can result in medication spread to the more inferior nerve root as opposed to the exiting nerve root.
- Connect contrast syringe and tubing. Inject and look for any vascular flow on AP and lateral views. If the needle is correctly positioned, contrast will typically be seen flowing under the pedicle and into the epidural space on the AP view (Figure 9-2H)
- Once accurate position is determined, inject dexamethasone/Bupivacaine. No significant flush is needed.

Complications

- Epidural hematoma
- Abscess
- Temporary lower-extremity paralysis if local anesthetic is inadvertently placed in the intrathecal or subdural space, although this is much more rare with nerve block than ESI
- Spinal headache if the needle is advanced through the dura
- Poststeroid facial flushing
- Worsening of blood glucose levels temporarily in diabetics
- Potential cord infarction, particularly if particulate steroids are utilized

Useful Hints

- When utilizing the curved needle technique, placing your index finger along the side of the needle shaft with the curve can have a fulcrum effect, causing the needle to curve towards the neural foramen even more abruptly
- If the needle tip is intrathecal, contrast will move anteriorly and flow with gravity if the table is tilted with contrast outlining nerve roots. If this pattern is seen, the needle should be removed. Injection can be re-attempted at a different level or the patient can come back on another day.

Postprocedure Care

- Same as ESI

Facet Injection

- See Interventional Pain Chapter for more details

Useful Hints

- The facet injection approach targets the inferior recess of the facet joint. Targeting the facet joint line directly using an oblique approach is possible but typically more challenging due to a high frequency of overhanging osteophytes.
- Some literature shows a similar degree of pain relief with extra-articular injection around the facet. If the facet cannot be accessed despite multiple attempts, perform a peri-facet injection instead.
- When a pars defect is the target, select the facet joint that is superior to the defect (ie, for an L5 pars select the L4–L5 facet). Approach the facet as above. The needle may fall into the pars defect itself. Contrast may be seen filling both the facet and the pars defect.
- For a facet joint synovial cyst rupture, briskly inject a mixture of contrast/Bupivacaine after the steroid/local anesthetic mixture. Pressure will build and injection may become difficult with development of patient pain, but further injection will result in loss of resistance and resolution of pain with bursting of the cyst. Once the cyst ruptures, contrast leakage should be seen in the epidural space.

CT GUIDED BONE PROCEDURES—GENERAL PRINCIPLES

Background

Needle biopsy of skeletal neoplasms was 1st introduced by Martin and Ellis in 1930 (*Br J Surg* 1947;34(135):240–61). Advances have been made in techniques and equipment since then.

Indications

- Differentiating true neoplasm from nonneoplastic entities
- Histopathologic analysis of primary and metastatic bone lesions
- Obtaining tissue sample for culture in cases of osteomyelitis
- Evaluating treatment response for diseases such as multiple myeloma and leukemia

Contraindications

- Hypersensitivity to any of the medications for regional anesthesia or moderate sedation. Try to replace medications with appropriate alternative substitutes (Table 9-2) or avoid applying moderate sedation. Discussion should be made with patient regarding this matter before performing the procedure.
- Overlying skin infection is a relative contraindication so as to avoid introduction of infection into an underlying noninfected tissues. Try a different approach or entry site that avoids obvious infection.
- Bacteremia and sepsis are relative contraindications.
- Coagulopathies and anticoagulation (Platelets <50000/mm^3 or INR >1.5), although little data exists regarding the actual risk. Biopsies are generally not emergent procedures. Anticoagulation may need to be stopped and abnormal INR and platelet counts corrected before biopsy. This depends on the type of medication and

indication for it. The risk of stopping the anticoagulation must be weighed against the potential risk of a hemorrhagic complication.
- Inaccessible tumor due to adjacent vital structures, intervening bowel, or other critical structures

Equipment
- CT scan is typically used for bone biopsy
- Bone lesions with cortical destruction and a soft tissue component can alternatively be biopsied under ultrasound with appropriate technique
- Fluoroscopy can be an alternative approach in select cases

Supplies
- Skin sterilization (1 × gauze for alcohol and 3 × gauze for iodine disinfectant like Betadine antiseptic solution OR a scrub with a chlorhexidine prep kit)
- Barrier gown, mask, cap
- Radiopaque marker or grid for CT-guided procedures
- Self-adhesive fenestrated drape
- Surgical drape sheath to cover body
- 16G–18G drawing needle
- 25G lidocaine needle
- 22G spinal needle for deep lidocaine injection and periosteal anesthesia
- 22G spinal needle for FNA (if needed)
- Disposable scalpel blade #11
- Bone core biopsy set (information to follow)
- Sample container
- Extra gauze pads
- Wound dressings
- Extra supplies needed for bone marrow aspiration:
  - Sodium heparin, Injection, 1000 USP Units/mL, 2 mL vials (for bone marrow aspiration)
  - 20 cc (for heparinized bone marrow aspirate) and 5 cc (for nonheparinized bone marrow aspirate) syringes
  - Vacutainers (heparinized × 1 and nonheparinized × 1)
  - Microscope slides, 1" × 3", frosted

Sedation
- Bone biopsies are generally performed under conscious (moderate) sedation using Fentanyl (a narcotic analgesic agent) and Midazolam (Versed®, and anxiolytic agent). Please refer to chapter on sedation techniques for further information.
- General anesthesia may be necessary in uncooperative patients or children
- Regional nerve block may be of use for painful lesions, such as neurogenic tumors, or lesions in the hand and foot
- Liberal periosteal anesthetic infiltration helps to minimize pain

Complications
Percutaneous needle biopsies have a very low complication rate (1.1%) compared to open biopsy (up to 16%) *(Cancer 2000;89:2677–86)*
- Risk of malignant cells seeding along the needle track, particularly if the lesion is a sarcoma. This could necessitate en bloc resection of the needle track with the tumor at limb-sparing reconstructive surgery and could make surgical approach more complicated. Therefore, radiologist and orthopedic oncologist team approach is crucial to choose the appropriate needle path prior to biopsies. Coaxial approach to biopsy may reduce this risk.
- Drug-induced allergic reactions
- Common complications of moderate sedation
- Infection
- Bleeding—Postbiopsy embolization of the needle track using an absorbable hemostatic agent may be helpful in hemorrhagic lesions
- Vascular injury
- Nerve injury

Useful Hints
- Thorough image analysis is critical before biopsy to evaluate the necessity of biopsy, percutaneous approach planning, and to determine the target point within the lesion. Additional imaging may be necessary. Anatomic imaging findings should be correlated with clinical scenario and findings on functional studies, such as diffusion-weighted images (DWI), MRI, PET, and bone scanning.
- When multiple lesions are present, select the lesion that is most amenable to biopsy and/or most suspicious, allowing the highest yield with the lowest complication risk.

- The radiologist and orthopedic oncologic surgeon should take a team approach, especially when limb-sparing surgery is planned for primary bone/soft tissue sarcoma. Lack of communication may result in preventable limb amputation or tumor recurrence along the trajectory of biopsy needle. Coaxial technique may reduce the chance of track seeding.
- If a destructive bone lesion is associated with a soft tissue mass, the biopsy may be taken from the soft tissue component. It is better to obtain a sample from the intraosseous part of the mass, if feasible.
- It is preferable to biopsy more viable, less necrotic and noncystic portions of the mass
- If tissue sampling of a destructive lesion is poor (ie, scant material), it can be helpful to biopsy the interface of the lesion with normal bone. This may help sampling viable tissue revealing the lesion well, and the support of the more normal bone may result in better sampling.
- It is preferable to obtain 2–3 biopsy samples from different parts of the mass, especially when dealing with a large mass
- In lesions with calcified/ossified components, sampling from the less mineralized parts often yields the least results
- Sampling should be performed form the enhancing portions of the mass or areas with more diffusion restriction on MRI or more metabolic activity on PET as seen on prebiopsy cross-sectional imaging. This avoids sampling necrotic areas of the mass, which have a lower pathologic yield.

Postprocedure Care
- Observe patient for 30–45 min after procedure
- Inform patient about the possibility of soreness at the needle puncture site and signs and symptoms of infection and bleeding
- Provide patient with the name and contact information of a physician who can help if any problem were to arise

---

CT-GUIDED BONE PROCEDURES—TECHNIQUE

- CT-guided bone biopsies are usually performed using a co-axial needle technique to gain a stable position through which the biopsy may be performed. More superficial lesions may be biopsied without coaxial needle technique. Coaxial technique may also be less damaging to intervening normal tissue, and reduces the likelihood of track seeding.
- For sclerotic lesions and osseous lesions with intact cortex, typically a standard "bone biopsy set" such as Bonopty®, Jamshidi®, or Arrow® OnControl® powered bone access system are required
- Different bone biopsy sets have different detailed technical specifications. Following, we describe step-by-step procedural techniques based on Bonopty® coaxial bone biopsy system as a prototype for these procedures, given the fact that this system is more commonly used among different institutes. More technical information regarding Jamshidi® and Arrow® OnControl® powered bone biopsy needles may be found at the official website of each device manufacturer (http://arrowoncontrol.com; https://www.bd.com/en-us/offerings/capabilities/interventional-specialties/jamshidi-bone-marrow-biopsy-needles).
- Bonopty® coaxial bone biopsy system (12G or 14G) includes a Penetration set (penetration cannula with stylet, drill, and depth gauge) and a biopsy set (biopsy cannula with stylet, core lock, ejector pin, depth gauge, and sample ejector guide)

1) Bone Marrow Aspiration and Biopsy

Sampling Site
- Posterior iliac crest (PIC) is the ideal site due to safety and ease of performance
- Anterior iliac crest (AIC) should be considered if the PIC is diseased or inaccessible because of morbid obesity or inability to position the patient
- Antero-medial tibia (<18 mo only). Not an ideal site in adults due to variable marrow cellularity and thickness of bony cortex.

Technique
Following, we explain bone marrow aspiration and biopsy technique using Bonopty® coaxial bone biopsy system via the PIC as the aspiration site
- Patient is prone position on CT table
- Obtain AP and lateral CT scout views of the pelvic region as indicated
- Adjust scan region to include the PIC and the anticipated region of needle placement. Obtain CT images, perhaps at 1–3 mm thickness or personal preference

- Select image location number where the posterior cortex is relatively flat and there is a parallel trajectory of intraosseous needle to the lateral bony cortices
- Utilize the measurement software of the CT scanner to measure the distance between skin and bone cortex. This is generally the depth needed for periosteal anesthesia and the coaxial cannula. Also, measure skin to intraosseous target depth whether random bone marrow or a discrete lesion. This is generally the length of the biopsy needle needed.
- A skin grid/marker could be placed to determine the exact penetration site on the selected image or alternatively measurement could be performed on CT images from midline by using the laser light of the CT machine
- Remove skin grid/marker
- Prepare and drape the skin in a sterile fashion
- Use drape sheath to provide larger sterile filed
- Cover CT machine control panel with sterile transparent plastic sheath
- Provide moderate (conscious) sedation
- Provide skin anesthesia with 25G needle. A 22G spinal needle may be needed to reach the deeper soft tissue and periosteum. Robust periosteal anesthesia is key for pain control during the procedure.
- The spinal needle can be removed or left in place to guide penetration cannula by a tandem needle technique
- Make a small skin incision (dermatotomy) at the puncture site with #11 scalpel blade
- Advance the penetration cannula and stylet under intermittent imaging along the same trajectory as anesthetized to reach the bony cortex. Stylet can be removed to provide more local anesthesia if needed.
- If unable to penetrate cortex with the diamond-tipped stylet, exchange the stylet with the drill stylet
- Apply pressure and advance the drill in a clockwise fashion to embed the drill and cannula within the cortex. The cannula should be pulled back slightly to reveal more of the drill tip for effective drill action. Image intermittently to see the drill breaching the inner cortex reaching the softer medullary region. Advance the penetration cannula a few millimeters into the bone.
- Slowly remove the drill stylet
- Attach 5-cc nonheparinized syringe and aspirate 3 cc of marrow over approximately 5 s. Hand this to technical assistant to prepare slides. Due to pressure change, this may be painful briefly for the patient, so warning them is advised.
- Attach 20-cc syringe preloaded with 1-cc heparin and aspirate 10–20 cc of marrow blood. The amount needed can vary depending on the tests that are planned. Pass this off to the technical assistant or heme/path tech. Clotting can occur, despite the heparin, so it's prudent to do this quickly. Consider inverting the syringe several times to the heparin. If aspiration is slow, the syringe may be intermittently removed and inverted for mixing.
- Place the biopsy needle and stylet into the penetration cannula slowly until you reach resistance
- Remove the stylet and advance the biopsy needle by applying pressure and rotating in a clockwise fashion. An ideal biopsy core is 2 cm or longer.
- Advance core lock wire (if available) through the biopsy needle to secure the sample
- Take the needle and core lock out by simultaneously rotating clockwise and withdrawing
- Attach sample ejector guide to the distal tip of biopsy needle and insert ejector pin to push out the sample retrograde through the Luer opening of the biopsy needle hub. This technique is associated with less crush artifact than pushing the sample out the biopsy end.
- Insert the sample into the relevant container. This is typically formalin, though certain tests may guide need for placement in another medium.

Useful Hints

- It is crucial to have the penetration set well aligned along the expected path before entering the bony cortex. Re-alignment could be very difficult when penetration cannula and drill are within the cortex.
- Drill is approximately 8 mm longer than penetration cannula and has an eccentric tip. This design provides a channel just wider than the external diameter of the penetration cannula of the coaxial system, so the cannula can be advanced into the cortex and can act as a coaxial introducer.
- Note that the bone is very sensitive to pressure changes. Reinsert or remove the stylet/drill gently. This could produce excruciating pain not controlled by local lidocaine due to sudden change in intraosseous pressure from a column of air being

pushed into the bone. Same situation could happen while quickly aspiration marrow to prevent clot formation. Be aware, alert the patient, and maintain sterility.
- In patients with extremely dense bone (or while sampling a sclerotic lesion) the tip of the beveled end of the needle may be bent during the procedure, making it difficult to insert the stylet or remove the sample. The device can be replaced midprocedure if indicated. Multiple attempts may be necessary.

1) Bone Lesion Biopsy

Primary Bone Lesions

Primary Bone Lesions
Seeding along the biopsy track is a serious concern while sampling primary bone sarcoma and other lesions in cases in which limb-sparing reconstructive surgery is being contemplated. The following notes will help prevent this phenomenon and its devastating consequences (AJR 1999;173:1663–71; AJR Am J Roentgenol 2008;190(5):W283–9).
- Consider biopsy as part of the surgical therapy and have a case-by-case discussion with the orthopedic oncologic surgeon
- The shortest path between the skin and lesion is usually preferred. A longer path may be taken to avoid a critical structure to be preserved after surgery
- Coaxial technique should reduce the possibility of track seeding
- The needle path must be close to the future surgical incision for limb-sparing surgery so that the needle track can be resected with the tumor
- Familiarity with compartmental anatomy is important to avoid contamination of a disease-free compartment. This is very important when these structures are needed for reconstructive surgery
- Avoid passing through intra-articular space or neurovascular structures
- Avoid the physes in skeletally immature patients to keep physis-sparing surgery an option
- A set of anatomically based guidelines is available that can help radiologists in decision making regarding biopsy pathways for lesions that may be treatable with limb-sparing surgery (Table 9-6) (Radiographics 2007;27(1):189–05). These guidelines are not applicable to all bone biopsy cases and are subject to variations based upon patients' clinical situations and surgeons' preferences.

Technique

Overall technique is basically the same as "Bone Marrow Aspiration and Biopsy." The main differences are as follows:
- There is no need for gross marrow aspiration
- After securing the penetration cannula through the bony cortex, advance the biopsy needle and stylet to reach the intraosseous lesion. Sequential CT imaging and/or use of depth gauge could control the penetrating depth of the needle.
- If indicated, remove the stylet and perform FNA by using an appropriate FNA needle, typically 22G. FNA may be interpreted near bedside by a cytopathologist to guide further decision making regarding sampling. Eg, if lymphoma is a consideration, a supportive preliminary reading may direct additional FNA for placement in RPMI solution for later flow cytometry. Or, the FNA result may be used to confirm satisfactory needle position for core biopsy. In cases where a cytopathologist is not available, or cases where FNA is not deemed necessary, then only core biopsies may be obtained.
- Follow the biopsy technique as described above

Useful Hints
- Lesions with an extraosseous soft tissue component or frank cortical loss can sometimes be biopsied under US
- If the bony cortex is destroyed, there is extraosseous soft tissue component, or the consistency of the intraosseous lesion is soft, then a standard "soft tissue biopsy needle" (eg, Temno) may be optimal or preferred for tissue sampling even though it's a "bone lesion." In cases with an intact cortex over a lytic lesion, the Bonopty penetration cannula can be used to access the lesion, and a soft tissue biopsy needle is then passed through the bone penetration cannula for tissue sampling.
- For dense sclerotic lesions, FNA could be performed after core biopsy, but may be low yield. Touch preps may also be made from core biopsies if onsite cytopathologic analysis is needed.
- The number of core samples needed for histopathologic analysis depends on the biopsy needle gauge, size of the core sample, size of the tumor, degree of necrosis or cystic changes, and whether there is request for additional testing (eg, cytogenetics). Typical histopathologic analysis is performed on samples preserved in formalin, while other testing may require placement in saline or RPMI solution.
- FNA can often differentiate a metastasis from a benign lesion; however, core biopsy is superior to FNA in determining tumor cell type and grade, which is necessary for the diagnosis of primary bone tumor/sarcoma.

Table 9-6 Recommended biopsy approach for musculoskeletal bone lesions

Location	Structure to Avoid	Approach	Positioning
Pelvis	Gluteus and rectus femoris m.	Anterolateral or posteromedial directly into iliac bone	Supine or prone
Femur: HN junction	GT bursa, femoral NV bundle, lateral femoral crx a.	Inferolateral subtrochanteric through the femoral neck	Decubitus partially abducted to align femoral neck with gantry plane
Shaft	Rectus femoris, Vastus intermedius, LIS, Sciatic n., Profunda femoris a.	Posterolateral just anterior to LIS	Prone or prone oblique
Distal	Joint capsule, NV bundle at popliteal fossa and adductor canal, medial and lateral superior geniculate a.	Lateral: Anterior to LIS avoid joint capsule Medial: Align with adductor tubercle through posteromedial vastus medialis	Supine with internal or external rotation
Tibia	Tibial tubercle; anterior, posterior, and peroneal NV bundles; deep peroneal n.; peroneus brevis and longus tendons	Anteromedial	Supine with internal or external rotation
Fibula	Same as in Tibia + CPN coursing around fibular neck	Proximal and distal; directly into bone through skin and subcutaneous fat. Shaft; just anterior or posterior to PIS	Supine with internal rotation
Humerus: Proximal	LHBT, radial n., cephalic v., deltopectoral groove, pectoralis m.	Anterior just lateral to cephalic v. and medial to LHBT through small portion of deltoid m.	Supine with external rotation
Shaft	Biceps m., cephalic v., spiral groove (radial n. and radial collateral a.)	Just posterior to biceps m. and cephalic v. through distal deltoid or brachialis m.	Supine with internal rotation
Distal	Cubital NV bundle, ulnar n., median n., recurrent radial a.	Directly into medal or lateral epicondyles or anterolateral through the brachialis m.	Supine with internal or external rotation
Radius	Radial and ulnar n. and a., median n., 1st extensor compartment tendons (AbPL, EPB)	HN junction: Posterolateral, distal; lateral through skin and subcutaneous tissue, Shaft: Lateral but variable case-by-case	Variable case-by-case based on tumor site
Ulna	Same as in radius + ECU tendon and m.	Olecranon: Direct posterior. Shaft: Posteromedial through small portion of flexor digitorum profundus m. Distal: Direct medial	Variable case-by-case based on tumor site
Spine	Spinal canal, NV bundle, aorta, SVC, IVC, uninvolved tissue compartments, peritoneal cavity, lung, trachea, esophagus	Cervical: Anterolateral for anterior lesions. Posterolateral for posterior element lesions. Thoracic: Costovertebral or Transpedicular Lumbar: Transpedicular Discitis: Posterolateral paravertebral	Prone for thoracic, lumbar and posterior elements of cervical spine. Supine for anterior cervical spine

Position to have needle entry site facing upward on the CT table.

HN, head–neck; GT, greater trochanter; Crx, circumflex; a, artery; n, nerve; v, vein; m, muscle; LIS, lateral intermuscular septum; CPN, common peroneal nerve; PIS, posterior interosseous septum; LHBT, long head of the biceps muscle tendon; AbPL, abductor pollicis longus; EPB, extensor pollicis brevis; ECU, extensor carpi ulnaris.

Metastatic Disease

Biopsy of metastatic lesions has different considerations compared with primary osseous lesions/sarcoma

Technique

Technique is generally same as "Primary Bone Lesion" biopsy. Attention to the following hints is recommended.

Useful Hints

- As a general rule, if the lesion is unlikely to be metastatic or if there is some doubt about the potential metastatic nature of the disease, plan the biopsy as if seeding of the biopsy track may occur. This way, if the lesion is a primary malignancy, surgical options are not affected.
- The biopsy track is less important in metastatic lesion biopsies because seeding is of questionable concern.
- When multiple lesions are present, select the lesion that is most amenable to biopsy, allowing the highest yield with the lowest complication risk.
- Use the shortest and most direct route, unless there's a critical intervening structure. Longer paths are worthwhile in these cases.
- Care should be taken to avoid vital structures such as neurovascular bundles

Osteomyelitis/Spondylodiscitis

Bone biopsy can be performed to confirm diagnosis and isolate organisms in cases of osteomyelitis/ spondylodiscitis. This may help with optimization of antibiotic therapeutic regimens. Although MRI has a high sensitivity and specificity for osteomyelitis and spondylodiscitis, tissue sampling remains the gold standard in diagnosis. However, recent reports have questioned the percentage yield of image-guided percutaneous biopsy (yield of approximately 41–48% (*Neurosurg Focus* 2014;37(2):E10; *AJR Am J Neuroradiol* 2017;38(10):2021–27) and only providing additional information to clinicians in 9.5% of spondylodiscitis cases (*Neurosurg Focus* 2014;37(2):E10) even when there is a high clinical suspicion for osteomyelitis. Therefore, the necessity for biopsy must be evaluated based on imaging and clinical findings on a case-by-case basis.

Technique

Technique is generally the same as for the "Primary Bone Lesion" biopsy. Attention to the following hints is recommended.

Useful Hints

Osteomyelitis

- Check clinical information such as presence of bacteremia/sepsis, other sources of infection, ESR and CRP trends, and WBC counts before approving the procedure. This will help to assess the medical necessity of the procedure.
- Attempts should be made to avoid overlying inflamed/infected soft tissues to decrease rate of sample contamination, especially in cases with large decubitus ulcers. You want to prevent soft tissue infection contaminating your bone sample.
- Specimen should be sent for microbiologic culture as well as histology, as the latter has higher positive yield (*AJR Am J Roentgenol* 2006;186(4):977–80)
- The more samples or greater volume of material obtained, the higher the diagnostic yield
- The effect of prebiopsy antibiotic treatment on culture results may have been exaggerated previously, but it is recommended to discontinue antibiotic therapy before the procedure for at least 24 h. However there is no consensus on this duration among different institutes.
- If there is a fluid component, this should be aspirated as it likely has a higher culture yield. Aspiration of 2 mL of pus has been shown to increase the diagnostic yield (*AJR Am J Roentgenol* 2007;188(6):1529–34), however, 2 mL aspirate is rarely obtained.

Spondylodiscitis

- The generally recommended sampling route for spondylodiscitis is a posterolateral paravertebral approach (Table 9-6)
- In planning the needle route, special attention should be made to avoid vital anatomical structures (Table 9-6)
- In suspected cases of spondylodiscitis, the adjacent subchondral bone should also be biopsied, in addition to the disc, as this is the expected site of origin of hematogenous discitis
- Prior antibiotic exposure, regardless of duration, does not significantly decrease diagnostic yield from percutaneous sampling for suspected active spondylodiscitis (*AJNR Am J Neuroradiol* 2017;38(10):2021–27; *Clin Radiol* 2016;71(3):228–34)

US Guided Procedures—General Principles

Indications
Ultrasound provides real time imaging of the pathologies and better visualization of soft tissues. This makes it an ideal procedural modality for pathologies related to nerves, tendons, and bursa.

Contraindications
Same as "Pain Management—General Principles"

Equipment
- Standard US machine with different probes based on depth of the target structure
- Generally, 12-MHz linear probe is used for global overview and 15-MHz "hockey stick" probe is used for higher resolution of small structures

Supplies
Same as "Arthrography-Supplies" with few changes:
- There is no need for 3-cc contrast syringe and the syringe for gadolinium mixture injection
- 10-cc syringes (×3–5) are needed for rotator cuff calcific tendonitis lavage, each filled with 4-cc sterile normal saline and 4-cc Lidocaine/Bupivacaine 0.25%
- Sterile probe cover

Medications
Different injectates are being utilized for bursal/perineural/peritendinous injections. There is no global consensus on the ingredients of these cocktails. Following recommended injectates follows clinical protocols at the University of Virginia, Department of Radiology and Medical Imaging.

Bursal/Peritendinous Injection
- 0.5 mL of Kenalog® 40 mg/mL + 1.5 mL of Bupivacaine 0.25%

Perineural Injection
- 0.5 mL of Kenalog® 40 mg/mL and 1.0 mL of Bupivacaine 0.25%

Complications
Same as "Pain Management—General Principles"

Useful Hints
- Adjust frequency output and focal depth to adequately assess both superficial and deeper structures
- Beam steering or compounding to avoid anisotropy and possible misdiagnosis

1) Bursal Injection

A) Greater Trochanteric Bursa
The greater trochanteric bursa is located posterolaterally along the hip subjacent to the gluteus maximus and superficial to the posterior facet of the greater trochanter

Technique
- Prepare the injectate (see above)
- Position patient in lateral decubitus, affected side up, and hip and knee joints flexed for patient comfort
- Place the transducer in transverse plane across the greater trochanter to obtain an image where the osseous landmarks include the anterior and lateral trochanteric facets, where the gluteus minimus and medius tendons insert, respectively
- Slide the transducer slightly posteriorly to see the more superficial large gluteus maximus muscle belly
- Insert a 22G spinal needle from a posterior to anterior approach and place the needle tip subjacent to the gluteus maximus muscle belly
- Take the stylet out, inject slowing, and observe distention of the bursa directly under ultrasound. Avoid injection and tracking of the injectate into the muscle belly.
- Take the needle out, clean the skin, and put on a small adhesive bandage

Useful Hints
- Do not use a smaller caliber needle, which can be difficult to direct and steer to deeper spaces under ultrasound
- Any intra-articular or periarticular injections of the hip are usually deep structures depending on body habitus. Using a curvilinear lower frequency transducer is recommended, such as 5–6 MHz.
- The other bursae around the trochanter are the subgluteus minimus, subgluteus medius, and ischiofemoral.

B) Ischial Bursa

The ischial bursa surrounds the hamstring complex tendon insertion onto the ischium. Pain associated with this bursa is usually associated with hamstring tendinosis or tearing. With ultrasound or MRI, findings of tendon abnormality are more often present than fluid within the bursa.

Technique

* Prepare the injectate (see above)
* Patient is placed in prone position
* Image the ischial tuberosity in both the transverse and longitudinal planes to evaluate for tendinosis or tears of the hamstring tendon complex
* Transverse plane:
  * Place the transducer across the ischium and hamstring tendon complex to obtain an ultrasound image where the bony cortex of the ischium is seen with tendon fibers
  * Introduce a 22G spinal needle from a lateral to medial or medial to lateral approach. Visualize the needle and place the needle tip superficial to the hamstring tendon complex.
* Longitudinal plane:
  * Place the superior aspect of the transducer at the ischial tuberosity and the inferior aspect along the proximal musculotendinous junction. The tendon fibers are seen as long linear array of fibers. On the ultrasound image, the ischium should be obtained as an osseous landmark, superiorly.
  * Introduce a 22G spinal needle from an inferior to superior approach and place the needle tip superficial to the hamstring tendon complex
* Take the stylet out, inject slowing, and observe distention of the bursa directly under ultrasound. Avoid intratendinous injection.
* Take the needle out, clean the skin, and put on a small adhesive bandage

Useful Hints

* To find the ischium, use the gluteal fold as a landmark. Place the transducer slightly above the fold and scan inferiorly with some mild added pressure to image just under the gluteal fold.
* The ischial attachment of the hamstring tendon complex is along the lateral and superior aspect of the ischium. The medial and inferior aspect of the ischium is the site of the adductor magnus insertion.
* Take care not to perform an intratendinous injection due to the possible risk of tendon rupture

C) Iliopsoas Bursa

The iliopsoas bursa is the largest bursa in the body and surrounds the iliopsoas tendon. Fluid from this bursa can extend into the pelvis along the tendon and iliacus muscle. It is typically an anterior hip joint collection.

Technique

* Prepare the injectate (see above)
* Place patient in supine position with the leg/hip in neutral to internal rotation
* Place the transducer across the anterior hip joint superiorly in transverse plane visualizing the superior aspect of the femoral head just inferior to the anterior acetabulum. The iliopsoas tendon is seen deep to its muscle belly sitting very close to the anterior hip joint capsule.
* Introduce a 22G spinal needle from a lateral to medial approach and place the tip just superficial to the tendon, along the superolateral aspect
* Take the stylet out, inject slowing, and observe distention of the bursa directly under ultrasound. Avoid intratendinous or intramuscular injection.
* Take the needle out, clean the skin, and put on a small adhesive bandage

Useful Hints

* Use the osseous landmark of the acetabulum and femoral head junction to find the best location
* It is easier to inject the iliopsoas bursa at the level of the anterosuperior hip. The inferior aspect of the tendon and bursa makes a deep oblique course to insert on the lesser trochanter, which is located deep and medial in the thigh.
* Abnormalities to the iliopsoas tendon and bursa can be related to a snapping hip where the tendon "pops or snaps" with contraction. Dynamic evaluation with ultrasound can be performed to directly visualize this abnormal motion with provocative maneuvers.

D) Subacromial–Subdeltoid (SASD) Bursa

The best way to locate and visualize the SASD bursa is to recognize that it is subjacent to the deltoid muscle

Technique
- Prepare the injectate (see above)
- Position the patient in lateral decubitus with the affected side up
- Place the transducer longitudinally along the anterolateral shoulder where the acromion, deltoid, greater tuberosity, and rotator cuff are visualized
- Introduce a 25G 4 cm needle (22G spinal needle if needed due to body habitus) from an inferior to superior approach
- Take the stylet out, inject slowing, and observe distention of the bursa directly under ultrasound. Avoid injecting into the rotator cuff tendons or deltoid muscle.
- Take the needle out, clean the skin, and put on a small adhesive bandage

Usual Hints
- Modified Crass maneuver (positioning the patient's hand along the posterior hip (hand in back pocket) with the elbow flexed and oriented posteriorly) could be used to locate the bursa and rotator cuff more anteriorly and not obscured under the acromion
- SASD bursitis is diagnosed on ultrasound by fluid and/or synovial thickening of the bursa

E) Baker's Cyst

The Baker's cyst (popliteal cyst/bursa) is bordered by the semimembranosus and the medial head of the gastrocnemius tendons. When this bursa is distended, it has a bilobed appearance between these two tendons. Baker's cysts are symptomatic due to pressure and size; however, can lead to severe pain/discomfort after rupture and extravasation. Ultrasound is used to diagnose, aspirate, and inject steroids/local anesthetic into a Baker's cyst.

Technique
- Prepare the injectate (see above)
- Place the patient in prone position
- Place the transducer transversely across the medial posterior knee at the level of the joint line/tibial plateau
- Confirm the presence of a fluid collection in the exact location between the semi-membranosus and the medial head of the gastrocnemius
- Perform cyst aspiration first with an 18G needle (4 cm or rarely spinal needle)
- Inject slowing and observing directly with ultrasound that there is fluid distension of the bursa, not into the surrounding muscles
- Take the needle out, clean the skin, and put on a small adhesive bandage

Useful Hints
- Confirming that the fluid collection is located between the semimembranosus and the medial head of the gastrocnemius makes the diagnosis of a Baker's cyst. Care must be made to confirm this by ultrasound or MRI. Other posterior knee fluid collections, bursae, ganglion cysts, and even tumors have been wrongly diagnosed as baker's cysts.

2) Perineural Injection

A) Morton's Neuroma Injection

Morton's neuromas are located most commonly in the third intermetatarsal space; however, it can be seen in the other intermetatarsal spaces

Technique
- Prepare the injectate (see above)
- Position the foot flat on the examination table with the knee flexed
- Place the transducer longitudinal along the affected intermetatarsal space
- Advance a 25G 4 cm needle from a distal to proximal approach, along the dorsal surface of the foot at the level of the metatarsal head–neck junction in-between the toes
- Inject slowing and observe the spread of the injectate in the intermetatarsal space
- Take the needle out, clean the skin, and put on a small adhesive bandage

Useful Hints
- Cold anesthetic spray is used for local anesthetic. Due to the added discomfort of lidocaine and the superficial location of the digital nerve, only cold anesthetic spray is used in our clinical practice.
- Color Doppler is used to visualize the artery and vein that course with the digital nerve to localize the injection site

B) Tarsal Tunnel (Tibial Nerve) Injection

The tarsal tunnel is a fibrosseous tunnel composed of the flexor retinaculum and the posteromedial tibia (Figure 9-3A). In this confined space, the tibial nerve can be

Figure 9-3 A: Transverse US image of the posteromedial ankle depicting normal structures within the tarsal tunnel from anterior to posterior including tibialis tendon (PTT), flexor digitorum longus (FDL) tendon, tibial artery and vein(s) (AV), tibial nerve (TN), and flexor hallucis longus (FHL) tendon covered by the flexor retinaculum (FR). White line shows the ideal needle route for TN block. **B:** Transverse US image of the anterior shoulder showing the long head of the biceps with the needle adjacent to the tendon within the tendon sheath. **C:** Shoulder radiograph shows hydroxyapatite deposition at the supraspinatus tendon. **D:** Longitudinal US image of the shoulder depicts area of calcification with posterior shadowing at the supraspinatus tendon with the tip of the needle approaching the area of calcification during rotator cuff calcific tendonitis lavage.

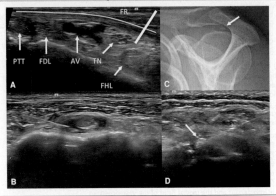

affected if there is increased mass effect on the nerve due to masses, cysts, varicosities, and tenosynovitis of the flexor tendons to name a few.

Technique
- Prepare the injectate (see above)
- Patient in supine position, place the affected foot is external rotation and the knee in flexion to scan the medial aspect of the ankle posterior to the medial malleolus
- Place the transducer in transverse plane superior to the medial malleolar tip (by approximately 2–3 cm). Place color Doppler to visualize the vessels that course with the tibial nerve.
- Advance a 25G 4 cm needle from a posterior to anterior approach into the tarsal tunnel. The needle is visualized coursing deep to the flexor retinaculum in close proximity to the tibial nerve.
- Inject slowing and observe the spread of the injectate surrounding the nerve
- Take the needle out, clean the skin, and put on a small adhesive bandage

Useful Hints
- To have maximum distribution of injectate along the nerve course, the volume of bupivacaine or lidocaine can be increased (by 3–5 mL)
- The tibial nerve is located superficial to the flexor hallucis longus (FHL) muscle. While scanning, the FHL can be located by flexing the great toe and observing the contraction of the muscle.
- Carefully observe that the needle tip is subjacent to the flexor retinaculum and not in the FHL muscle. Otherwise, the injectate will not distribute along the tarsal tunnel.
- Inject the tibial nerve proximally before it divides into the lateral and medial plantar nerves
- The nerve can be located in variable locations in relationship to the vessels. In addition to color Doppler, looking for the honeycomb multi-fasciculated appearance of the nerve is another distinction.

3) Peritendinous/Periligamentous Injection

A) Plantar Fasciitis
The thickening of the central band of the plantar fascia (PF) (>4–5 mm) is used to diagnose plantar fasciitis on ultrasound. The maximal area of tenderness is along the medial aspect of the plantar surface of the heel.

Technique

- Prepare the injectate (see above)
- Patient is prone with the foot on the table and not hanging off the edge to keep the plantar surface of foot as parallel to the examination table surface, as possible
- Place the transducer in the longitudinal plane to see the osseous landmark of the calcaneus with the PF attachment. A calcaneal enthesophyte (spur) is commonly present. Now the PF is localized, transverse plan imaging is performed by turning the transducer 90° at the area of maximal thickness of the PF.
- Introduce a 25G 4 cm needle from a medial to lateral approach and place the needle tip along the medial border of the PF
- Half of the injectate is placed superficial to the PF and the other half deep to the PF
- Take the needle out, clean the skin, and put on a small adhesive bandage

Useful Hints

- With US, confirm that the area of maximal tenderness is also the area of maximal thickness
- Measure the depth of the PF from the skin surface on the ultrasound image to localize where to place the skin entrance site of the needle along the medial heel
- In addition to steroid injections, chronic plantar fasciitis can also be treated nonoperatively with platelet rich plasma, dry needling, and percutaneous needle tenotomy with variable success

B) Biceps Tendon

The long head of the biceps tendon is injected within the proximal extra-articular groove

Technique

- Prepare the injectate (see above)
- Patient in supine position with external rotation of the arm
- Place the US transducer along the anterior superior aspect of the humeral head in the transverse plane with the biceps tendon and groove visualized in axial cross section (Figure 9-3B)
- Advance a 25G 4 cm needle (lateral to medial or medial to lateral approach). The needle tip is placed within the bicipital groove adjacent to the tendon.
- Inject slowing and observe the spread of the injectate within the groove and not intrasubstance in the tendon
- Take the needle out, clean the skin, and put on a small adhesive bandage

Useful Hints

- Check with color Doppler to determine the presence of vessels along the groove prior to the placement of the needle. Occasionally, a vessel is present along the lateral aspect of the bicipital groove.

C) Rotator Cuff Calcific Tendonitis

Calcific deposition of the rotator cuff have been treated with ultrasound guided barbotage or lavage

Technique

- 10 mL syringes (×3–5) are filled with 8 mL with lidocaine/bupivacaine and sterile normal saline (1:1 ratio). These syringes are used to pulse the fluid into the calcific deposit for lavage.
- Position the patient in lateral decubitus with the affected side up
- Advance an 18G 4 cm needle in the center of the deposition. Pulsations are performed with the syringe. The calcific material will return into the syringe due to the pressure within the calcific deposit.
- Leaving the needle in place, a new syringe can be exchanged when needed until the calcific deposit has been removed
- Fenestration of the area can also be performed once the lavage is complete
- After the lavage, a SASD steroid injection is performed to decrease post procedural pain (See above)
- Take the needle out, clean the skin, and put on a small adhesive bandage

Useful Hints

- The calcific deposition will appear on US as an area of globular echogenicity that usually shadows (Figure 9-3C and D)
- Only pass the needle once into the calcific deposit so that the pressure of the pulsing lavage flows back into the syringe. If multiple needle holes are created, a sieve is produced and the lavage is not effective.
- This technique is not an aspiration. The calcium will not pass through the needle with suction only.

D) Peroneal Tendons
The peroneus brevis and longus tendons share a common peroneal tendon sheath

Technique
- Prepare the injectate (see above)
- The lateral malleolus/distal fibula is scanned posteriorly along the retromalleolar groove, distal to the malleolar tip, and to the level of the cuboid for the peroneus longus and base of the fifth metatarsal for the peroneus brevis tendon
- Place the transducer in the transverse plane
- Advance a 25G 4 cm needle under the peroneal tendon sheath
- Inject slowing and observe the spread of the injectate within the sheath and not intratendinous
- Take the needle out, clean the skin, and put on a small adhesive bandage

Useful Hints
- When scanning the peroneal tendons, understand the oblique course of these tendons to optimize tracking the tendons while imaging. It is helpful to start at the retromalleolar groove of the distal fibula. Within the retromalleolar groove, the peroneus brevis is located closest to the fibula.

E) Posterior Tibialis Tendon (PTT)
The PTT is the largest tendon within the tarsal tunnel. It can be associated with medial ankle/foot pain and pes planus.

Technique
- Prepare the injectate (see above)
- Patient in prone position with the feet drape of the edge of the table
- Place the transducer in the transverse plane along the posterior medial ankle posterior to the medial malleolus. The first tendon just posterior to the medial malleolus is the PTT.
- Advance a 25G 4 cm needle from the posterior to anterior approach going through the flexor retinaculum
- Inject slowing and observe the spread of the injectate within the tendon sheath and surrounding the tendon and not intratendinous
- Take the needle out, clean the skin, and put on a small adhesive bandage

F) Common Extensor and Flexor Tendons of the Elbow
Common extensor and flexor tendons of the elbow are a frequent site of pain and tendinosis due to overuse or injury. Ultrasound guided injections can ensure precise placement of the needle and administration of steroids and local anesthetic.

Technique
- Prepare the injectate (see above)
- Place the patient in prone position. For visualization of the common extensor tendon origin, the arm is abducted, elbow flexed, and the forearm is down, and the thumb is directed up. To visualize the common flexor tendon origin, the arm is abducted, elbow flexed and the arm is up, and the small finger is directed up.
- For both tendons, place the transducer in the longitudinal plane. The osseous landmarks to look for are the epicondyles with their respective tendon attachment sites.
- Advance a 25G 4 cm needle from a distal to proximal approach with the needle tip placed along the superficial surface of the tendon near the osseous attachment
- Inject slowing and observe the spread of the injectate along the tendon and not intratendinous
- After the injection, needle tenotomy or fenestration can be performed. This time the needle is placed through the tendon and the tip contacts bone. Numerous fenestrations can be made.
- Take the needle out, clean the skin, and put on a small adhesive bandage

Useful Hints
- In addition to steroid injections, chronic epicondylitis can also be treated nonoperatively with ultrasound-guided platelet rich plasma, dry needling, and percutaneous needle tenotomy with variable success.

ARTERIAL INTERVENTIONS

PERIPHERAL VASCULAR DISEASE

Definition
- Reduction in tissue perfusion most commonly 2° to atherosclerosis (*Essentials of General Surgery.* 5 ed. Diseases of the Vascular System. 2013: Wolters Kluwer)
- Emboli and thrombi can incite significant morbidity/mortality (limb loss)
- Varying degrees/locations of lower-extremity (LE) vasculature stenoses

Etiology & Risk Factors
- Aortoiliac: Smoking, hypertension (HTN), hyperlipidemia (HPL). Often appears in 45–65-year-old patients (pts)
- Tibial occlusive: Diabetes (DM), chronic kidney disease (CKD), Age
- Vasculitides—Eg, Buerger's (thromboangiitis obliterans): Male, heavy smokers
  - Often concomitant with Raynaud phenomenon
- Cystic adventitial disease (85% of these cases affect popliteal artery) (*Overview of Acute Occlusion of the Extremities (Acute Limb Ischemia), in UpToDate.* 2017, UpToDate)
- External arterial compression (eg, thoracic outlet, entrapment syndromes)

Pathophysiology: Mechanisms of vessel lumen occlusion
- Atherosclerosis
  - Endothelial/Intimal injury → Macrophage & LDL recruitment manifests as foam cells → Fatty streak (intracellular lipid accumulation) → Smooth muscle cell migration via upregulation of PDGF & FGF → extracellular lipid accumulation (intermediate lesion) → intracellular + extracellular lipid encased by thin fibrous cap (atheroma) → fibrous cap becomes more proteinaceous and calcified to form a fibroatheroma (*Overview of Acute Occlusion of the Extremities (Acute Limb Ischemia), in UpToDate.* 2017, UpToDate)
  - Complications: Rupture, hemorrhage, thrombosis
- Thrombosis
  - Hemodynamic: Sepsis, hypotension, low cardiac output
  - Anatomic: Dissection, bypass graft, narrowing
- Emboli
  - 80% cardiac origin
    - Plaque, tumor, iatrogenic (*Vascular/Endovascular Surgery Combat Manual,* ed. G. Associates. 2013: Flagstaff)
  - Emboli destination: Femoral > iliac > aorta > popliteal
  - Highest morbidity and mortality due to acuity

Clinical Manifestation
- Intermittent claudication: Pain w/ increased use, relieved by rest
  - 50% recovery w/ conservative tx (*J Vasc Interv Radiol* 2006;17(9):1383–97; quiz 1398)
- Cramping
- Position-dependent ischemia—gravity aids in perfusion
  - Arterial lesions present with symptomatology one muscle compartment inferior
- Leriche syndrome: Impotence, LE claudication, buttock muscle wasting, and rest pain
  - If untreated, 50% need amputation for symptomatic relief (*J Vasc Interv Radiol* 2006;17(9):1383–97; quiz 1398)
- Ulceration: Insufficient arterial flow impeding wound healing

Fontaine Classification	
Grade	Symptoms
I	Insignificant occlusion
II	Mild claudication/limb pain (IIA >200 m tolerance, IIB <200 m tolerance)
III	Rest pain
IV	Gangrene/tissue death

- Gangrene
  - Dry: Gangrene with mummified tissue
  - Wet: Gangrene with purulence/infection

Physical Exam
- 6 P's: Pain, pallor, pulselessness, paresthesia, poikilothermia, paralysis
- Extremity alopecia
- Atrophic skin

- Muscle atrophy
- Ulceration/gangrene
- Position-dependent perfusion

Noninvasive Studies
Doppler Study
- Triphasic waveform: Normal vascular anatomy Systole -> vascular recoil -> diastole
- Biphasic/monophasic waveform: Stenotic arteries
  Loss of vascular recoil -> forward flow
- Upper extremity: Brachial, radial, ulnar
- Lower extremity: Femoral, popliteal, dorsalis pedis, posterior tibialis
- Always mark previously discovered Doppler signals to aid in future exams!

ABI	PAD Severity	Clinical Symptom
>1.3	Variable	Noncompressible arteries, severe atherosclerosis, claudication
0.9–1.3	Normal	None
0.7–0.9	Mild	Little/no claudication
0.4–0.7	Moderate	Claudication
<0.4	Severe	Rest pain/Tissue damage

Ankle–Brachial Index (ABI)
- Highest systolic blood pressure at which Doppler signals are audible after calf pressure cuff deflation divided by highest systolic brachial pressure measurement in similar fashion (Vascular/ Endovascular Surgery Combat Manual, ed. G. Associates. 2013: Flagstaff)
- Utilized for diagnosis/surveillance
- Limited utility in patients with less severe stenosis and calcified vasculature (Vasc Med 2006;11(1):29–3)
  - May underestimate PAD severity with incompressible vessels or patients with microvascular disease

Toe–Brachial Index (TBI)
- TBI utilized in PAD pt w/ noncompressible arteries
- TBI >0.65 normal & TBI <0.40 severe PAD (J Vasc Surg 1997;26(3):517–38)

Exercise Treadmill
- Measure degree of claudication functional limitation
  - Uncover claudication on normal ABIs
- Gardner protocol
  - Standard exercise regimen 2 mph, 12° incline, for 5 min/symptom limitation
- Pre/post-ABI measurements

Segmental Pressures
- ABI blood pressure cuffs placed throughout lower extremity (superior thigh, inferior thigh, calf, ankle)
- Pressure difference of 20 mmHg between cuffs is clinically significant (Vascular/ Endovascular Surgery Combat Manual, ed. G. Associates. 2013: Flagstaff; J Vasc Interv Radiol 2016;27(7):947–51)
- Limited utility in proximal limb stenosis

Pulse Volume Recordings
- Inflation of pressure cuffs to the point of venous occlusion but arterial patency, with subsequent Doppler auscultation of blood flow (J Vasc Interv Radiol 2016;27(7):947–51; J Vasc Interv Radiol 2003;14(9 Pt 2):S495–S15)
- ABI >1.30 (ie, calcified vasculature)
- Localize disease in reproducible manner
  - Not affected by calcium
- Most powerful noninvasive study
  - Continuous-wave Doppler testing as complement

Reflection Photoplethysmography
- Detection of optical radiation from peripheral blood pulsations
- Pulse wave transit time a measurement of arterial compliance
  - Delay of 23 mm ± 9 indicative of LE PAD (J Vasc Interv Radiol 2016;27(7):947–51)
- Diabetic/CKD patient subgroup

Imaging

Doppler Ultrasonography

- Localize region of occlusion, degree of occlusion, and blood flow characteristics (direction/peak flow velocity/flow turbulence)
  - Color Doppler, pulse Doppler
  - Waveform broadening indicative of stenosis
- Evaluation of native vessels, bypass grafts, areas of endovascular intervention
  - Aid in operative/endovascular planning
- Further evaluation of other arterial pathologies (aneurysms, dissections, malformations, embolisms, etc.)

CT Angiography (CTA)

- Less invasive, expedient, prevalent, inexpensive
- Static image of stenotic/aneurysmal areas (does not demonstrate flow dynamics)
  - Visualize calcific plaques
- 3D imaging of vasculature via computer reconstruction
- Diagnostic utility diminishes as contrast travels distally along lower extremities
- Iodine contrast may exacerbate renal insufficiency
- Radiation exposure

Magnetic Resonance Angiography (MRA)

- High-diagnostic accuracy for soft tissue vascular lesions
- Flow MRI an alternative to CTA in renal failure/CKD patients (*J Vasc Interv Radiol* 2016; 27(7):947–51)
- Static image of stenotic/aneurysmal areas (does not demonstrate flow dynamics)
- Scarce, expensive, prone to artifact due to acquisition time
- Risk of subcutaneous fibrosis with gadolinium contrast in CKD patients

Angiography

- Invasive dynamic imaging of vasculature
- Allows for simultaneous intervention
- Risk of procedural complications

Treatment of PAD

Medical

- Behavior modification (tobacco cessation, diet, & exercise)
- Nicotine replacement
- Podiatry, meticulous foot/wound care
- Rigorous glycemic control (HbA1C <7%) (*J Vasc Interv Radiol* 2006;17(9):1383–97; quiz 1398; *J Vasc Interv Radiol* 2003;14(9 Pt 2):S495–S15; *Arterial Interventions: Peripheral Arterial Disease. Interventional Radiology Procedures* 2017 5/10/2017]; Available from: https://www.irprocedures.com)
- Statin therapy (Goal LDL <70 mg/dL) (*J Vasc Interv Radiol* 2006;17(9):1383–97; quiz 1398; *J Vasc Interv Radiol* 2003;14(9 Pt 2):S495–S15; *Arterial Interventions: Peripheral Arterial Disease. Interventional Radiology Procedures* 2017 5/10/2017]; Available from: https://www.irprocedures.com)
- Antihypertensive medication (β-Blockers, ACEI)
  - Goal BP 140/90 or 130/80 in DM/CKD (*J Vasc Interv Radiol* 2006;17(9):1383–97; quiz 1398; *J Vasc Interv Radiol* 2003;14(9 Pt 2):S495–S15; *Arterial Interventions: Peripheral Arterial Disease. Interventional Radiology Procedures* 2017 5/10/2017]; Available from: https://www.irprocedures.com)
- Antiplatelet therapy (Aspirin, clopidogrel, cilostazol, pentoxifylline, prasugrel, dipyridamole)

Endovascular

- Balloon angioplasty, stenting, atherectomy
- Iliac and femoropopliteal lesions
  - Stenting for failed balloon/laser atherectomy/thermal interventions
- Pre- and postprocedural pressure gradient measurement

Surgical

- Endarterectomy
  - Limited application in PAD due to lesion size/extent
- Bypass procedure
  - Extensive plaques not amenable to endovascular intervention or endarterectomy (TASC C/D lesions)
  - Aortoiliac disease
    - Aortofemoral bypass initial approach
      - Femoral–femoral/Axillofemoral bypasses considered in patients with contraindications to abdominal surgery (hostile abdomen)
      - Extrabdominal bypasses with decreased patency rates

- Iliac endarterectomy, aortoiliac bypass, and iliofemoral bypass in cases with contraindication to aortofemoral bypass
- Infrainguinal disease
  - Use of autogenous veins ideal
    - Synthetic grafts if autogenous not available
  - Distal tibial/ pedal artery for distal anastomosis

ACUTE OCCLUSIVE DISEASE OF UPPER EXTREMITY

Background
- Diseases of the brachiocephalic vessels
  - Frequently asymptomatic
    - UE with extensive collateral circulation
    - Frequently incidental finding

Etiologies

Structural	Vascular	Iatrogenic	Trauma

– Thoracic outlet syndrome (see below)
 – Embolic
 – Cardiac: Afib, Valve Vegetations
 – Septic: Fever + multiple emboli (shower, varying temporally)
 – Paradoxical: PFO, VSD
	– Atherosclerosis
	   • Most common in US
	   • Tobacco
	   • Generally affects LEs
	 – Vasculitis
	   • Buerger's Disease
	   • Takayasu
	 – Connective tissue disease
	   • Scleroderma
	   • CREST
	 – Aneurysm
	 – Hypercoagulable state
	 – Fibromuscular dysplasia
	 – Raynaud's
		– Dialysis graft/fistula steal syndromes
		 – Radial or brachial artery caths
			– Blunt
			 – Penetrating
			 – Overuse (vibration, occupational, recreational)
			 30% of trauma to brachial art

- Thoracic outlet syndrome
  - Anomalous cervical ribs, muscular hypertrophy, external compression, trauma
  - Compression of neurovascular bundle
    - Interscalene triangle most common
  - Poor posture, repetitive abduction/external rotation
    - Baseball, swimming, tennis, etc.
  - Worsening with abduction and external rotation

Presentation
- UE claudication
- Rest pain
- Neurological symptoms
  - Affected extremity-inducing symptoms
  - TIA/Stroke
  - Vertebrobasilar insufficiency: Ataxia, vertigo, drop attacks *(Overview of Acute Occlusion of the Extremities (Acute Limb Ischemia), in UpToDate. 2017, UpToDate)*
- Coronary symptoms
  - Subclavian steal: Insufficiency symptoms in setting of UE activity *(Overview of Acute Occlusion of the Extremities (Acute Limb Ischemia), in UpToDate. 2017, UpToDate)*
  - Can induce coronary or vertebrobasilar symptoms depending on location/history
- History of repetitive UE use (occupational/recreational)
- Iatrogenic
  - UE arterial instrumentation
  - Sternal surgical history
  - Vasoconstricting medication

Physical Exam
- 6 P's (affected extremity): Pain, pallor, pulselessness, paresthesia, poikilothermia, paralysis
- Gangrene
- UE pulse asymmetry
- Blood pressure asymmetry
- Temperature/color changes in affected extremity
  - Allen test: Occlusion of radial/ulnar arteries with clenched fist, with subsequent occlusion of hand perfusion. Selective release of vessels will re-perfuse hand in complete palmar arch.

Diagnosis
- Inflammatory vessel disease
  - History
  - ESR, ANA, RF
- Hypercoagulable
  - PT, PTT, INR, Protein C&S, Factor V Leiden
- Cardiac
  - EKG
  - TTE/TEE: Central embolic etiologies
  - CXR
- Structural/ trauma
  - CTA—Calcium lesions visible
  - MRA—Soft tissue resolution
  - Doppler—Altered blood flow waveforms, reversal of flow in steal
  - Angiography—Gold standard dx w/ tx

Treatment

Medical
- Risk factor modification (smoking, diet, rest)
- Inflammatory—Prednisone, methotrexate
- Embolic—Antiplatelet therapy (aspirin, clopidogrel), anticoagulation (warfarin), antilipid (statin, niacin, fibrates)
- Arterial spasm—Nifedipine, prazosin, hydralazine

Endovascular
- Angioplasty/stenting
  - Atherosclerosis
  - Acute occlusion/trauma

Surgery
- Thoracic outlet—Neurovascular decompression
- Vertebrobasilar insufficiency—Carotid-subclavian bypass, subclavian transposition
- Acute occlusion/trauma—Bypass grafting, embolectomy
- Atherosclerosis—Endarterectomy, reconstruction, bypass
- Aneurysm—Coil, thrombin injection, resection

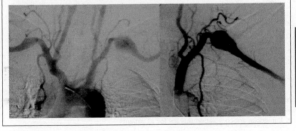

Figure 10-1 Thoracic Outlet Syndrome. Arterial aneurysmal dilatation of the left subclavian artery. Courtesy of Preet Kang.

ACUTE OCCLUSIVE DISEASE OF THE LOWER EXTREMITY

Background
- Ischemia to limb with immediate presentation (<2 w)
- Temporality of symptoms precludes compensatory collateral circulation response
  - Pts with chronic disease have more developed collateral circulation for compensation
- Urgent diagnosis and treatment warranted to reduce already significant morbidity and mortality
  - >4–6 h ischemia may lead to irreversible effects
- Emboli/thrombi occlude areas of arterial bifurcation/narrowing
  - Femoral > Arm > Aortoiliac > Popliteal > Visceral (*Essentials of General Surgery.* 5 ed. Diseases of the Vascular System. 2013: Wolters Kluwer)

Etiology

Cardiac	Vascular	Iatrogenic	Trauma
– Afib	– Arterial emboli	– Stent thrombosis	– Blunt
– MI	– Arterial thrombi	– Bypass thrombosis	– Penetrating
– Paradoxical emboli	– Atherosclerosis	– Prosthetic valve migration	
– Septic emboli	– Dissection	– Endovascular	
– Atrial myxoma	– Aneurysm	– Surgical	
– Valvular vegetations	– Hypercoagulable state	– Vasoconstricting meds	
	– Arteritis		

Presentation
- 6P's: Pain, pulselessness, pallor, paresthesia, poikilothermia, paralysis
- Claudication/rest pain
- Ulceration/gangrene
- Thromboemboli produce large vessel ischemia, atheroemboli produce microvascular ischemia
- Blue toe syndrome: Atheroemboli producing end small vessel occlusion commonly in digital arteries
  - Cholesterol shower embolism
  - Palpable/dopplerable DP/PT
- Bilaterality indicates more proximal source

Diagnosis

Rutherford Clinical Classification Acute Limb Ischemia (*J Vasc Surg* 1997;26(3):517–38)		
Viable	Threatened	Nonviable
– Mild pain	– Severe pain	– Insensate
– Neurovascularly intact	– Neurovascular deficits	– Complete neurovascular loss
– Intact arterial/venous flow	– Diminished venous flow	– No blood flow

(Reprinted from Rutherford RB, Baker JD, Ernst C, et al. Recommended standards for reports dealing with lower extremity ischemia: revised version. *J Vasc Surg* 1997;26(3):517–38. Copyright © 1997 Society for Vascular Surgery and International Society for Cardiovascular Surgery, North American Chapter, with permission.)

- Classification determines urgency of diagnosis vs. workup
  - Viable needs STAT workup to define location/severity of blockage
  - Threatened limbs need urgent operative management, with intraop arteriography for diagnosis
- Physical exam
  - Limb physical appearance
  - Femoral, popliteal, posterior tibialis, dorsalis pedis pulses
- Doppler US
- CT angiography
  - Intraluminal defect without contrast constitution distally
- Arteriography
  - Failure of contrast to flow distally

Treatment
- Management urgency dictated by classification of ischemia
- Immediate anticoagulation therapy for all patients

Viable extremity
- Percutaneous thrombolytic therapy for distal lesions
- Embolectomy for proximal lesions
- Recommendations based on the thrombolysis or peripheral artery surgery (TOPAS) and Surgery vs. Thrombolysis for Ischemia of Lower Extremity (STILE) (*Ann Surg* 1994; 220(3):251–66; discussion 266–8; *J Vasc Surg* 1996;23(1):64–73; discussion 74–5)
  - Percutaneous thrombolysis for ALI <14 d
    - Graft thrombus
    - Decreased amputation/complication of subsequent open procedure
    - Risk of intracranial hemorrhage
  - Mechanical thromboembolectomy as adjunct in <14 d
    - Primary tx in >14 d
    - 40% of thrombolysis pts need eventual embolectomy

Threatened
- Immediate operative revascularization
  - Aortobifemoral bypass ideal in aortoiliac disease *(Vascular/ Endovascular Surgery Combat Manual, ed. G. Associates. 2013: Flagstaff)*
  - With autogenous vein in infrainguinal bypasses if possible
- Embolectomy followed by completion angiogram
- Intraoperative lytic therapy for lesions nonamenable to embolectomy
- 4-compartment fasciotomy to prevent compartment syndrome in extended ischemia

Nonviable
- Systemic antibiotics
- Joint preserving amputation for prosthetic considerations

ACUTE MESENTERIC ISCHEMIA

Background
- Acute occlusion of visceral vasculature in patients usually with previously compromised vasculature
- Significant morbidity and mortality

Etiology

Cardiac	Vascular	Iatrogenic
– Arrhythmias (Afib)	– Arterial emboli (50%)	– Endovascular
– MI (hypokinesis)	– Arterial thrombi (25%)	– Surgical
– Paradoxical emboli	– Atherosclerosis	– Vasoconstricting
– Septic emboli	– Dissection	meds
– Atrial myxoma	– Aneurysm	
– Valvular vegetations	– Hypercoagulable state	
	– Arteritis	
	– Vasospasm	

Clinical Presentation
- Sudden onset of abdominal pain
- Intestinal angina
- Nausea/vomiting
- Hematochezia

Physical Exam
- Normal initially
- Progressive distension
- Progressive pain out of proportion to exam
- Nonlocalized abdominal pain
- Peritonitis associated with grave prognosis

Diagnosis
- Classic history and exam findings

Laboratory
- Leukocytosis
- Hemoconcentration (due to fluid shifts)
- Metabolic acidosis
- Elevated lactate

Imaging
- KUB—Ileus, Thickened bowel, Pneumatosis (advanced disease), Free air (grave)
- CT w/wo contrast
  - STAT confirmation
    - Delayed contrast study to evaluate vasculature
  - Diagnose arterial vs. venous etiology
    - Atherosclerosis
  - Thickened bowel
    - Pneumatosis (late grave sign)
    - Portal venous gas
  - Intraluminal contrast blush sign of bleeding
    - Intraoperative angiography
- ECHO (to investigate cardiac etiologies, when stable)

Treatment
Medical
- Fluid resuscitation
  - Correction of acidosis
  - Tx low flow states

- Vascular medications
  - Vasodilation
  - Removal of vasoconstrictive agents
- NGT decompression
- IV pain control
- Broad spectrum antibiotics
- Systemic anticoagulation
  - Heparin to prevent thrombus propagation

Surgical
- Immediate to prevent severe morbidity/mortality
- Emergent surgical resection of compromised bowel
  - Bowel exploration with intra-operative Doppler examination of visceral blood supply
  - Embolectomy
  - 2nd look procedure 24 h after for further evaluation/resection
- Endovascular thrombolysis/stenting/plasty interventions in less critical patients
  (Overview of Intestinal Ischemia in Adults. In: UpToDate. 2017, UpToDate)
- Arterial bypass

Figure 10-2 Acute Mesenteric Ischemia—Pneumatosis annotated by arrow.
Courtesy of Mohammed Al-Natour.

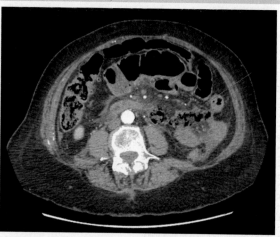

CHRONIC MESENTERIC ISCHEMIA

Background
- Compromised blood flow to vessels supplying visceral organs (Celiac, SMA, IMA)
- Collateral circulation may compensate for single major branch occlusion (gastroduo-denal/marginal artery)
  - 2-vessel disease/poor collateral circulation prone to symptoms
- Chronic symptoms with propensity for acute occlusion
- 15–20% in elderly >65 y *(Essentials of General Surgery. 5th ed. Diseases of the Vascular System. Wolters Kluwer; 2013)*

Etiology
- Atherosclerosis
  - Consistent with PAD risk factors (DM, tobacco, CKD)
  - Concurrent with CAD, CVD, PAD
- Median arcuate ligament syndrome: celiac trunk compression by median arcuate ligament
- Fibromuscular dysplasia
- Vasculitis (Takayasu, polyarteritis nodosa)

Clinical Presentation
- Postprandial intestinal angina
- Anorexia (pain/anxiety)
- Malabsorption
- Diarrhea
- Weight loss

Physical Exam
- Cachexia
- Pain out of proportion to physical exam
- Abdominal bruit

Diagnosis
- Classic H&P

Duplex US—Initially (Overview of Intestinal Ischemia in Adults. In: UpToDate. 2017, UpToDate)
- Limited by body habitus/bowel gas pattern
- Retrograde hepatic artery flow diagnostic

US Velocity Criteria

Artery	% Stenosis	Criteria
SMA	>70%	Peak systolic velocity >275 cm/s
Celiac	>70%	Peak systolic velocity >200 cm/s
Renal	>60%	Renal aortic ratio >3.5 (PSV in renal artery/PSV in adjacent aorta)
	>80%	Renal aortic ratio >3.5 & renal artery end-diastolic velocity >150 cm/s

CTA
- Concurrent evaluation of other abdominal processes
- Atherosclerotic burden
- Operative planning for clamping/bypass locations

Angiography
- Diagnostic/therapeutic utility
- AP/Lateral views for visuospatial anatomic identification and endovascular intervention

Treatment

Medical
- Risk factor modification (smoking cessation, HTN/HPL/DM management, etc.)
- Anticoagulation (ASA, clopidogrel, warfarin, cilostazol)
- Nutritional support/consult

Endovascular
- Balloon expandable stenting
  - Restenosis/continued symptoms common (70% patency 3 y vs. 90% bypass)
  (Overview of Intestinal Ischemia in Adults. In: UpToDate. 2017, UpToDate)
  - For ill patients not amenable to surgical bypass
    - Poor nutrition and foreseeable poor wound healing/postoperative course
  - Heavily calcified ostia may require retrograde stenting

Surgical
- Definitive treatment
- Endarterectomy
  - Disease concentrated in ostia
- Surgical bypass
  - Synthetic grafts standard therapy
    - Vein grafts in cases of infection concern
  - Bypass origin and destination need healthy vessel segments for implantation
  - Anterograde bypass
    - Origin superior to destination
    - Decreased kinking
    - Mimics physiologic arterial flow
    - Intraoperative morbidity due to aortic clamping
  - Retrograde bypass
    - Origin inferior to destination
    - Advantageous in patients with previous superior abdominal operations
    - Kinking risk
    - Intraoperative ease

Figure 10-3 Celiac and SMA Stenosis—Courtesy of Mohammed Al-Natour.

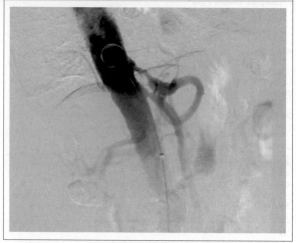

Figure 10-4 Chronic Mesenteric Ischemia—Vasculopath status post aortobifemoral bypass surgery with chronic mesenteric ischemia. CTA with celiac and SMA stenosis (**Left**). Angioplasty and stenting of celiac and SMA (**Right**). Courtesy of Preet Kang.

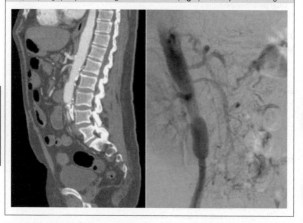

MANAGING BYPASS GRAFTS

- Neurovascular checks in immediate postoperative period
  - Q15m for 1 h, q30m for 1 h, q2h in PACU, q4h on floor
  - Mark audible Doppler sites for easy re-examination
  - Complications of bleeding, graft failure, compartment syndrome, reperfusion injury, swelling
- ABI/Duplex ultrasound examination on outpatient basis 1 mo, 3 mo, 6 mo, and 1 y postoperatively (*Vascular/ Endovascular Surgery Combat Manual*, ed. G. Associates. 2013: Flagstaff; *J Vasc Interv Radiol* 2016;27(7):947–51)
  - Subsequent annual surveillance with ABI/duplex ultrasound

- Lifelong medical therapy
  - Per case basis
  - Dual antiplatelet therapy (Aspirin, clopidogrel)
  - Anticoagulation (Heparin, warfarin)
- Acute thrombosis of graft
  - Clinical worsening w/ ABI confirmation
  - Requires immediate thrombolytic intervention
  - Continuous local thrombolysis via angiographically directed catheter infusion
  - Continuous fibrinogen monitoring
    - Fibrinogen >150: tPA at 1 μg/kg
      Fibrinogen 100–150: tPA at 0.5 μg/kg
      Fibrinogen <100: No tPA and initiate high intensity heparin ggt w/ bolus
  - Daily angiographic evaluation for resolution
  - Complications
    - Bleeding at catheter entry
      - Reinforce
      - Manual pressure
      - Pressure dressing
    - Hematoma
      - Discontinue tPA infusion

BASIC ENDOVASCULAR PRE-, PERI-, & POSTOP MANAGEMENT

Preoperative Management

Revised Cardiac Risk Index for Pre-operative Risk (N Engl J Med 1977;297(16):845–50)		
Factors	Scoring & Risk	
	0 pts	0.4%
+ High Risk Surgery	+1 pt	0.9%
+ History of Ischemic Heart Disease	+2 pts	6.6%
+ History of CHF	+3 pts	11%
+ History of CVD	+4 pts	11%
+ Preop tx with insulin	+5 pts	11%
+ Preop Cr >2 mg/dL	+6 pts	11%

History and Physical
- Indication for procedure
- Previous contrast allergies
- Renal failure
  - CKD highest risk factor for contrast nephropathy
  - Diabetes increasing cause of renal disease
  - Elderly with decreased renal function
- History of thrombotic/hemophilic disorders
- Current medications (namely antiplatelet/ anticoagulation)
- Pulse exam (dorsalis pedis, posterior tibialis, popliteal, femoral)

Laboratory Testing
- CBC
- BMP
- PT/PTT/INR
- Creatinine/GFR

Pre-Procedural Imaging
- Duplex ultrasound: PAD, DVT, AV fistula
- Arterial–brachial index (ABI): PAD
- Computed tomography: Aortoiliac disease, cerebrovascular disease, coronary artery disease
- Magnetic resonance: PAD, cerebrovascular disease

Preprocedural Orders
- NPO after midnight
- Hold antiplatelet/anticoagulation
- IV hydration (in renal failure/contrast allergy)
- Preop N-acetylcysteine in pt with Cr >2.0 mg/dL (*Arterial Interventions: Peripheral Arterial Disease. Interventional Radiology Procedures 2017 5/10/2017]; Available from: https://www.irprocedures.com*)

Intraop Care
- Continuous cardiac monitoring
- Blood pressure monitoring
- Conscious sedation with continuous pulse oximetry
- IV pain medication PRN

Complications

Vasospasm
- Vessel reaction to catheter/contrast irritation
- Treated with phentolamine, nitroglycerine (NTG)

Percutaneous Site Bleeding
- Immediate or delayed manifestation
- Bleeding complications prone to pseudoaneurysm/hematoma *(Arterial Interventions: Peripheral Arterial Disease. Interventional Radiology Procedures 2017 5/10/2017]; Available from: https://www.irproce- dures.com; Interventional Radiology: A Survival Guide. 4th ed. Principles of Angioplasty. Edinburgh: Elsevier; 2017)*
- Apply manual pressure and/or pressure dressing

Pseudoaneurysm
- Potential manifestation from post procedure bleeding, inadequate pressure post-procedurally, catheter trauma, poor healing
- 1% of diagnostic procedures, 3–7% of interventional procedures *(Int J Angiol 2007;16(3): 119–20)*
- Treated with observation (<1 cm), ultrasound-guided compression (1–2 cm), ultra-sound-guided thrombin injection (>2 cm), endovascular stent occlusion, surgical repair *(Int J Angiol 2011;20(4):235–42)*
- 1-mo followup after intervention

Hematoma
- Acute mass near percutaneous access site
- Size/location may cause compression of nearby vasculature or nerves
  - Paresthesia, pain, weakness
- Location/evolution dictates management
- Initial management with pressure application
  - Contained hematomas may tamponade
  - Severely symptomatic/rapidly evolving hematomas require urgent embolic/operative intervention

Radiocontrast-induced nephropathy (RCIN): Increased in serum creatinine of 0.5 mg/dL or 25% increase within 48 h after contrast administration *(World J Cardiol 2012;4(5):157–72)*
- 12–14% of procedures requiring radiographic contrast (prevalence in diabetic patients) *(World J Cardiol 2012;4(5):157–72)*
- Prevention via review of history, hydration, minimizing contrast load, alternative contrast agents (CO_2)
  - Gadolinium risk in renal dysfunction
- Maximum radiographic contrast dose (MCD): 5 mL contrast/kg (maximum 300 mL)
- Preprocedural hydration, steroid/antihistamine administration

Dissection
- Intimal tear creating intraluminal flap
  - Propagation of dissection may occlude nearby vessels
- Aortic dissection during diagnostic/interventional cardiology procedures was approximately 0.06% *(Circulation 2015;131(24):2114–9)*
- Treated with 3–5 min of balloon inflation, or stenting in refractory cases
  - Completion angiography to confirm resolution
- Surgical intervention in refractory cases

Rupture
- Contrast extravasation with angiography
- Traumatic advancement of catheter/guidewire or excessive angioplasty inflation
- Monitor hemodynamic status, check coagulation screen, T/S, resuscitate as needed
- Treated with 3–5 min of balloon expansion
  - Apply stent over extravasation site if balloon fails
  - Repeat angiogram for extravasation evaluation
- Surgical intervention in refractory/emergent cases

Embolism
- Via thrombosis/foreign body
- Catheter directed heparin ggt, aspiration catheter
- Vascular surgical intervention in refractory cases

Postoperative Care
- Strict supine bed rest for 4 h
- Neurovascular checks (q15 min for 1 h, q30 min for 2 h, q1h >3 h)
- Hemodynamic monitoring: BP, CBC, Op site surveillance for hematoma
- Kidney function monitoring: UOP, BMP
- ± Hospital admission
  - Hypertensive
  - Coagulopathic
  - Oliguria
  - Unstable diabetes
  - Metabolic derangements
  - Concerning clinical symptoms (nausea/vomiting)

ANGIOGRAPHY

Introduction
- The injection of radiopaque contrast agent in blood vessel lumen to dynamically visualize arterial/venous blood flow.
- Use to delineate arterial/venous anatomy
- Visualize areas of blood extravasation

Indications

Obstructions
- Cerebrovascular stenosis, ischemic stroke
- Coronary artery disease, angina, myocardial infarction
- Mesenteric ischemia (*Essentials of General Surgery.* 5 ed. Diseases of the Vascular System. 2013: Wolters Kluwer; *Overview of Intestinal Ischemia in Adults.* In: *UpToDate.* 2017, UpToDate)
- Renal stenosis, fibromuscular dysplasia, renal artery hypertension
- PAD, aortoiliac disease, acute limb ischemia (*Overview of Acute Occlusion of the Extremities (Acute Limb Ischemia),* in *UpToDate.* 2017, UpToDate)

Hemorrhage
- Trauma (*Essentials of General Surgery.* 5 ed. Diseases of the Vascular System. 2013: Wolters Kluwer; *Vascular/Endovascular Surgery Combat Manual,* ed. G. Associates. 2013: Flagstaff; *Interventional Radiology: A Survival Guide.* 4 ed. Principles of Angioplasty. 2017, Edinburgh: Elsevier)
- Hemorrhagic stroke
- Gastrointestinal bleeding
- Retroperitoneal bleeding

Tumor Blood Supply for Embolization
Fistula Evaluations (*Arteriovenous Fistulas: Etiology and Treatment.* Endovascular Today 2012 7/25/2017]; Available from: http://evtoday.com/2012/04/arteriovenous-fistulas-etiology-and-treatment.)
- Hemodialysis
- Aortoenteric
- Arteriovenous fistulas (carotid-cavernous, dural, pulmonary, hepatic, gastrointestinal)
  - Increase in size if untreated
- Arteriovenous malformations (cerebral, hepatic, pulmonary, gastrointestinal)
- High flow resistance, pain, ulceration, ischemia (*Interventional Radiology: A Survival Guide.* 4 ed. Principles of Angioplasty. 2017, Edinburgh: Elsevier)
  - Hemorrhagic Telangiectasia
  - Osler–Weber–Rendu syndrome

Basic Vascular Access and Angiography Operative Technique

Positioning and Prep
- Supine positioning
- Sterile preparation of groin—Prior to percutaneous access
- Localization of desired vessel—Via palpation or ultrasound guidance (Femoral: Middle of medial 1/3 femoral head)
- Analgesia—Infiltration of skin with 2% lidocaine with 22G needle

Seldinger Technique (*Handbook of Interventional Radiologic Procedures.* 2nd ed. New York: Little, Brown and Company; 1996)
- Seldinger needle-guided access of blood vessel (21G, 2.75 in, angled 40°)
- Remove stylet to visualize return of blood to confirm access
- Introduction of 0.018" guidewire into vessel via implanted needle lumen. **Do not** force guidewire.
- Removal of implanted needle with guidewire securing access
- Introduction of vessel 5F transitional dilators with subsequent placement of working sheath (6F–7F)

- Serial introduction of guidewires under fluoro guidance as needed via sheath lumen (Bentson or hydrophilic to reduce plaque disruption)
- Catheter selection depends on vasculature and access.

Catheter Access of Desired Vessel (*PocketRadiologist: Inventional Top 100 Procedures.* 1st ed. A. Inc. 2003, Salt Lake City, Utah: W.B. Saunders Company)

- Perform thoracic or abdominal aortogram with branch/bilateral extremity runoffs using a pigtail or multi-side hole catheter.
  - Thoracic aorta: 45°–60° LAO and PA views, 25 cc/40 s for 40 cc contrast non-trauma with digital subtraction angiography (DSA), 30 cc/s for 60 cc trauma with DSA
  - Abdominal aorta: PA view for extremities, lateral view for viscera, oblique view for renal, 15 cc/s for 30 cc contrast
- Selective vessel catheterization using hydrophilic 0.035" angled/3 mm J-tip guidewire and curved 4F–5F supporting catheter, subsequent contrast injections for further characterization of distal extremity occlusions.
  - Upper extremity: Subclavian/brachial catheter access, 100–200 µg intra-arterial nitroglycerine (NTG) for vasodilation, Visipaque contrast (less pain/movement), warm extremity
  - Iliac: Contralateral percutaneous access, 10 cc/s for 20 cc contrast
  - Infrapopliteal: Contralateral percutaneous access, 150–200 µg intra-arterial NTG and Visipaque contrast
  - Foot: Use DSA and collimation, Visipaque contrast, 100–300 cc NTG, warm extremity
- Depending on level of disease outlined in previous imaging
  - Utilize known bony anatomic landmarks for vascular branch points to minimize contrast and radiation
- Multiple views required for evaluation of peripheral stenosis
  - Iliac: 30° RAO/LAO
  - Infrapopliteal: Selective angiography, oblique images to open intraosseous space
  - Trans-stenotic pressure gradients in uncertain cases
- Superselective catheterization allows for decreased contrast dosage and improved study sensitivity

Closure

- Manual compression of closure site for 20 min without closure device. (*Arterial Interventions: Peripheral Arterial Disease.* Interventional Radiology Procedures 2017 5/10/2017]; Available from: https://www.irprocedures.com; *Interventional Radiology: A Survival Guide.* 4 ed. Principles of Angioplasty. 2017, Edinburgh: Elsevier) Do not occlude vessel flow.
- Refer to closure device manufacturer recommendations for indications, deployment, and compression time.

Figure 10-5 Endovascular Complications—Iliac artery rupture with contrast extravasation (**Left**), Dissection of left external iliac (**Right**). Courtesy of Preet Kang.

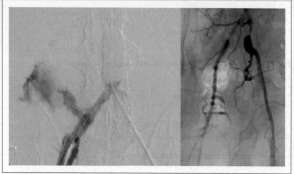

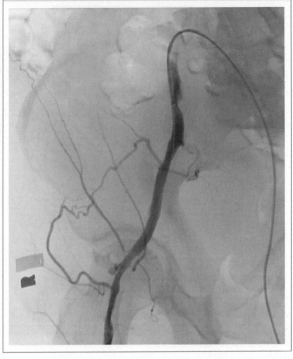

Figure 10-6 Right Common Femoral Artery Pseudoaneurysm—Pseudoaneurysm seen during right iliac stenting from left CFA access a day later. Courtesy of Preet Kang.

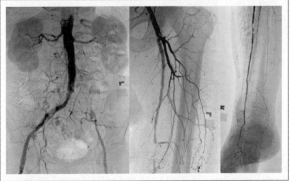

Figure 10-7 Peripheral Vascular Disease—Aortoiliac disease (Left), superior femoral artery occlusion (Middle), anterior tibial artery occlusion (Right). Courtesy of Preet Kang.

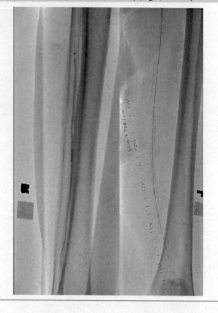

Figure 10-8 Endovascular Interventions—Angioplasty of anterior tibial artery (**Left**), stent placement of superficial femoral artery (**Right**). Courtesy of Preet Kang.

Angioplasty

Trans-Atlantic Inter-Society Consensus (TASC) II Classification for Aortoiliac and Femoropopliteal Disease and Preferred Treatment *(J Vasc Surg 2007;45(Suppl S):S5–S67)*			
Type A – Stenosis (**sten**) of common iliac artery (CIA) – Single ≤3 cm external iliac artery (EIA) stent	Type B – ≤3 cm sten infra-renal aorta – Unilateral CIA occlusion (**occl**) – Sten 3–10 cm of EIA distal to CIA – Unilateral EIA occl beyond CIA/internal iliac artery (IIA) orifice	Type C – Bilateral CIA occl – 3–10 cm bilateral EIA occl – EIA sten/occl extending into CIA/IIA – Calcified EIA occl	Type D – Infrarenal aortoiliac occl – Diffuse aortoiliac disease – Multiple diffuse sten – CIA/EIA occl – Bilateral EIA occl – Iliac sten with AAA
Endovascular	Endovascular	Surgery > Endovascular	Surgery
Type A – Single lesion ≤10 cm in length – Single occl ≤5 cm length	Type B – Mult sten/occl ≤5 cm – Single sten/occl ≤15 cm excluding infrageniculate popliteal artery – Heavily calcified occl ≤5 cm – Single popliteal sten	Type C – Multiple sten/occl totaling >15 cm – Recurrent stenosis/occl after failing treatment	Type D – Chronic total occl CFA/SFA (>20 cm, involving popliteal artery) – Chronic total occl popliteal artery and trifurcation vessels
Endovascular	Endovascular	Surgery > Endovascular	Surgery

(Reprinted from Norgren L, Hiatt WR, Dormandy JA, et al. Inter-Society Consensus for the Management of Peripheral Arterial Disease (TASC II). *J Vasc Surg* 2007;45(1 Suppl):S5–67. Copyright © 2007 The Society for Vascular Surgery, with permission.)

Background

Angioplasty: Mechanical disruption of plaque allowing for intimal remodeling and restoration of blood flow (*Vascular/ Endovascular Surgery Combat Manual, ed. G. Associates. 2013: Flagstaff; J Vasc Interv Radiol 2006;17(9):1383–97; quiz 1398; Arterial Interventions: Peripheral Arterial Disease. Interventional Radiology Procedures 2017 5/10/2017]; Available from: https://www.irprocedures.com*)

- Mechanically induced fissures allow for increased diameter
- Does NOT change plaque volume

Results

- Faglia et al. studied 993 diabetic CLI pts w/ infrapopliteal disease treated with angioplasty primarily, with 8.8% symptom recurrence and 1.7% major amputation at 26.2 months. (*Eur J Vasc Endovasc Surg 2005;29(6):620–7*)
- Better endovascular outcomes in diabetics over ESRD pts w/ wound healing and limb salvage, no difference in 1–3 y survival. ESRD vessel calcinosis suspected for poor results.
- Poor endovascular outcomes with chronically ill/immobile or dementia pts (mortality, mobility, independence) (*J Vasc Surg 2006;44(4):747–55; discussion 755–6*)
- Cutting balloon angioplasty (CBA), cryoplasty, and Excimer laser-assisted angioplasty may offer superior results to bare angioplasty in select pts (*Catheter Cardiovasc Interv 2004; 61(1):1–4;l; Chill trial J Endovasc Ther 2009;16(2 Suppl 2):II19–II30; Semin Vasc Surg 2006;19(2):96–101; Semin Vasc Surg 2007;20(1):29–36; J Vasc Surg 2007;46(2):289–95*)

Indications

Nonulcerated/nongangrenous extremity

Failed conservative therapy (*J Vasc Interv Radiol 2006;17(9):1383–97; quiz 1398; J Vasc Interv Radiol 2003; 14(9 Pt 2): S495–S15*)

- Symptoms despite behavioral modification/pharmacologic interventions

Poor Surgical Candidates

Single infrarenal aortic stenosis (*J Vasc Interv Radiol 2006;17(9):1383–97; quiz 1398; J Vasc Interv Radiol 2003;14(9 Pt 2):S495–S15*)

- <3 cm lesions
- 90% short-term success, long-term outcomes unknown.
- Exclusive angioplasty a historical practice, current knowledge favors stenting

Iliac Stenosis

- <5 cm lesions
- 95% short-term success, >80% 5-y patency (*J Vasc Interv Radiol 2006;17(9):1383–97; quiz 1398; J Vasc Interv Radiol 2003;14(9 Pt 2): S495–S15*)
- Stenting for failed balloon dilation/recurrent lesions
- Best results with focal lesions, nondiabetic
- Exclusive angioplasty a historical practice, current knowledge favors stenting

Femoropopliteal Stenosis

- <5 cm lesions
- Best results w/ nondiabetic, minimal vascular disease, stenosis
- Stenting for failed balloon dilation/recurrent lesions
- Limitations of stenosis near SFA origin/distal popliteal

Infrapopliteal Stenosis

- <1 cm lesions
- Reserved for significant rest pain
- Poorer outcomes

Focal Stenosis of Bypass Grafts

Contraindications (*J Vasc Interv Radiol 2003;14(9 Pt 2):S495–S15*)

- Multifocal stenosis
- Total occlusion
- Eccentric stenosis
- Long-segment stenosis/occlusion
- Distal vessels

Angioplasty Operative Technique (*Interventional Radiology: A Survival Guide. 4th ed. Principles of Angioplasty. Edinburgh: Elsevier; 2017; PocketRadiologist: Inventional Top 100 Procedures. 1st ed. A. Inc. 2003, Salt Lake City, Utah: W.B. Saunders Company; Atlas of Vascular Anatomy: An Angiographic Approach. 2th ed. Philadelphia, PA: Lippincott Williams & Wilkins; 2007*)

Positioning and Prep

- Supine positioning
- Sterile preparation of skin—Contralateral to site of pathology
- Analgesia—2% lidocaine, 22G needle

- Localization of desired vessel—Via palpation or ultrasound guidance

Seldinger Technique Vascular Access—21G 2.75-in needle, 0.018" guidewire, 6F–7F sheath introduction

Intraoperative Angiogram—For lesion assessment and planning
- Save angiogram imaging to mark monitor for lesions
  - Do NOT move after marking
- Compare marked lesions against live fluoroscopy during wire/balloon advancement throughout case
- Utilize for lesion measurement and balloon selection
- Short and concentric lesions favorable to angioplasty. Long/multifocal and eccentric lesions favor stenting/surgery

Proximal-Distal Tracking
- Advance 0.035" angled tip/steerable hydrophilic guidewire and angled-tip catheter beyond lesion to attain tracking
- Exchange catheter for extra stiff Amplatz for balloon support

Introduce Balloon
- Over guidewire with markers encompassing lesion
- Common iliac balloon size: 7–10 mm
  External iliac balloon size: 5–8 mm

Anticoagulate—Prior to intervention with heparin (3000–5000 units), APTT >250 s

Inflate Balloon—Under fluoroscopic guidance to monitor for dilation and balloon migration

Inflation Pressures (Atmospheres (atm))
- Upper extremity: 2–4 atm
- Iliac: 8–10 atm

Inflation Times
- Stenosis: 1–2 min, until waist resolves
- Occlusion: 2–3 min
- Dissection: 3–5 min

Balloon Deflation and Removal

Completion Angiography/Pressure Gradient Measurement
- Goal of <30% residual stenosis, <5 mmHg pressure gradient
- Evaluation of complications (dissection, rupture, embolization)

Intraoperative Difficulty (*Arterial Interventions: Peripheral Arterial Disease.* Interventional Radiology Procedures 2017 5/10/2017]; Available from: https://www.irprocedures.com; *Interventional Radiology: A Survival Guide.* 4 ed. Principles of Angioplasty. 2017, Edinburgh: Elsevier)

Vasospasm
- Vessel reaction to catheter/contrast irritation
- Treated with phentolamine, NTG

Difficult Proximal-Distal Access
- Utilizing stiffer guidewires/smaller catheters
- Do NOT force access—Risk vascular injury and embolism

Balloon Migration During Inflation
- Guidewire fixation
- Longer balloons for traction

Balloon Rupture
- Removal of defective balloon and repeat attempt
- Trial with more durable balloon

Dilation Resistant Stenosis
- Attempt with high-pressure balloon
- Cutting balloon trial

Nondeflating Balloon
- Syringe aspiration
- Tap system removal
- Chiba needle puncture

Difficult Balloon Extraction
- Ensure full deflation
- Anterograde/retrograde insertion of larger sheath to fully reduce balloon
- Embolized balloon fragments need to be recovered endovascularly or surgically

Complications

- Stenosis recoil
  - Recoil after angioplasty
  - Re-attempt angioplasty with full inflation if safe
  - Stenting in refractory case

STENTING

Background

- Stenting: Insertion of long term exogenous cannula to maintain luminal patency
- Primary stenting: Stent placement is primary goal of procedure Secondary stenting: Stent placement as a result of an uncertain angioplasty outcome
- Use covered stents to manage aneurysms/leaks
- Use self-expanding/balloon expanding for vascular stenosis

Aortoiliac Disease Results

- Dutch Iliac Stent Trial (DIST) compared primary angioplasty with secondary stent placement vs. primary stent placement
  - No difference short-/long-term patency, but primary PTA w/ 43% secondary stenting and 7% complication rate (*Lancet* 1998;351(9110):1153–9; *Radiology* 2006;238(2):734–44)
- Meta-analysis of 2116 patients showed superior technical success (96% vs. 90%) and 4-y patency (77% vs. 64%), without significant complication difference, of stenting over angioplasty (*Radiology* 1997;204(1):87–96)

Indications	Contraindications
– Restenosis	– Tortuous anatomy
– Refractory to angioplasty	– Stenting site adjacent to vital vessels
– Iliac occlusion	– High migration risk
– Aneurysm	
– Stricture	
– High-risk lesion	
– Embolization	
– Renal artery stenosis	
– Carotid artery stenosis	

Femoropopliteal Disease Results

- RESILIENT trial compared stenting vs. PTA (*Results of the RESILIENT trial: a randomized comparison of PTA to Lifestent.* Transcathetr Ther.; 2008)
  - 1-y patency 80% vs. 38%
  - Freedom from revascularization (FFR) 87% vs. 46%
  - Initial PTA success with similar outcomes to stenting
- Femoral Artery Stenting Trial (FAST) showed no difference in FFR (18.3% vs. 14.9%) or restenosis (38.6% vs. 31.7%)
- Current knowledge favors femoropopliteal PTA first with lifestyle modification, exercise, and medical therapy. 21%–35% with PTA failure can be stented. (*Handbook of Interventional Radiologic Procedures.* 4th ed. Lippincott Williams & Wilkins; 2011)

Infrapopliteal Disease Results

- Drug-eluting stents (DES) showed superior results to bare metal stents (BMS) with 1-y restenosis (63.3% vs. 21.4%), major amputation (0% vs. 10%), and FFR (0% vs. 23.3%) (*J Endovasc Ther* 2007;14(2):241–50; *Comparison of sirolimus-eluting vs. bare-metal stents for the treatment of infrapopliteal obstructions.* Eurointervention; 2006)
- Self-expanding nitinol stents demonstrated 95.9% limb salvage and restenosis rate of 20.45% at 1 y (*J Cardiovasc Surg (Torino)* 2007;48(4):455–61)

Stenting Operative Technique (*Arterial Interventions: Peripheral Arterial Disease.* Interventional Radiology Procedures 2017 5/10/2017]; Available from: https://www.irprocedures.com; *Interventional Radiology: A Survival Guide.* 4 ed. Principles of Angioplasty. 2017, Edinburgh: Elsevier)

Analysis of Preoperative Imaging—For planning and stent selection

- Small stent at risk for migration, large stents at risk for occlusion/thrombus
  - For aneurismal disease, implantation site diameters must be 10–20% larger. For stenosis, oversize by 1 mm.
- Selection of appropriate stent for pathology

Supine positioning and sterile prep/drape—Contralateral groin

Localization of desired vessel—Via palpation or ultrasound guidance

Seldinger technique vascular access—21G 2.75-in needle, 0.018" guidewire, introduction 6F–7F working sheath

Intraoperative angiogram—For lesion assessment and operative course, similar to angioplasty
- Save angiogram imaging to mark monitor for lesions. Compare during live fluoroscopy w/ wire/balloon advancement.

Proximal-distal tracking—Advance of 0.035" angled tip/steerable hydrophilic guidewire and angled-tip catheter beyond lesion to attain proximal and distal tracking. Prepare stent according to manufacturer instructions.

Anticoagulate—Prior to intervention with heparin, APTT >250 s

Introduce stent—Over guidewire w/ markers encompassing lesion

Deploy stent—Under continuous fluoroscopy
- Self-deploying stents automatically expand to form
- Balloon-deployed stents require angioplasty for form expansion

Angioplasty—To fully secure and form stent to vessel wall

Complete balloon deflation and removal

Completion angiography/pressure gradient measurement

Intraoperative Difficulty (Arterial Interventions: Peripheral Arterial Disease. Interventional Radiology Procedures 2017 5/10/2017]: Available from: https://www.irprocedures.com; Interventional Radiology: A Survival Guide. 4 ed. Principles of Angioplasty. 2017, Edinburgh: Elsevier)

Vasospasm
- Vessel reaction to catheter/contrast irritation
- Treated with phentolamine, NTG

Difficult Proximal-Distal Access
- Utilizing stiffer guidewires/smaller catheters (Amplatz, Lunderquist)
- Do NOT force access—Risk vascular injury and embolism
- Presenting angioplasty if feasible
- Proximal–distal rendezvous

Stent Insecure on Balloon
- Do not deploy stent if intrainflation migration occurs
- Attempt stent retrieval via balloon deflation/inflation
  - Pin the migrating stent against stenosis (if safe) when recapturing
- Attempt with new stent

Stent Does not Deploy from Balloon
- Attempt complete reinflation
- Attempt with new stent

Stent Migration
- Check catheter shaft/groin sheath
  - Withdraw stent into sheath and replace apparatus
- Distal migration
  - Locate stent and pass guidewire through it
  - Retrieval via angioplasty balloon or GooseNeck snare
- Stent migrates on lesion
  - Do not fully deploy stent
  - Apply traction/pressure to adjust stent for optimal coverage in partially deployed stents
  - May consider additional stent placement if optimal coverage not possible with one stent
- Insufficient stent diameter risk factor for migration

Complications

"Jailing a Vessel"—Options
- Aberrant vessels can be sacrificed
  - Eg, small renal accessory
- Risk ischemia if an essential vessel is compromised
  - Stent-graft repair (extra-anatomical grafting)
    - Fem–fem crossover
  - Increase length of anchorage in more complex cases involving carotid/subclavian bypass grafts or mesentery/renal bypass
    - Use fenestrated/branched grafts
- Unwanted vessels may perpetuate pathology
  - Eg, vessel feeding into Type II endoleak

ABDOMINAL AORTIC ANEURYSMS

Background
- Aorta diameter ~3 cm
- Definition: 1.5 factor diameter increase of vessel compared to native vessel (Vascular/Endovascular Surgery Combat Manual, ed. G. Associates. 2013: Flagstaff; Management of Asymptomatic Abdominal Aortic Aneurysm. In: UpToDate. 2017, UpToDate)

- ~10% growth/y or 0.3 cm/y *(Management of Asymptomatic Abdominal Aortic Aneurysm. In: UpToDate. 2017, UpToDate)*. Growth associated w/ increasing aortic tortuosity/increasing branch involvement
- Aneurysmosis: Multiple aneurysms. AAA associated with 16% unilateral and 12% bilateral iliac aneurysms
- Rupture risk: <2% w/ <4 cm, 25–41% w/ >5 cm. Female predilection. *(Handbook of Interventional Radiologic Procedures. 4th ed. Lippincott Williams & Wilkins; 2011)*
- Nearly all AAAs infrarenal
- Incidence: Elderly (4–7% in 65–80) and male (5M:1F)

Classification
- True: Involving 3-vessel layers (intima, media, adventitia)
  False: Involving 1–2 layers of vessel
- Fusiform: Diffuse dilation along vessel
  Saccular: Concentrated outpouching of vessel

Etiology

Vascular/Structural	Inherited	Arteritis
– Atherosclerosis	Connective tissue	– Takayasu arteritis
– Smoking	Disease	– Syphilitic
– Vessel–vessel	– Marfan	– Polyarteritis nodosa
anastomosis	– Ehler–Danlos	– SLE
– Trauma/iatrogenic	– Cystic medial necrosis	
	Familial: 20% w/ 1st-degree relative	

Clinical Presentation
- Majority asymptomatic (<5 cm)
- Abdominal fullness
- Abdominal pain
  - Radiating to back with rupture
- Advanced aneurysms can project emboli distally
- Severe hypotension in rupture

Physical Exam
- Pulsatile abdominal mass
- Popliteal aneurysms
  - 50% have concurrent aortic aneurysm *(Management of Asymptomatic Abdominal Aortic Aneurysm. In: UpToDate. 2017, UpToDate)*

Diagnosis *(Ann Intern Med 1997;126(6):441–9)*
- Ultrasound
  - Fast and cost-effective diagnosis and surveillance
  - Screening males >65 y w/ smoking history, or strong FHx
  - Upon discovery of popliteal aneurysms
- CT
  - Aneurysm measurement/monitoring
  - Location
  - Operative planning

Treatment

Medical
- Behavioral modification (tobacco cessation, diet modification)
- Nicotine replacement
- Statin therapy
- Strict BP control
  - β-Blockers, hydralazine, ACEI, ARB
  - Decrease progression/rupture
  - Decrease risk of dissection
- Rupture
  - Aggressive fluid resuscitation
  - IV pain control
  - Immediate endovascular/operative intervention
- <5.5 cm observation only *(J Vasc Surg 2001;33(2):443)*
  - Serum lipids/blood pressure monitoring
  - Ultrasonography every 2–3 y <4 cm
  - Ultrasound or CT scanning every 6–12 mo 4.0–5.4 cm
- >5.5 cm/symptomatic warrant immediate repair (UK Small Aneurysm Trial, Aneurysm Detection And Management (ADAM)) *(J Vasc Surg 2001;33(2):443)*
  - Despite lower risk EVAR not indicated <5.5 cm

Open Repair

- Transperitoneal
  - Operative ease (ruptured aneurysm)
  - Exposure of peritoneal contents
  - Virgin abdomen
- Retroperitoneal
  - Previous abdominal surgeries
  - Decreased ileus/pulmonary dysfunction
  - Difficulty accessing R iliac

Endovascular Aneurysm Repair (EVAR)

- Indications
  - Aortic rupture/dissection
  - Symptomatic or rapidly expanding aneurysm (>0.5 cm/6 m)
  - Asymptomatic fusiform aneurysm (>5.5 cm, men; 4.5 cm, women)
  - Embolic complications from aneurysm
  - Inflammatory aneurysms (increased risk rupture)
- Contraindications
  - Unfavorable anatomy—Excessive aortic tortuosity, inadequate vasculature collaterals in mesenteric involvement, femoral/iliac tortuosity/atherosclerosis, poor graft landing zones, significant thrombus in expected landing zones
  - Prognostic—Short life expectancy, renal insufficiency
- Results demonstrate EVAR associated with fewer complications, less hospital days/intensive care days, and overall mortality (N Engl J Med 2004;351(16):1607–18)

EVAR OPERATIVE TECHNIQUE

Operative Planning/Graft Selection (Handbook of Interventional Radiologic Procedures. 4th ed. Lippincott Williams & Wilkins; 2011)

- Careful review of preoperative CTA with 3D reconstructions
- Measure proximal native vessel (NV) diameter, distal NV diameter, proximal NV graft junction length (NVGJL), distal NVGJL, aneurysm length, total treatment length, and aortic angulation
  - Proximal NVGJL of 10–15 mm to reduce Type 1A endoleak
  - Proximal/distal graft diameter should be 10% larger than outer NV diameters. Consider tapered grafts with differing diameters.
  - Aortic angulations <60 degrees preferable
  - Distal aortic diameter of >18 mm in bifurcated systems to accommodate iliac stent components
- Bifurcated deployment: Measure diameter and NVGJL distally
  - Proximal CIA lesions can have distal CIA landing zone
  - Predeployment embolization of ipsilateral hypogastric arterial trunk in aneurysms extending beyond CIA (necessitating EIA landing) to reduce endoleak
- Favorable anatomy: No prohibitive thrombus/calcification, no significant vessel tortuosity, sufficient renal and mesenteric vasculature/collaterals, and adequate femoral access
  - May need to consider angioplasty of contralateral femoral/iliac artery to allow for device sheath advancement

Procedure (Handbook of Interventional Radiologic Procedures. 4th ed. Lippincott Williams & Wilkins; 2011)

- Supine positioning with sterile prep and drape of bilateral groins
- Percutaneous femoral access under image guidance/surgical exposure on side ipsilateral to graft extension
- Sheath placement and guidewire access to abdominal aorta
- Multi-side hole pigtail catheter advancement to level of renal arteries
- PA abdominal aortogram performed (30 cc/s for 60 cc contrast). Mark screen and compare preop imaging to angiographic findings. Adjust plan as needed.
- Exchange pigtail catheter with super stiff 0.035″ Amplatz wire above proximal landing zone
- Anticoagulate patient for goal APTT of 250–300 s
- Prepare stent graft per manufacturer guidelines and then advance device under fluoroscopic guidance to the proximal landing zone utilizing opaque device markers, inferior to lowest renal artery
- Deployment of graft trunk and ipsilateral limb extension under continuous fluoroscopic guidance; consider breath-holding maneuvers during deployment to increase accuracy
  - Inferior limb of ipsilateral graft extension must reside proximal to internal iliac artery

- On contralateral side (location of absent endograft extension) the aortic graft is cannulated with a second guidewire and pigtail catheter. Perform aortogram to confirm intragraft placement.
  - Alternative confirmation via IVUS in contrast-sensitive pts
- Super stiff 0.035" Amplatz wire passed into pigtail catheter for repositioning, and then retrograde contralateral sheath angiogram is performed to assess potential hypogastric artery coverage
- Pigtail catheter is removed and contralateral limb extension device is advanced under continuous fluoroscopic guidance, ensuring adequate graft–graft overlap
- Endograft extension is deployed under continuous fluoroscopic guidance; consider respiratory maneuvers during deployment to improve accuracy
  - Inferior limb of extension proximal to internal iliac artery
- Guidewire balloon expansion of graft–vessel and graft–graft junctions to ensure security
- Reintroduction of pigtail catheter superior to most proximal graft portion and completion aortogram is performed for evaluation of endoleaks
- Further interventions as needed for complications/graft failures
- Guidewires removed
- Closure of femoral access sites with angioseal, application of 30 min of pressure

EVAR Postoperative Care

ICU Surveillance
- 24-h postop monitoring of neurovascular status
- Renal function monitoring via labs and US

Complications
- Graft failure—Migration, endoleak, malposition
- Graft stenosis/thrombosis/infection
- Postimplantation syndrome—Fever, leukocytosis, abdominal/back pain

CT Surveillance—At 1, 6, and 12 mo, then annually *(Management of Asymptomatic Abdominal Aortic Aneurysm. In: UpToDate. 2017, UpToDate; Ann Intern Med 1997;126(6):441–9)*

Figure 10-9 Abdominal Aortic Aneurysm and Repair—CTA reconstruction preintervention (**Upper Left**), FEVAR main body and renals (**Upper Right**), Iliac limb extension of endograft (**Bottom Left**), CTA postreconstruction (**Bottom Right**). Courtesy of Preet Kang.

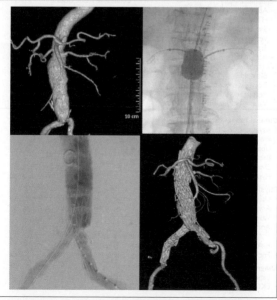

THORACIC AORTIC ANEURYSMS

Background
- Normal thoracic aorta ~3–3.5 cm
- 1/3 of aortic aneurysms
  - Ascending aorta 60%, descending 40% (*Management of Thoracic Aortic Aneurysm in Adults, in UpToDate.* 2017, UpToDate)
  - 80% Fusiform, 20% saccular (*Handbook of Interventional Radiologic Procedures.* 4th ed. Lippincott Williams & Wilkins; 2011)
  - Male: Female ratio 1.5:1 (*Handbook of Interventional Radiologic Procedures.* 4th ed. Lippincott Williams & Wilkins; 2011)
- Definition: 1.5 factor diameter increase of vessel compared to native vessel
  - Natural ~10 mm/y growth
  - Risk of rupture when diameter reaches 6 cm
- Normal thoracic aorta ~3–3.5 cm

Classifications (*Essentials of General Surgery.* 5 ed. Diseases of the Vascular System. 2013: Wolters Kluwer; *Management of Thoracic Aortic Aneurysm in Adults, in UpToDate.* 2017, UpToDate)
- Thoracic
  - Ascending: Aortic valve to innominate artery
  - Arch: Brachiocephalic involvement
  - Descending: Distal to L subclavian
  - Thoracoabdominal
- Thoracoabdominal
  - Type I: Superior to 6th intercostal space to suprarenal aorta (infrarenal arteries)
  - Type II: Superior to 6th intercostal space to infrarenal aorta
  - Type III: Inferior to 6th intercostal space to abd. aorta
  - Type IV: Abdominal aortic aneurysm
  - Type V: Inferior to 6th intercostal space to visceral abdominal aorta
- Fusiform: Diffuse dilation along vessel
- Saccular: Concentrated outpouching of vessel

Etiology

Vascular/Structural	Inherited
Endothelial Injury	Connective Tissue Disease
– Atherosclerosis	– Marfan
– HTN	– Ehler–Danlos
– Smoking	– Cystic medial necrosis
– Vessel–vessel anastomosis	
– Trauma	**Arterides**
– Iatrogenic	
Aortic Valve Disease	– Takayasu arteritis
– Bicuspid	– Syphilitic
– Aortic stenosis	– Polyarteritis nodosa
– Vegetated valves	– Turner syndrome
– Valve replacement	– SLE

Clinical Presentation
- Asymptomatic, incidental finding
- Previous aneurysms/dissections
- Upper chest pain
- Back pain
- Distal emboli in advanced aneurysms
- Hypotension in rupture

Physical Exam
- Usually no physical signs
- Asymmetric pulses
- Vascular bruits
- Aortic heart murmurs
  - AS: R 2nd intercostal crescendo–decrescendo systolic murmur
  - AR: R 2nd intercostal diastolic murmur
- Focal neurologic deficits

Diagnostic Studies
- Laboratory: CBC, BMP, D-Dimer, Troponins, Lactate
- EKG

- TTE/TEE
  - Expedient study in suspected rupture
  - Evaluation of valvular pathologies
- Chest X-ray
  - Mediastinal widening
  - Tracheal deviation
  - Aortic calcifications
  - Enlarged aortic knob
- CTA
  - Initial definitive diagnostic modality
    - Diameter measurement, progression
    - Evaluation of entire aorta for concurrent AAAs
  - 3D rendering of analogous radiographic findings
  - Operative planning with vessel anatomy and graft measurement
- MRA
  - Evaluation of aortic vessel inflammatory/connective tissue pathologies

Treatment
- >6 cm or symptomatic aneurysms
- Surgical repair
  - Sternotomy access
- Thoracic endovascular aneurysm repair (TEVAR)
  - Indications (Handbook of Interventional Radiologic Procedures. 4th ed. Lippincott Williams & Wilkins; 2011)
    - For symptomatic, fast growing (>1 cm/y), or penetrating atherosclerotic ulcers
    - For posttraumatic or postsurgical pseudoaneurysms
    - Off-label use in intramural hematomas, mycotic aneurysms, aortic fistulas, and acute rupture
  - Contraindications (Handbook of Interventional Radiologic Procedures. 4th ed. Lippincott Williams & Wilkins; 2011)
    - Graft infection or rejection risk
    - Tortuous/difficult thoracic/abdominal aortic anatomy
    - If significant risk of occlusion to vital vasculature occurs (carotid, subclavian, celiac)

TEVAR Operative Technique

Operative Planning/Graft Selection (Handbook of Interventional Radiologic Procedures. 4th ed. Lippincott Williams & Wilkins; 2011)
- Measure proximal NV diameter, distal NV diameter, proximal NVGJL, distal NVGJL, aneurysm length, total treatment length, and radius of treated thoracic arch
  - Proximal/distal graft diameter is 10–20% greater than NV
  - Longer graft/NV junctions preferable. 5 mm overlap in graft/graft junctions.
  - Elongate NVGJL if acute aortic angles are incurred
- Favorable anatomy: No prohibitive thrombus/calcification, no significant vessel tortuosity, neck diameters <40 mm, <60-degrees aortic angulation, and adequate femoral access
  Spinal drainage w/ possible endograft coverage of T8–L2 and periop hypotension

Procedure (Handbook of Interventional Radiologic Procedures. 4th ed. Lippincott Williams & Wilkins; 2011)
- Supine positioning with sterile prep and drape of bilateral groins
- Percutaneous femoral access under image guidance/surgical exposure
- Initial femoral artery access contralateral to stent-graft deployment site
- Sheath placement and subsequent guidewire access to proximal thoracic aorta
- Advance multi-side hole pigtail catheter over guidewire to proximal thoracic aorta
  Perform aortogram w/ 30 cc/s for 60 cc contrast at 45–75 degrees LAO. Mark screen and compare preop imaging to angiographic findings.
- Percutaneous femoral access of stent-graft deployment site with advancement of 0.035" stiff Amplatz wire to proximal aorta
- Anticoagulate patient for goal APTT of 250–300 s
- Prepare stent graft per manufacturer guidelines and then advance device under fluoroscopic guidance to the proximal landing zone utilizing opaque device markers
- Deploy under continuous fluoroscopy; consider breath-holding maneuvers during deployment to increase accuracy
- Withdraw deployment catheter under fluoroscopic guidance
- Deploy extension grafts under similar fashion
- Angioplasty expansion of graft–vessel and graft–graft junctions
- Completion aortogram/evaluation of endoleaks
- Remove guidewires/intravascular hardware
- Closure of femoral access sites with Angioseal, application of 30 min of pressure

TEVAR Postoperative Care

ICU Surveillance
- 24-h postop with continuous neurovascular monitoring
- BP surveillance with mean arterial pressure of 100 mmHg

Complications
- Graft failure—Migration, endoleak, malposition
- Cerebrovascular accident
- New aortic perforation, dissection
- Postimplantation syndrome: Fever, leukocytosis, chest/back pain
- Spinal cord ischemia

Spinal Drain
- Indications
  - Post AAA repair
    - Hypogastric artery embolization
  - Extensive graft coverage (>20 cm) or T8–L1 coverage
  - TEVAR concurrent with AAA repair
  - Planned occlusion of L subclavian arteries
- Management (*J Vasc Surg* 2009;49(4):1089; author reply 1090; *J Vasc Interv Radiol* 2010;21(9):1343–6)
  - Obtain complete baseline neurologic examination
  - Goal mean perfusion pressure >60 mmHg
    - Mean perfusion pressure = MAP − Spinal pressure
    - CSF pressure <10–20 mmHg
  - Maintain spinal drain for 48 h
  - May discontinue after 24-h clamp trial
  - Continue spinal drain for progressive neurological deficit

Endoleaks

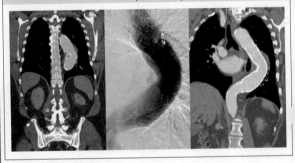

Figure 10-10 Endoleak—Gore thoracic endograft placement in 2008 (**Left**). Endoleak detected in 2017, likely graft tear (**Middle**). Relining of tear with new endograft (**Right**). Courtesy of Preet Kang.

- 20–25% of patients
- Diagnostic studies
  - Lifelong surveillance/maintenance
    - 1 m, 6 m, 12 m, and annual surveillance
  - Duplex ultrasonography
    - Initial, fast, cheap
  - CTA
    - Most routine diagnostic modality
    - Static image of contrast extravasation
    - Diameter growth evaluation
  - Angiography
    - Dynamic image to evaluate endoleak flow directionality

Type	Description	Intervention
1A/1B	Graft–vessel junction failure A: Leakage at proximal junction B: Leakage at distal junction	Endovascular repair: Angioplasty -> bare metal balloon expandable stent -> stent graft insertion -> open repair

Type	Description	Intervention
2	Retrograde flow from nonoccluded arteries (IMA > lumbar > accessory renal)	Observe if stable: (Spontaneous thrombosis) Repair if growing: Trans lumbar coil embolization of feeding vessels and aneurysm sac
3	Graft–graft junction failure	Endovascular repair: Stent graft placement with angioplasty
4	Leakage through endograft material	Uncommon with new generation endografts, usually self-limiting
5	Endotension	Open repair

AORTIC DISSECTIONS

Background
- Definition: Tear of aortic intima into media
  - Creation of intimal flap and false lumen in which diverted blood flow can propagate tear proximally or distally
  - Ascending aorta most frequent (Overview of Acute Aortic Syndromes. In: UpToDate. 2017, UpToDate)
  - Significant tears can occlude true lumen of aorta or vital branch points
- Stanford Classification (Clinical Features and Diagnosis of Acute Aortic Dissection, in UpToDate. 2017, UpToDate)
  - Type A: Involve ascending thoracic aorta
  - Type B: Involve descending thoracic aorta distal to L subclavian
- Elderly male: 65–80 y

Etiology

Vascular/Structural	Connective Tissue Disorders
– HTN	– Marfan
– Atherosclerosis	– Ehler–Danlos
– Aortic coarctation	– Cystic medial necrosis
– Prior aneurysm	– Turner syndrome
Iatrogenic/Trauma	**Inflammatory**
– Surgical valve repair	– Takayasu arteritis
– Cardiac catheterization	– Syphilitic
– Vascular anastomosis	– Rheumatoid

Clinical Presentation
- Depending on extent of propagation along aortic tree
- Abrupt onset tearing chest pain radiating to back
  - Ascending with anterior chest pain
  - Descending with back pain
- Proximal propagation
  - MI
  - Syncope
  - Tamponade
  - Stroke/upper neurologic symptoms
- Distal propagation
  - AKI/low UOP
  - Mesenteric ischemia
  - Groin pain (via occlusion of gonadal arteries)
  - Lower neurological symptoms (via spinal artery occlusion)
  - Critical limb ischemia

Physical Exam
- Clue into extent of propagation, highly variable

Cardiac
- Diaphoresis
- Muffled heart sounds
- Diastolic murmur
- Widened pulse pressure

Vascular
- Asymmetric carotid/brachial/radial pulses
- Peripheral ischemia: 6 P's

- High mortality with inc. number of pulse asymmetries and/or carotid pulse asymmetry

Neurologic
- Upper: Contralateral weakness/numbness/paralysis, facial droop, AMS, syncope
- Lower: Bilateral LE weakness/numbness/paralysis, warm extremity (not peripheral ischemia)

Renal
- Decreased UOP, flank pain

Diagnosis
- Laboratory/imaging workup highly variable, dependent on propagation location/extent

Laboratory
- CBC, BMP, LFTs
- Troponin
- PT/INR/PTT

EKG
- MI: ST elevation
- Tamponade: Pulsus alternans/low QRS voltage

TEE
- Initial diagnostic modality in unstable patients
  - Color Doppler delineate true vs. false lumen
  - Requires intubation
- Evaluate ascending dissection extent/aortic involvement
- Large pericardial effusion
- Regurgitation
- Hypokinesis

Chest X-ray
- Aortic silhouette widening
- Pleural effusion
- Aortic kinking

CTA
- Initial diagnostic modality in stable patients
- Evaluation of aortic dissection extent
- Evaluation of aortic branch involvement
- "Double barrel" sign—True and false lumen
  - False lumen commonly with thrombus
- Aortic widening
- Surveillance for aneurysm expansion/endoleak

Aortography
- Intraoperative diagnosis, treatment planning
- Characterization of false lumen blood flow

Treatment

Medical
- Stable Type B dissections
- Blood pressure control
  - Fast-acting β-blockers (esmolol ggt), long-acting β-blockers (labetalol, propranolol) w/ strict SBP goal 100–120 mmHg
  - CCB alternative (verapamil/diltiazem)
  - Nitroprusside prn extra control
- Pain control: IV PCA (dilaudid, morphine)

Endovascular
- Reserved for Type B dissections
- EVAR/TEVAR. See previous section for procedural details

Surgical
- All Type A dissections or Type B dissections threatening blood flow (emergent)
- Type B dissections with impending aneurysm rupture
- Replacement of aorta, resection of intimal tears/aneurysmal sac, repairing aortic valve

Background

- IVC Filter is used in the management of deep venous thrombosis (DVT) and/or pulmonary embolism (PE)
- Primary role is prevention of thromboembolic migration from lower extremities to the lungs
- Reduces risk of PE, increases risk of DVT *(Circulation 2005;112(3):416–22)*
- Primary treatment of venous thromboembolism (VTE) remains anticoagulation (AC)
- Indications for IVC filtration are controversial. Generally, their utility is greatest when anticoagulation has either failed or resulted in complications (bleeding).

Categories of IVC Filters *(Handbook of Interventional Radiologic Procedures. 2011: Lippincott Williams & Wilkins; Semin Intervent Radiol 2016;33(2):75–8)*

- Permanent: Nonretrievable; have been around the longest, thus they have the most data regarding their use. Eg, Greenfield (Fig. 11-1), Vena Tech LP, Bird's Nest, Trap Ease, Simon Nitinol

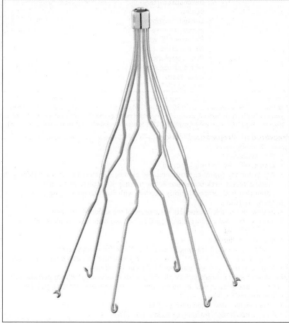

Figure 11-1 Greenfield IVC filter. (Image provided courtesy of Boston Scientific. ©2018 Boston Scientific Corporation or its affiliates. All rights reserved.)

- Optional (retrievable): Typically designed with hook at the top of the filter allowing for easy retrieval through transjugular approach; but all are FDA approved for permanent use. Eg, Celect, Gunther-Tulip, Option, ALN, Denali (Fig. 11-2)
- Optional (convertible): Device is altered after placement so that it no longer functions as a filter but remains in the cava as a stent. Eg, VenaTech Convertible
- Temporary: Attached to catheter or tether exiting the skin

Indications and Contraindications for IVC Filter Placement *(J Vasc Intervent Radiol 2011;22(11):1499–06; J Vasc Interv Radiol 2009;20(6):697–707; Semin Intervent Radiol 2016;33(2):65–70; J vasc Intervent Radiol 2006;17(3):449–59)*

- Controversial and vary among professional medical societies. The following is adapted from most recent (2006) SIR consensus guidelines *(Vasc Intervent Radiol 2006;17(3):449–59)*

Absolute Indications (Proven VTE)	Relative Indications (Proven VTE)	Prophylactic Indications (No VTE; Primary Prophylaxis not Feasible*)	Contraindications to Filter Placement
• Recurrent VTE (acute or chronic) despite adequate anticoagulation • Contraindication to anticoagulation • Complication of anticoagulation • Inability to achieve/maintain therapeutic anticoagulation	• Large, free-floating proximal DVT • High risk of complication of anticoagulation (eg, ataxia, frequent falls) • Massive PE treated with thrombolysis • Difficulty establishing therapeutic anticoagulation • Chronic PE treated with thromboendarterectomy • Limited cardiopulmonary reserve • Recurrent PE with filter in place • Poor compliance with anticoagulant medications • Iliocaval DVT	• Trauma patient with high risk of VTE • Surgical procedure in patient at high risk of VTE • Medical condition with high risk of VTE	• No access route to vena cava • No location available in vena cava for placement of filter

*Primary prophylaxis not feasible due to high bleeding risk, inability to monitor patient for VTE, etc.
(Adapted from Kaufman JA, Kinney TB, Streiff MB, et al., Guidelines for the use of retrievable and convertible vena cava filters: report from the society of interventional radiology multidisciplinary consensus conference. J Vasc Interv Radiol 2006;17(3):449–59. Copyright © 2006 Society of Interventional Radiology, with permission.)

Preprocedure Preparation/Workup (Handbook of Interventional Radiologic Procedures. 2011: Lippincott Williams & Wilkins)
• Patient evaluation:
  • Ensure IVC filter is truly indicated
  • Assess for any special circumstances (eg, existing catheters that may interfere with vascular access, neck braces preventing transjugular access, restrictions in positioning, back braces that may interfere with fluoroscopic imaging, etc.)
• Imaging evaluation:
  • Review all available cross-sectional imaging of the abdomen and pelvis
  • Identify any caval variants and/or caval thrombosis prior to procedure and plan accordingly
• Laboratory evaluation:
  • Guidelines vary, but are typically similar to those for venous access
  • Many patients will be on AC so procedure should not be delayed for correction
  • In general, INR <3.0 and platelets >30,000/μL is sufficient
• Informed consent should include all of the usual risks associated with percutaneous venous procedures as well as the following (J Vasc Intervent Radiol 2011;22(11):1522–30):
  • Recurrent PE (5%)
  • Symptomatic caval thrombosis (1–5%)
  • Filter embolization, fracture, or malposition (1%)
  • Symptomatic perforation by a filter element (<1%)

Anatomical Variants (Handbook of Interventional Radiologic Procedures. 2011: Lippincott Williams & Wilkins)
• Ideally these may be identified in cross-sectional imaging prior to the procedure; however, these may commonly be seen for the first time on preplacement cavogram
• Duplicated IVC (<1%): Usually joins at the left renal vein, may join lower
• Left-sided IVC (<1%)
• Circumaortic left renal vein (3–4%): Inferior component of venous ring lies posterior to aorta, drains into the IVC inferior to normal left renal vein
• Retroaortic left renal vein (2–3%): Usually drains into IVC inferior to right renal vein (or rarely at the confluence of the iliac veins)
• Mega cava (<1%) normal anatomy but IVC diameter >28 mm

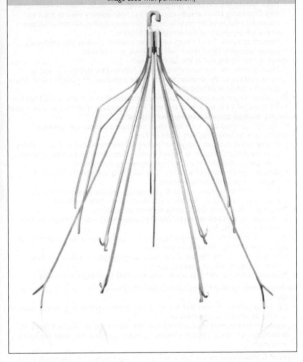

Figure 11-2 Denali IVC filter. (From http://www.bardpv.com/?portfolio=denali#pretty Photo. ©2018 BD. BD, the BD Logo, are trademarks of Becton, Dickinson and Company. Image used with permission.)

Fluoroscopic-Guided Technique (*Handbook of Interventional Radiologic Procedures. 2011: Lippincott Williams & Wilkins*)

- Obtain access:
  - Preferred approach is through the right common femoral vein or right internal jugular vein
  - Can be through a variety of approaches (subclavian, translumbar) in complex scenarios
- Advance wire and catheter/sheath to common iliac vein (preferably left) and perform high-quality cavogram
  - 4F catheter or greater pigtail catheter; some providers may simply inject through introducer sheath and achieve adequate images
  - Use same positioning and field of view that will be used during filter deployment
  - Injection rate of 15–20 mL/s for 2 s
  - Digital subtraction angiography (DSA) filming at 4–6 frames/s; suspended respiration in anterior–posterior projection
  - If poor renal function, CO_2 angiography can be utilized as necessary
  - Contralateral iliac vein and renal veins should be identified as inflow of unopacified blood or by reflux of contrast into vein orifices
- *Goals of venography:*
  - Define IVC and renal vein anatomy (see variants discussed above)
  - Determine cava size (most filters designed for cava <28 mm)
  - Confirm patency of IVC
- After adequate cavography, filter deployment should be planned so that tip/hook of filter is at level of the lowest renal vein inflow

- Use reference points such as the spine for reliability
- If needed, exchange catheter for introducer sheath over guidewire (avoid moving patient or image intensifier)
  - Major benefit of performing venogram through introducer sheath is avoiding this step. Decreasing time between cavogram and filter delivery ensures accurate placement relative to the renal veins and decreases patient discomfort/motion
- Position delivery sheath at the desired final location
  - Femoral approach: Tip of sheath will be just superior to renal vein confluence
  - Jugular approach: Tip of sheath will be inferior to renal veins
- Advance filter to the end of the delivery sheath
  - Most systems have radiopaque markers for fluoroscopic guidance as well as visual markers on the exterior portion of the introducer to guide the filter to the correct location within the sheath
- Reposition the entire system so that the constrained filter is in the desired location
  - Tip/hook will be at the level of the renal veins regardless of which approach is taken
- Deploy the filter per manufacturer's instructions
  - Usually a "pin and pull" technique under continuous fluoroscopic guidance
- Deployment technique can vary based on filter
  - In general this requires a very firm "pinning" of the introducer with one hand in order to hold the filter in its desired location. Sometimes gentle forward pressure is needed to keep the filter from migrating during deployment
  - Sheath is gently retracted with the other hand over the filter/introducer in one steady motion until filter is deployed
  - If filter appears to migrate or tilt during deployment, the system can usually be repositioned as long as the filter is still constrained within the sheath
- Retract introducer into sheath under fluoroscopic guidance
  - This may have a hook or "teeth"-like mechanism which may get caught on filter if not carefully retracted
- Remove introducer and may repeat cavogram through delivery sheath using same injection and filming rate as described above
  - Many providers skip this step if the final nonangiographic images of the filter demonstrate it to be in adequate position
- Remove sheath and hold pressure at venotomy until hemostasis is achieved

Bedside Intravascular Ultrasound-Guided Technique (Vasc Endovasc Surg 2013;47(2): 97–101)
- Can be considered in cases where patient is unable to travel to angiography suite, or in order to avoid iodinated contrast
- Single-puncture technique (ie, without real-time ultrasound visualization) has been demonstrated to be as safe and effective as double puncture (real-time ultrasound visualization)

Special Considerations (Handbook of Interventional Radiologic Procedures. 2011: Lippincott Williams & Wilkins)
- IVC thrombosis: Filter needs to be cranial to the thrombus
  - If thrombus does not extend to renal veins, place filter as low as possible in infrarenal IVC, even if body of the filter lies entirely within the infrarenal IVC
  - If thrombus extends to renal veins, place filter in suprarenal segment, either just above the renal veins or in the intrahepatic IVC
  - If there is a filter already in place but thrombus extends superior to existing filter, a second filter could be placed above the thrombus, usually in the suprarenal IVC
- Duplicated IVC: Both cavae need to be filtered; multiple options depending on anatomy
  - Place one filter in each IVC, just below renal veins, OR
  - Place a single suprarenal filter
  - If the second IVC is an accessory cava (ie, it is small and communicates with the main IVC at the levels of the common iliac and renal veins), consider occluding it with coils or a plug followed by filter placement in the main IVC
- Circumaortic left renal vein: Risk of embolization via the venous ring if filter is placed between the two orifices
  - Place filter feet below orifice of retrocaval component, OR
  - Place filter in suprarenal location
- Retroaortic left renal vein:
  - Place filter below orifice of left renal vein if there is room, OR
  - Place filter with its apex at the level of the right renal vein (in cases of very low left renal vein orifice), OR
  - Place one filter in each common iliac vein

- Mega Cava:
  - Vena Tech LP approved for IVC diameters up to 35 mm
  - Bird's Nest filter approved for IVC diameters up to 40 mm
  - If neither of these are possible, place filters in each common iliac vein
- Currently pregnant patients:
  - Suprarenal placement minimizes fetal radiation exposure

Problem Solving (*Handbook of Interventional Radiologic Procedures. 2011: Lippincott Williams & Wilkins*)
- Kinked sheath (*Am J Roentgenol 1992;158(4):875–80*): Can occur if filter is delivered without a guidewire, or when dealing with a tortuous delivery course, such as accessing from a location other than the right internal jugular vein or right common femoral vein
  - Attempting to push the filter against a kink can result in perforation of the sheath and extrusion of the filter
  - To correct, the operator can try advancing/withdrawing the filter and sheath as a unit centrally or peripherally to straighten the kink
  - If the kink is unable to be straightened by manipulation, exchange for a larger sheath that can accommodate the filter delivery system without kinking
  - If all else fails, abandon the access site and consider a more in-line direct approach
- Incompletely opened filter (*Handbook of Interventional Radiologic Procedures. 2011: Lippincott Williams & Wilkins*): 1st step is to perform cavogram to assess caval coverage, confirm stability and evaluate for thrombus
  - If there is concern for incomplete caval coverage or if the filter has been misplaced into a small branch, intervention likely warranted
  - Manipulation with an angled catheter can sometimes open the filter
  - If retrievable, simply remove the filter and insert a new device
  - If permanent, place a second filter central to the 1st
- Guidewire entrapment (*Radiology 1996;198(1):71–6*): Can occur with over-the-wire deployment
  - Pulling hard on the guidewire will often make entrapment worse or may dislodge filter
  - Advance a catheter over the guidewire to attempt to disengage
  - If catheter manipulation is unsuccessful, consider engaging the wire from opposite access and pulling past the point of entrapment

Complications
- Few comparative studies have been completed to prospectively compare different devices, so complication rates are often reported for filtration devices as a group, although they vary considerably depending on the filter being studied
- The following complication rates are compiled from the most recent quality improvement guidelines published in JVIR (*J Vasc Intervent Radiol 2011*):
  - Death: 0.12%
  - Filter embolization: 0.1%
  - Deployment outside target area: 1–9%
  - Access site thrombosis/occlusion: 3–10%
- Trackable events may or may not be clinically significant, but are reported in all cases since filters are implanted devices (*J Vasc Intervent Radiol 2011*):
  - IVC penetration: 0–41%
    - Very rarely (0.4%) clinically significant
  - Filter movement: 0–18%
    - Also rarely significant clinically
  - Filter fracture: 2–10%
  - Recurrent PE: 0.5–6%
  - Access site thrombus (all types): 0–25%
  - IVC occlusion: 2–30%
  - Insertion problems: 5–23%
  - Other complications: 1–15%

Postprocedural Care (*J Vasc Intervent Radiol 2011*)
- Primary pharmacologic treatment or prophylaxis for VTE should commence at the 1st safe opportunity (*Handbook of Interventional Radiologic Procedures. 2011: Lippincott Williams & Wilkins*)
- For permanent filters, regular abdominal films should be obtained every 3–5 y to monitor filter position and integrity (*Handbook of interventional radiologic procedures. 2011: Lippincott Williams & Wilkins*)
- For retrievable filters, a rigorous followup and tracking is recommended so that retrieval and/or anticoagulation can be planned as soon as feasible (*Handbook of interventional radiologic procedures. 2011: Lippincott Williams & Wilkins*)
  - Initial followup should occur 1 mo after placement to assess for retrieval

- Indications (*Handbook of Interventional Radiologic Procedures.* 2011: Lippincott Williams & Wilkins):
  - Absolute: Filter is documented source of major morbidity that will be relieved by retrieval
  - Relative: Adequate primary therapy or prophylaxis of VTE
- Contraindications (*Handbook of Interventional Radiologic Procedures.* 2011: Lippincott Williams & Wilkins):
  - Significant retained thrombus within the filter
  - Inadequate primary therapy or prophylaxis of VTE
  - Life expectancy less than 6 mo
- Preprocedure preparation (*Handbook of Interventional Radiologic Procedures.* 2011: Lippincott Williams & Wilkins):
  - Labs: Coagulation studies and blood counts for patients on therapeutic anticoagulation to ensure they are in therapeutic range. Serum creatinine should also be assessed in patients with impaired renal function
  - Imaging: Preprocedure diagnostic imaging for VTE is only indicated in therapeutically anticoagulated patients if there is clinical concern for new, recurrent or progressive VTE
    - If filter was placed for VTE prophylaxis (ie, patient is not on therapeutic AC), duplex venous ultrasound of the lower extremities is indicated prior to retrieval
  - Prior imaging should be reviewed to assess filter type, location, presence of trapped thrombus, filter integrity, caval penetration, and filter migration
- Procedure (*Handbook of Interventional Radiologic Procedures.* 2011: Lippincott Williams & Wilkins)
  - Access is typically transjugular but can also be transfemoral
  - High-quality preretrieval cavogram is performed to assess for position, complications, or thrombus
  - Retrieval technique depends on the device, but the most common approach involves introducing a snare and catheter through a large sheath toward the hook of the filter
  - After the filter hook is snared, the sheath is advanced over the filter until the entire filter is captured within the sheath
  - Once all filter hooks are completely within the sheath, the snare and filter can be pulled out through the sheath. The filter should be carefully inspected to assess its integrity
  - Postretrieval cavography may be performed but is not required in cases of noncomplicated retrieval
  - Complicated retrieval methods are diverse and beyond the scope of this text. When the filter apex or struts are firmly adherent to the wall or the filter is significantly tilted, techniques for retrieval include reverse curve catheter and wire–loop snare technique, balloon inflation to align filter, endobronchial forceps dissection, or laser ablation to free the filter from the wall. Using a larger sheath (>14F–16F) is of utmost importance in any complex retrieval technique utilized.
- Complications (*Handbook of Interventional Radiologic Procedures.* 2011: Lippincott Williams & Wilkins):
  - Failure to retrieve the filter: 5–20%
  - Filter migration: <1%
  - Filter fracture: <1%
  - Symptomatic laceration or perforation of the vena cava: <1%
  - Vena caval thrombosis: <1%
  - Hemodynamically significant arrhythmia: <1%
- Postprocedural care (*Handbook of Interventional Radiologic Procedures.* 2011: Lippincott Williams & Wilkins):
  - Immediate postprocedure period includes routine monitoring similar for venous access procedures
  - Primary treatment of prophylaxis for VTE should continue until no longer clinically indicated

VENOUS THROMBOLYSIS

Background

- The primary treatment for deep vein thrombosis (DVT) and pulmonary embolism (PE), collectively referred to as venous thromboembolism (VTE), is anticoagulation (AC). Its purpose is to prevent the progression of thrombosis and/or prevent pulmonary embolism (*Handbook of Interventional Radiologic Procedures.* 2011: Lippincott Williams & Wilkins)
- However, anticoagulant drugs do not actively eliminate venous thrombus, so their use may not be sufficient to prevent serious complications of DVT (*Handbook of Interventional Radiologic Procedures.* 2011: Lippincott Williams & Wilkins)
- Postthrombotic syndrome (PTS) is a debilitating late complication occurring in a minority (20–50%) of patients with acute DVT. PTS can present as several

- manifestations ranging from swelling and chronic leg pain to stasis dermatitis and skin ulceration (*Cardiovasc Diagn Ther 2016;6(6):623–31*)
- The development of PTS is directly related to continued presence of thrombus in the deep venous system resulting in valvular damage and/or obstruction (*Cardiovasc Diagn Ther 2016;6(6):623–31*)
- Catheter-directed thrombolysis (CDT) during the acute presentation of DVT can relieve venous outflow obstruction, maintain valvular function, and prevent PTS by rapid thrombus elimination (*Handbook of Interventional Radiologic Procedures. 2011: Lippincott Williams & Wilkins; Cardiovasc Diagn Ther 2016;6(6):623–31*)

Indications (*Handbook of Interventional Radiologic Procedures. 2011: Lippincott Williams & Wilkins; J Vasc Intervent Radiol 2014;25(9):1317–25*)
- The following criteria are from SIR QI guidelines and should be met when considering endovascular thrombus removal for lower-extremity DVT (*J Vasc Intervent Radiol 2014;25(9): 1317–25*):
  - Recently ambulatory patient
  - Imaging proven symptomatic DVT in inferior vena cava (IVC) or iliac, common femoral, and/or femoral vein
  - Symptomatic <28 d or strong clinical suspicion that DVT has formed within the past 28 d (*J Vasc Intervent Radiol 2014;25(9):1317–25*)
    - Thrombolysis is much more likely to be successful when initiated within 14 d of symptom onset. This 14-d cutoff is often used in clinical practice.

Contraindications (*J Vasc Intervent Radiol 2014;25(9):1317–25*)
- Absolute:
  - Active internal bleeding or disseminated intravascular coagulation
  - Recent (within 3 mo) cerebrovascular event (including TIA), neurosurgery (intracranial, spinal), or intracranial trauma
- Relative:
  - Recent (within 7–10 d) cardiopulmonary resuscitation, major surgery, obstetrical delivery, organ biopsy, major trauma, or cataract surgery
  - Intracranial tumor, other intracranial lesion, or seizure disorder
  - Uncontrolled hypertension (systolic >180 mmHg or diastolic >110 mmHg)
  - Recent (within 3 mo) major gastrointestinal bleeding or internal eye surgery
  - Serious allergic or other reaction to thrombolytic agent, anticoagulant, or contrast media (not controlled by steroid/antihistamine pretreatment)
  - Severe thrombocytopenia
  - Known right-to-left cardiac or pulmonary shunt or left heart thrombus
  - Severe dyspnea or severe acute medical illness precluding safe procedure performance
  - Suspicion for infected venous thrombus
  - Renal failure (GFR <60 mL/min)
  - Pregnancy or lactation
  - Severe hepatic dysfunction
  - Bacterial endocarditis
  - Diabetic hemorrhagic retinopathy

Preprocedure Preparation/Workup (*Handbook of Interventional Radiologic Procedures. 2011: Lippincott Williams & Wilkins*)
- Patient evaluation: Assess symptomatology and whether CDT is truly indicated, with particular attention to:
  - Risk factors for bleeding complications
  - Baseline ambulatory status
  - Life expectancy
  - If chronically nonambulatory or low life-expectancy, there may be very little benefit to CDT
- Imaging evaluation:
  - Review duplex venous ultrasound to confirm diagnosis or DVT
  - Cross-sectional imaging of the central veins may be obtained prior to invasive venography at the discretion of the operator
- Laboratory evaluation:
  - Ensure INR is below 2.0 (preferably 1.5) and stop any irreversible anticoagulants at least 24 h prior to CDT
  - Pregnancy test should always be obtained in women of childbearing potential
- Consent should discuss the risks of bleeding as well as the uncertainties surrounding CDT and should also address any adjunctive measures such as angioplasty or stent placement
  - IVC filter placement prior to CDT is sometimes performed and should be anticipated during the consent process

Procedure Technique (*Handbook of Interventional Radiologic Procedures. 2011: Lippincott Williams & Wilkins*)

- Obtain ultrasound-guided access peripheral to the extent of thrombus:
  - Lower extremity: Popliteal vein or posterior tibial vein
  - Upper extremity: Brachial or basilic veins
  - Consider size of sheath that will be necessary to accommodate infusion catheter when deciding how peripheral to access
  - Use angled catheter-wire manipulation to obtain central access through thrombus burden
- Perform central venogram to confirm central patency and if desired/required pullback venogram through diagnostic catheter to define thrombus extent:
  - Typically done with serial hand injections of 5–10 cc iodinated contrast and digital subtraction imaging
- Infusion-first CDT (*Handbook of Interventional Radiologic Procedures. 2011: Lippincott Williams & Wilkins*):
  - Select either a traditional multi-side–hole infusion catheter or an ultrasound-emitting infusion catheter (EkoWave, EKOS corporation, Bothell, WA) of appropriate length to match the thrombosed venous segment
  - Advance catheter into position and start infusing thrombolytic drug (*Handbook of Interventional Radiologic Procedures. 2011: Lippincott Williams & Wilkins; J Vasc Surg 2013;57(1):254–61*)
    - Recombinant tissue plasminogen activator (rt-PA at 0.01 mg/kg, not to exceed 1.0 mg/h)
    - Urokinase (UK) at 120000–180000 U/h
    - Reteplase at 0.50–0.75 U/h
    - Tenecteplase (TNK) at 0.25–0.50 mg/h
  - Simultaneously administer anticoagulant therapy by infusing subtherapeutic unfractionated heparin through the peripheral venous access
  - May elevate the treated extremity during infusion
  - Monitor the patient in stepdown unit or intensive care unit during infusion and obtain peripheral laboratory studies (including CBC and PTT) at least every 4–6 h. Fibrinogen level may also be monitored but data is insufficient to support its efficacy in preventing complications
  - Frequently assess for sentinel bleeding such as epistaxis, ear bleeding, or profuse access site bleeding
  - After 6–18 h of infusion, bring back to the angiographic suite and repeat the venogram
- Single-session pharmacomechanical CDT (PCDT): Involves rapid dispersion of significant dose of thrombolytic as well as mechanical thrombolysis using one of the following devices (*Handbook of Interventional Radiologic Procedures. 2011: Lippincott Williams & Wilkins*)
  - Trellis (Bacchus Vascular/Covidien/Medtronic, Santa Clara, CA): Two balloons are inflated to isolate the thrombosed venous segment, followed by mechanical maceration with a sinusoidal oscillating wire
  - AngioJet Rheolytic Thrombectomy (Boston Scientific Corp, Minneapolis, MN): Power-pulse thrombolysis with powerful delivery of the thrombolytic drug into the thrombus, followed by aspiration of the softened residual clot. AngioJet Zelante (8F) for vessels >6 mm. Monitor for bradyarrhythmia during Angiojet use close to the heart.
- Following infusion-first CDT or single-session PCDT, repeat venogram is performed
  - If near-complete (>90%) lysis and good anterograde flow are observed with no venous stenosis or obstruction, treatment may be stopped
  - If residual thrombus is present, adjunctive measures may be used to remove it
- Balloon maceration:
  - Advance a standard angioplasty balloon catheter (6–10 mm for the femoral vein, 10–14 mm for the common femoral vein or iliac vein) into the thrombus. Repeatedly inflate and deflate the balloon in different parts of the thrombus to macerate the thrombus
- Aspiration thrombectomy:
  - Advance standard catheter central to the thrombus, and vigorously aspirate as the catheter is withdrawn. Repeat as needed
  - Penumbra Indigo Cat8 aspiration system (Alameda, CA): Continuous high level circumferential aspiration with mechanical clot separation
- Rheolytic thrombectomy:
  - Performed with AngioJet in aspiration mode
- Infusion end point: Any one of the following is observed
  - Near-complete (>90%) thrombolysis
  - Clinically overt bleeding
  - Minimal progress is seen on two subsequent venograms

- Treatment of obstructive lesions:
  - Balloon angioplasty and stent placement for areas of stenosis or obstruction
  - Self-expanding stents for iliac vein and/or common femoral vein if needed
  - Balloon angioplasty alone for femoral or popliteal vein stenosis
  - Patients with Paget–Schroetter syndrome should have thoracic outlet decompressed surgically
  - Subclavian stenting is contraindicated

Postprocedural Care (Handbook of Interventional Radiologic Procedures. 2011: Lippincott Williams & Wilkins)

- Immediate postprocedure period:
  - Bed rest for at least 4 h, followed by early ambulation
  - Therapeutic anticoagulation should be initiated as soon as hemostasis is obtained
- Followup:
  - Always counsel patient for reddish-brown discoloration of urine and encourage aggressive hydration
  - Consider retrieval of IVC filter (if placed) at any time following PCDT
  - Offer graduated compression stockings to reduce lower-extremity swelling
  - Patient should be seen in clinic within 1 mo of procedure, with focused evaluation for postthrombotic syndrome
    - Villalta score: Considered gold standard for diagnosis and classification of PTS
      (J Vasc Surg 2013;57(1):254–61)

Villalta Scoring System (J Vasc Surg 2013;57(1):254–61)

Symptoms	None	Mild	Moderate	Severe
• Pain	0	1	2	3
• Cramps	0	1	2	3
• Heaviness	0	1	2	3
• Paresthesia	0	1	2	3
• Pruritis	0	1	2	3
Signs				
• Pretibial edema	0	1	2	3
• Skin induration	0	1	2	3
• Hyperpigmentation	0	1	2	3
• Redness	0	1	2	3
• Venous ectasia	0	1	2	3
• Pain on calf compression	0	1	2	3
• Venous ulcer	Absent			Present

Score <5: Negative for PTS
Score 5–9: Mild PTS
Score 10–14: Moderate PTS
Score >15 or venous ulcer present: Severe PTS
(Adapted from Soosainathan A, Moore HM, Gohel MS, et al. Scoring systems for the post-thrombotic syndrome. J Vasc Surg 2013;57(1):254–61. Copyright © 2013 Society for Vascular Surgery, with permission.)

Complications (J Vasc Intervent Radiol 2014;25(9):1317–25)

- Major bleeding: 2.8%
- Symptomatic PE: 0.5%
- Intracranial bleeding: 0%
- Overall major complications: 3.9%

Landmark studies (Handbook of Interventional Radiologic Procedures. 2011: Lippincott Williams & Wilkins; Lancet 2012;379(9810):31–8; N Engl J Med 2017;377(23):2240–52)

- CaVenT: Catheter-directed venous thrombolysis in acute iliofemoral vein thrombosis (N Engl J Med 2017;377(23):2240–52)
  - Used infusion-only CDT with anticoagulant therapy in patients with iliac and/or upper femoral DVT
  - Demonstrated 26% relative reduction in risk of PTS over 2-y followup (41.4% vs. 55.6%, p = 0.04) compared with anticoagulation alone
  - Limitations: Sample size of 189 patients (92 of whom received CDT); geographical limitation to southern Norway
- Acute Venous Thrombosis: Thrombus Removal with Adjunctive Catheter-Directed Thrombolysis (ATTRACT) trial (N Engl J Med 2017;377(23):2240–52)
  - NIH-funded multicenter randomized clinical trial evaluating the ability of PCDT to prevent PTS Assessed Trellis and AngioJet systems as well as infusion-first thrombolysis

- Incidence of PTS unchanged with PCDT (46.7%) vs. anticoagulation alone (48.2%); $p = 0.56$
- Recurrent VTE actually higher in PCDT than anticoagulation alone (12.5% vs. 8.5%, $p = 0.09$)
- Major and any bleeding rates statistically higher with PCDT (1.7% vs. 0.3% for anticoagulation alone); no intracranial or fatal hemorrhages in either group
- Leg pain and swelling significantly improved with PCDT ($p = 0.019$ and $p = 0.05$)
- Moderate or severe PTS less likely with PCDT (17.9% vs. 23.7%; $p = 0.035$); difference was greater for iliofemoral DVT than femoropopliteal DVT
- PCDT less effective in patients >65 y of age
- Various subanalyses of data from ATTRACT trial are ongoing

PULMONARY THROMBOLYSIS/THROMBECTOMY

Background

- Acute pulmonary embolism (PE) increases pulmonary vascular resistance and thus the load on right ventricle (RV). RV dilatation results in tachycardia and increased contractility
- Increased intramural pressure can lead to reduced coronary blood flow. RV dilatation and bowing of interventricular septum can lead to left ventricle (LV) underfilling which in turn can contribute to systemic hypotension
- Hypoxemia in PE is multifactorial, but mostly due to ventilation–perfusion mismatch
- Primary treatment of acute pulmonary embolism (PE) is anticoagulation in hemodynamically stable patients (*Handbook of Interventional Radiologic Procedures.* 2011: Lippincott Williams & Wilkins; *Circulation* 2011;123(16):1788–30)
- Classification of Pulmonary Emboli (*Circulation* 2011;123(16):1788–30):

Massive	Acute PE with sustained hypotension (<90 mmHg systolic) > 15 min or requiring inotropic support
Submassive	Acute PE with either RV dysfunction (CT, BNP/proBNP, ECG changes) or myocardial necrosis (elevated troponins)
Low Risk	Absence of hypotension, RV dysfunction, and myocardial necrosis

- Massive and submassive PE are associated with an increased mortality rate compared to smaller PE; thus additional treatment is sometimes warranted in these cases
- Systemic thrombolytic therapy is indicated in patients presenting with shock, hypotension, or other signs of systemic hypoperfusion caused by acute massive PE and in patients presenting with RV dysfunction with submassive PE (*Handbook of Interventional Radiologic Procedures.* 2011: Lippincott Williams & Wilkins; *Circulation* 2011;123(16):1788–30; *Am J Cardiol* 2013;111(2):273–77)
- Systemic thrombolytic therapy has been studied for over 30 y, and has been shown to rapidly reduce clot burden, improve hemodynamic parameters, and reduce mortality in appropriately selected patients (*Handbook of Interventional Radiologic Procedures.* 2011: Lippincott Williams & Wilkins; *Circulation* 2011;123(16):1788–30)
  - MOPETT (2013): Submassive PE; low-dose tPA vs. anticoagulation alone (randomized nonblinded); reduced pulmonary hypertension and recurrent PE with low-dose tPA (*Am J Cardiol* 2013;111(2):273–77)
  - PEITHO (2014): Submassive PE; placebo vs. tenecteplase (double blind); decrease in hemodynamic decompensation with tenecteplase, but increased rates of major extracranial bleeding and strokes (*N Engl J Med* 2014;370(15):1402–11)
  - TOPCOAT (2014): Submassive PE; placebo vs. tenecteplase (double blind); increased probability of "favorable composite outcome" with tenecteplase; limited by early termination and underpowered data (*J Thromb Haemost* 2014;12(4):459–68)
- Catheter-directed thrombolysis (CDT) attempts to maximize thrombolytic effects while minimizing the required dose of the drug and its complications, however is less extensively studied than systemic thrombolysis (*Handbook of Interventional Radiologic Procedures.* 2011: Lippincott Williams & Wilkins)
- Mechanical fragmentation, aspiration thrombectomy, rheolytic thrombectomy, sonographic disruption, and stent recanalization are all adjuncts to thrombolysis
- No single catheter-directed technique has been established as superior, thus the approach to treatment depends on the individual experience of the operator and the availabilities of the treating institution

- Goals of catheter-based therapy include rapidly reducing pulmonary artery pressure, RV strain, and pulmonary vascular resistance; increasing systemic perfusion; and facilitating RV recovery (Circulation 2011;123(16):1788–30)

Indications for Catheter-Directed Therapy (Circulation 2011;123:1788–30; Chest 2012;141(2 suppl):7S–47S; Eur Heart J 2014;35(43):3033–69)
- The following recommendations are adapted from the American Heart Association (AHA) scientific statement on massive and submassive pulmonary embolism. These recommendations are for either catheter embolectomy/fragmentation or surgical embolectomy depending on local expertise in patients with the following indications (Circulation 2011;123(16):1788–30):
  - Massive PE and contraindication to systemic thrombolysis
  - Massive PE and continued hemodynamic instability after receiving systemic thrombolysis
  - Submassive acute PE with clinical evidence of adverse prognosis (new hemodynamic instability, worsening respiratory failure, severe RV dysfunction, or major myocardial necrosis)
- The AHA recommends transfer to an institution experienced in either catheter embolectomy or surgical thrombectomy if these procedures are not available locally and the patient can be safely transferred
- Catheter embolectomy and surgical thrombectomy are not recommended for patients with low-risk PE or submassive acute PE with minor RV dysfunction, minor myocardial necrosis, and no clinical worsening
- Recommendations from the American College of Chest Physicians (ACCP) are similar to those above with the addition of the following indication for catheter-directed therapy (Chest 2012;141(2 suppl):7S–47S):
  - Acute PE with hypotension and shock likely to cause death before systemic thrombolysis can take effect (eg, within hours), if appropriate expertise and resources are available
- The following list of contraindications to systemic thrombolysis is adapted from the European Society of Cardiology (ESC) and is based on data derived from ST-elevated myocardial infarction guidelines (Chest 2012;141(2 suppl):7S–47S; Eur Heart J 2014;35(43):3033–69):
  - Hemorrhagic stroke or stroke of unknown origin at any time
  - Ischemic stroke in the preceding 6 mo
  - Central nervous system damage or neoplasms
  - Recent major trauma/surgery/head injury in the preceding 3 w
  - Severe gastrointestinal bleeding within the last month
  - Known bleeding risk
- Relative contraindications to systemic thrombolysis (Eur Heart J 2014;35(43):3033–69):
  - Transient ischemic attack in the preceding 6 mo
  - Pregnancy, or within 1 w postpartum
  - Traumatic resuscitation
  - Refractory hypertension (systolic blood pressure >180 mmHg)
  - Advanced liver disease
  - Infective endocarditis
- It should be noted that catheter-directed therapy often includes local administration of thrombolytic. Although the dose is significantly lower than that used for systemic thrombolysis, there is still a risk of bleeding with catheter-directed thrombolysis.
- Society of Interventional Radiology recently released its own recommendations, including (J Vasc Intervent Radiol 2018;29(3):293–97):
  - CDT is recommended in carefully selected patients with proximal acute massive PE, especially in highly compromised or rapidly deteriorating PE patients who have failed systemic thrombolysis
  - Available data is insufficient to recommend routine use of CDT for patients with submassive PE, but these patients should be closely monitored for deterioration and/or progression to massive PE physiology
  - For patients undergoing CDT for PE, SIR recommends close monitoring in an advanced care unit, routine ultrasound guidance for venous puncture, avoidance of AngioJet rheolytic thrombectomy and avoidance of mechanical interventions in patients with submassive PE in stable condition
  - If heparin is given during thrombolysis, subtherapeutic dosing is recommended to reduce bleeding risk
- There are no standardized guidelines regarding catheter-directed therapy, thus the assessment of the benefits and risks of treatment must be individualized and is ultimately in the hands of the provider (Ther Adv Drug Saf 2015;6(2):57–66)
  - In the setting of high-risk PE, some argue that absolute contraindications should be interpreted as relative (Eur Heart J 2014;35(43):3033–69; Ther Adv Drug Saf 2015;6(2):57–66)

Preprocedure Preparation/Workup (Handbook of Interventional Radiologic Procedures. 2011: Lippincott Williams & Wilkins)

- Patient evaluation:
  - Assess cardiopulmonary status through history, physical exam, electrocardiography, echocardiography, prior right-sided hemodynamics and imaging
  - Remember if there is evidence of left bundle-branch block, transvenous pacer should be placed prior to pulmonary angiography to prevent complete heart block
- Imaging evaluation (Handbook of Interventional Radiologic Procedures. 2011: Lippincott Williams & Wilkins; Eur Heart J 2014;35(43):3033–69):
  - Echocardiogram: RV dilation, increased RV–LV diameter ratio, hypokinesia of the free RV wall, tricuspid regurgitation (Eur Heart J 2014;35(43):3033–69)
  - Chest X-ray: Rapid assessment for other cardiopulmonary conditions (pneumothorax, pneumonia, aortic dissection, etc.) that may mimic PE; also an adjunct to lung scintigraphy (V/Q scan)
  - Computed tomography pulmonary angiography (CTPA): Evaluating thrombus burden, RV enlargement, RV–LV diameter ratio, ventricular septal bowing, etc.
  - Lung scintigraphy (V/Q): In cases where CTPA is contraindicated or unavailable, can offer general perspective on clot burden
  - Venous duplex: Not required, but can be helpful to diagnose concurrent lower-extremity DVT
- Laboratory evaluation:
  - Peripheral blood counts and coagulation panel, renal function panel, brain natriuretic peptide (BNP) and troponins to assess bleeding risk, ability to tolerate intravenous contrast, and evidence of right heart strain, respectively
- Consent should address the uncertainty involved with catheter-directed pulmonary thrombolysis. As discussed previously, the decision to treat is fairly nonstandardized; thus, a thorough discussion of the risks, benefits, and alternatives of the procedure is especially important

Pulmonary Angiography Technique (Handbook of Interventional Radiologic Procedures. 2011: Lippincott Williams & Wilkins)

- Access through the right common femoral or right internal jugular vein, latter preferred if evidence of iliofemoral thrombosis
- Place venous sheath capable of accommodating treatment device. Two adjacent sheaths can be placed for bilateral pulmonary access. Longer sheaths can be placed into the PA to obtain stability of subsequently placed infusion catheters.
- Advance preshaped catheter (eg, Grollman) or pigtail catheter through right heart to main pulmonary artery (PA). Measuring baseline pressures of PA, right atrium (RA), and RV is important.
  - Normal RA pressures are 0–5 mmHg
  - Normal RV pressures are 20–25 mmHg
  - Normal PA pressures are 20–25 mmHg systolic and 10–15 mmHg diastolic, with a mean pressure of 9–18 mmHg
  - Use caution when manipulating the catheter or wire in the right ventricle as irritation of the endocardium can induce arrhythmias
  - When RV end-diastolic pressure >20 mmHg, the mortality associated with pulmonary angiography approaches 2–3% (Handbook of Interventional Radiologic Procedures. 2011: Lippincott Williams & Wilkins)
    - If evidence of pulmonary hypertension, use subselective technique with low ionic contrast load (Handbook of Interventional Radiologic Procedures. 2011: Lippincott Williams & Wilkins)
- Perform arteriography based on baseline PA pressure and expected location of embolism as seen on CTPA or V/Q scan
  - Injection rates may be reduced to 10–15 mL/s for a total volume of 20–30 mL for the right and left PA
  - Minimize contrast load since most patients have received prior CTA which can be used for assessing distribution of clot burden
  - Obtain images with maximal inspiration, and at least two different projections, with magnification views if necessary

Endovascular Techniques

- Most techniques can be grouped into the following general categories, and are commonly used in conjunction with one another:
  - Proximal infusion of thrombolytic
  - Mechanical fragmentation
  - Rheolytic thrombectomy
  - Aspiration thrombectomy

- Local administration of thrombolytic proximal to the thrombus: historical relevance (*Circulation* 1988;77(2):353–60; *J Vasc Intervent Radiol* 2012;23(2):167–79)
  - This technique has actually been studied for decades, and confers no additional benefit to systemic thrombolysis (*Circulation* 1988;77(2):353–60)
  - Obstructing embolus actually causes proximal vortex formation, which prevents proximally administered thrombolytic from even reaching the embolus
  - Thus, catheter-directed thrombolysis requires direct intrathrombus injection and/or embolus fragmentation to be effective (*J Vasc Intervent Radiol* 2012;23(2):167–79). Catheter can be exchanged for a multi-side hole infusion catheter after traversing the thrombus (rheolytic therapy, discussed below)
- Rotating pigtail fragmentation (mechanical fragmentation): Most common method (*J Vasc Intervent Radiol* 2012;23(2):167–79; *J Vasc Intervent Radiol* 2009;20(11):1431–40; *J Am Coll Cardiol* 2000;36(2):375–80)
  - Used in 69% of CDT cases in meta-analysis of 594 patients. Often used in conjunction with other techniques (*J Vasc Intervent Radiol* 2009;20(11):1431–40)
  - Widely available, low cost
  - Effectively debulks proximal emboli
  - Can result in distal embolization with pulmonary artery pressure elevation
    - Requires adjunctive aspiration thrombectomy, which can be performed with virtually any large bore end-hole catheter
    - Balloon fragmentation may also be used as adjunct for more distal emboli (*J Vasc Intervent Radiol* 2012;23(2):167–79)
- Additional mechanical fragmentation devices:
  - Helix Clot Buster thrombectomy device (ev3/Covidien, Plymouth, MN)
  - Arrow-Trerotola PTD (Teleflex Medical, Wayne, PA)
- EkoSonic Endovascular System (EKOS, Bothell, WA): Rheolytic
  - Ultrasound-assisted catheter-directed low-dose fibrinolysis (USAT): 0.5–1 mg TPA/catheter/h
  - Combines low-intensity high-frequency ultrasound with thrombolytic infusion; which separates fibrin strands without fragmenting thrombus
  - ULTIMA (2013): Randomized controlled trial comparing USAT to anticoagulation alone (*Circulation* 2014;129(1):479–86)
    - Reduced RV/LV ratio after 24 h of treatment, statistically significantly better than heparin alone
    - No increase in bleeding complications
  - SEATTLE II (2015): Prospective single-arm multi-center trial (*JACC: Cardiovasc Intervent* 2015;8(10):1382–92)
    - Treatment with USAT decreased RV dilatation, reduced pulmonary hypertension, decreased anatomic thrombus burden, and minimized intracranial hemorrhage in patients with acute massive and submassive PE
    - Only compared these values in patients at presentation vs. 48 h posttreatment
    - Limited by no comparator group
  - OPTALYSE PE (2017): Randomized patients with submassive PE to 4 cohorts with different duration and dose of USAT (*Am J Respir Crit Care Med* 2017;195:A2835)
    - Significant reduction in RV/LV ratios in all cohorts at 48 h posttreatment
    - All cohorts had zero to very low bleeding rates
    - Significant in that the effective dose for reduction in RV/LV ratios is lower than that used in prior studies
  - PERFECT (2015): Multicenter registry of patients with massive and submassive PE treated with CDT (*Chest* 2015;148(3):667–73)
    - Clinical success rate of 85%
    - Improvement in pulmonary arterial pressure, improvement in RV strain on followup echocardiography compared to presentation
    - No major complications, hemorrhages, or strokes
    - Subgroup analysis showed no significant different between USAT and standard CDT
- AngioJet Rapid thrombectomy system (Boston Scientific, Natick, MA): Rheolytic
  - Associated with bradyarrhythmia-related complications (*Handbook of Interventional Radiologic Procedures*. 2011: Lippincott Williams & Wilkins)
- Aspiration thrombectomy
  - Any large-bore (22F) cannula can be used to remove fresh thrombi; typically requires clinical perfusionist and general anesthesia
  - AngioVac (AngioDynamics, Albany, NY), Penumbra CAT 6-8 (Penumbra, Alameda, CA)

Complications (*Handbook of Interventional Radiologic Procedures*. 2011: Lippincott Williams & Wilkins)
- Refractory or recurrent cardiopulmonary arrest
- Hemoptysis and pulmonary edema as a result of reperfusion
- Hemolysis (with rheolytic devices)
- Hemorrhage (with lytic enzymes and anticoagulants)

CHRONIC VENOUS SYNDROMES

Background
- Venous occlusion/stenosis can occur due to a variety of causes including anatomic compression, chronic thrombosis, and/or long-standing central venous catheters
- The approach to treatment of venous occlusion depends on the etiology, anatomic site, symptomatology, chronicity, and comorbidities of each individual patient
- Most venous syndromes require some combination of percutaneous transluminal angioplasty (PTA), stenting, catheter-directed thrombolysis (CDT), and/or definitive surgical management
- This section will address several syndromes of venous occlusion individually and focus on the unique aspects of each
- The technique for crossing occluded venous segments is similar in each syndrome, and typically requires the use of hydrophilic-coated guidewires with curved catheters
- A dual-access approach from both proximal and distal to the occlusion can aid in traversing the occluded segment. Once the occlusion is crossed from one access, the other access can be used to snare the crossed wire/catheter and secure access for venography and/or stenting

Paget–Schroetter Syndrome (Effort Thrombosis) (Cardiovasc Diagn Ther 2016;6(6):582–92)
- Usually seen in dominant arm of young, physically active male patients and is due to anatomic abnormalities involving the thoracic outlet such as cervical ribs, congenital bands, or hypertrophic scalene muscles among others
- Presents with unilateral arm swelling, pain, discomfort, erythema, cyanosis, and varicosities, usually in an acute or subacute setting following a recent sports-related event
- Paget–Schroetter syndrome (PSS) is more likely to cause postthrombotic syndrome (PTS) than likely to cause pulmonary embolism (PE) when compared to catheter-related upper-extremity deep vein thrombosis (UEDVT)
- Cross-sectional venography (CTV or MRV) is often helpful to determine the cause and site of anatomical compression
- Gold standard for diagnosis is positional venography (digital subtraction venography while manipulating the patient's affected arm), although this has largely been replaced with cross-sectional imaging
- Treatment with conservative measures alone such as bed rest, limb elevation, warm compresses, and anticoagulation often results in high rates of residual symptoms, recurrent thrombosis, and long-standing disability
- Systemic thrombolysis is more effective than conservative measures, but does carry a risk of major bleeding
- Catheter-directed mechanical and TPA thrombolysis is recommended in all patients with acute to subacute presentation, ideally within 2 w of symptom onset
- A peripherally inserted central venous (PICC) catheter can be left in situ to maintain access
- Principles and tools of venous thrombolysis are similar to those described in the lower-extremity venous thrombolysis chapter
- Aggressive balloon angioplasty must be avoided prior to surgical intervention. Therapeutic anticoagulation should be continued.
- Due to the persistent anatomical compression associated with Paget–Schroetter syndrome, the condition requires definitive surgical management, often involving a combination of decompression with patch angioplasty or (in cases of long-standing occlusion) bypass of the subclavian vein
- Any attempts at primary angioplasty or stenting prior to surgery should be avoided as these endovascular techniques will only cause further endothelial damage and complicate future surgical intervention
- Following surgical decompression, the interventional radiologist can play a role in venoplasty or stenting of the stenotic subclavian segment or bypass graft

Secondary Upper-Extremity Deep Vein Thrombosis (Catheter-Related)
- Much more common than primary upper-extremity deep vein thrombosis (Paget–Schroetter syndrome)
- Rate of clinically overt UEDVT after central venous catheter placement varies between 5% and 28%, and is higher in patients with underlying malignancy or history of thrombosis or thrombophilia (Circulation 2012;126(6):768–73; J Thomb Haemost 2011;9(2):312–19)
- Catheter-related risk factors include subclavian venipuncture, technically difficult or left-sided catheter placement, location of catheter tip not at cavoatrial junction, prior central venous catheterization, and large-lumen catheters (J Thomb Haemost 2011;9(2):312–19)

- Treatment-related risk factors include radiation therapy to the chest, bolus chemotherapy, and parenteral nutrition (*J Thomb Haemost* 2011;9(2):312–19)
- Other noncatheter-related causes of UEDVT include malignant venous compression, prior trauma or surgery, pregnancy and oral contraceptive use (*Circulation* 2012;126(6):768–73)
- Signs and symptoms include heaviness, discomfort, pain, paresthesia, and swelling of the affected arm, with pitting edema, redness, collateral veins, and/or cyanosis on physical exam (*Cardiovasc Diagn Ther* 2016;6(6):582–92)
- As stated above, the risk of PE is higher with catheter-associated UEDVT than with PSS, although the risk of PE from UEDVT in general is much lower than that of lower-extremity DVT (*Circulation* 2012;126(6):768–73)
- Compression ultrasonography is usually sufficient for diagnosis, although cross-sectional venography can be helpful to better assess the etiology and extent of venous stenosis/occlusion, as well as guide future treatment endeavors
- American College of Chest Physicians (2012) consensus guidelines for acute UEDVT treatment (*Chest* 2012;141(2):e419S–e494S)
  - Distal UEDVT: Anticoagulation alone or surveillance
  - Proximal UEDVT: Acute anticoagulation
  - Severe UEDVT involving most of subclavian/axillary vein: CDT or pharmacomechanical thrombectomy
  - Superior vena cava (SVC) syndrome: Urgent angioplasty/stent (see below)
  - Catheter associated UEDVT: No routine catheter removal (except in certain cases, described below)
  - Idiopathic UEDVT: Perform cancer screening
  - PSS: Surgical decompression
- Routine removal of the central venous catheter is not recommended, but may be considered in the following cases (*Chest* 2012;141(2):e419S–94S):
  - Catheter malfunction or infection
  - Contraindication to anticoagulation
  - Persistent symptoms or signs of UEDVT during initial treatment
  - Catheter no longer needed
- Catheter-directed thrombolysis is recommended for patients with proximal UEDVT of recent onset and severe symptoms, low risk of bleeding complications, and good functional status (*Circulation* 2012;126(6):768–73; *Chest* 2012;141(2):e419S–94S)
  - Pharmacomechanical techniques such as rheolytic thrombectomy or ultrasound-assisted thrombolysis can reduce thrombolytic infusion time, duration of hospital stay, and costs. Some of these techniques are discussed in more detail in the venous and pulmonary thrombolysis sections.
- Following CDT if there is still residual stenosis on venography, primary angioplasty should be attempted (*Handbook of Interventional Radiologic Procedures*. 2011: Lippincott Williams & Wilkins)
  - Recoil of >50% suggests a predisposition to recurrence and thrombosis
  - Primary stenting is usually not advised unless there is an arteriovenous fistula sustaining adequate flow to the stent (see dialysis interventions chapter)
  - Secondary stenting should only be utilized if there is significant elastic recoil and only after repeated failure of angioplasty

Superior Vena Cava Syndrome (*J Roentgenol* 2009;193(2):549–58)
- Caused by underlying malignancy in 95% of cases (*J Roentgenol* 2009;193(2):549–58)
- Syndrome includes congestion and edema of the face and upper thorax, as well as dyspnea, hoarseness of voice, dysphagia, severe headache, and cognitive dysfunction resulting from cerebral venous hypertension
- Traditional treatment for malignant SVC syndrome includes radiation therapy and/or chemotherapy (*J Roentgenol* 2009;193(2):549–58)
- Stent placement had once been considered an adjunct to chemoradiation; however, in the past decades there has been a paradigm shift toward self-expanding stent placement as 1st-line treatment due to its ability to provide urgent relief of symptoms without interfering with subsequent antitumor treatments (*J Roentgenol* 2009;193(2):549–58)
- Malignant SVC syndrome: Endovascular stent technical success >95% with relief of symptoms in 24–72 h. Primary patency of >83% at 3 mo; secondary patency of >93%. (*Handbook of Interventional Radiologic Procedures*. 2011: Lippincott Williams & Wilkins; *J Roentgenol* 2009;193(2):549–58)
  - There is a risk of mediastinal and pericardiac bleeding/hemopericardium and anesthesia/surgical support must be considered during this intervention.
- Benign SVC syndrome: Endovascular treatment effective for duration of up to 3 y; frequent requirements of repeat intervention. Primary patency 77–91% at 1 y; 85% secondary patency at 17 months. Limited data in assessing long-term effectiveness

(Handbook of Interventional Radiologic Procedures. 2011: Lippincott Williams & Wilkins; Catheter Cardiovasc Interv 2005; 65(3):405–11)

Iliocaval Thrombosis and May–Thurner Syndrome (Cardiovasc Diagn Ther 2016;6(6): 582–92)

- May–Thurner: Compression of the left common iliac vein by the right common iliac artery; predominantly seen in young to middle-aged females; present in 18–49% of patients with left-sided lower-extremity DVT (Cardiovasc Diagn Ther 2016;6(6):582–92)
- Inferior vena cava (IVC) stenosis/obstruction can occur due to a variety of causes including extrinsic tumor compression, indwelling IVC filter, and extension of iliac vein thrombosis. The management is similar to May–Thurner syndrome so these entities are discussed together
- Doppler ultrasound: Lack of respiratory variations or absence of response to Valsalva maneuver can suggest proximal (iliac) DVT in the setting of common femoral vein patency
- CT or MR venography is especially useful to demonstrate extent of proximal thrombosis and/or occlusion
- Intravascular ultrasound (IVUS) is also helpful in May–Thurner syndrome and typically is performed in conjunction with thrombolysis
- Standard of care in acute iliofemoral DVT: Urgent catheter-directed thrombolysis with mechanical thrombectomy, venoplasty, and common iliac vein stenting (Cardiovasc Diagn Ther 2016;6(6):582–92; J Vasc Intervent Radiol 2000;11(10):1297–02; J Vasc Surg 2011;53(3):706–12)
- Typically performed with popliteal access in the prone position. Preprocedure placement of retrievable IVC filter may be considered in high-risk patients to reduce periprocedural morbidity from pulmonary embolism
- Early thrombolytic therapy (pharmacologic or mechanical) is thought to play a major role in preventing postthrombotic syndrome (J Vasc Intervent Radiol 2000;11(10):1297–02)
- In cases of chronic occlusion without acute DVT, there is little role for thrombolysis, so venoplasty and stenting can be performed electively
- After 12–48 h of thrombolysis, venoplasty, and stenting is typically performed using a large self-expanding nitinol or stainless steel stent across the stenosis and into the IVC (J Vasc Intervent Radiol 2000;11(10):1297–02)
- If the IVC is uninvolved, the iliac stent should extend <1 cm into the IVC to minimize effects on contralateral flow (Handbook of Interventional Radiologic Procedures. 2011: Lippincott Williams & Wilkins)
- In cases of IVC stenosis/occlusion it may be necessary to place bilateral "kissing" stents extending from the IVC into both common iliac veins
- While self-expanding stents are preferred for iliac veins, balloon expandable stents can be used in the vena cava (Handbook of Interventional Radiologic Procedures. 2011: Lippincott Williams & Wilkins)
- Patients will typically be placed on oral anticoagulation after stenting for at least 6 mo, and are followed with clinic visits and duplex sonography at 3–6-mo intervals. Revascularization in the event of stent occlusion or in-stent stenosis are typically successfully (J Vasc Surg 2011;53(3):706–12)
- For May–Thurner syndrome, primary and secondary stent patency at 2-y followup has been reported as high as 78% and 95%, respectively (Cardiovasc Diagn Ther 2016;6(6): 582–92; J Vasc Intervent Radiol 2000; J Vasc Surg 2011;53(3):706–12)

Portal Vein Thrombosis (J Vasc Intervent Radiol 2017;28(12):1714–21)

- Occurs in 10–25% of patients with cirrhosis, and is considered a relative contraindication to liver transplantation due to its contribution to intraoperative and perioperative morbidity and mortality
- Portal vein recanalization can often be performed in conjunction with transjugular intrahepatic portosystemic shunt (TIPS) creation in order to provide a patent portal vein at the time of transplant
- In addition to transjugular access for TIPS (discussed separately in hepatobiliary section), the portal vein is accessed via transhepatic or transplenic approach
- After deployment of TIPS stent (typically peripherally within the portal vein to maximize length of main portal vein that can be used for transplantation), venoplasty of the entire portal system and TIPS is performed until adequate flow is established
- Embolization of varices or shunts can also be performed to maximize flow through the TIPS
- High technical success rate (98%) and 5-y overall survival rate in recent cohort (J Vasc Intervent Radiol 2017;28(12):1714–21)

RENAL AND GENITOURINARY INTERVENTIONS

Background
- Many endovascular and percutaneous treatment options exist to treat common renal pathologies
- Percutaneous options offer decreased morbidity compared with surgical approaches
- Surgical techniques continue to improve in renal interventions; therefore a discussion should always be had with the surgical team prior to intervention to discuss the best option for each patient
- Kidney is considered a "high-risk" organ for bleeding—INR and platelet requirements for intervention should be more strictly followed compared to similar procedures in other organs
- Renal artery interventions are commonly performed with ipsilateral common femoral arterial access. Radial/brachial access may be easier if the renal artery has an acute takeoff on preprocedural imaging but this may limit the size of the catheters/sheaths used
- Percutaneous nephrostomy access is safest through the relatively avascular zone between the posterior one-third and anterior two-third of the kidney (Brodel's line). Lower pole access is commonly used for nephrostomy tube placement. Upper pole access may be required to provide support to urology for anterograde stone treatment.
- Preprocedural imaging should be reviewed prior to any intervention to plan the ideal approach and evaluate for altered anatomy; variant vascular and parenchymal anatomy is commonly seen in the kidney (including duplicated collecting systems, accessory renal arteries, or ectopic kidneys)
  - Ultrasound—Quick, inexpensive, best for evaluating the collecting system for obstruction and vasculature for flow/stenosis
  - CT—Best to evaluate the vascular anatomy from the aorta and see surrounding structures; contrast is helpful to evaluate pathology/anatomy and may be necessary in the workup of vascular stenosis/pathology; however, remember that many interventions require contrast and may result in significant contrast nephrotoxicity if imaging and intervention are done within a short interval
  - MR—Most time consuming and expensive, best to use for evaluation of malignancy or urodynamics

Kidney Disease
- Stages are defined by the Kidney Disease Outcomes Quality Initiative (KDOQI) from the National Kidney Foundation
- Chronic Kidney Disease (CKD)—Kidney damage or decreased GFR less than 60 mL/min/1.73 m^2 for at least 3 mo, regardless of etiology
- Most common cause—DM: 45%

Staging

Stage	Kidney Status	GFR
1	Mild kidney damage	>90
2	Mild GFR reduction	60–89
3	Moderate reduction	Subdivided: a) 45–59 b) 30–44
4	Severe reduction	15–29
5	Kidney failure	<15

Contrast-induced Kidney Disease
- Risk factors—CKD 4–5, diabetes, CHF, hypotension
- Defined as a rise of creatinine by 25% or by 0.5 mg/dL within 48 h of contrast load
- Often resolves within 1 w
- Contributor to morbidity associated with IR procedures—Interventionalist should attempt to reduce risk prior to giving large contrast volume for necessary procedures—Avoid nephrotoxic medications whenever able (ACE inhibitors, NSAIDs, etc.)
- Patients on dialysis can undergo hemofiltration after procedure
- Meds to prevent:
  - Hydration—Regimen given by JAMA isotonic IV sodium bicarb 3 cc/kg/h for 1 h before and 1 cc/kg/h for 6 h after (JAMA 2004;291(19):2328–34); hydration with IV NS has been found to be equally effective (Ann Int Med 2009;151(9):631–38)
  - N-acetylcysteine—1200 mg PO BID 1 d before and day of procedure (N Engl J Med 2006;354(26):2773–82)

Nephrolithiasis

- Common indication for IR-guided renal intervention
- Types
  - Calcium oxalate: 70–90%
  - Uric acid: 5–10%, associated with gout and chronic diarrhea; not seen on X-ray
  - Struvite: Related to chronic UTI, Proteus
  - Cystine: Congenital
- May present with hematuria, pain due to obstruction, and/or infection
- Workup: Noncontrast CT, UA
- IR involvement will center on degree of hydronephrosis and likelihood of stone passage—Larger stones or patients with pyonephrosis require nephrostomy for decompression
  - Discuss the procedure with urology to determine if access is needed for decompression + stone retrieval or decompression alone
  - Indications for urgent intervention—Hydronephrosis with AKI, intractable pain (esp for solitary or transplant kidneys)
  - Indication for emergent intervention—Sepsis

Renal oncologic treatment and renal biopsy are discussed in separate chapters

---

NEPHROSTOMY AND NU PLACEMENT

Background

- Percutaneous nephrostomy (PCN) provides rapid relief of urinary obstruction
- Used in the management of multiple genitourinary pathologies and to provide access for urologic surgical procedures such as lithotripsy
- May decrease the mortality of patients with urosepsis and urinary obstruction from 40–8% (Eur Radiol 2006;16(9):2016)
- High success rates: 99% PCN success rate in dilated collecting systems, 85% PCN success rate in nondilated collecting systems; 88–96% success rate for ureteral stenting (Radiology 2004;230(2):435–42; J Vasc Intervent Radiol 2003;14(9):S277–81.

Indications to Intervene

- Relief of urinary obstruction in patients where retrograde ureteral cannulation is unsuccessful or contraindicated, particularly in cases of urosepsis due to obstruction
- Acute renal failure related to obstruction
- Urinary diversion in cases of ureteral injury or urine leak
- Postsurgical or radiation-induced ureteral stricture
- Urinary diversion for severe refractory hemorrhagic cystitis (check history of chemotherapy)
- Preprocedural access for lithotripsy or ureteral stenting

Indications for Stent Placement (Yonsei Med J 2003;44(2):273–8; J Endourol 2010;24(7):1189–93; J Endourol 2000;14(7):583–87)

- Benign ureteral strictures—Iatrogenic, postradiation, extrinsic compression—Patency rates from balloon dilation and stenting 57% at 36 mo; better patency rates for shorter segment strictures
- Malignant strictures—Less successful, 36-mo patency rate 14%; failure rate 36% over 95 d for plastic stents—Reserve stenting for palliative cases when surgical intervention not possible

Workup of the Patient Requiring Nephrostomy/NU Placement

- Evaluate patient's history and prior imaging to identify the cause and location of ureteral/bladder obstruction—Enlarged prostate, cervical/ovarian malignancies, iatrogenic ureteral injuries, etc.
- Evaluate patient's current treatment course including history of antibiotics. Patients require preprocedural antibiotics in cases of obstructive pyonephrosis or high-risk procedures such as staghorn calculi
- Determine degree of hydronephrosis and presence of infection/pyelonephritis/pyelitis
- Creatinine including history of renal failure
- WBC in cases of suspected pyonephrosis
- Hemoglobin, platelet count, and coagulation factors in preparation for procedure
- Evaluate potassium—High potassium may require dialysis prior to the procedure to reduce the risk of cardiac arrhythmias
- Obtain or review preprocedural imaging to plan the optimal procedural approach—Ultrasound to evaluate the collecting system; CT to evaluate for stones; MR to evaluate for malignant causes of obstruction
- Determine the size, location, and orientation of the kidneys

- Evaluate for bowel, adjacent organs, or large vessels near the planned nephrostomy access site
- Evaluate kidney for masses or cysts that may interfere with needle placement or be confused with the renal pelvis on ultrasound
- Evaluate the location of stones if the procedure is being done prior to lithotripsy
- Recognize presence of duplicated systems which may require placement of catheters in multiple parts of the collecting system
- In cases of unilateral chronic obstruction, consider determining how much the kidney contributes to overall renal function—If no contribution, no indication to intervene. Can be assessed using Whitaker test or nuclear renogram
- If a patient is morbidly obese, ultrasound may be severely limited. Plan ahead for additional methods of visualizing and cannulating the collecting system. Make sure the patient has working central venous access or peripheral IV for this (see Technical Notes below).

Contraindications (J Vascu Intervent Radiol 1997;8(5):769–74; AJR Am J Roentgenol 1998;170(5):1169–76)
- Severe coagulopathy or anticoagulation unable to be discontinued
- Severe hyperkalemia
- Uncontrolled hypertension

Whitaker Test (Am J Roentgenol 1980;134(1):9–15)
- Used to evaluate a dilated renal collecting system for functional obstruction—Can help determine need for urinary diversion
- Invasive—Used as a second resort to CT/MR/ultrasound
- Can be used to determine results of treatment—Done before and after ureteral stenting to determine success
- Pressure measurements are taken within the renal collecting system through a pressure wire or catheter as well as within the bladder using a Foley and manometer. Differential pressure measurements are calculated during fluid infusion into the collecting system. Degree of pressure elevation in the pelvis correlates with obstruction through the collecting system (degree of pressure elevation in a system is proportional to resistance/degree of obstruction and rate of flow—Poiseuille equation)

Determining the Catheter Type
- Nephrostomy Tube (PCN)—Locking pigtail is in the renal pelvis and drains external to the patient
  - Best for ureteral obstructions, urine diversion, and rapid decompression of hydronephrosis
  - Best for patients with pyonephrosis—Allows for rapid decompression with lower risk of sepsis compared to ureteral stenting
- Nephroureterostomy Catheter or Nephroureteral Stent (NU)—A long internal/external drainage catheter with locking pigtail in the renal pelvis
  - The externally drainage portion is similar to a nephrostomy tube and can be connected to a drainage bag or capped
  - The internal drainage portion is similar to a ureteral stent and allow urine to drain through a ureteral stricture to the bladder (or ileostomy)
  - With the external portion capped, it can serve as a trial for how the patient would do with an internal stent without losing percutaneous access
  - Exchanged percutaneously, which may be easier or preferred by some patients
  - More secure than a nephrostomy—Better if patient is prone to pull on the tube—Harder to dislodge
  - Often used in patients with ileal conduits
- Ureteral (double J) stent—Entirely internal ureteral stent with no external component
  - Most comfortable option for the patient; however adequate flow from the kidney to the bladder must be established
  - Commonly placed retrograde by urologists. Can be percutaneously placed antegrade as well.
  - PCN or NU can be internalized and exchanged for a ureteral stent

Procedure Technique (Machan. *Handbook of Interventional Radiologic Procedures.* Lippincott Williams & Wilkins; 2011)
- For cases of obstructive pyonephrosis, antibiotics should be given if not already given—Single IV dose of cephalosporin such as cefazolin (Ancef) is commonly used; if penicillin allergy, consider ciprofloxacin, levofloxacin, or vancomycin—Consult infectious disease specialist to determine local sensitivities and hospital policy. Coverage should be against *E. coli*, Klebsiella, Enterococcus, and Pseudomonas.

- Identify the kidney using a low-frequency 3.5 MHz transducer. Plan the appropriate site of entry into the kidney. This will depend on the indication—For relief of obstruction, lower pole access is preferred. Attempt to approach through the relatively avascular zone at the junction between the posterior one-third and anterior two-third of the kidney (Brodel's line—approximately 30–45° from midline in the prone position). For stone retrieval or ureteral interventions, a mid or upper pole approach may be preferred to allow for a more direct path to the ureter.
- Place a 21G or 22G needle with stylet under ultrasound or fluoroscopic guidance into the target calyx. Entry through a posterior calyx is preferred. If the initial access is too central or directly into the renal pelvis, a 2-stick technique after opacifying the collecting system with contrast should be considered before dilating the tract and placing a nephrostomy tube to avoid a higher risk of complications.
- Remove the stylet and advance a 0.018" wire into the collecting system under fluoroscopy. Advancing the wire down the ureter will provide the most secure access for exchange.
- Exchange the needle over the wire for a 6F coaxial introducer sheath over the wire and into the collecting system. Advance the plastic catheter over the metallic inner stiffener once the system is through the renal cortex to prevent injury to the pelvis.
- Inject contrast to opacify the collecting system, understand anatomy, and confirm positioning. Consider aspiration of contents as well to prevent overdistention and sepsis, particularly in cases of infected obstructions.
- Remove inner dilators/stiffeners from the outer sheath and exchange the 0.018" wire for a 0.035" wire. An angled catheter and hydrophilic guidewire may be helpful to navigate past stones, ureteral strictures, or other obstructions. A stiff wire such as an Amplatz wire may be useful to provide stability during catheter placement; however, this wire has a risk of damaging the pelvis due to its stiffness—Use cautiously.
- Exchange the 6F sheath for a nephrostomy tube over the guidewire. Depending on the size of the tube placed, additional dilators may be required prior to tube placement to facilitate easy placement. 8F tubes are often used for initial drainage. 10F–12F tubes may be required if there is purulent urine or significant debris within the collecting system. Larger tubes may also be requested by urology referring providers based on the size of the tubes/devices they plan to use for stone retrieval or stent placement. Discuss with multidisciplinary team to determine appropriate tube to place in each case.
- Form the locking pigtail on the catheter within the renal pelvis. A final contrast injection confirms appropriate positing of the tube.
- If a nephroureterostomy or double J stent is being placed, the guidewire must be advanced through the ureter and into the bladder. This can be accomplished using an angled catheter and hydrophilic guidewire. Gently flushing saline or dilute contrast into the renal pelvis can help distend the collecting system to navigate past stones within the collecting system—Be careful with this technique in patients with infection as overdistention can precipitate bacteremia and sepsis.

Technical Notes

- In challenging cases such as when the collecting system is nondilated or difficult to see with ultrasound due to the patient's body habitus, 2 other techniques to consider include:
    - **Double stick method:** Advance a 21G or 22G needle under fluoroscopic or ultrasound guidance into the central renal collecting system and inject contrast to opacify the collecting system. A second needle can be advanced into the desired calyx for nephrostomy tube placement under fluoroscopic guidance and the procedure completed as above.
    - **Intravenous contrast injection:** In patients with preserved renal function, injecting 50 mL iodinated contrast intravenously at the beginning of the procedure will opacify the collecting systems as it is excreted by the kidneys. This a good technique to visualize a nondilated collecting system. When the collecting system is opacified with excreted contrast, the desired calyx can be accessed under fluoroscopy.
- Injecting a combination of contrast and air can be considered to differentiate between anterior and posterior calyces, since posterior calyces will fill with air and anterior calyces will fill with contrast when the patient is prone
    - Injecting air will distort visualization of the renal collecting system on ultrasound and should be reserved for cases when ultrasound is no longer needed
- No difference has been shown in the success rates or complication rates between single- and double-stick methods. (N Engl J Med 2006;354(26):2773–82; Machan. Handbook of Interventional Radiologic Procedures. Lippincott Williams & Wilkins; 2011)

- Entry sites that are too medial will traverse the paraspinal muscles and cause significant patient discomfort
- Entry sites that are too lateral risk injury to the colon. If planned trajectory appears too lateral or medial, re-evaluate if other access windows are available and double-check for any intervening bowel.
- In certain situations of anterior/upper pole tube placement, the approach may require intercostal needle placement. Remember to place needles above the rib to avoid injury to the intercostal artery or nerve.
- CT can be used for access; however, this requires significant radiation exposure. It is generally reserved for cases of abnormal anatomy such as horseshoe kidneys or renal ectopia. It can also be considered if the patient cannot be positioned prone or decubitus.
- Placement of nephrostomy tubes requires support from the stiffer parts of the wires used—Attempt to place the wire into the ureter to provide stability and reduce buckling of the catheters

Special Notes about NU/double J
- In cases where NU or ureteral stent placement is desired, percutaneous nephrostomy and ureteral stent placement can be performed in a single session; however, a staged procedure should be considered in the setting of pyonephrosis, if the ureter cannot be easily catheterized, or if significant bleeding occurs during percutaneous nephrostomy. After placement of a percutaneous nephrostomy tube and external drainage to decompress the collecting system, the patient can return after several days to convert the nephrostomy tube to a double J ureteral stent or nephroureteral stent.
- Catheter manipulation within an infected collecting system may increase the risk of systemic infection or sepsis
- A long sheath (23 cm, 6F sheath) can be placed over the wire into the renal pelvis to secure access into the collecting system and increase pushability when attempting to cannulate the ureter or cross a ureteral stricture. Glide catheters (4F) may be needed to cross a tight ureteral stricture that a standard catheter cannot.
- Balloon dilation may be required prior to ureteral stent placement if a stricture is difficult to cross with a catheter. Dilation with a 4–6 mm balloon is usually sufficient to allow ureteral stent placement. The balloon can also be used to push ureteral stones into the bladder if obstruction is due to stones.
- The proximal pigtail of a ureteral stent should be in the renal pelvis and the distal pigtail should be in the bladder. The ureteral length can also be estimated by the patient's height (*Image-Guided Interventions E-Book: Expert Radiology Series.* Elsevier Health Sciences; 2013):
  - Patient height less than 5'10"—22 cm ureteral stent segment
  - 5'10"–6'4"—24 cm
  - Greater than 6'4"—26 cm
- Double J stent placement similar to NU placement. A pusher is used to advance the stent over a wire into position. The stent is released from the pusher and the wire is then removed. Consult manufacturer instructions for the type of stent available at your institution.
- A safety nephrostomy tube may be placed following antegrade double J stent placement to maintain access to the renal pelvis and ensure the stent is working. The PCN is capped for several days to evaluate creatinine and urine flow and removed if the stent is functioning adequately. Antegrade nephrostogram can be performed through the PCN after the procedure and several days later to ensure stent patency prior to removal.

Nephrostomy Exchange
- Done routinely in 6–12-w intervals to prevent tubes from becoming clogged
- Antibiotics are not required for all routine exchanges but may be required if a patient routinely becomes bacteremic during exchanges (*Tech Vasc Interv Radiol* 2009;12(3):193–204)
- A small amount of contrast is injected through the indwelling nephrostomy tube to confirm positioning
- The catheter is cut to release the locking pigtail. The indwelling tube is removed over a guidewire and a new catheter is advanced into its place. Contrast is then injected through the new tube after placement to confirm positioning.
- If unable to advance a wire through an occluded or encrusted nephrostomy tube, consider using a hydrophilic wire or stiffer wire to cross the obstruction. A stiff wire, such as an Amplatz wire may also be helpful to straighten the pigtail as the catheter is removed.

- If a wire is still unable to be advanced, consider placing a peel-away sheath over the occluded tube (for instance, an 8F–9F peel-away sheath over an 8F tube). The sheath must be long enough to reach the renal collecting system. Remove the occluded tube and advance a guidewire followed by the new tube through the sheath. Inject contrast to document intrarenal placement and then remove sheath by peeling. Secure new tube with locking pigtail.

Dislodged Catheters

- If a PCN tube becomes pulled out, re-establishing access into the renal collecting system through the existing tract may be possible if it remains patent and intact
- An older established tract will remain patent longer than a recently placed nephrostomy tube
- A Kumpe catheter and hydrophilic guidewire are advanced within a patent tract into the renal pelvis. Contrast injection is then performed to confirm access within the renal pelvis. Once access is confirmed, a guidewire can be advanced into the ureter or coiled within the renal pelvis and a new PCN subsequently placed.
- If a partially dislodged PCN is unable to be immediately replaced (such as overnight), secure the dislodged catheter to the skin with gauze and tape to maintain the tract as much as possible
- Catheter dislodgment is more common in patients who are obese. Mobility of the skin or pannus may pull on the catheter as the patient sits up or changes from the prone to supine position following the procedure. Evaluate the patient's body habitus and skin site when determining the best place to secure the catheter and try to find less mobile areas of skin.

Special Cases of PCN

- Transplant kidneys are generally located in the iliac fossa; therefore, an anterolateral calyx is usually the easiest and safest site for nephrostomy access. Avoid a transperitoneal access as bowel injury is possible with this approach. Note that in cases where NU or double J stents are intended, shorter ureteral length tubes are needed (8–10 cm). A biliary drainage catheter with multiple side holes may be useful.
- Pediatrics—Most common indications = UPJ obstruction and posterior urethral valves bridging to surgery; use smaller tubes and shorter ureteral segments; use smaller amounts of contrast; kidney is very mobile and tube displacement is a serious concern–Monitor output more frequently in these patients
- Pregnancy–Patient may present with obstructive uropathy due to ureteral compression by the gravid uterus. Right-sided obstruction is more common. Retrograde stent placement through the bladder should be attempted first as it involves less radiation; however, PCN may be faster. The patient may not be able to lie prone when pregnant and preprocedural planning for optimal positioning is essential; discuss the risks of radiation exposure with the patient.

Complications

- Overall complication rate—10%
- Bleeding is the most common 1–4%—Can manifest as perinephric hematoma, retroperitoneal hemorrhage, or bleeding into the collecting system causing hematuria or catheter/stent obstruction by clots
- Infection and sepsis—1–3%
- Vascular injury, pseudoaneurysm formation, AV fistula
- Bowel perforation
- Ureteral injury/rupture
- Pneumothorax (for superior pole access that traverses the pleura)
- Catheter dislodgement
- Catheter obstruction—Due to urine sediment or noncompliance with regular exchanges
- Ureteral fistulization—More commonly related to radiation

Postprocedural Care

- Intraoperative hypotension, rigors, or other indications of sepsis induced by manipulation of the collecting system should be treated with antibiotics, IV fluids, and consideration of ICU monitoring for 24–48 h after the procedure
- Evaluate creatinine—Changes in creatinine could indicate renal damage
- Ultrasound or noncontrast CT can be used to evaluate for postprocedural bleeding/perinephric hematoma
- CTA may be considered to evaluate for active bleeding or vascular injury
- Evaluate hemoglobin to ensure there are no rapid decreases; hematuria is common after the procedure and should progressively improve. Clots in the urine are normal for the 1st 24 h.

- Monitor WBC—Should go down after procedure in cases of infection; if going up, may indicate additional source of infection and/or urosepsis from the procedure
- Monitor urine output from the tubes and track changes—Sudden decrease in output may suggest a dislodged catheter or continued obstruction
- Make sure patient is scheduled for routine exchanges in short intervals. Waiting too long may result in catheter obstruction and make exchange more difficult
- Patient education about drain maintenance is essential to prevent infection and dislodgement. Drains can be flushed 2–3 times/d with sterile saline to maintain patency in cases of hematuria, high stone burden, or infection

Tips and Tricks

- Remember that most renal catheters are placed with the patient in a prone position—This may be difficult, especially in larger patients where this position can precipitate apnea and airway compromise. Preprocedural planning is essential and alternate positioning or access sites should be considered. If the patient is unable to tolerate prone positioning and no alternative can be performed, airway support with anesthesia and intubation may be needed.
- If the pigtail does not form correctly in the renal pelvis or bladder, twist the catheter after pulling the pigtail drawstring and holding gentle tension on the string. Continuously twist in 1 direction—Do not twist back and forth as this can irritate the mucosa.
- Remember that the drawstring for a pigtail on a renal catheter can break if too much tension is applied
- When inserting a renal catheter over a glidewire through the skin, the metal stiffener is helpful for greater support during a fresh nephrostomy/NU placement. The plastic stiffener usually provides sufficient support for nephrostomy tube exchange through an established tract.
- Make sure the catheter is wet either with saline or lubricant when inserting through the skin to prevent buckling within the skin
- Make sure that the initial incision in the skin is well dissected to prevent buckling of the catheter in the subcutaneous tissues
- The major source of patient pain during a procedure is at the skin as well as at the renal pelvis, with dilation/distention of the pelvis causing significant discomfort. During initial placement, the renal capsule should also be adequately anesthetized with lidocaine or equivalent.

RENOVASCULAR STENTING

Background (Abrams' Angiography: Interventional Radiology. 2006: Lippincott Williams & Wilkins)

- Renovascular hypertension (RVH) accounts for 5% of all cases of HTN; 75% of these are due to atherosclerotic disease or fibromuscular dysplasia (FMD) (Handbook of Interventional Radiologic Procedures. 2011: Lippincott Williams & Wilkins)
- Annual mortality rate from cardiovascular disease related to atherosclerotic renovascular disease—16% (Vasc Surg 2010; Springer: 293–304)
- Blood pressure control in patients is essential. Studies show doubling of mortality from ischemic heart disease and stroke for every 20 mmHg increase in systolic pressure (Lancet 2003;361(9366):1391–92)
- Renal artery stenosis (RAS) is a frequent and potentially reversible cause of RVH. Presence of RAS does not always indicate a cause of hypertension—Essential benign hypertension can cause atherosclerosis of the arteries and present with RAS. Optimal evaluation of causes of hypertension and knowledge of when intervention will play a role is essential.
- RAS is independently associated with cardiovascular mortality in patients with CAD
- 4-y survival with 75% stenosis is 68%; bilateral disease has a 4-y survival of 47% (Kidney Int 2001;60(4):1490–7)
- Hemodynamically significant RAS resulting in hypertension is better controlled on fewer medications after intervention than without. Renal function is improved in 40% of patients who present with renal insufficiency (RI) related to RAS.
- Understanding when to intervene with angioplasty and stenting is essential as only 40% of patients with renal insufficiency due to RAS will show improvement in renal function after intervention
- 3 separate studies have shown no significant benefit in overall outcomes and mortality between angioplasty/stenting vs. optimal medical management; however, the study designs have been questioned.
  - CORAL (Cardiovascular outcomes in renal atherosclerotic lesions)—947 pts with RAS randomized to stenting vs. meds—No significant difference in the rate of adverse cardiac/renal events (N Engl J Med 2014;370(1):13–22)

- ASTRAL (angioplasty and stenting for renal artery lesions)—806 pts with atherosclerosis undergo revascularization + meds vs. meds only—Primary outcome renal function/creatinine or cardiovascular event rates (N Engl J Med 2009;2009(361):1953–62)
- STAR—140 pts with low GFR randomized to stent +meds or meds only—No significant difference in cardiac events (Ann Int Med 2009;150(12):840–48)
- Intervention is usually reserved for patients who fail medical management or have reversible causes of hypertension such as FMD
- RAS is associated with increased age, female gender, reduced GFR, increased BP, and CAD

Demographics (J Am Coll Cardiol 2004;43(9):1606–13; Kidney Int Suppl 1975:S153–60; JAMA 1972;220(9):1209–18)
- Atherosclerotic RAS—Average age 52, more common in male smokers; usually left sided, 30% bilateral
- FMD—Average age 38–40, more common in females, although males present younger; no race predilection; usually right sided, 25% bilateral

Workup of Patients with RVH
- Obtain patient history of BP treatment—History of medications used, dosages, and responses to treatment
- Obtain baseline parameters of renal function and size—Size is most appropriately measured by ultrasound due to lack of radiation
- Imaging evaluation of renal vasculature—CTA/MRA to look for origin of renal arteries and degree of stenosis; ultrasound to look for Doppler waveforms and vessel patency/velocities
- If one-imaging modality is not convincing for RAS, another should be ordered prior to invasive imaging if RVH/RAS is clinically suspected
- Creatinine
- Hemoglobin, platelets, and coagulation factors to determine eligibility of procedures
- Baseline physical exam of the extremities including color, sensation, pulses, and capillary return—Important for comparison after the procedure to identify complications such as distal embolization of plaque
- Transplant arterial stenosis—Indicated by tardus parvus waveforms distally on ultrasound; usually occurs due to neointimal hyperplasia and/or iatrogenic injury
- Additional signs of RVH that should prompt noninvasive imaging for RAS (J Vasc Intervent Radiol 2010;21(4):421–30):
  - Onset of HTN after age 55
  - Abdominal bruit
  - Resistant HTN
  - Recurrent flash pulmonary edema (indicates severe bilateral RAS)
  - Renal failure without cause with normal urine sediment
  - Diffuse atherosclerotic disease in other areas
  - Smoking history with new HTN
  - AKI caused by anti-HTN meds
  - Malignant HTN (end-organ damage, LVH, CHF, neurologic disturbance related to HTN)
  - Unilateral small kidney with new HTN
  - Unstable angina in the setting of suspected RAS (UA symptoms improve after renal revascularization)

Specific Imaging Features to Evaluate
- Location of the renal artery origins (level in relation to the spine, are they more anterior or lateral)
- Angle of takeoff of the renal arteries—Will determine catheter used
- Number of renal arteries on each side
- Presence of aneurysms
- Location of stenosis, length of stenosis, and approximate degree of stenosis (ostial lesions are better evaluated on coronal and sagittal reconstructions than on axial images); determine if main or accessory branches are involved
- Number of stenotic lesions
- Presence of additional renal pathology such as infarct, infection, hydronephrosis, masses
- Are the stenoses calcified? Calcifications make angioplasty more difficult
- Size of the kidney
- Presence of atherosclerotic disease, narrowing, and tortuosity in the bilateral iliac vessels (or subclavian/brachial arteries if using radial access)

Fibromuscular Dysplasia
- Most common cause of RVH in younger patients due to a structural cause
- Due to abnormality of the smooth muscle in the arterial wall

- 3 main types—Medial fibroplasia (most common, string of beads with beads larger than parent artery); medial hyperplasia (least common, concentric stenosis); perimedial fibroplasia (string of beads with beads smaller than parent)
- Beaded nature makes visual inspection of vessels unreliable—Pressure measurements encouraged to determine clinical significance of stenoses
- Studies show 75% improvement rate following angioplasty of FMD stenoses and 44% cure rate (Seminars in Interventional Radiology 2009;26(3):245–252)

Indications to Not Intervene
- Normotensive on 2 or fewer medications
- Imaging with conclusive evidence of normal renal arteries
- Normal renal function by lab markers and imaging
- No evidence of renal mass loss
- Long-segment complete occlusion (relative contraindication)
- Severe atheromatous disease in the aorta making embolization risk high or history of severe peripheral arterial disease (relative)

Indications for Intervention
- Understand the goals of intervention—Ideally to restore normal BP without antihypertensive medications or to reduce the amount of medications needed for BP control; additional endpoints include preservation of renal function
- Studies do not show percutaneous approach to be statistically significantly different from surgical treatment—Decision to intervene should be discussed with the patient and multidisciplinary team
- Treatment failure—Defined as uncontrolled hypertension despite use of three medications, loss of renal function, loss of renal mass on imaging, or unexplained flash pulmonary edema (baseline parameters for mass and function are essential in the initial workup)
- Younger patient with imaging suggestive of FMD
- Noninvasive imaging showing RAS >50% (indicated cross-sectional area reduced by 75%)
- New onset HTN in younger patient even without imaging of FMD (imaging may have inadequate sensitivity)
- Unilaterally increased renin secretion and contralateral suppression of renin secretion on renal vein sampling.

Indications for Stenting
- All stenoses should be evaluated for their hemodynamic significance and degree of narrowing.
- >75% narrowing of the diameter of a vessel lumen results in >90% cross-sectional area reduction and is clinically significant; visual inspection is enough to guide intervention
- <50% narrowing of the vessel lumen results in <75% cross-sectional area reduction and is usually not significant; pressure gradients may be required to determine importance
- 50–75% narrowing always requires pressure measurements
- Technique used for measuring pressure across a stenosis should be reproducible and accurate without blocking flow through the vessel—Large catheters will give falsely low pressure measurements; use 0.014 pressure-sensing wires whenever possible; especially true in FMD where catheters can stent open the stenoses and cause false readings
- Gradient >21 mmHg across has highest accuracy in predicting improvement in HTN after stenting (Vascular Diseases: Surgical & Interventional Therapy. 3rd ed. New York: Churchill Livingstone; 1994:721–41)
- Mean arterial pressure gradient of at least 10% across stenosis
- Do not stent lesions that are over 2 cm, at branch points, or with arterial diameters less than 4 mm
- Balloon expandable stents are the most common used—Allow for precise deployment

Preprocedural Care
- Hydration is essential to avoid contrast nephrotoxicity (CIN)—Start isotonic NS at 1–2 cc/kg/h 3–12 h prior and 6–24 h after
- If patient is allergic to contrast, premedicate with steroids and antihistamine—Consult your department policy on this. If contrast allergy is severe or risk of CIN is high, CO_2 can be used as a contrast agent.
- Prophylactic hemodialysis has not been shown to be useful
- Pharmacologic prophylaxis against CIN is not effective
- Discontinue all nonessential nephrotoxic and renally excreted drugs for 24–48 h prior to and after procedure

Procedure Technique (Handbook of Interventional Radiologic Procedures. Lippincott Williams & Wilkins; 2011:205–213)
- Evaluate the site of access using fluoroscopy (locate the position of the femoral head), ultrasound (to evaluate for plaque and high takeoff of common femoral artery), and palpation

- Consider ipsilateral common femoral access for the renal artery being treated—This will allow the catheter selecting the renal artery to be stabilized against the opposite wall
- Access the common femoral artery at the level of the femoral head with a 21G needle and advance a 0.018" guidewire through the needle
- Exchange the needle for a 5F transitional dilator set over the guidewire and remove the inner dilator and wire. Occlude the outer sheath with a finger to limit blood loss through the transitional sheath.
- Advance a 0.035" guidewire into the aorta (Bentson guidewire or hydrophilic glidewire to help avoid plaque disruption in heavily atherosclerotic vessels)—An angled glidewire may be required to maneuver through heavily calcified and tortuous vessels
- Exchange the 5F outer sheath over the guidewire for the working sheath (usually 6F or 7F). Remember to aspirate through the sheath to remove bubbles and then start a saline drip or flush frequently to avoid sheath clotting.
- Access the renal artery by placing a catheter over the wire and through the sheath and selecting the renal artery. The catheter used will depend on the anatomy and proceduralist preference. A C2 catheter is commonly used for renal arteries.
- Perform angiography to evaluate the anatomy. Images generally require 5–10° LAO for evaluation of the left side and 20–30° LAO for evaluation of the right side.
- Consider the "no touch" technique to allow the base catheter and additional microwire to sit in the aorta without scraping the wall—particularly useful in cases of significant aortic plaque
- Use a 0.035" wire or switch to a microwire to cross the stenosis and anchor catheter if there is appropriate landing room
- A pressure wire can be advanced across the stenosis identified by angiography to determine its clinical significance
- If the stenosis is significant visually or by pressure measurement, advance a wire across the stenosis
- Position an angioplasty balloon across the stenosis and inflate to dilate the stenosis. Leave inflated for 1–2 min with intermittent fluoroscopy. 5–8 mm diameter balloons are often used.
- Remove balloon and perform followup angiogram to see if stenosis is improved. Make decision to stent based on success of angioplasty and place stent across the area as indicated.
- Consider postangioplasty and poststenting pressure measurements to document improvement. This is not always necessary based on the visual appearance.
- Remove all catheters and wires and consider a femoral arterial closure device, especially in patients who are unable to lay flat for prolonged periods and obese patients where manual compression can be difficult

Types of Stents

- Covered stent—better for treatment of pseudoaneurysms or to treat complications such as dissection or rupture; not as useful for primary RAS
- Bare metal stent—good radial force and low cost options for ostial narrowing
- Drug-eluting—may help to limit restenosis in theory; however, they are more expensive and further studies are needed
- Cutting balloon angioplasty—for stenoses not able to be treated with conventional balloons. May be useful for in-stent restenosis or transplant artery stenosis.
- Avoid stents if vessels are less than 4 mm or in nonostial locations
- Generally 1–2 cm lengths, 4–8 mm diameters

Intraoperative Notes

- Learn to recognize the "accordion sign" of a wire buckling under fluoroscopy. This means the wire is stuck on a plaque and further pushing can cause plaque dislodgment and distal embolization.
- Recognize the shape of a J-wire—if the J portion of the wire appears to change shape, this means the wire is stuck in a small branch and further advancement can cause vessel injury.
- Consider using CO_2 or small amounts of gadolinium contrast in patients with severe iodinated contrast allergies or severe CIN
- Heparin should be given during the procedure to make sure catheters do not clot and intimal disruption caused by angioplasty does not lead to thrombosis
- Vasodilator use is encouraged during procedures in small vessels such as renal arteries to prevent vasospasm caused by wire manipulation
- As patients with RAS/RVH often have significant aortic atherosclerotic plaque, consider trying to select the renal artery with a small amount of a soft guidewire such as a Bentson guidewire extending from the catheter tip to avoid scraping the aortic lumen. A stiffer wire may be required once the renal artery ostium is entered in order to anchor the catheter and cross the stenosis.

- Delayed washout of contrast through the renal vasculature is suggestive of residual stenosis, arterial injury, or embolization of plaque; renal blood flow should be rapid
- Patients should not experience significant pain during balloon dilation. If there is significant pain, reevaluate with contrast for vessel damage.

Intraoperative Images that Should be Taken
- Ultrasound or fluoroscopic image of the access site
- Angiographic run from the renal artery ostium
- Evaluation of the artery stenosis in at least two planes
- Fluoroscopic image with balloon up
- Followup angiogram after angioplasty or stenting

Complications
- 30-d all-cause mortality—<1%
- Most common: Access site complications including hematoma and pseudoaneurysm/fistula formation—5%
  - Avoid by properly selecting route of entry (see chapter on Access)
- CIN—rise in creatinine is expected for 1–2 d after procedure, should go down after this
- Infection
- Stent fracture or migration
- Vessel dissection—treated by placing a balloon across the injury—important to leave a wire through the artery until the conclusion of the procedure in order to quickly treat this complication; stent placement is controversial for nonflow limiting dissection due to the risk of in-stent stenosis; flow limiting dissections require surgical consultation and prolonged balloon reinflation ± stent
- Vessel thrombosis—usually due to insufficient anticoagulation; treat with intra-arterial tPA infusion (5 mg loading over 30 min + 0.5 mg/h for 24 h) ± abciximab (0.25 mg/kg loading dose + 20 cc/h for 12 h)
- Vessel rupture—can lead to rapid loss of blood; place balloon across the site immediately and reverse anticoagulation with protamine 1.5 mg for every 100 units of heparin; give ample fluid resuscitation; covered stent placement may be required as a last resort
- Embolization of plaque distally—3%
- Renal infarction, perinephric hematoma
- Myocardial infarction—1%
- Compartment syndrome—more commonly due to bleeding when attempting brachial/radial artery access

Endpoints of Procedure (Handbook of Interventional Radiologic Procedures. Lippincott Williams & Wilkins; 2011:205–213)
- Improved or cured blood pressure—90–100% in FMD, 50–90% in atherosclerosis, 70–100% in transplant stenosis
  - Cured—BP below 140/90 without meds
  - Improved—decrease in diastolic BP of 15 or more on same or fewer meds; decrease in diastolic BP of 15 with normal BP on meds
  - Stable—diastolic BP decrease less than 15
  - Failure—no change in BP, no change in meds
- Improvement in renal function
  - Improved—decrease in creatinine 20% or more
- 13% restenosis rate

Postprocedural Care
- Important to encourage lifestyle modifications to prevent and delay recurrence (smoking cessation, weight/lipid control)
- Frequent checks of creatinine for 1st 24–48 h
- BP diary—have patients log their blood pressures to evaluate how effective treatments were and whether medications can be titrated down
- Monitor postoperative BP for 48 h—if it drops, administer IV NS, if it goes high, start ACEI
- Postoperative anticoagulation with aspirin 81 mg ± Plavix 300 mg if stented
- Frequent groin/arm checks for arterial access site
- Neurologic checks to determine distal embolization of plaque
- Scheduled renal imaging at several month intervals with ultrasound can determine early stent thrombosis
- Increase in HTN med doses or number of medications can indicate restenosis
- Restenosis is more difficult to treat than primary stenosis; may require larger balloons/stents and lead to more complications; re-treatment is reserved for severe cases

RENAL VEIN SAMPLING

Background
- Generally performed prior to planned renal artery revascularization to determine whether renal artery stenosis (RAS) seen on imaging is significant and contributes to HTN
- Renal vein sampling has a 65% sensitivity for improvement in HTN after revascularization; 89% negative predictive value for RAS being clinically significant
- Elderly patients—21% specificity, 16% negative predictive value—not as useful in this population

Indications
- RAS seen on noninvasive imaging
- To determine if tumors secrete renin or other substances

Contraindications
- RAS for which intervention is not planned anyway
- Venous anatomic abnormalities
- Alternative known causes of HTN or renal dysfunction for which additional workup has low utility
- Coagulopathy

Physiology
- Low perfusion pressure of the kidney and decreased sodium levels → kidney releases renin → liver secretes angiotensin 1 → converted to angiotensin 2 by ACE (lung)
- Angiotensin 2 = vasoconstrictor
- → Aldosterone release from zona glomerulosa (adrenal gland)
- → Na and H_2O retention (kidney)
- Kidney will increase renin secretion to maintain its perfusion pressure when the pressure in the renal artery decreases due to RAS
- The kidney that is not affected by RAS will have hyposecretion of renin due to suppression—differential measurements between the two kidneys is needed to understand significance of elevated renin
- Captopril challenge—giving captopril prior to the procedure will accentuate differences in renin between each kidney
- Renin ratio of 1.5:1 or greater—sensitivity 63%, specificity 60%

Workup of Patients Undergoing Renal Vein Sampling
- Review preprocedure imaging to identify the number and location of renal veins and vascular anomalies/obstructions (circumaortic/retroaortic path)
- If no prior imaging available, consider CT with venous phase imaging to evaluate for venous anomalies
- Consider if the patient is a candidate for renovascular revascularization—if the patient is not a candidate, then renal vein sampling may not be useful.
- CBC with platelets, coagulation factors to prepare for procedure
- Creatinine to evaluate renal function prior to contrast use
- Patient should discontinue anti-HTN meds for 2 w to increase sensitivity of the procedure—especially B blockers and ACEI

Procedure Technique
- Give captopril (1 mg/kg) PO 60–90 min prior
- Access the right common femoral vein (left common femoral vein or right jugular vein could also be considered) with micropuncture system and dilate up to 5F catheter to access the renal veins. The Cobra C2 catheter is commonly used to select the renal veins.
- Position the tip of the catheter within the main renal vein. In the left renal vein, the catheter tip should be beyond the origin of the gonadal vein. Obtain a blood sample from each renal vein.
- Samples should be obtained from each main renal vein on each side. This may require selecting more than one vessel based on the patient's anatomy.
- Obtain a blood sample in the main IVC as a comparison sample. Always discard 5–10 cc of blood prior to obtaining the sample to ensure sample is uncontaminated.

Complications
- Small risk of bleeding, infection, or injury to the renal vein or kidney—more common with larger catheters

Postprocedural Care
- Monitor site of access for bleeding—lower risk as procedure is done with venous access, not arterial

- Evaluate creatinine—changes can suggest complications like perinephric hematoma
- Postprocedural imaging is generally not needed unless patient exhibits prolonged pain, hypotension, acute drops in hemoglobin, or elevated creatinine

---

RENAL ARTERY EMBOLIZATION

Background (*Image-Guided Interventions E-Book: Expert Radiology Series.* Elsevier Health Sciences; 2013:404–410)

- Total embolization is rarely required now due to improved surgical techniques that have lower bleeding rates
- 1% rate of iatrogenic hemorrhage following renal interventions requiring embolization or treatment
- 2% clinically significant bleeding rate after partial nephrectomy requiring intervention (*Urology* 2011;78(4):820–26)
- Some studies have shown a limited survival benefit for preoperative or palliative renal artery embolization for renal malignancies (*Seminars in Interventional Radiology* 2014;31(1):70–81)
- Embolization may be performed to decrease the size and bleeding risk of sporadic angiomyolipomas. The technique is not as effective in treatment of tuberous sclerosis related AML.
- Several studies have shown very few or no major complications when using a partial embolization technique compared to total embolization.

Indications
Complete Renal Artery Embolization
- Inoperable renal malignancies—patient must have persistent hypercalcemia (paraneoplastic syndrome), hematuria, or intratumoral bleeding
- Tumor debulking in patients with venous extension of tumors prior to surgery—helps reduce bleeding risk
- Reduce operative bleeding risk in patients who cannot receive blood transfusions (Jehovah's witness, ABO incompatibility)
- Significant nephrotic syndrome
- Persistent urine leaks (usually iatrogenic or traumatic) without surgical options
- Transplant kidney intolerance—renal isolation in lieu of surgical removal

Selective Renal Artery Embolization
- Angiomyolipoma: Bleeding risk increases with size. Embolization is recommended for lesions >4 cm or in pregnancy where the lesion may grow and has an increased rupture risk
- Bleeding renal tumors or blunt trauma with active arterial extravasation
- Large renal pseudoaneurysms/AV fistula causing hemodynamic instability in cases where anatomy precludes stenting/coiling of the shunt

Workup of the Patient Undergoing Embolization
- CBC, INR in preparation for procedure
- WBC—embolization in patients with active pyelonephritis or UTI can precipitate abscess
- UA
- Creatinine/GFR
- Review preprocedural imaging for ectopic or duplicated kidneys. Evaluate the renal artery anatomy for accessory arteries, location of the origins (approximate vertebral level), and any stenoses.
- Evaluate the iliac vessels for stenoses/atherosclerosis along the intended path—will dictate safety of using specific catheter/wire combinations
- In cases of impaired renal function or single functional kidney requiring total embolization, remember that the patient may require dialysis after the procedure. Consider the need for a temporary or tunneled dialysis catheter.

Special Note about Aneurysms
- Renal artery aneurysms predispose to several complications including spontaneous bleeding and distal infarction due to thrombus formation within the aneurysm sac and distal embolization of clot
- Predisposing factors: Connective tissue disorders, trauma, vasculitis (polyarteritis nodosa)
- Threshold to treat—2 cm. The treatment of smaller aneurysms should be considered in higher-risk patients with connective tissue disorder, malignant HTN, or prior to pregnancy which may predispose to aneurysm growth or rupture (*Cardiovasc Surg* 1996;4(2):185–89)

- Treatment options (main artery): Exclusion by covered stent 1st option, otherwise coils
- Treatment options (side branches or distal aneurysm): Coil, stent, glue

Contraindications
- Active infection (of any source but particularly urinary tract and pyelonephritis)
- Single kidney, impaired renal function, uncorrectable coagulopathy or contrast allergy are relative contraindications

Complications
- Bleeding
- Infection (higher risk in diabetes)
- Renal infarct due to renal artery branch occlusion or nontarget embolization
- Arterial rupture/injury
- Development of hypertension

Embolization Equipment
- Absolute ethanol—for total embolization
- Bucrylate (glue)—total or partial embolization
- Ethiodized oil—total or partial, usually mixed with glue
- Particles—Polyvinyl alcohol (PVA) or embolic microspheres—for total or partial embolization
- Coils—for proximal or selective embolization—detachable coils may be used for precise placement, visible throughout deployment

Technique (Handbook of Interventional Radiologic Procedures. Lippincott Williams & Wilkins; 2011)
- Procedural technique is very similar to the embolization procedures described in the Trauma section. See this section for more details.
- Use micropuncture system to access the common femoral artery (or radial/brachial artery in upper-extremity access. Exchange for a 5F or 6F sheath over the wire and place 5F selective catheter into the aorta to select the renal artery ostium (a Cobra C2 catheter is commonly used for the renal arteries).
- Perform angiography to evaluate the anatomy and plan embolization approach
- 4F or 5F catheters can be used catheterize the main artery for total embolization. Microcatheters are used for subselective catheterization of smaller branches for partial embolization.
- For total embolization with ethanol, a balloon catheter may be positioned in the proximal renal artery to occlude the origin and prevent nontarget embolization. Ethanol is then injected distal to the balloon. Wait for 10 min and reassess flow through the artery by taking down the balloon and injecting small amounts of contrast. Repeat the process until distal blood flow has stopped. Ethanol injection can also be done without a balloon; however, the amount injected must be smaller and slower to prevent reflux, and the process is generally repeatedly performed until stasis. Absolute maximum used should be less than 50 cc.
- In using glue or particles, an occlusion balloon may also be considered to prevent reflux and nontarget embolization. Remember that all embolic therapies, but particularly glue, can become clogged inside catheters. Once clogged, you will have to remove the catheter and obtain a new one. 5% dextrose in sterile water is used before and after glue administration to reduce the risk of intracatheter polymerization. Additionally, the tip of the catheter (higher risk with microcatheter) can become stuck to the vessel due to the glue—remember to withdraw the catheter into the base catheter as soon as administration is done to prevent the catheter sticking to the patient. If the catheter becomes stuck, attempt flushing with 5% dextrose—do NOT pull on the catheter with force as this can cause significant arterial injury. Surgical consultation may be required in severe cases.
- See arterial interventions section for more information on treatment of AV fistulas.

Postoperative Management
- Complication rate—4%
- Mortality rate—0.07%
- Embolization of the entire kidney has a high predisposition to post-embolization syndrome (nausea, fever, pain). Treat with IVF, Tylenol (antipyretic), and Zofran (antiemetic).
- Pain management is also important for the postoperative care of a patient with postembolization syndrome. Prophylactic or post-procedural epidural anesthesia has been shown to be very effective. Alternatives can include patient controlled analgesia pump or short interval IV doses of opioids such as fentanyl or dilaudid for the initial postoperative period (24–48 h). Oral pain medications generally do not work as well for this indication.
- Risk of postoperative symptoms, particularly pain, are reduced with partial embolization.
- Postembolization syndrome can last for up to 4–6 w

- Expect rises in creatinine immediately and for 24–48 h after procedure. Reassess frequently, especially in cases of single functional kidney.
- Postoperative imaging can show gas within the kidney in cases of total embolization. This does not necessarily indicate infection—correlate with symptoms, fever, and WBC.

DIALYSIS ACCESS INTERVENTIONS

Background *(Image-Guided Interventions E-Book: Expert Radiology Series. 2013: Elsevier Health Sciences; Abrams' angiography: interventional radiology. 2006: Lippincott Williams & Wilkins)*
- The prevalence of renal failure requiring hemodialysis (HD) is extremely high—almost 400,000–500,000 patients receive HD each year with a growing incidence due to diabetes
- Growth of dialysis population 12% over 75 y
- Average wait time for renal transplant after being declared dialysis dependent—2 y
- Multiple types of dialysis access—tunneled/temporary dialysis catheters, graft, fistula
- NKF KDOQI (National Kidney Foundation Kidney Disease Outcomes Quality initiative)—dictates guidelines for management of dialysis patients both in the hospital and in dialysis centers
- AV fistula—preferred method—robust, longer-lasting, more natural (no internal devices/synthetic objects), less infection risk, lower stenosis rates with less frequent intervention requirements
  - Downside—takes longer to mature and become usable after formation (up to 4–5 mo); technically more challenging; highly dependent on favorable extremity arterial/venous anatomy; complications often have to be managed surgically, more difficult to treat percutaneously
  - NKF KDOQI—"Fistula First Initiative"—fistula should be first line treatment and is preferred over grafts
  - Fistulas are started as distally in the extremity as possible so if another one is needed it can be created more proximally
- AV graft—easier to create, uses a synthetic sheath-like material to bridge the gap between the artery and vein; graft is directly punctured during dialysis; easier to declot through percutaneous approach
  - Downside—higher infection rates, still requires a short amount of time to mature before using
  - Primary patency rate (at 3 y)—40–60% *(Kid Internat 2002;62(4):1109–24)*, although some studies show patency around 20–28%
- Tunneled dialysis catheters—can be used long term, do not require any time for maturation (can be used immediately after placement); most malfunctions are due to positioning, not due to the device
  - Downside—uncomfortable for patients, higher infection rates, requires daily care
- For patients on dialysis, 15–20% of hospitalizations are related to HD access—much of KDOQI focus is for regular outpatient management to prevent need for hospitalization
- Most problems with graft/fistulas are at the venous anastomosis or in the outflow vein
- Goal is to maintain access through existing graft/fistula for as long as possible and avoid having to place new access elsewhere

Additional Notes About Grafts/Fistulas
- Upper arm AVF compared to AVG—fistula has 38% rate of early failure, graft has a failure rate of 15%—graft easier to use early on *(Clin J Am Soc Nephrol 2009;4(1):86–92)*
- Mean AVF survival—3.4 y before treatment required
- Mean AVG survival—1.6 y
- Terms upstream/downstream can be confusing depending on the anatomy—to avoid confusion, can use terms peripheral and central to describe direction of blood flow—central is usually venous side, peripheral is usually arterial side
- In patients expected to receive HD access in an extremity, venipunctures including PICCs and central lines should be avoided in this extremity to preserve the native veins
- Preference in creation of fistulas—radiocephalic, then brachiocephalic, transposed brachiobasilic, and lastly graft

Dialysis Access Surveillance (guidelines by KDOQI) *(Clin J Am Soc Nephrol 2009;4(1): 86–92)*
- Monitoring—examination by physical exam to detect signs of stenosis; preferred monthly; can include difficulty in cannulation or difficulty in hemostasis after cannulation; mandated by CMS
- Surveillance—examination by ultrasound or other noninvasive testing; can include flow measurements during access done in dialysis unit; mandated by CMS
- Diagnostic testing—further evaluation performed due to abnormalities on surveillance

Indications for Intervention (*ACR-SIR Practice Guideline for Endovascular Management of the Thrombosed or Dysfunctional Dialysis Access. Digest of Council Actions*)

- Low flow—flow rate less than 600 cc/min (grafts), 400 cc/min (fistula), although flow rates between 800–1,000 cc/min are preferred
  - Single low value should not prompt intervention—evaluate trend—decrease of 25% or more from a stable baseline flow rate is significant (*J Vasc Interv Radiol* 1999;10(8):1141)
  - Increased risk of stenosis occurs within 3 mo for flows between 600–800 cc/min in grafts (*J Vasc Interv Radiol* 1998;9(3):532–3)
- Imaging showing evidence of stenosis: high velocities, altered waveforms (tardus parvus centrally, elevated RI proximally)
- Physical exam and imaging findings of stenosis (greater than 50%)
- Enlarging pseudoaneurysms
- Fistula/graft clotting
- Graft infection—indication for surgical management, not percutaneous
  - Percutaneous treatment of infected graft can cause sepsis and has been associated with endocarditis
- Significantly delayed maturation of a fistula (failure to mature within 3 mo)—indication mainly to determine if angioplasty would be possible (*Seminars in dialysis*. Wiley Online Library: 2005:1–21)
  - Reasons for failure of maturation—outflow or AV anastomosis stenosis (managed with angioplasty); competitive outflow with collaterals (managed with surgical or endovascular ligation/embolization); small outflow vein (<6 mm)
  - Can be treated by balloon dilation of the fistula every few weeks/months to enlarge the vessel

When to Stent (KDOQI guidelines)
- Acute elastic recoil of vein and greater than 50% residual stenosis status post angioplasty (although surgical intervention is stated as preferable over stenting)
- Restenosis within 3 mo after angioplasty
- Acute repair of vascular injury/rupture
- Exclusion of pseudoaneurysm

Workup for Intervention
- CBC, INR for coagulation parameters—ideally INR <2, plt >50K
- WBC—if high, may indicate graft infection (which is a contraindication)
- Evaluate imaging, particularly ultrasound, to look for the site of stenosis. This can be suggested by visual inspection and physical exam.
  - Ultrasound evaluation of AVF/AVG—determine flow velocities, luminal sizes and areas of stenosis, areas of atherosclerotic disease, surrounding hematoma/aneurysm
  - Peak systolic velocity > 2× upstream velocity—indicates downstream (more central) stenosis
  - Tardus parvus waveform—suggestive of upstream (peripheral) stenosis
- Look up the patient's surgical history to determine the expected anatomy to encounter in the procedure
- Check patient's dialysis history to determine how long the problem has existed and whether flow was lost abruptly or over a prolonged period of time (prolonged—likely gradually forming stenosis; abrupt—likely thrombosis)
- Evaluate for underlying cardiopulmonary disease with evaluation of chest imaging if available; look for underlying SVC or other venous stenosis of aberrant anatomy
- Check surgical date from fistula/graft creation—early complications (within 1st 30 d) often require surgical repair. Percutaneous options should only be attempted after careful discussion with the operating surgeon.
- Evaluate prior history of intervention to identify prior sites of stenosis
- Remember that the procedure may not be successful, therefore plans should be discussed for a backup method of dialysis until the procedure can be reattempted or surgical intervention can be performed. The patient may require central venous access placement for HD (see chapter on venous access)—consent patient for this and workup as stated.
- Perform physical examination (see below)

Contraindications
- Infection—overlying erythema is usually thrombophlebitis in fistulas and not a true infection; more likely to have a true infection in grafts
- Contrast allergy (relative)
- Coagulopathy
- Graft/fistula formation within the past 30 d—angioplasty can induce rupture and delay maturation

- Long-segment stenoses or multiple areas of stenosis (relative contraindication due to time involved and risk of prolonged intervention)—greater than 7 cm—associated with reduced long-term patency
- Existing ischemia of the distal extremity—increasing flow into the fistula/graft will worsen vascular steal and ischemia.
- Right to left shunts—relative contraindication– potential for thrombus dislodged from the graft to enter the CNS
- Severe cardiopulmonary comorbidities—due to the pulmonary emboli created by the procedure
  - Returning a large amount of blood to the heart can also precipitate congestive failure—in these cases, leaving a slight stenosis to the HD access may be preferable

Physical Examination
- It is important to understand how to perform physical examination of a fistula/graft. This can help to identify the vascular anatomy and location of stenoses.
- AVG/AVF are made of an arterial inflow, arteriovenous anastomosis, a cannulation component (the graft or a segment of the outflow vein), and the venous outflow
- As good as ultrasound in detecting significant stenosis
  - Positive predictive value—69–93% (Clin J Am Soc Nephrol 2007;2(4):786–800)
- Inflow—upper extremity arterial system and arteriovenous anastomosis (fistula) or anastomosis of artery with synthetic tubing (graft)
  - Usually lost in early AVF/AVG failure
  - Will have decreased palpable flow in the venous segment that is used for cannulation
- Outflow—venous anastomosis of the graft to the native vein (graft) or anastomosis of a native vein to a central vein (fistula)
  - Usually the cause of delayed failure
  - Loss of "thrill," increased pulsatility in the cannulation component
- Enlarged collateral veins in the chest or extremity suggest central venous stenosis (subclavian, innominate vein, or SVC)
- Evaluate and document the radial, brachial, ulnar pulses within the extremity, the capillary refill, skin color, sensation, and strength. Compare to the opposite extremity. Ideally the same person should evaluate this before and after the procedure in order to detect subtle changes.
  - Evaluate for steal—decreased perfusion to the arm indicated by poor capillary refill, pallor, decreased pulses
- Evaluate graft for overlying skin erythema and tenderness
- Palpate the graft to determine presence of thrill. This can also be auscultated—high pitched bruits indicate a site of stenosis.

Types of Dialysis Access (Am J Roentgenol 2015;205(4):726–34)

Type	Advantages	Disadvantages	Site of Stenosis
Radiocephalic fistula	Most distal type—good for future fistula creation Less vascular steal distally	Lower flow rates—difficult to mature	Juxta-anastomotic
Brachiocephalic fistula	Easier to create	Increased risk of poor flow to the hand	Cephalic arch (subclavian, axillary)
Brachial-to-transposed basilic	High flow rates, easy to mature	Difficult to create, increased risk of poor flow to the hand	Proximal swing segment (portion that is reconnected to the axillary vein)
Grafts (PTFE)	Mature faster	Faster rates of thrombosis; foreign body	Venous anastomosis

Technique (Handbook of Interventional Radiologic Procedures. Lippincott Williams & Wilkins: 2011)
- The technique varies based on whether you are performing a fistulogram and intervention on a patent fistula or also performing a declot on a thrombosed fistula
- 3000–5000 IU of heparin should be given through a peripheral IV if intervention is planned. Heparin may also be given immediately after sheath placement if there is suspicion for thrombus from the fistulogram to help treat PE that might occur from dislodging
- Single-dose antibiotics (Ancef 1 g IV) is occasionally given to prevent infection, especially if stenting is planned, but is not standard or research supported
- "Antegrade" refers to aim toward the direction of blood flow (toward the venous out-flow). "Retrograde" refers to aiming against the blood flow (toward the arterial inflow).

Fistulogram

- Start with palpating and/or evaluating the graft with ultrasound to get a sense of the anatomy and to locate the venous and arterial components. Sterilize the planned entry site and use a 21G micropuncture system to gain access.
- For suspected venous anastomotic or outflow vein stenosis, antegrade access should be obtained initially within the venous component of the graft/fistula and aimed toward the body (direction of blood flow). Upsize the micropuncture access to a 6F–7F short sheath (usually 4–6 cm in length). The sheath should be as short as possible to visualize the most amount of graft without having to reposition. Access should be made as close to the arterial anastomosis as possible. Most balloons/stents used in declotting/angioplasty are able to go through a 5F or 6F system; however, a larger sheath allows for contrast to be injected while devices are inside. Anticipate if intervention will be required and what sized devices will be used to minimize sheath changes.
- For suspected arterial anastomotic or inflow stenosis, initial retrograde access toward the anastomosis should be considered
- Avoid placing access directly adjacent to a stenosis as the subsequent sheath placed will block visualization of the finding
- Inject contrast through the sheath to image the fistula/graft, outflow vein, and central venous system
- Findings on fistulogram to look for: Greater than 50% narrowing of a vessel suggests a hemodynamically significant decrease in lumen; assess for additional collateral vessels suggestive of stenosis, altered anatomy, pseudoaneurysms, spasm, and thrombus (filling defects in the lumen). Pressures can be measured for equivocal findings with a 10 mmHg or greater gradient indicating a significant stenosis.
- To subsequently visualize the portion of the venous outflow that is proximal to the sheath as well as the arterial segments, compress the venous portion distal to the sheath to reflux contrast across the arterial anastomosis. This can be achieved manually with a hemostat on the skin or via a balloon placed in the venous portion to occlude the outflow with contrast then injected in the antegrade sheath. Alternatively, a retrograde sheath can be placed distal to the antegrade venous sheath within the outflow tract and a wire and Kumpe advanced in a retrograde fashion past the arteriovenous anastomosis. The wire is then removed and contrast injected within the artery to evaluate the inflow artery and arteriovenous anastomosis. Remember to have enough space between the access sites so the sheaths do not block each other or the vessel.

Technique: Declotting/Stenting

- For percutaneous declotting of a fistula or graft, dual antegrade and retrograde access is typically required as described previously
- Make sure heparin has been administered prior to starting interventions
- Antegrade access is obtained initially to clear the venous portion of thrombus
- Place a 0.35″ wire (Bentson is preferred but glidewire can help maneuver through chronic clots/stenosis) through the sheath and advance it to the SVC through the antegrade access
- Advance a Kumpe catheter or glide catheter over the glidewire through the sheath toward the central venous system to the level of the SVC. Subsequently remove the wire and inject contrast as you retract the catheter to determine the extent of thrombus within the graft/fistula. Be careful that the sheath is not dislodged while retracting the catheter.
- Readvance the guidewire back through the venous sheath past the site of stenosis or thrombosis seen on fistulogram. All interventions should be performed over a wire to make sure access is maintained in the event of a complication.
- Mechanical thrombectomy devices may be required if there is significant thrombus within the fistula/graft. These include Trerotola (rotating sieve), AngioJet (clot fragmenter/aspirator), and Helix. These are preferred for extensive clot management.
- Pharmacologic thrombolysis (tPA) may be used as an adjunct to mechanical thrombectomy and can be injected directly into the clot. tPA does not work on the platelet plug/thrombus formed at the arteriovenous anastomosis. tPA rarely works as the sole method of declot.
  - Direct tPA (2–4 mg) injection into the fistula prior to the procedure has not been shown to be effective (*J Vasc Interv Radio* 2001;12(10):1157–65)
- Balloon maceration of thrombus with sequential inflation and advancement of an angioplasty balloon or Fogarty balloon can also be used to clear the outflow vein of thrombus
- Once the outflow vein is cleared of thrombus, followup fistulogram is performed to evaluate for residual sites of stenosis

- For treatment of stenoses as well as clots not responding to mechanical or pharmacologic thrombectomy, an appropriate size angioplasty balloon is advanced across the stenosis/clot. The size of the balloon is determined by the parent vessel and should be 20% larger than the normal vein (often 7–8 mm). Dilate for 1–3 min (longer inflation times associated with increased success). The length of the balloon should cover the stenosis without significantly covering normal vessel. Occasionally, angioplasty of the entire graft/fistula is required for significant thrombus or multiple stenoses. Be aware that overdilation of a vein or artery can cause significant injury including pseudoaneurysm formation and vessel rupture—do not overdilate. Also be aware that dilation often causes patient discomfort—this can be treated with intravenous medications or local lidocaine. Also remember to provide heparin prior to balloon dilation of a vessel to avoid thrombosis.
- Remove the balloon and repeat fistulogram with contrast to assess for improvement.
- If there is residual stenosis despite prolonged angioplasty, placement of a self-expanding stent should be considered. Due to the superficial nature of grafts/fistulas, there is a risk of external compression which can become problematic and crush balloon-expanding stents. Self-expanding stents offer greater flexibility and radial force for areas prone to external compression. A balloon may be used after initial stent placement to expand and secure the stent.
- Resistant or recurrent stenoses can be treated with cutting balloons. These have a reduced rate of vessel recoil and generally do not need stenting.
- After the venous side has been treated, place a second retrograde access in the venous component of the graft/fistula using micropuncture technique upsized to a 6F–7F sheath. The sheath should be distal to the antegrade sheath and point toward the arterial anastomosis (opposite direction of flow). The sheath should not be placed too close to the original antegrade sheath or there may be obstruction to flow.
- The platelet plug at the anastomosis and thrombus in the proximal aspect of the fistula/graft is then removed to restore blood flow into the fistula. Place a Fogarty balloon from the retrograde access into the artery and inflate. Inflate the balloon with dilute contrast to allow it to be visualized. If the contrast is not diluted, the balloon may be slow to deflate. Pull the Fogarty back across the anastomosis into the fistula/graft. Repeat this procedure until normal blood flow into the fistula is restored. The platelet plug can be very adherent and require some force or several passes with the Fogarty for complete removal. Remember to keep a hand on the sheath as it can become dislodged with this maneuver. Also remember to evaluate the extent of disease in the artery and at the anastomosis—if there is significant thrombus, this can embolize distally into the hand and cause ischemia. Alternatively, a mechanical thrombectomy device such as the Arrow-Trerotola Percutaneous Thrombectomy Device can be used to remove the arterial platelet plug.
- Repeat angiographic runs from the artery throughout the fistula via the retrograde approach to re-evaluate the fistula for improved flow, residual stenosis, and assess for complications (pseudoaneurysm, rupture, dissection). Ideally these runs should be done with the wire in place and the balloon ready to be deployed in case of visualized vessel damage. Dissections can be treated by expanding a balloon for an extended period of time—this has to be balanced with the effects of cutting off flow distally. Occasionally, stent placement may be required to treat complications.
- Stent placement may also be required for treatment of stenoses that do not resolve with angioplasty or reappear after balloon expansion. Stents should be sized based on the size of the vessel and positioned to cover the extent of the stenosis without involving a significant amount of normal vein as longer stents can interfere with puncturing of the vessel during dialysis access. Stents should also not be placed too close to the arteriovenous anastomosis as this can block the inflow and lead to graft/fistula failure.
- Backbleeding—used to treat an arterial embolus distal to the AV anastomosis. A Fogarty balloon is used to occlude the inflow artery proximal to the AV anastomosis. Physiologic reversal of blood flow in the arteries distal to the anastomosis causes the clot to enter the fistula/graft where it can then be aspirated through the sheath or macerated with a balloon (*J Vasc Interv Radiol* 1998;9(1):141–43)

Closing the Access
- Due to the use of sheaths within a high flow vascular system, obtaining appropriate hemostasis is important after the procedure. This is done with manual compression or placing pressure-stitches over the venotomy sites: Create a Z using nonabsorbable sutures with the diagonal portion of the Z going across the incision; cinch the suture to close the puncture site and tie or place the two ends of the suture through a stopcock—this will allow the suture to maintain tension without having to hold the suture manually and can be removed in 6–12 h.

- Purse-string suture can also be used to create tension on the skin and close the puncture sites
- Always remember to create the desired suture configuration prior to removing the sheath. Place a finger over the venotomy site to provide hemostasis while you cinch the suture.
- Create the suture close to the skin to avoid damaging the graft/fistula
- Longer time to hemostasis will be required in patients who received heparin or tPA
- Remember not to cover the skin entry site during manual compression as this can make it difficult to know when hemostasis has been achieved and blood will cause a subcutaneous hematoma when it cannot leave the extremity
  - Remember to not compress the fistula/graft too much—this can cause the vessel to thrombose

Goals and Outcomes
- Success rate at improving flow—96%
- Re-establishing a palpable thrill is associated with the most long-term success compared to visual improvement in stenoses or other physical exam findings
- 12–24 mo patency rate—23–51%; 6 mo—40–50% after angioplasty, 50% after stent
- 6 mo instent stenosis rate—28% (Am J Kidney Dis 2002;39(5):966–71), although depends on size, type of stent used
- Nitinol stents have better patency than wall-stents
- Restenosis is usually due to neointimal hyperplasia
- Patency rates are lower in patients who received Angiojet for thrombectomy—15% at 3 mo (only device that has this in evidence)
- The primary goal of intervention is to preserve the graft/fistula access and delay surgical intervention
- Recurrent stenosis requiring repeat intervention within 6 mo is very common regardless of the procedure technique
- Physical exam can be sufficient to determine satisfactory improvement following the procedure—extensive postprocedure gradient measuring or angiography is not necessary if physical exam is convincing of improved flow
- Patency rate with stents is similar to angioplasty alone
- Stenosis caused by atherosclerosis has better patency rates than stenosis caused by neointimal hyperplasia (JAMA 2004;291(19):2328–34; Ann Int Med 2009;151(9):631–38)
- Success after intervention defined by SIR/KDOQI:
  - Less than 30% residual stenosis
  - Normalization of hemodynamics across a previous stenosis
  - Improvement in flow rates through the access

Types of Patency	Definition
Primary	Graft/fistula stays open after initial creation
Assisted primary	Intervention performed to improve flow; however graft never stops working due to stenosis/occlusion
Secondary	Graft/fistula develops stenosis/thrombosis and intervention is performed to reestablish flow

Complications and Management
- Total complication rate—10%
- Vessel rupture or dissection, 5%—treated with balloon tamponade—if not successful despite prolonged tamponade, place stent across the injury
  - Note that if the site of injury is close to the arteriovenous anastomosis, a stent can occlude the inflow of the vessel—consult vascular surgery prior to placement to discuss surgical options to preserve the access
  - 70% of venous ruptures will respond to balloon alone; arterial ruptures are more serious and more likely to require a stent
- Pseudoaneurysm formation—can occur with damage to the vein or artery, but is more worrisome with arterial injury as it can expand rapidly due to high inflow—treated by compressing the aneurysm neck for a prolonged period of time (usually with ultrasound guidance to find the exact location of the neck)—if unsuccessful, can be treated with a covered stent across the neck
  - If the aneurysm neck is small, thrombin injection into the sac with compression of the neck can be performed; however, there is a risk of embolization of thrombin which can cause devastating distal ischemia—this should be reserved as a last resort
- Bleeding—usually worsened due to the use of heparin required during angioplasty—treated with compression
  - Small postprocedural hematomas are common and usually insignificant; however, important to evaluate for signs of compartment syndrome within the arm/leg

- Distal ischemia—due to thrombus dislodged during treatment—may require systemic or localized tPA and thrombolysis or urgent surgical intervention—important to frequently assess pulses/sensation and capillary refill in the hand/feet after procedure
  - Backbleeding technique—balloon inflated in the arterial inflow to occlude flow; patient then asked to exercise the hand to promote retrograde blood flow from the distal hand into the graft and pushing of clot into the outflow centrally; balloon then taken down and repeat angio performed
  - May also be able to access the radial artery distal to any blockages and retrograde push clots back into the fistula/graft using a balloon
  - Thrombectomy/aspiration can be attempted, however this has the risk of causing further distal emboli and clot impaction and should be reserved as a last resort
- Steal—reestablishing high flow through the graft/fistula can divert too much blood away from the native distal artery—this can cause ischemia in the hand/feet and can be seen on fistulogram showing minimal flow distal to the HD access—this may be treated by reducing the size of the access with smaller/tapered stents or may require surgical intervention with ligation of the vessel
- Pulmonary embolism—when pushing clots with the Fogarty or moving the balloons through the venous system, thrombus can become dislodged and travel centrally—usually the size of clots is too small to cause significant hemodynamic compromise; however, this can become important with underlying cardiac or pulmonary disease—may require more prolonged anticoagulation in this case
- Infection—should be considered as an endocarditis equivalent—treatment with antibiotics for 6 w minimum, potentially longer for grafts; can also cause bacteremia by disrupting infected clot

Postoperative Care

- Patients should be frequently evaluated (at least every 1–2 h) for signs of vessel compromise in the arm/leg—check pulses, sensation, strength, and skin color/capillary refill
- Evaluate the arm for size to determine if there is an expanding hematoma or aneurysm
- Monitor breathing and pulse rates to determine if dislodged thrombus centrally is causing problems—may require CT to evaluate for hemodynamically significant PE
- Postoperative hydration is important due to the large amounts of contrast used
- Nonabsorbable sutures can generally be removed 6–12 h after the procedure once hemostasis is achieved and puncture sites are no longer bleeding
  - Persistent bleeding from the venotomy sites indicates residual or recurrent stenosis causing high pressures in the AVF/AVG
- Continue to evaluate the graft/fistula for the physical exam signs of patency
- Patients should be told of the symptoms to look out for to evaluate for early infection—erythema/tenderness over the graft, fevers
- Restoring flow in a graft/fistula with untreated or recurrent central venous stenosis can result in venous HTN—upper-extremity swelling, facial edema, tenderness/pain (don't confuse with infection)

Tips and Tricks

- Remember that during balloon manipulation such as Fogarty pull through, both the retrograde access sheath as well as the antegrade venous sheath can become dislodged during the abrupt pull movement. Secure the sheaths using hemostats attached to the drapes, tape the sheaths down, or have an assistant hold the sheaths in place.
- Due to low flow in the venous component, sheaths can become clotted if not actively being used—when using one of the sheaths consider regular flushes to the sheath not being used or consider attaching a flush bag.
- When treating outflow stenosis with a single antegrade sheath, the fistula proximal to the sheath and the AV anastomosis can be evaluated by compressing the outflow during contrast injection to reflux contrast across the anastomosis. This is best accomplished with a large hemostat directly onto the vein. This also helps avoid radiation to the hand.
- Initial evaluation may reveal multiple stenotic lesions throughout a dialysis access and deciding which to treat can be difficult. Often addressing the most significant stenosis is enough to reinitiate appropriate flow. Evaluating pressures across an indeterminate stenosis is an effective way to determine whether intervention is warranted.

SUPRAPUBIC BLADDER CATHETERIZATION

Background
- Chronic indwelling Foley placement is often necessary in patients who are unable to have regular Foley placement through the urethra. Suprapubic catheter placement is a safe long-term alternative solution.

Indications
- Paraplegia—suprapubic catheters have been shown to have lower rates of infection and are considered more comfortable (Aust J Surg 1987;57(1):33–6)
- Atonic bladder
- Urethra obstruction—prostate hypertrophy/cancer, strictures
- Acute urinary retention with urosepsis

Contraindications
- Abnormal bladder location precluding safe catheter trajectory
- Coagulopathy—relative
- Temporary catheterization requirement—relative, although suprapubic options have been shown to be effective in patients with acute and temporary urinary retention

Workup
- Lab markers—check INR/platelets/hematocrit to determine preoperative transfusion needs
- Check UA for signs of infection
- Check prior imaging to determine safe trajectory
- Discuss with urology and other involved providers whether needs are temporary—smaller tubes can be placed if catheterization is expected to be temporary

Technique
- Use ultrasound for visualization of the bladder
  - Evaluate for intervening structures along the planned trajectory such as bowel or vessels
  - If patient is too large or good ultrasound window cannot be obtained, bladder can be targeted by its outline on fluoroscopy or after giving the patient contrast to highlight the bladder
  - CT also be used to access the bladder in large patients or if there is small window for safe access to avoid bowel or other structures
- Prep the skin using sterile technique. The standard access site is near midline above the pubic bone.
- Use a 21G micropuncture needle and advance into the bladder. Place a 0.018" Cope wire through the needle and exchange for a 4F or 5F microdilator over the wire. Remove wire.
- Once access dilator is in place, inject contrast to confirm bladder access.
- Place a 0.035" guidewire through the dilator and exchange for subsequently larger dilators up to the size of the Foley being used
  - Bentson wires may be sufficient, but Amplatz wires can offer more stability especially in larger patients and are recommended
  - An 8F–10F pigtail catheter may be placed initially or for temporary bladder access
  - For longer term bladder access, the initial catheter can be exchanged and upsized for a 16F–20F Foley catheter with retention balloon
- Place Foley over the wire and into the bladder. Due to the flimsiness of the Foley, a peel-away sheath may be required for additional stability.
- Suture the Foley in place and remove wire. Confirm positioning with additional contrast. Inflate Foley balloon.

Complications
- Bleeding—rare, particularly if ultrasound is used to identify nearby vessels
- Infection of the skin or urinary tract—usually a delayed complication due to poor maintenance/cleaning of the catheter
- Bowel injury—rare with proper preoperative planning
- Bladder rupture—often due to overdilation or losing access during the procedure

Postoperative Care
- Patient and caregivers should be given instructions on how to flush the catheter and wash the skin to reduce risk of infection or blocked catheter
- Catheters can be left in place for months to years if properly maintained

Tips and Tricks
- Remember that the bladder wall can be compliant and entering the bladder with a needle can be difficult if the bladder is not distended. Waiting until the bladder is full

- and distended can help with the procedure. Avoid entering the bladder at an angle to prevent the needle bouncing off the wall.
- Multiple visits for progressive dilation and upsizing to the final desired Foley size may be required in patients with neurogenic bladder or chronic outlet obstruction and thickened bladder wall.

PROSTATE ARTERY EMBOLIZATION (PAE)

Background
- Benign prostate hyperplasia (BPH) is one of the most common diagnoses in men over 50 and affects an estimated 14 million patients in the US
- An estimated 90% of men over 90 have some level of BPH symptoms
- Current approaches to treatment include medical management with alpha blockers and 5a-reductase inhibitors or surgical options such as transurethral prostate resection (TURP) or prostatectomy
  - Medical management has been shown to be effective in a large proportion of patients but rarely leads to complete resolution of symptoms. Medical management is also associated with issues of polypharmacy in elderly patients and elevated long-term costs.
  - TURP is the current gold standard of treatment but has the potential for severe complications including bleeding, sexual dysfunction, and incontinence

Indications
- Minimally invasive alternative for patients with lower urinary tract symptoms (LUTS) related to BPH that are causing issues with quality of life
- Poor surgical candidates due to large prostate sizes or medical comorbidities
- Failure of medical management
- Bleeding after biopsy/prostatectomy

Contraindications
- Active infection, particularly urinary tract infection
- Abnormal vascular anatomy that prevents embolization
- Coagulopathy
- Severe contrast allergy—relative
- PAE not shown to be effective for other causes of LUTS—prostatitis, strictures, prostate/bladder cancer, atonic/hyperactive bladder (*J Vasc Interv Radiol* 2011;22:11–19)
- Severe femoral artery atherosclerosis or tortuosity—relative, makes procedure technically difficult but not contraindicated

Workup
- Evaluate lab markers for INR, platelets, hemoglobin—ideally INR <2, platelets >50K
- PSA levels should be determined
- Review prior CT scans or other imaging if available to determine abnormal anatomy and plan surgical approach and site of vessel entry
  - Although preoperative MRI is not required, it can be helpful to further evaluate the prostate for contraindications and determine anatomy
- Determine preoperative symptoms to determine if procedure is effective. Investigate urinary symptoms, pain level, sexual function/history, and overall quality of life metrics.
  - International Prostate Symptom Score (IPSS)—score of 0 to 5 for seven symptoms; 0–7 total score = mild LUTS, 8–19 moderate, 20–35 severe

Advantages of PAE Over Surgery
- Single femoral or radial artery puncture required—quicker recovery
- Shorter hospital stay—can be done as an outpatient
- No requirement for general anesthesia
- Technical success achieved in over 95% of patients in most studies
- No upper limit of prostate size for eligibility

Technique
- Start with single dose antibiotics—400 mg IV ciprofloxacin (also given as oral form for 1 w after)
- Foley should be placed if not already present as contrast in the bladder during the procedure can obscure visualization of pelvic arteries
- Obtain arterial access with micropuncture technique and upsize to 5F sheath
- Perform pelvic and internal iliac angiography to evaluate the anatomy:
  - Evaluate for the inferior vesical artery which gives rise to prostatic arteries—may arise from the internal pudendal, internal iliac, or obturator arteries
  - Arteries are best evaluated at a 40–50° oblique view

- Through the base catheter, place a microcatheter and microwire into the internal iliac artery and pass it into the identified inferior vesical/prostatic artery on one side of the pelvis
- Begin embolization after using contrast to confirm appropriate catheter placement into the prostatic artery
  - Embolization materials used—Embozene microspheres, Embospheres, PVA particles (300–500 μm size)
- The procedure is then repeated on the opposite side of the pelvis
- Embolization is performed until complete hemostasis is obtained in each prostatic artery
- Remove devices and obtain hemostasis at the arterial access site

Postoperative Care
- Patients can be discharged within 2–6 h depending on type of arterial hemostasis
- Postembolization syndrome—can occur within 2–4 d—treat with NSAIDs
- Oral antibiotics are prescribed for 1 w

Results and Complications
- Main goal is improvement in LUTS—important to have a baseline and compare long-term
  - Studies shown to improve IPSS score, quality of life metrics, urinary peak flow rate, and reduce prostate volume (Radiology 2013;266:668–77; J Vasc Interv Radiol 2016;27(8):1115–22)
  - Procedure is fairly new and long-term data over 2–3 y is lacking
  - Repeat procedures for recurrent symptoms have been reported
  - Ability to remove an indwelling bladder catheter can be considered a success even with no change in other parameters
- Complication rate—21% (3% major complication rate)
- Smaller studies have shown no significant complications
- No studies reporting erectile dysfunction or urinary incontinence
- Major complication of procedure—bleeding at access site and UTI
- Additional milder and rarer complications—urinary frequency, dysuria, hematuria, hematospermia
  - May suggest nontarget embolization that is not detected in the procedure
  - Dysuria—suggests prostatitis
  - Self-limited and does not require further workup/treatment unless symptoms persist or worsen
- PSA levels often rise within the 1st 1–2 d
- Study of 200 patients with large prostate (over 100 cm^3), 84% had improvement in symptoms that was sustained over 6 mo; improvement rate 76% at 1 y (J Urol 1976;115:692–95)
- Prostate volume reduction of 40% and improvement in IPSS scores seen in studies at 12 mo (Radiology 2014;270:920–8)
- Study looking at patients with acute urinary retention showed improvement in symptoms and ability to remove bladder catheters in 95% of patients. At long-term followup, 79% had no recurrence of symptoms
- 114 patients with severe LUTS comparing PAE versus TURP—both showed similar improvements in IPSS, quality of life, and urinary flow rate
  - TURP complications—significant bleeding 3.8%, transurethral resection syndrome 1.9%
  - PAE complications—technical failure 5.3%, no improvement in symptoms 9.4%
  - PAE shown to have a shorter hospital stay
- 25% of patients shown to have no improvement in symptoms in one small study
- Success rate 75–94% if bilateral embolization is achieved. Clinical success rate drops to 50% if only unilateral embolization is possible.
- SIR Position Statement on PAE: "PAE for BPH is a novel and promising therapy that appears safe and efficacious based on short-term followup. Patient satisfaction is high, and repeat interventions are low"

ADDITIONAL RESOURCES

1. Aruny JE, Lewis CA, Cardella JF, et al. Quality improvement guidelines for percutaneous management of the thrombosed or dysfunctional dialysis access. J Vasc Intervent Radiol 2003;14(9):S247–S53.
2. Bergqvist D, Björck M, Lundgren F, et al. Invasive treatment for renovascular disease. A twenty year experience from a population based registry. J Cardiovasc Surg 2008;49(5):559–63.

3. Bissler JJ, Racadio J, Donnelly LF, et al. Reduction of postembolization syndrome after ablation of renal angiomyolipoma. *Am J Kidney Dis* 2002;39(5):966–71.
4. Burnett AL, Wein AJ. Benign prostatic hyperplasia in primary care: What you need to know. *J Urol* 2006;175:S19–S24.
5. Carnevale FC, da Motta-Leal-Filho JM, Antunes AA, et al. Quality of life and symptoms relief support prostatic artery embolization for patients with acute urinary retention due to benign prostatic hyperplasia. *J Vasc Interv Radiol* 2012; 24:535–42.
6. Chang YH, Wang LJ, Chuang CK, et al. The efficacy and outcomes of urgent superselective transcatheter arterial embolization of patients with ruptured renal angiomyolipomas. *J Trauma* 2007;62(6):1487–90.
7. Das CJ, Neyaz Z, Thapa P, et al. Fibromuscular dysplasia of the renal arteries: a radiological review. *Int Urol Nephrol* 2007;39(1):233–38.
8. De Baere T, Lagrange C, Kuoch V, et al. Transcatheter ethanol renal ablation in 20 patients with persistent urine leaks: an alternative to surgical nephrectomy. *J Urol* 2000;164(4):1148–52.
9. Funaki B, Szymski GX, Leef JA, et al. Wallstent deployment to salvage dialysis graft thrombolysis complicated by venous rupture: early and intermediate results. *AJR Am Jf Roentgenol* 1997;169(5):1435–37.
10. Gao YA, Huang Y, Zhang R, et al. Benign prostatic hyperplasia: prostatic arterial embolization versus transurethral resection of the prostate—a prospective, randomized, and controlled clinical trial. *Radiology* 2014;270:920–28.
11. Golwyn DH Jr, Routh WD, Chen MY, et al. Percutaneous transcatheter renal ablation with absolute ethanol for uncontrolled hypertension or nephrotic syndrome: results in 11 Patients with end-stage renal disease. *J Vasc Interv Radiol* 1997;8(4):527–33.
12. Gray RJ. Angioplasty and stents for peripheral and central venous lesions. *Tech Vasc Interv Radiol* 1999;2(4):189–98.
13. Hirsch, AT, Haskal ZJ, Hertzer NR, et al. ACC/AHA 2005 Practice Guidelines for the management of patients with peripheral arterial disease (lower extremity, renal, mesenteric, and abdominal aortic). *Circulation* 2006;113(11):e463–e54.
14. Ichsan J, Hunt Dr. Suprapubic catheters: a comparison of suprapubic versus urethral catheters in the treatment of acute urinary retention. *Aust N J Surg* 1987; 57(1):33–6.
15. Iqbal S, Sharma A, Wicky ST. Arterial interventions for renovascular hypertension. *Semin Intervent Radiol* 2009;26(3):245–52.
16. Kanterman RY, Vesely TM, Pilgram TK, et al. Dialysis access grafts: anatomic location of venous stenosis and results of angioplasty. *Radiology* 1995;195(1):135–39.
17. Kariya S, Tanigawa N, Kojima H, et al. Percutaneous transluminal cutting-balloon angioplasty for hemodialysis access stenoses resistant to conventional balloon angioplasty. *Acta Radiol* 2006;47(10):1017–21.
18. Leesar MA, Varma J, Shapira A, et al. Prediction of hypertension improvement after stenting of renal artery stenosis: comparative accuracy of translesional pressure gradients, intravascular ultrasound, and angiography. *J Am Coll Cardiol* 2009;53(25):2363–71.
19. Lewington S, Clarke R, Qizilbash N, et al. Age-specific relevance of usual blood pressure to vascular mortality. *Lancet* 2003;361(9366):1391–92.
20. Martin LC, Rees, O'Bryant T, *Percutaneous angioplasty of the renal arteries. Vascular diseases: surgical & interventional therapy.* 3rd ed. New York: Churchill Livingstone; 1994:721–41.
21. Mccarley P, Wingard RL, Shyr Y, et al. Vascular access blood flow monitoring reduces access morbidity and costs. *Kid Internat* 2001;60(3):1164–72.
22. McWilliams J, Kuo MD, Rose SC, et al. Society of Interventional Radiology Position Statement: Prostate artery embolization for treatment of benign disease of the prostate. *J Vasc Interv Radiol* 2014;25:1349–51.
23. Mitchell ME, Waltman AC, Athanasoulis CA, et al. Control of massive prostatic bleeding with angiographic techniques. *J Urol* 1976;115:692–95.
24. Morse SS, Sniderman KW, Strauss EB, et al. Postbiopsy renal allograft arteriovenous fistula: therapeutic embolization. *Urol Radiol* 1985;7(1):161.
25. Nikolic B. Hemodialysis fistula interventions: Diagnostic and treatment challenges and technical considerations. *Tech Vasc Intervent Radiol* 2008;11(3):67–74.
26. Pappas J, Vesely T. Vascular rupture during angioplasty of hemodialysis graft-related stenoses. *Graft* 2002;3(3):120–6.
27. Pisco JM, Bilhim T, Pinheiro LC, et al. Medium and long term outcome of prostate artery embolization for patients with benign prostatic hyperplasia: Results in 630 patients. *J Vasc Interv Radiol* 2016;27(8):1115–22.

28. Pisco JM, Pinheiro LC, Bilhim T, et al. Prostatic arterial embolization to treat benign prostatic hyperplasia. *J Vasc Interv Radiol* 2011;22:11–19.

29. Pisco JM, Pinheiro LC, Bilhim T, et al. Prostatic arterial embolization for benign prostatic hyperplasia: short- and intermediate-term results. *Radiology* 2013; 266:668–77.

30. Rooke TW, Hirsch AT, Misra S, et al. 2011 ACCF/AHA Focused update of the guideline for the management of patients with peripheral artery disease (updating the 2005 guideline): A Report of the American College of Cardiology Foundation/American Heart Association Task Force on Practice Guidelines Developed in Collaboration With the Society for Cardiovascular Angiography and Interventions, Society of Interventional Radiology, Society for Vascular Medicine, and Society for Vascular Surgery. *J Vasc Surg* 2011;54(5):e32–e58.

31. Scolari F, Ravani P, Gaggi R, et al. The challenge of diagnosing atheroembolic renal disease. *Circulation* 2007;116(3):298–04.

32. Sharafuddin MJ, Hicks ME. Current status of percutaneous mechanical thrombectomy. Part III. Present and future applications. *J Vasc Intervent Radiol* 1998; 9(2):209–24.

33. Shin SW, Do YS, Choo SW, et al. Salvage of immature arteriovenous fistulas with percutaneous transluminal angioplasty. *Cardiovasc Intervent Radiol* 2005; 28(4):434–8.

34. Simon N, Franklin SS, Bleifer KH, et al. Clinical characteristics of renovascular hypertension. *Jama* 1972;220(9):1209–18.

35. Swan TL, Smyth SH, Ruffenach SJ, et al. Pulmonary embolism following hemodialysis access thrombolysis/thrombectomy. *J Vasc Intervent Radiol* 1995;6(5):683–6.

36. Tacke J, Mahnken A, Bucker A, et al. Nephron-sparing percutaneous ablation of a 5 cm renal cell carcinoma by superselective embolization and percutaneous RF-ablation. in *RöFo-Fortschritte auf dem Gebiet der Röntgenstrahlen und der bildgebenden Verfahren.* © New York: Georg Thieme Verlag Stuttgart; 2001.

37. Tisi PV, Callam MJ. Treatment for femoral pseudoaneurysms. *The Cochrane Library,* 2013.

38. Tsao BE, Wilbourn AJ. The medial brachial fascial compartment syndrome following axillary arteriography. *Neurology* 2003;61(8):1037–41.

39. Trerotola SO, Kwak A, Clark TW, et al. Prospective study of balloon inflation pressures and other technical aspects of hemodialysis access angioplasty. *J Vasc Interv Radiol* 2005;16(12):1613–8.

40. Vesely TM. Use of a purse string suture to close a percutaneous access site after hemodialysis graft interventions. *J Vasc Interv Radiol* 1998;9(3):447–50.

41. Vesely TM. Use of stent grafts to repair hemodialysis graft–related pseudoaneurysms. *J Vasc Interv Radiol* 2005;16(10):1301–7.

42. Villalta JD, Sorensen MD, Durack JC, et al. Selective arterial embolization of angiomyolipomas: a comparison of smaller and larger embolic agents. *J Urol* 2011;186(3):921–27.

43. Wu S, Ahmad I, Qayyum S, et al. Paradoxical embolism after declotting of hemodialysis fistulae/grafts in patients with patent foramen ovale. *Clin J Am Soc Nephrol* 2011;6(6):1333–6.

44. Zaleski GX, Funaki B, Gentile L, et al. Purse-string sutures and miniature tourniquet to achieve immediate hemostasis of percutaneous grafts and fistulas: a simple trick with a twist. *Am J Roentgenol* 2000;175(6):1643–5.

PORTAL HYPERTENSION

Definition (*J Hepatol 2012;57:458–61; World J Gastroenterol 2017;23(10):1735–46; Clin Liver Dis 2001;5:617–27; Semin Liver Dis 1986;6:309–17*)
- Elevation of blood pressure within the portal venous system defined as portosystemic/hepatic venous pressure gradient (HVPG) >5 mmHg
- **HVPG** = wedged hepatic vein pressure − free hepatic vein pressure
- HVPG ≥10 mmHg can lead to clinically significant portal hypertension → complications

Epidemiology and Etiology (*J Hepatol 2012;57:458–61; World J Gastroenterol 2017;23(10):1735–46; Clin Liver Dis 2001;5:617–27; Semin Liver Dis 1986;6:309–17; Clinics in liver disease 2014;18(2):281–91; Int J Hepatol 2012;2012:895787; Child CG, Turcotte JG. The liver and portal hypertension. In: CG Child, ed. Surgery and Portal Hypertension. Philadelphia, PA: Saunders; 1964:50–4; Expert Rev Gastroenterol Hepatol 2013;7:141–55*)
- Most common cause of portal hypertension in Western countries is cirrhosis
- Worldwide, noncirrhotic causes of portal hypertension are more common such as hepatic schistosomiasis and portal venous thrombosis

Causes	Diseases
Prehepatic	Portal vein thrombosis, splenic vein thrombosis
Intrahepatic	Presinusoidal: Portal tract fibrosis or infiltration: Idiopathic, primary biliary cirrhosis, schistosomiasis, myeloproliferative disease, Wilson's, amyloidosis
	Sinusoidal: Liver cirrhosis (independent of etiology)
	Postsinusoidal: Veno-occlusive disease
Posthepatic	Budd–Chiari Constrictive pericarditis IVC obstruction Right-sided heart failure Severe tricuspid regurgitation

Pathophysiology: Result of ↑ vascular resistance aggravated by ↑ collateral vascular flow
- Increased vascular resistance from cirrhosis is due to **structural** factors from fibrosis at the level of the hepatic microcirculation causing sinusoidal portal hypertension as well as **dynamic** factors resulting from vasoconstriction mediated by endothelial dysfunction
- Portal hypertension is associated with ↑ cardiac output and ↓ systemic vascular resistance resulting in hyperdynamic circulatory state with splanchnic and systemic arterial vasodilation → increases portal blood flow → leads to more severe portal hypertension
- Portosystemic collateral vessels develop from dilatation of pre-existing anastomosis and angiogenesis in response to the elevated portal pressures → shunts blood away from the liver into the low-pressure systemic venous system as a means for reducing portal venous pressure (not enough to normalize portal pressures)

Portosystemic Collateral Pathways (*Expert Rev Gastroenterol Hepatol 2013;7:141–55; J Clin Exp Hepatol 2012;2(4):338–52; Clin Liver Dis 2005;9(4):685–13, vii.; CMAJ 2006;174(10):1433–43; Dig Dis 2016;34(4):382–6; Clinical radiology 2015;70(10):1047*)
- **Esophageal varices:** Coronary vein → azygos/hemiazygos veins
- **Gastric fundal varices:** Splenic vein → azygos vein
- **Splenorenal shunt:** Splenic or short gastric → left adrenal/inferior phrenic → left renal vein
- **Mesenteric varices:** SMV or IMV → iliac veins
- **Caput Medusa:** Umbilical vein → epigastric veins
- **Hemorrhoids:** IMV → inferior hemorrhoidal veins

Diagnostic Studies (*World J Gastroenterol 2017;23(10):1735–46; Clin Liver Dis 2001;5:617–27; Semin Liver Dis 1986;6:309–17; Clin Liver Dis 2014;18(2):281–91; Int J Hepatol 2012;2012:895787; Child CG, Turcotte JG. The liver and portal hypertension. In: CG Child, ed. Surgery and Portal Hypertension. Philadelphia, PA: Saunders; 1964:50–4; Expert Rev Gastroenterol Hepatol 2013;7:141–55; J Clin Exp Hepatol 2012;2(4):338–52; J Clin Exp Hepatol 2012;2(4):338–52*)
- **Transjugular hepatic vein catheterization:** Portal pressure can be estimated indirectly by the hepatic venous pressure gradient → the gradient between the wedged (or occluded) hepatic venous pressure and the free hepatic venous pressure

- Normal hepatic venous pressure gradient (HVPG) <5 mmHg
- **Ultrasonography:** Ascites, splenomegaly, nodular liver, portal vein diameter > 13 mm, portal flow mean velocity <12 cm/s, reversal of portal venous flow directionality, portosystemic collaterals, portal or splenic vein thrombosis if present
- **CT:** Ascites, splenomegaly, portosystemic collaterals, recanalization of the umbilical vein, nodular liver

Clinical Manifestations/Prognosis (Clin Liver Dis 2001;5:617–27; Hepatology 2007;45(3):797–05; World J Gastroenterol 2012;18(11):1166–75; J Hepatol 2002;36(4):494–500)
- Many of the clinical manifestations are related to the underlying cause of portal hypertension (ie, cirrhosis related cardiomyopathy and coagulopathy)
- Asymptomatic until complications develop (HVPG ≥10–12 mmHg)

Complications
Gastroesophageal varices → rupture, bleeding
Portal hypertensive gastropathy
Ascites
Spontaneous bacterial peritonitis (SBP)
Hepatorenal syndrome
Hepatic hydrothorax
Hepatopulmonary syndrome
Portopulmonary hypertension

- **Child–Turcotte–Pugh (CTP)** score and the **model for end-stage liver disease (MELD)** score are prognostic models used for the assessment of liver disease severity and survival → helps guide management

Child–Turcotte–Pugh (CTP) Model			
	Points		
Parameters	**1**	**2**	**3**
Ascites	Absent	Slight	Moderate
Hepatic encephalopathy	None	Grade 1–2	Grade 3–4
Bilirubin mg/dL	<2	2–3	>3
Albumin g/dL	>3.5	2.8–3.5	<2.8
Prothrombin time Seconds over control INR	<4 <1.7	4–6 1.7–2.3	>6 >2.3

Child A: Score 5–6 (well compensated) → 100% 1-y survival
Child B: Score 7–9 (significant functional compromise) 80% →1-y survival
Child C: Score of 10 (decompensated) → 45% 1-y survival
- Interobserver variability for the subjective parameters in the CPS classification led to the development of MELD system

Model for End-stage Liver Disease (MELD)
$$MELD = 9.57 \times \log_e(creatinine) + 3.78 \times \log_e(total\ bilirubin) + 11.2 \times \log_e(INR) + 6.43$$

3-mo Mortality
MELD score >40: 71.3% mortality
MELD score 30–39: 52.6% mortality
MELD score 20–29: 19.6% mortality
MELD score 10–19: 6.0% mortality
MELD score <9: 1.9% mortality
- Increasing MELD score is associated with increasing severity of hepatic dysfunction and increased 3-mo mortality risk
- MELD was originally developed to predict 3-mo mortality following transjugular intrahepatic portosystemic shunt (TIPS) placement
- MELD is also used in United Network for Organ Sharing (UNOS) to prioritize patients on the liver transplant waitlist
- Certain studies show MELD score to be superior to CTP in predicting 3-mo mortality. However, reliability decreases for long-term prediction

Treatment and Management (Clin Liver Dis 2005;9(4):685–13, vii.; CMAJ 2006;174(10):1433–43; Dig Dis 2016;34(4):382–6; Clinical radiology 2015;70(10): 1047; Clin Liver Dis 2014;18(2):451–76; Hepatology 2007;45(3):797–05; World J Gastroenterol 2012;18(11):1166–75; J Hepatol 2002;36(4):494–500)
- Directed at the underlying cause of portal hypertension and complications

- Reducing HVPG <12 mmHg, decreases complications associated with portal hypertension
- Variceal hemorrhage: Pharmacologic therapy w/beta blockers (propanol and nadalol), endoscopic procedures such as sclerotherapy and variceal ligation, transhepatic portosystemic shunt (TIPS), balloon-occluded retrograde transvenous obliteration (BRTO), plug-assisted retrograde transvenous obliteration (PARTO), coil-assisted retrograde transvenous obliteration (CARTO)
- Ascites w/o variceal hemorrhage →low sodium diet + diuretics, paracentesis
- SBP → antibiotics
- Hepatic encephalopathy → lactulose +/– rifaximin

TRANSJUGULAR INTRAHEPATIC PORTOSYSTEMIC SHUNT (TIPS)

Background (Semin Intervent Radiol 2014;31(3):235–42; Am J Roentgenol 2012;199(4):746–55)
- **Procedural Overview:** Form a tract between the hepatic vein and the portal vein (Figure 13-1) to shunt blood away from liver sinusoids thereby reducing portal venous pressure
- **Objective** → reduce **portal** pressure in patients with complications related to **portal hypertension**
- Portal hypertension is most commonly the result of cirrhosis which can cause complications resulting in → variceal bleeding, ascites, hepatic encephalopathy, hepatorenal syndrome, and hepatic insufficiency (J Hepatol 2006;44(1):217–31)
- Portal hypertension → reduction in survival from a median of 12 y to just 2 y (J Hepatol 2006;44(1):217–31)
- TIPS → direct reduction of portal venous pressure, to achieve an ideal portosystemic gradient <12 mmHg required for adequate portal decompression and reduction in variceal bleeding
- Reduces the filtration into the peritoneal space → allowing lymphatic absorption of ascitic fluid and thereby control of ascites and hydrothorax (Gut 2010;59(7):988–1000)
- Increases glomerular filtration and urine output, promotes natriuresis, and reduces the plasma rennin activity, aldosterone levels, and noradrenaline levels → improving the renal function that is altered from advanced cirrhosis (Hepatology 1998;28(2):416–22)
- TIPS is most commonly used for secondary prevention of bleeding and as salvage therapy in acute variceal bleeding
- Treatment options for the management of acute variceal bleeding: Endoscopic therapy, vasoactive drugs, balloon tamponade, and esophageal transaction → effective 80–90% patients
- Patients who do not respond are referred for TIPS
- Meta-analysis demonstrated decrease in the risk of recurrent bleeding after insertion of a TIPS compared with various forms of endoscopic therapy
- Embolization of the esophageal varices at the time of the TIPS is controversial → indeterminate whether the combination of TIPS and variceal embolization is more effective than TIPS alone
- Some recommend transjugular embolization of the varices to increase the effect of the shunt with respect to acute hemostasis
- Variceal embolization is also indicated for patients with recurrent esophageal bleeding despite a patent shunt
- The varices may be embolized with coils, cyanoacrylate glue, onyx, vascular occlude, or sclerosants such as sodium tetradecyl sulfate

Patient Selection (Semin Intervent Radiol 2014;31(3):235–42; Am J Roentgenol 2012;199(4): 746–55; Am J Gastroenterol 2003;98:1167–74; J Vasc Interv Radiol 2016;27(1):1–7; J Vasc Interv Radiol 1997;8(5):733–44; Semin Intervent Radiol 1995;12:337–46; Semin Intervent Radiol 2015;32(2):123–32; AJR 2006;186:1138–43; J Hepatol 2006;44(1):217–31)
- **Indications** → **variceal hemorrhage not controlled by endoscopy or medical management, secondary prophylaxis of variceal bleeding, refractory ascites**, hepatic hydrothorax, portal hypertensive gastropathy or intestinopathy, Budd–Chiari syndrome, hepatorenal syndrome, hepatopulmonary, hepatic veno-occlusive disease
- **Contraindications**
Absolute → Severe or rapidly progressive liver failure, severe or uncontrolled encephalopathy, primary prevention of variceal bleeding, congestive heart failure, severe tricuspid regurgitation, severe pulmonary hypertension, multiple hepatic cysts, uncontrolled systemic infection or sepsis, unrelieved biliary obstruction
Relative → Hepatocellular carcinoma (central), obstruction of all hepatic veins, portal vein thrombosis, moderate pulmonary hypertension, severe coagulopathy (INR > 5), thrombocytopenia of <20,000 cells/cm^3, hepatic encephalopathy

- **Increased risk of post-TIPS mortality 3 mo following TIPS:** Childs–Pugh class C, **MELD score > 18** (Am J Gastroenterol 2003;98:1167–74)

Preprocedural Work-Up (J Vasc Interv Radiol 2016;27(1):1–7; J Vasc Interv Radiol 1997;8(5):733–44; Semin Intervent Radiol 1995;12:337–46)

- Endoscopy should be performed before TIPS consultation both to confirm variceal bleeding and to attempt endoscopic management
- **Obtain informed consent for the procedure**
- **Labs within 24 h of procedure** → CBC, coagulation screen, CMP including LFTs, type, and screen
- Thrombocytopenia (platelet count <50,000 cells/mL), anemia (hematocrit, <25%), or coagulopathy may potentially need to be corrected
- IV hydration for patients with renal insufficiency
- Cross-matched blood products should be available for the patient in the blood bank
- **Imaging** → **Cross-sectional** (CT) for evaluation of vasculature and anatomy, ultrasound w/ Doppler for further evaluation of patency of vasculature
- Preprocedure echocardiography → to assess for elevated right-sided heart pressures and pulmonary hypertension
- Large volume paracentesis and/or thoracentesis (if hydrothorax) performed prior to the procedure (ascites moves the liver medially and caudally)
- IV antibiotic prophylaxis → ceftriaxone, ampicillin/sulbactam; if penicillin-allergy then levofloxacin, ciprofloxacin, clindamycin, or vancomycin. (Kandarpa K. *Handbook of Interventional Radiologic Procedures.* Lippincott Williams & Wilkins; 2011)
- Conscious sedation with intravenous fentanyl and midazolam. Alternatively, general anesthesia or monitored anesthesia care (MAC) with propofol administration particularly in variceal bleeders with hepatic encephalopathy should be considered.

Anatomic Considerations (Radiology 1994;191:705–12; Gut 2010;59(7):988–1000; Hepatology 2009;51:306; AJR 2005;85:89–91)

- Right hepatic vein (RHV) is largest, preferentially used (minimize risk of stenosis, safer, easier due to posterior location); if absent or small use middle hepatic vein (MHV) (J Vasc Interv Radiol 1997;8(5):733–44)
- MHV risk capsular injury due to anterior position and angulation
- Budd–Chiari hepatic veins are occluded → use remnant RHV or TIPS directly from the intrahepatic inferior vena cava (IVC) to the portal vein (PV)
- Variable portal anatomy → absence of right portal vein (RPV) trunk with trifurcation of PV into left portal and right anterior and posterior branches of RPV
- Accessory HVs and anomalous origins to PV branches are common

Technical Procedure (Kessel D. Robertson I. Interventional Radiology: A Survival Guide. 4th ed. Elsevier; 2016; Radiology 1994;191:705–12; Gut 2010;59(7):988–1000; Hepatology 2009;51:306; AJR 2005;185:89–91)

- **Equipment**
  - Basic angiography set
  - Guidewires: 3-mm J, curved hydrophilic wire (regular and stiff), Amplatz wire (regular and short tip)
  - Multipurpose angled catheter, angioplasty balloons 8, 10, and 12 mm by 4 cm
  - TIPS set (Haskal, Rösch–Uchida, or Ring sets)
    - 40-cm 10F sheath with end marker
    - 51-cm curved guide-catheter with metal stiffener
    - 60-cm long sheathed needle
  - TIPS stents and stent grafts 8, 10, and 12 mm. FDA approved—WALLSTENT (bare stent) and the VIATORR [ePTFE]-lined stent graft)
  - Vascular pressure transducer (to measure portosystemic pressure gradient)
  - Ultrasound for right IJV puncture
  - Intravascular ultrasound for portal vein access

Procedure (Kandarpa K. Handbook of Interventional Radiologic Procedures. Lippincott Williams & Wilkins; 2011; Kessel D. Robertson I. Interventional Radiology: A Survival Guide. Elsevier; 2016)

1. **Access:** Obtain right IJ access using direct ultrasound guidance
2. **Catheterization:** Pass the J wire and catheter into the IVC. Rotate the catheter to the patient's right to direct the catheter into the right hepatic vein. Guidewire and catheter should be advanced into the vein.
3. **Runs:** Wedged hepatic venogram of the distal and peripheral tributary of the hepatic vein using a gentle injection of contrast or CO_2 to help visualize portal system. If fails → carbon dioxide portography by gas injection directly through the TIPS needle into the hepatic parenchyma.

4. **Catheterization of hepatic vein:** Amplatz guidewire is placed through the catheter into the selected hepatic vein, the diagnostic catheter removed, and the transjugular puncture needle and sheath is advanced into the hepatic vein. Exchange the catheter for the curved guide-catheter and advance this just beyond the tip of the sheath.

5. **Portal vein puncture:** Remove the guidewire and turn the guide-catheter so it points anteriorly and slightly to the right (RPV lies anterior to RHV) with its tip 2–3 cm into the RHV. Advance the sheathed needle through the guide-catheter aiming to hit the RPV 1–3 cm from the portal bifurcation. Attach a syringe and aspirate during slow needle and sheath withdrawal until fluid or bubbles are seen. Perform short contrast run:
   i. Contrast flows toward the right atrium → still in hepatic vein
   ii. Contrast flows toward the periphery of the liver → either in portal vein or hepatic artery
   iii. Contrast flows toward the portal bifurcation there is reversed flow in the portal vein. If it doesn't clear → in bile duct.

6. **Catheterization portal vein:** Introduce a hydrophilic wire through the portal vein and advance the entire guide-catheter and sheath into the portal vein. Exchange the hydrophilic wire for the Amplatz wire and remove the catheter and guide-catheter over the wire.

7. **Measure pressures:** Place the catheter into the portal vein and pull the sheath back into the right atrium. Measure the portosystemic pressure gradient between the portal vein and right atrium.

8. **TIPS tract formation and stenting:** Dilate the tract with an 8-mm angioplasty balloon. Perform venogram by simultaneously injecting into the portal and hepatic veins and measure the length of stent (cover from the origin of the hepatic vein → parenchymal tract → project about 2 cm into the portal vein); usually 10-mm stent graft for bleeding and an 8-mm stent graft for ascites. Tract dilation is based on the pressure gradient → dilate to 8 mm and then measure the portosystemic gradient. Gradient > 12 mmHg → dilate tract to 10 mm and then 12 mm until gradient decreases

9. **Venogram:** Gradient <12 mmHg → perform a completion venogram hopefully showing almost all portal vein flow passing through the stent into the hepatic vein.

10. **Embolization:** Embolization of esophageal varices during an acute active bleed as clinically indicated

---

Figure 13-1 A **TIPS** is a percutaneously created connection within the liver between the portal and systemic circulations.

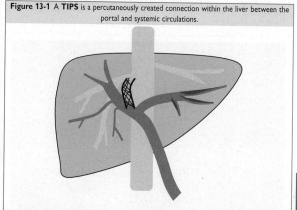

Postprocedural Management (Kandarpa K. *Handbook of Interventional Radiologic Procedures.* Lippincott Williams & Wilkins; 2011)

- Monitor RA pressures after procedure (expected increase sometimes up to 1 mo); if mean RA pressure is >10 mm → overnight diuresis of >1 L
- Excessively high final right atrial pressures (esp. acutely bleeding patients receiving fluid resuscitation → limits the decompressive effects of the shunt → preventable secondary pulmonary edema)

Procedural Complications (Kandarpa K. *Handbook of Interventional Radiologic Procedures.* Lippincott Williams & Wilkins; 2011; *Hepatology* 1998;28(2):416–22; *J Vasc Interv Radiol* 2009;20:180–85)

- Threshold for major complications is 5% as per Quality Improvement Guidelines for TIPS (*J Vasc Interv Radiol* 2016;27(1):1–7)
- **Major complications:** Hemoperitoneum (intracapsular puncture), stent malposition, hemobilia, radiation skin burn, hepatic infarction, renal failure requiring dialysis, encephalopathy, death
- **Minor complications:** Transient contrast-induced nephropathy, hepatic artery puncture injury, fever, entry site hematoma

Long-Term Complications (Kandarpa K. *Handbook of Interventional Radiologic Procedures.* Lippincott Williams & Wilkins; 2011; *Hepatology* 1998;28(2):416–22; *J Vasc Interv Radiol* 2009;20:180–85; *Eur J Gastroenterol Hepatol* 2006;18:1135; *Semin Intervent Radiol* 2012;29(2):118–28; *Semin Intervent Radiol* 2011;28(3):303–13)

- Post-TIPS encephalopathy (greatest prognostic factor is pre-existing encephalopathy)
- Liver failure
- Shunt malfunction is the result of narrowing or occlusion caused by intimal hyperplasia or in situ thrombosis
- Shunt stenosis (bare metal stents → 25–50% of cases within 6–12 mo postprocedure; longer patency with PTFE-covered stent)
- Stenosis of the hepatic vein at the margin of the TIPS is the most common site of pathology, followed by an intra-TIPS stenosis → treat with balloon angioplasty

Surveillance (*AJR Am J Roentgenol* 2008;191(6):1751–7; *Eur J Gastroenterol Hepatol* 2006;18:1135–41; *Semin Intervent Radiol* 2012;29(2):118–28; *Semin Intervent Radiol* 2011;28(3):303–13)

- Postprocedure baseline TIPS sonography → within 1 wk of initial placement for Wallstents and 1 mo for covered stents (detects stent occlusion initially after procedure)
- F/u at 3 mo, 6 mo, and every 6–12 mo thereafter
- If US is nondiagnostic → CT or venography to assess shunt patency
- Shunt thrombosis: Absent flow at color Doppler US and has an aphasic spectral waveform
- Stenosis on US: Abnormally high (>190 cm/s) or abnormally low (<90 cm/s) velocity within the shunt. Other evidence includes an abnormal change in velocity (increase or decrease >50 cm/s) compared with the prior examination.
- Intrahepatic portal venous flow that was hepatofugal on the prior examination and has changed to hepatopetal flow
- When sonographic findings suggest shunt dysfunction, TIPS angiography with portosystemic gradient measurement is warranted (*Semin Intervent Radiol* 2015;32(2); Thieme Medical Publishers)

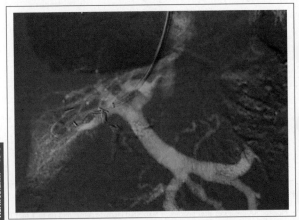

Carbon dioxide–wedged hepatic venography during TIPS procedure.

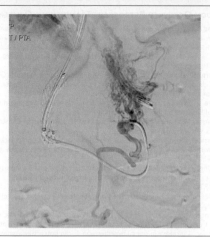

Coil embolization of gastric varices after TIPS placement.

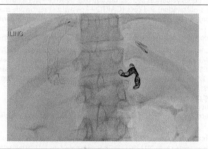

Status post-TIPS and coil embolization of gastric varices after refractory acute variceal bleeding.

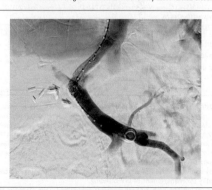

Status post-TIPS placement with communication of the portal and systemic system.

BALLOON-OCCLUDED RETROGRADE TRANSVENOUS OBLITERATION

Background (Kandarpa K. *Handbook of Interventional Radiologic Procedures*. Lippincott Williams & Wilkins; 2011; *Semin Intervent Radiol* 2012;29(2):118–28; *Semin Intervent Radiol* 2011;28(3):303–13 © Thieme Medical Publishers, 2011; *Semin Intervent Radiol* 2011;28(3):333–8; *Am J Roentgenol* 2012;199(4):721–9; *Radiol Case Rep* 2016;11(4):365–9; *J Gastroenterol Hepatol* 2016;31:727e33; *Semin Intervent Radiol* 2011;28:288–95; *Am J Gastroenterol* 1989;84(10):1244–9)

- **Procedural Overview:** Treatment and prevention of gastric variceal (GV) bleeding via occlusion of the portosystemic outflow veins with a balloon catheter, followed by injection of a sclerosing agent into the varix
- **Objective** → complete obliteration of gastric varices with preservation of the anatomical hepatopetal flow of the splenoportal circulation
- Gastric varices (GV) are submucosal venous saccules in the wall of the stomach—20% of patients with portal hypertension
- Gastric variceal bleeding occur due to left-sided spontaneous portosystemic shunt (gastrorenal [80–85%], direct gastrocaval, and gastrocaval shunts via the inferior phrenic vein)
- GV bleeding → greater hemorrhage and transfusion requirements, increased risk of rebleeding and higher mortality rate than esophageal variceal bleeding
- TIPS or BRTO can be performed
- BRTO is less invasive, can be performed on patients with low hepatic reserve and encephalopathy
- BRTO → occlusion of spontaneous gastrorenal (a natural portosystemic decompressive) shunt resulting in diversion of blood flow toward the portal circulation and in turn the liver → increase in portal hypertension → can potentially aggravate esophageal varices and ascites
- Permanent occlusive devices such as vascular plug (PARTO—plug assisted retrograde transvenous obliteration) and coils (CARTO—coil assisted retrograde transvenous obliteration) can be used instead of an indwelling balloon catheter → permanent shunt occlusion → terminates procedure in 1 stage → shortened procedure time without potential complications associated with the use of indwelling balloon catheter

Indications (Kandarpa K. *Handbook of Interventional Radiologic Procedures*. Lippincott Williams & Wilkins; 2011; *Semin Intervent Radiol* 2012;29(2):118–28; *Semin Intervent Radiol* 2011;28(3):303–13 © Thieme Medical Publishers, 2011; *Semin Intervent Radiol* 2011;28(3):333–8; *Am J Roentgenol* 2012;199(4):721–9; *Radiol Case Rep* 2016;11(4):365–9; *J Gastroenterol Hepatol* 2016;31:727e33; *Semin Intervent Radiol* 2011;28:288–95; *Am J Gastroenterol* 1989;84(10):1244–9)

- Impending, prior, or active gastric variceal bleeding
- GV with hepatic encephalopathy refractory to medical management
- Bleeding ectopic varices (eg, duodenal). must have a catheter-accessible efferent drainage

Contraindications (Kandarpa K. *Handbook of Interventional Radiologic Procedures*. Lippincott Williams & Wilkins; 2011; *Semin Intervent Radiol* 2012;29(2):118–28; *Semin Intervent Radiol* 2011;28(3):303–13 © Thieme Medical Publishers, 2011; *Semin Intervent Radiol* 2011;28(3):333–8; *Am J Roentgenol* 2012;199(4):721–9; *Radiol Case Rep* 2016;11(4):365–9; *J Gastroenterol Hepatol* 2016;31:727e33; *Semin Intervent Radiol* 2011;28:288–95; *Am J Gastroenterol* 1989;84(10):1244–9)

Absolute	Relative
Uncorrected coagulopathy	Refractory ascites
Unstable to tolerate procedure	Severe liver dysfunction
Varices that do not drain into the renal or caval systems	High-risk esophageal varices
	Portal vein thrombosis
	Uncontrolled esophageal variceal bleeding

Preprocedural Work-Up (*Semin Intervent Radiol* 2011;28(3):303–13 © Thieme Medical Publishers, 2011; *Semin Intervent Radiol* 2011;28(3):333–8; *Am J Roentgenol* 2012;199(4):721–9; *Radiol Case Rep* 2016;11(4):365–9; *J Gastroenterol Hepatol* 2016;31:727e33; *Semin Intervent Radiol* 2011;28:288–95; *Am J Gastroenterol* 1989;84(10):1244–9; *Hepatology* 1992;16(6):1343–9; *Gastroenterology* 2004;126(4):1175–89; *Semin Intervent Radiol* 2011;28:288e95; *J Gastroenterol* 2007;42:663e72; *Dig Dis Sci* 2015;60:1543e53; *J Gastroenterol Hepatol* 2016;31:727e33; *Hepatology* 1989;9(6):808–14; *Hepatology* 2001;33(4):821–25; *Semin Intervent Radiol* 2011;28(3):325–32; *Semin Intervent Radiol* 2011;28(3):303–13)

- Endoscopy to distinguish between an esophageal and gastric source of bleeding. First-line modality for management of GV bleeding.
- Preprocedure imaging with 3-phase contrast-enhanced CT or magnetic resonance angiography/venography (MRA/MRV) to evaluate the portal vein and the extent of

portosystemic shunts → evaluate the size of the gastrorenal shunt for suitability of the procedure and device selection, understand the portal inflow to the shunt (some of these shunts can have multiple small inflow veins), identify collateral veins that may require embolization prior to instillation of sclerosants (eg, phrenic or pericardiophrenic veins)

- If draining veins are too large to be occluded by a balloon → ineligible for BRTO → but may consider PARTO or CARTO
- Patients with contiguous gastric or portal branch veins that do not contribute to the shunt balloon occlusion of the draining vein → hemodynamic shift within the varices and result in shunting of the sclerosant away from the varices through the contiguous gastric veins (AJR Am J Roentgenol 2012;199(4):746–55; Am J Gastroenterol 2003;98:1167–74)
- Obtain informed consent for the procedure
- Patients with known or suspected portal hypertension, medical therapy is required → antiportal hypertension medications and antibiotic prophylaxis
- Acutely bleeding patients with hemodynamic instability → aggressive resuscitation with (packed red blood cells, fresh-frozen plasma, platelets, cryoglobulin, pressor support, IV fluids)
- However, avoid over aggressive fluid resuscitation → can exacerbate portal hypertension → volume expansion increases portal vein pressure→ therefore systemic blood pressures lower than normal are acceptable
- Lower target hematocrit (21%) with packed red blood cell transfusions, optimize platelet count and function
- Preprocedure laboratory studies: Serum electrolytes, complete blood cell count, coagulation panel, and liver and kidney function tests
- Hemodynamic monitoring with electrocardiography, blood pressure, and oxygen saturation
- Conscious sedation using IV fentanyl and midazolam is suitable for most patients

Technical Procedure (Kandarpa K. *Handbook of Interventional Radiologic Procedures*. Lippincott Williams & Wilkins; 2011)

- **Equipment:**
  - Basic angiography set
  - Guidewires: 3-mm J, curved hydrophilic wire
  - Embolic vs. sclerosant agent

Embolic/Sclerosant Agents
Ethanolamine oleate
Polidocanol foam
n-Butyl cyanoacrylate
Sodium tetradecyl sulfate
Gelfoam for PARTO

  - Balloon-occlusion catheters
  - Plug for PARTO (Amplatzer plug of various sizes)
  - Coils for CARTO (pushable vs. detachable, metallic, or polymer embolization coils)

Procedure (Kandarpa K. *Handbook of Interventional Radiologic Procedures*. Lippincott Williams & Wilkins; 2011)

1. **Access:** Obtained usually through the femoral or internal jugular veins. Typically, 7–9F, 50–70 cm long vascular sheath placed based on estimated size of the shunt ostium and the occlusion balloon needed (Figure 13-2).
2. **Catheterization:** Catheterization of gastrorenal shunt arising from the left renal vein
   - A 4F or 5F catheter (Cobra, reverse curve, Simmons 1, or Headhunter) is used to select the left renal vein. It is advanced toward the renal hilum and then gently rotated while being drawn back, directed at the cephalic wall of the left renal vein. The gastrorenal vein empties into the left renal vein through the enlarged adrenal vein along its central cephalic aspect.
   - A soft Teflon-coated metallic or hydrophilic guidewire is advanced into the gastrorenal shunt after which the long sheath advanced over the diagnostic catheter and guidewire beyond the junction of the shunt and renal vein. A parallel, "buddy wire" or catheter may be placed alongside the original guidewire. After shunt venography, the catheter is exchanged for an appropriately sized occlusion balloon. The balloon is positioned in a secure caudal location within the shunt, gently inflated and retrograde contrast venography performed, to begin to map the shunt. Iodinated contrast and carbon dioxide can be used as well as cone-beam CT.

- Reverse curve single and double balloon BRTO occlusion catheters are available in Asia; these can potentially reduce the number of steps in gastrorenal vein catheterization.

3. **Balloon occlusion venography:** Evaluation of shunt anatomy can reveal collateral veins, for example, paravertebral, pericardial, pericardiophrenic, or inferior phrenic veins, that may warrant coil embolization before instillation of the sclerosant. When using liquid sclerosants, these large veins may otherwise thwart contrast filling the entirety of varix, hence the need to skeletonize the shunt. The "inflow" of the shunt should be identified (ie, its path toward the splenic vein) so that the proper amount of embolic solution is instilled, both sufficient to occlude the majority of the varix but not spill into the splenic vein.

4. Advance a microcatheter through the balloon lumen into the varix as far as feasible. The intent is to expose the majority of the varix to the occlusive agent or sclerosant, without reflux into the splenic vein.

5. The sclerosant agent of choice is mixed with air and contrast agent. The following preparation of Sotradecol can be used: 2 mL of sodium tetradecyl sulfate (STS) 3%, 1 mL of Lipiodol, and 3 mL of air. Carbon dioxide can be used and may be preferable.

6. The sclerosant is injected under fluoroscopic guidance, while the occlusion balloon remains inflated in place

7. The balloon is typically deflated ~4 h later, although shorter protocols have been reported. Should flow persist, reinflation and re-sclerosis can be performed.

Plug/Coil-Assisted Retrograde Transvenous Obliteration (*J Vasc Interv Radiol* 2016; 27(1):1–7)

(Advantages: Single-session only, lesser need for collateral embolization, and decreased risk of sclerosis to nontarget vessels)

1. **Access** into the shunt as described earlier. Use a long vascular sheath of sufficient caliber to allow delivery of a suitable plug (or coil mass) and parallel (para-axial) catheter for delivering the embolic solution.

2. Perform shunt venography

3. Advance a microcatheter or diagnostic catheter deep into the shunt

4. For plug-assisted retrograde occlusion, an oversized AMPLATZER Vascular Plug II (AVP-II) (available in sizes up to 22 mm diameter) is extruded into the shunt *but not detached from its delivery mandrill.* If coils are used, these are deployed alongside the microcatheter.

5. Again the sclerosant agent of your choosing can be used. For example a thick slurry of Gelfoam, sclerosant, and iodinated contrast can be injected into the varix via the catheter within the shunt. The occlusive plug prevents egress of this solution. Relatively large volumes of this solution may be required. The static column can be readily visualized as the varix is progressively filled. Once a sufficient extent of varix stasis has been achieved, the plug is released at the distal "base" of the varix and the procedure is concluded.

Figure 13-2 Conventional BRTO procedure through transfemoral approach with balloon in the gastrorenal shunt. (SV, splenic vein; GV, gastric vein; PGV, posterior gastric vein; SGV, short gastric vein).

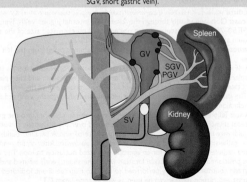

Postprocedural (Kandarpa K. *Handbook of Interventional Radiologic Procedures.* Lippincott Williams & Wilkins; 2011; *J Gastroenterol Hepatol* 2008;23:1702–9; *AJR Am J Roentgenol* 2007;189:W365–72)

- Elective BRTO patients should be admitted for overnight observation
- Laboratory evaluation in the first 48 h may demonstrate a mild increase in total bilirubin and liver function tests, usually self-limited, perhaps related to increased portal flow and pressure. Persistent deterioration in liver function should prompt a liver Doppler ultrasound to exclude portal vein thrombosis.
- Monitor patient's fluid status due to increased portal pressures (ie, ascites, hepatic hydrothorax, lower-extremity edema)
- Monitor renal function (hemoglobinuria, contrast, renal vein thrombosis, or the development of hepatorenal syndrome)
- Patients should be closely monitored with upper endoscopy post-BRTO for detection and management of esophageal varices
- Complications post-BRTO include fever, epigastric, chest and/or back pain, transient systemic hypertension, pleural effusion, and hemoglobinuria
- Less common complications have been observed in the first 7–10 d including pleural effusion (HH: 12%), and pulmonary infarction (2%), which usually resolves within the first 10 d

Follow-up (Kandarpa K. *Handbook of Interventional Radiologic Procedures.* Lippincott Williams & Wilkins; 2011; *J Gastroenterol Hepatol* 2008;23:1702–9; *AJR Am J Roentgenol* 2007;189:W365–72)

- Cross-sectional imaging (computed tomography venography [CTV] or magnetic resonance venography [MRV]) should be performed at least once during outpatient clinic follow-up at 3–6 mo and then as clinically indicated
- Technical success reported between 80% and 100%
- Recurrent GV bleeding between 0% and 9%

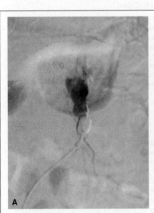 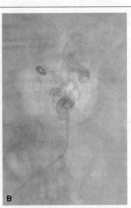

Conventional BRTO of splenorenal shunt: A. Balloon occlusion of the shunt; B. Status post BRTO

TRANSJUGULAR LIVER BIOPSY

Background (Kandarpa K. *Handbook of Interventional Radiologic Procedures.* Lippincott Williams & Wilkins; 2011; *J Hepatol* 2007;47:284–94; *J Vasc Interv Radiol* 2001;12:583–7; *J Vasc Interv Radiol* 2007;18:237–41; *J Vasc Interv Radiol* 2008;19:351–8; *Indian J Radiol Imaging* 2008;18(3):245–8; *J Vasc Interv Radiol* 2015:26(2):S84)

- Liver biopsy is the gold standard for the evaluation of chronic liver disease
- Transjugular liver biopsy (TJLB) is performed in patients with diffuse liver disease when liver biopsy is essential for the diagnosis and management but percutaneous image guided biopsy is contraindicated—most commonly due to concern for excessive bleeding or in coagulopathic patients
- **Procedural overview:** Transjugular approach → biopsy needle is inserted into the liver via the hepatic vein → core needle biopsy of liver parenchyma obtained. Hemodynamic pressure measurements may or may not be obtained in the same setting, dependent on the clinical scenario.

- Avoids the peritoneum and puncturing liver capsule → any bleeding related to procedure needle tract will be contained within the liver or autotransfuse into the hepatic vein
- Indirect portal pressures may be obtained when performing TJLB for hemodynamic evaluation
- Measurement of HVPG is a useful clinical tool, serves as a surrogate of clinical events in liver diseases
- Specimen obtained via transjugular liver biopsy is equivalent to specimen obtained by percutaneous liver biopsy (PLB)

Indications (Kandarpa K. *Handbook of Interventional Radiologic Procedures.* Lippincott Williams & Wilkins; 2011; Kessel D, Robertson I. *Interventional Radiology: A Survival Guide.* Elsevier; 2016; *J Hepatol* 2007;47:284–94; *J Vasc Interv Radiol* 2001;12:583–7)

- Coagulopathy (prolonged PT or PTT or a low platelet count)
- Ascites
- Morbid obesity
- Peliosis hepatis
- Small cirrhotic liver
- Requires portal pressure measurements as part of diagnostic work-up
- Failed PLB

Relative Contraindications (Kandarpa K. *Handbook of Interventional Radiologic Procedures.* Lippincott Williams & Wilkins; 2011; Kessel D, Robertson I. *Interventional Radiology: A Survival Guide.* Elsevier; 2016; *J Hepatol* 2007;47:284–94; *J Vasc Interv Radiol* 2001;12:583–7)

- Uncorrectable coagulation parameters
- Right internal jugular thrombosis
- Limited venous access (ie, SVC obstruction, transfemoral approach can be considered)
- Thrombosis of the hepatic veins (ie, Budd–Chiari)

Preprocedural Evaluation (Kandarpa K. *Handbook of Interventional Radiologic Procedures.* Lippincott Williams & Wilkins; 2011; Kessel D, Robertson I. *Interventional Radiology: A Survival Guide.* Elsevier; 2016)

- Obtain informed consent for the procedure
- Review cross-sectional imaging to examine anatomy (particularly in transplant patients)
- Labs: Prothrombin time (PT)/international normalized ratio (INR), partial thromboplastin time (PTT), platelet count, and serum creatinine level/GFR
- Attempts should be made to correct the underlying coagulopathy before the procedure
- Paracentesis should be performed prior to the procedure → Ascites can cause shifting of the liver

Anatomy (*J Hepatol* 2007;47:284–94; *J Vasc Interv Radiol* 2001;12:583–7; *J Vasc Interv Radiol* 2007;18:237–41; *J Vasc Interv Radiol* 2008;19:351–8)

- Hepatic veins join the IVC just below the right atrium
- Safest approach: Right hepatic vein while angling the sheath anteriorly → biopsy is taken from the maximum volume of parenchyma thereby decreasing chances of capsular perforation
- Avoid: Anterior biopsy from the middle hepatic vein (MHV) which increases risk of capsular injury, if need to take sample from MHV → lateral or posterior approach
- Can safely performed in patients with orthotopic liver transplant (OLT) → however, piggyback hepatic vein anastomosis: May be difficult to cannulate hepatic vein and obtain sufficient tissue sample for diagnosis

Transvenous Pressure Measurements (*Indian J Radiol Imaging* 2011;21(4):291–3; *Clin Mol Hepatol* 2014;20(1):6–14; *Clin Liver Dis* 2006;10:499–512; *Semin Liver Dis* 2006;26:348–62)

- Transvenous pressure measurements obtained during the procedure:
  - Right atrial pressure (RAP)
  - Free hepatic venous pressure (FHVP)
  - Infrahepatic vena cava pressure (IVCP)
  - Wedged hepatic venous pressure (WHVP)
- Hepatic venous pressure gradient (HVPG) represents the gradient between pressures in the portal vein (indirectly) and the hepatic vein → evaluates the presence and severity of portal hypertension
- Normal HVPG value is 1–5 mmHg, anything above → portal hypertension
- HVPG ≥ 10 mmHg → clinically significant portal hypertension
- HVPG = WHVP – FHVP
- WHVP obtained by blocking hepatic vein via balloon or "wedged" catheter, the static column of blood transmits the pressure from hepatic sinusoids → reflects sinusoidal pressure ≈ portal venous pressure in the setting of liver fibrosis

- Right atrial pressure → important in patients s/p liver transplantation and for evaluation of Budd–Chiari syndrome to exclude hemodynamic IVC stenosis
- Right atrial pressure ≈ infrahepatic IVC pressure → Ascites can elevate intra-abdominal pressure compared to right atrial pressure
- HVPG is a strong independent prognostic indicator in compensated and decompensated cirrhosis
- **Prognostic implications of HVPG thresholds:** The risk of developing complications of portal hypertension and mortality rates increase as HVPG values increase. Various HVPG thresholds have been noted to have prognostic significance among patients with cirrhosis:
- In patients with compensated cirrhosis:
  - HVPG 10 mmHg: Development of gastroesophageal varices, development of hepatocellular carcinoma, decompensation after surgery for hepatocellular carcinoma
  - HVPG 12 mmHg: Variceal bleeding
  - HVPG 16 mmHg: First clinical decompensation in patients with varices, mortality
- In patients with decompensated cirrhosis:
  - HVPG 16 mmHg: Variceal rebleeding, mortality
  - HVPG 20 mmHg (in patients with active variceal hemorrhage): Failure to control active variceal hemorrhage, low 1-y survival
  - HVPG 22 mmHg: Mortality in patient with alcoholic cirrhosis and acute alcoholic hepatitis
  - HVPG 30 mmHg: Spontaneous bacterial peritonitis

Equipment (Kandarpa K. Handbook of Interventional Radiologic Procedures. Lippincott Williams & Wilkins; 2011; Kessel D, Robertson I. Interventional Radiology: A Survival Guide. Elsevier; 2016)
- Basic angiography set
- Micropuncture access needle set
- 9F × 35-cm vascular sheath
- 0.035-in × 180-cm guidewire (Amplatz/Rosen/Bentson)
- FDA approved biopsy sets:
  TLAB Set (Argon Medical)
  LABS-100/200 set (Cook Medical)
  Both sets contain: A 7F × 49-cm sheath over angled metal sheath stiffener, 5F multipurpose catheter for hepatic vein catheterization, 8F dilator, and the biopsy needle

TLAB Set (Argon Medical)	LABS-100/200 set (Cook Medical)
7F stiff cannula/sheath	7F stiff cannula/sheath
18 or 19G Flexcore biopsy needle	18- or 19G F Quick-core biopsy needle
60-cm trocar length	68-cm trocar length
15-mm needle notch	15-mm needle notch
20-mm needle throw length	20-mm needle throw length

Procedure (Kandarpa K. Handbook of Interventional Radiologic Procedures. Lippincott Williams & Wilkins; 2011; Kessel D, Robertson I. Interventional Radiology: A Survival Guide. Elsevier; 2016)
- **Access:** After local anesthesia with 1% lidocaine, right internal jugular access is obtained using an 18G needle-catheter under ultrasonographic guidance. A 5F introducer catheter is replaced for a 9F vascular sheath over a 0.035-in guidewire.
- **Catheterization:** Pass the guidewire and catheter into the IVC. During the transit through the right atrium, the patient should be monitored for arrhythmias.
- Rotate the catheter so that the tip points toward the patient's right; slowly withdraw the catheter until the tip engages the RHV. Advance the wire and the catheter into the vein.
  If the hepatic venous angle is acute→ reverse curve catheter can be helpful to obtain access into the hepatic veins
  As needed selection of the RHV can be confirmed on oblique views verifying that the wire is directed posteriorly.
- **Runs:** Perform a hepatic venogram to evaluate for patency of the vein. The RHV is the target vein and typically has a shallow angle that allows easier sheath entry. If the RHV cannot be catheterized, the MHV can be attempted.
- **Pressure Measurements** (optional) (Clin Liver Dis 2005;9(4):685–913, vii; CMAJ 2006;174(10):1433–43; Clin Radiol 2015;70(10):1047–59)
  - **RAP** → via larger access sheath
  - **IVCP** → inserting the catheter in the infrahepatic IVC
  - **FHVP** → placing the tip of the catheter inside the hepatic vein, ~3–4 cm from its opening into the IVC
  - **WHVP** → either by inflation of a balloon-tipped catheter into the right hepatic vein (record after pressure tracing is stable, ~2 min) or by adequate occlusion of

the distal-most peripheral hepatic vein—which can be confirmed by inability to withdraw blood or with slow injection of contrast demonstrating a sinusoidogram (no reflux of contrast or washout through communications with other hepatic veins)

- Venous pressures should be allowed to stabilize over a period of at least 1 min for WHVP
- After pressure measurements are properly obtained, the balloon/catheter is exchanged over a stiff wire for the biopsy needle and stiff cannula/sheath
- *Biopsy:* 7F curved-end stiff cannula/sheath is placed over a 0.035 in guidewire (ie, Amplatz) and passed ~3–4 cm into the hepatic vein. Use the directional indicator on the hub to direct the sheath anteriorly (for RHV access) until it abuts the vein wall. The cutting needle is then advanced until the needle tip is beyond the end of the sheath and within the liver parenchyma. The inner stylet is depressed, taking the biopsy. Place mild forward pressure on the cannular during biopsy passes to prevent retraction of the cannula/sheath into the IVC. Repeat biopsy until adequate samples have been taken (Figure 13-3).
- **Catheter removal:** Stiff-angled guide cannula and vascular sheath are now removed. Hemostasis is achieved by applying manual pressure at the venotomy site.

Specimen is delivered to appropriate lab.

Figure 13-3 The biopsy needle is advanced through the right hepatic vein into the hepatic parenchyma.

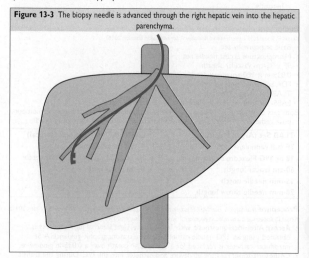

Complications (*J Hepatol* 2007;47:284–94; *J Vasc Interv Radiol* 2001;12:583–7; *J Vasc Interv Radiol* 2007;18:237–41; *J Vasc Interv Radiol* 2008;19:351–8; *Indian J Radiol Imaging* 2008;18(3):245–8; *J Vasc Interv Radiol* 2015;26(2):S84)

- **Major (0.56%):** Hepatic hematoma, liver capsule puncture → intraperitoneal hemorrhage, pseudoaneurysm, IVC injury, arterial laceration, hepatobiliary fistula, arterial–portal fistula
- **Minor (6.5%):** Access site hematoma, accidental carotid puncture

Postprocedural management (Kessel D, Robertson I. *Interventional Radiology: A Survival Guide.* Elsevier; 2016)

- Generally, well tolerated
- Acetaminophen prn for pain
- Monitor access site for bleeding (esp. if coagulopathic)
- Vital signs q15 min for 1 h, q30 min for 1 h, and then every hour postprocedure until discharge
- Clear liquid diet 1 h post procedure, regular diet thereafter
- Observation typically for 2–4 h post procedure
- Typically resume normal activity 24–48 h after discharge

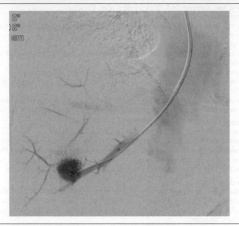

Transjugular liver biopsy: End-hole catheter was wedged into the right hepatic vein and wedge hepatic pressure was measured.

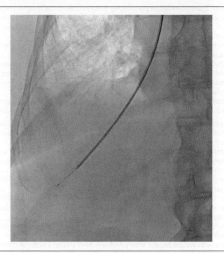

Transjugular liver biopsy: Anterior puncture was performed from the right hepatic vein into the liver parenchyma.

LIVER TRANSPLANTATION

Background (Kandarpa K. *Handbook of Interventional Radiologic Procedures.* Lippincott Williams & Wilkins; 2011; Kessel D, Robertson I. *Interventional Radiology: A Survival Guide.* Elsevier; 2016; *Am J Transplant* 2013;13(9):2384–94; *Cold Spring Harb Perspect Med* 2014;4(5). pii: a015602; *Transplantation* 1997;63(2):250–5; *AJR Am J Roentgenol* 1995;165(5):1145–9; *Transplantation* 1994;57(2):228–31; *AJR Am J Roentgenol* 1986;147(4):657–63)

- Definitive treatment for patients with liver failure
- Long-term survival rates: 1 y (99.5%), 5 y (97.6%), 10 y (93.2%), 15 y (87.2%), and 20 y (78.9%)
- Liver cirrhosis caused by chronic viral hepatitis and alcohol abuse account for ~70% of liver transplantation

- Baseline liver Doppler performed 24–48 h after transplant
- Normal postoperative Doppler findings:
  - Normal hepatic artery Doppler waveform: Rapid systolic up stroke with continuous diastolic flow
  - Systolic acceleration time should be <1 s
  - Resistive Indices (RI): 0.5–0.8 (may be elevated early postoperative period due to reperfusion edema)
  - Normal hepatopetal portal venous flow with a velocity <50 cm/s
  - Normal portal vein Doppler waveform: Continuous flow pattern toward the liver with mild respiratory-induced velocity variations
  - Normal hepatic vein Doppler appearance of the hepatic veins and IVC: Phasic flow pattern, reflecting the physiologic changes in the blood flow during the cardiac cycle

Indications
- **Acute liver failure:** Hepatitis A/B, intoxication, Budd–Chiari
- **Chronic liver failure:** Hepatitis B/C, alcohol-induced cirrhosis, primary biliary cirrhosis (PBC), autoimmune hepatitis, Wilson's, cystic fibrosis, HCC within Milan criteria, alpha 1 antitrypsin deficiency
- **Pediatric:** Biliary atresia, neonatal hepatitis, Byler disease, Alagille syndrome

Contraindications
- **Absolute:** Active alcohol abuse, uncontrolled systemic infections (ie, AIDS-defining symptoms in HIV patients), uncontrolled extrahepatic infections, extrahepatic malignancy, life-limiting medical conditions such as advanced cardiovascular, pulmonary, or neurologic disorders
- **Relative:** Advanced age, severe obesity, severe malnutrition, psychosocial conditions resulting in poor compliance, severe hepatopulmonary or hepatorenal syndrome

Types of Liver Transplantation (Am J Transplant 2013;13(9):2384–94; Cold Spring Harb Perspect Med 2014;4(5). pii: a015602; Transplantation 1997;63(2):250–5; AJR Am J Roentgenol 1995; 65(5):1145–9; Transplantation 1994;57(2):228–31; AJR Am J Roentgenol 1986;147(4):657–63; J Gastroenterol Hepatol 2013;28:18–25; Am J Surg 1991;161(1):76–83; Liver Transpl 2006;12:330–51; AJR Am J Roentgenol 2004;183(6):1577–84)
- Orthotopic liver transplant (OLT): (Most common) native liver is replaced by donor liver (deceased donor – **DDLT**) in the same anatomic position
- Living-donor liver transplantation (**LDLT**): Either right lobe (for adult recipient) or left lobe (for pediatric recipient) is removed from the donor and transplanted into the recipient → both the remnant liver in the donor and the transplanted liver regenerate over time
- Split donation: Donated liver is split into the left and right lobes → larger right lobe transplanted into the adult, smaller left lobe transplanted into pediatric patient

Liver Transplant Anatomy (Am J Transplant 2013;13(9):2384–94; Cold Spring Harb Perspect Med 2014;4(5). pii: a015602; Transplantation 1997;63(2):250–5; AJR Am J Roentgenol 1995;165(5):1145–9; Transplantation 1994;57(2):228–31; AJR Am J Roentgenol 1986;147(4):657–63)
- Prior to performing catheter angiography, review of the operative record is critical to understand how the transplantation was performed. This includes the site of the vascular anastomoses and how much of the donor liver was used.
- Knowledge of the surgical approach allows the angiogram to be tailored to the individual patient.
- Orthotopic liver transplantation requires donor-to-recipient surgical anastomosis of the hepatic artery (HA), portal vein (PV), inferior vena cava (IVC), and bile duct (BD)
- **HA anastomosis:**
  - Donor celiac axis is anastomosed to the recipient hepatic artery at either the bifurcation into left and right hepatic arteries or the takeoff of the gastroduodenal artery
  - Recipients with variant hepatic artery anatomy have smaller caliber of common hepatic artery which can predispose to stenosis
  - Small or diseased hepatic artery → donor iliac artery interposition graft can be anastomosed directly to the recipient aorta
- **IVC anastomosis:**
  - **Conventional technique:** Native retrohepatic IVC is removed en bloc with the liver → end-to-end/end-to-side or side-to-side anastomosis of the donor vena cava to both the suprahepatic and infrahepatic IVC (Figure 13-4)
  - **Piggyback technique:** Donor suprahepatic cava is anastomosed in an end-to-side fashion to the common cuff of recipient hepatic veins. The retrohepatic donor vena cava is ligated. Advantage → improved hemodynamics (Figure 13-5).
- **PV anastomosis:** End-to-end anastomosis
- **Biliary anastomosis:** Duct-to-duct between the donor and recipient common bile ducts, if unacceptable duct size mismatch or the recipient bile duct is unusable →

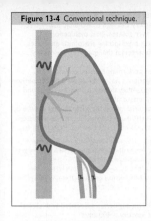

Figure 13-4 Conventional technique.

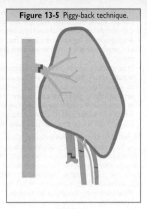

Figure 13-5 Piggy-back technique.

hepaticojejunostomy with Roux-en-Y or choledochocholedochostomy with end-to-end anastomosis of the donor CBD to the recipient CBD.

Liver Transplant Complications (Kessel D, Robertson I. *Interventional Radiology: A Survival Guide.* Elsevier; 2016; *Am J Transplant* 2013;13(9):2384–94; *Cold Spring Harb Perspect Med* 2014;4(5). pii: a015602; *Transplantation* 1997;63(2):250–5; *AJR Am J Roentgenol* 1995;165(5):1145–9; *Transplantation* 1994;57(2):228–31; *AJR Am J Roentgenol* 1986;147(4):657–63; *J Gastroenterol Hepatol* 2013;28:18–25; *Am J Surg* 1991;161(1):76–83; *Liver Transpl* 2006;12:330–51; *AJR Am J Roentgenol* 2004;183(6):1577–84; *HPB (Oxford)* 2004;6(2):69–75; *World J Hepatol* 2016;8(1):36–57; *Transplant Proc* 1997;29:2853–55; *Liver Transpl* 2001;7:75–81)

- Vascular and biliary complications usually occur at the anastomosis (Figure 15-6)
- Ultrasound with Doppler evaluation: First-line screening of liver transplant vascular complications → allows selection of patients who might benefit from direct catheter angiography

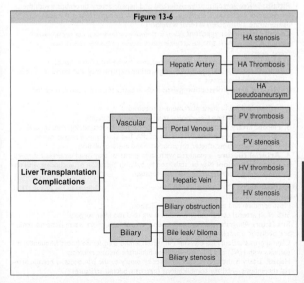

Figure 13-6

Liver Transplantation Complications
- Vascular
  - Hepatic Artery
    - HA stenosis
    - HA Thrombosis
    - HA pseudoaneurysm
  - Portal Venous
    - PV thrombosis
    - PV stenosis
  - Hepatic Vein
    - HV thrombosis
    - HV stenosis
- Biliary
  - Biliary obstruction
  - Bile leak/ biloma
  - Biliary stenosis

- Hepatic artery provides blood supply to liver parenchyma and biliary tree; therefore, complications associated with the hepatic artery can lead to ischemic biliary tree complications → bile duct necrosis, biloma, liver abscess, graft dysfunction
- Angiography → definitive diagnosis, may detect predisposing anatomical anomalies +/− possible therapeutic management (**Intra-arterial** therapy [IAT], angioplasty, stent)
- Due to disruption of collateral sources when performing hepatectomy for OLT, hepatic artery thrombosis (HAT) or acute ligation is not well tolerated (in comparison to native liver w/intact collaterals) → ischemia. Allograft may survive by portal and arterial inflows *via* portal and hepatic artery anastomoses.
- In cases of HA complications affecting the arterial inflow, the allograft may survive by portal inflow, but only if arterial collaterals exist (Kessel D, Robertson I. *Interventional Radiology: A Survival Guide.* Elsevier; 2016; J Vasc Interv Radiol 1997;8(5):733–44; Semin Intervent Radiol 1995;12:337–46).

Hepatic Arterial Stenosis (Kessel D, Robertson I. *Interventional Radiology: A Survival Guide.* Elsevier; 2016; Am J Transplant 2013;13(9):2384–94; Cold Spring Harb Perspect Med 2014;4(5). pii: a015602; Transplantation 1997;63(2):250–5; AJR Am J Roentgenol 1995;165(5):1145–9; Transplantation 1994;57(2):228–31; AJR Am J Roentgenol 1986;147(4):657–63; J Gastroenterol Hepatol 2013;28:18–25; Am J Surg 1991;161(1):76–83; Liver Transpl 2006;12:330–51; AJR Am J Roentgenol 2004;183(6):1577–84; HPB (Oxford) 2004;6(2):69–75; World J Hepatol 2016;8(1):36–57; Transplant Proc 1997;29:2853–5; Liver Transpl 2001;7:75–81)

- Most commonly occurs at anastomosis
- Narrowing of the transverse diameter > 50% on angiogram associated with clinical suspicion and an RI <0.5 and a peak systolic velocity > 400 cm/s
- **Treatment** for transplant hepatic artery stenosis is balloon angioplasty → stenting reserved for recurrent stenosis or treatment of severe dissections following PTA (stenting may limit future surgical options—revision, retransplant)
- Causes of hepatic artery stenosis: Clamp injury, intimal trauma from a perfusion catheter, disruption of the vasa vasorum causing ischemia of the arterial ends
- Low-grade narrowing of the hepatic artery may not demonstrate Doppler waveform abnormalities. If clinical suspicion is high, follow-up cross-sectional imaging or angiography can be obtained for further evaluation.
- **US findings**
  - High velocity >200 cm/s or 3× velocity of prestenotic segment at the point of stenosis with poststenotic turbulence
  - Tardus parvus waveform of intrahepatic arteries
  - Low RI <0.5
  - Delayed systolic acceleration time > 0.1 s
- **Pitfalls:** Severe aortoiliac atherosclerosis and hepatic artery thrombosis with the formation of intrahepatic collateral vessels → flow through collateral vessels may demonstrate a dampened arterial waveform
- **Complications/Management** (Kandarpa K. *Handbook of Interventional Radiologic Procedures.* Lippincott Williams & Wilkins; 2011; Kessel D, Robertson I. *Interventional Radiology: A Survival Guide.* Elsevier; 2016)
  1. **Hepatic artery spasm:** If untreated, may evolve into thrombosis. Administer 100–200 μg of IV nitroglycerine. Heparin may also be administered to prevent thrombosis.
  2. **Hepatic artery dissection** (particularly in cases of sharp arterial turns and kinks)
     - Flow-limiting → stent placement is required
     - Non-flow-limiting dissection→ treat with anticoagulation
  3. Hepatic artery thrombosis is likely secondary to dissection. Intraprocedural thrombosis → immediate IV 1–3 mg of tPA. Refractory thrombosis can be treated with transcatheter thrombolysis and anticoagulation.
  4. **Arterial rupture** → managed with stent grafts or may need emergent surgery
  5. **Stent migration:** May be stabilized by balloon dilatation or anchoring with an overlapping stent depending on the location

Hepatic Arterial Thrombosis (HAT) (Liver Transpl 2001;7:75–81; Transplant Proc 2006;38:2111–6; Transpl Int 2011;24:949–57)

- Most common and severe vascular complication
- 50% of all arterial complications, within 6 wk to 3 mo after surgery
- Risk factors: Allograft rejection, end-to-end anastomosis, short warm ischemia time, and pediatric transplantation
- Clinical presentation: Mild elevation in serum amino transferase (most frequently in patients with HAT) and bilirubin levels to fulminant hepatic necrosis
- Hepatic artery is the only source of vascular supply to the bile ducts → hepatic arterial thrombosis → biliary complications (necrosis, biloma, stricture)

- Postoperative US Doppler (↑ sensitivity ↑ specificity): Nonvisualization of hepatic artery (decreased blood flow from vasospasm or ↓ cardiac output can mimic similar findings)
- Endovascular angiogram is definitive diagnosis
- Tx: Revascularization (endovascular or surgical) or retransplantation

Hepatic Artery Pseudoaneurysm (Kessel D, Robertson I. *Interventional Radiology: A Survival Guide.* Elsevier; 2016; *Transpl Int* 2011;24:949–57)

- Extrahepatic pseudoaneurysm most commonly occurs at the arterial anastomosis de novo or arises as a complication of angioplasty
- Intrahepatic pseudoaneurysm may result from percutaneous biopsy, biliary procedures, or infection
- Rupture of a pseudoaneurysm has the potential to cause major arterial hemorrhage
- Fistula can develop between the aneurysm and the biliary tree or the GI tract → hemobilia or upper GI bleed
- US: Cystic structure, usually near the course of the hepatic artery; its interior is color-filled, demonstrating a turbulent arterial flow
- Contrast enhanced CT or MRA: Arterial enhancing vascular lesion
- Extrahepatic pseudoaneurysm tx: Include surgical resection, embolization, and exclusion with stent placement
- Intrahepatic pseudoaneurysms tx: Endovascular coil embolization or stenting to exclude the pseudoaneurysm if technically feasible

Technical Procedure (Kessel D, Robertson I. *Interventional Radiology: A Survival Guide.* Elsevier; 2016; *AJR Am J Roentgenol* 1995;165(5):1145–9; *Transplantation* 1994;57(2):228–31; *AJR Am J Roentgenol* 1986;147(4): 657–63; *J Gastroenterol Hepatol* 2013;28:18–25)

- **Access:** Usually the right common femoral artery, but sometimes a brachial artery approach will be necessary due to the angulation of the celiac axis
- **Catheterization:** Select the celiac axis arising anteriorly from the aorta at T12/L1
- **Angiogram:** Perform a diagnostic angiogram to evaluate the arterial anatomy. Delay imaging into the venous phase to image the portal anastomosis. For patients with an aorta to hepatic artery conduit → begin with an aortogram.
- Evaluate the vascular anatomy. The transplant hepatic artery may be anastomosed to the recipient hepatic artery or via a conduit to the aorta or iliac artery.
- Selective catheterization of the common hepatic artery and its branches may be required based on transplant anatomy
- Position a larger guide-catheter or sheath in the celiac axis or the aortohepatic artery conduit
- Hepatic artery thrombosis → Systemic anticoagulation with intravenous heparin is employed. Intra-arterial nitroglycerin can be administered to prevent arterial spasm.
- Hepatic artery stenosis → angioplasty; perform using the 0.014 and 0.018-in guidewire–balloon–stent systems → oversizing of the balloon should be done with caution, transplant hepatic arteries are more prone to rupture than native, atherosclerotic arteries. Limitations to stenting: Restenosis and the impact on surgical reconstruction if needed.
- Hepatic artery pseudoaneurysm → coil embolization

Follow-up (Kandarpa K. *Handbook of Interventional Radiologic Procedures.* Lippincott Williams & Wilkins; 2011; *Semin Intervent Radiol* 2004;21(4):221–33)

- Obtain baseline Doppler ultrasound shortly after PTA, detect changes in waveforms and flow velocities over time. Baseline examination is obtained shortly after PTA, and then changes in the waveforms and flow velocities can be easily detected over time.
- Reserve stenting to nonsurgical candidates with recurrent hepatic artery or to treat severe post-PTA dissections

Portal Venous Stenosis (PVS) (Kessel D, Robertson I. *Interventional Radiology: A Survival Guide.* Elsevier; 2016; *Am J Transplant* 2013;13(9):2384–94; *Cold Spring Harb Perspect Med* 2014;4(5). pii: a015602; *Transplantation* 1997;63(2):250–5; *AJR Am J Roentgenol* 1995;165(5):1145–9; *Transplantation* 1994;57(2):228–31; *AJR Am J Roentgenol* 1986;147(4):657–63; *J Gastroenterol Hepatol* 2013;28:18–25; *Am J Surg* 1991;161(1):76–83; *Liver Transpl* 2006;12:330–51; *AJR Am J Roentgenol* 2004;183(6):1577–84; *HPB (Oxford)* 2004;6(2):69–75; *World J Hepatol* 2016;8(1):36–57; *Transplant Proc* 1997;29:2853–5; *Liver Transpl* 2001;7:75–81; *Transplant Proc* 2006;38:2111–6; *Transpl Int* 2011;24:949–57; *Radiographics* 2003;23:1093–114; *Ann Ital Chir* 2001;72(2):187–205; *Semin Intervent Radiol* 2004;21(4):221–33; *J Vasc Interv Radiol* 1990;1:17–22)

- Clinical presentation: Portal hypertension, hepatic failure, edema, and massive ascites
- Reported incidence of 1% after liver transplantation

- Result of technical problems (vessel misalignment, differences in the caliber of the anastomosed vessels, or stretching of the portal vein at the anastomotic site), previous portal vein surgery or previous thrombosis, increased downstream resistance due to a suprahepatic stricture of the inferior vena cava (IVC), decreased portal inflow, and hypercoagulable states
- Stenosis of the portal vein usually occurs at the donor–recipient anastomosis
- US: Focal narrowing of portal vein, aliasing, and increased flow velocity at the site of stenosis
- Hemodynamically significant: Velocity gradient ↑ 3–4× relative to prestenotic segment w/ focal color aliasing on color and pulsed Doppler images
- Poststenotic dilatation and portal hypertension demonstrated by ↑ number or caliber of collateral vessels
- Venography → direct injection of the portal vein allows better assessment of the lesion. Can be performed transhepatic or transjugular approach
- Transhepatic approach, usually from the right side → better control and more direct approach to cross difficult, tight lesions
- Many patients with portal vein stenosis have significant ascites → perform paracentesis prior to procedure or use a stiff sheath to bridge the gap between the abdominal wall and liver
- Paracentesis may be performed before the procedure
- Treatment includes balloon angioplasty while stenting reserved for stenosis resistant to dilatation or recurrent lesions
- Adjunct thrombolytic therapy, either mechanical or pharmacologic, may be required to achieve satisfactory portal vein flow
- Success rates → 70% have been reported (Clin Radiol 2015;70(10):1047–59; Clin Liver Disease 2014;18(2):451–76)

Technical Procedure (Kessel D, Robertson I. Interventional Radiology: A Survival Guide. Elsevier; 2016)
1. **Access:**
   - **Transjugular access:** Used if there is a coagulopathy, extrahepatic anastomotic stenosis, possibility of using thrombolysis. Using transjugular access, the portal vein is accessed, similar to a TIPS.
   - **Direct percutaneous transhepatic access:** Access is in-line with the long axis of the portal vein allowing for easier manipulation of devices across the lesion. Useful in cases where the intrahepatic portal radicals are small or target stenosis is close to the porta hepatis (ie, split liver grafts), anastomotic stenosis is at the branch point of the right anterior and right posterior portal vein branches in split right lobe hepatic grafts.
2. **Portal venogram:** Assess for stenosis
3. **Obtain pressure gradients:** 5 mmHg gradient is the cutoff for significant stenosis
4. Once the stenotic lesion is traversed, therapeutic IV heparin is administered
5. If thrombus burden is significant, mechanical and/or pharmaceutical thrombolysis over 12–48 h can be performed prior to angioplasty
6. **Angioplasty:** Starting with smaller diameter balloon, perform balloon dilatation serially increasing incrementally by 2 mm to 110% of the adjacent normal portal vein diameter
7. **Stenting:** If there is immediate recoil (or >30% residual stenosis), stent deployment should be considered
8. **Postdilatation venogram** and repeat pressure measurement
9. Kissing balloon/stent technique is used if an anastomotic stenosis is at the branch point of the right anterior and right posterior portal vein branches in a split right lobe hepatic graft → requires 2 separate transhepatic portal access sites
10. If access is via the transhepatic route, prior to withdrawing the catheter, obtain an activated clotting time (ACT) assessment. ACT <180 → safe to remove the transhepatic sheath.
11. Remove sheath out of the portal vein while injecting contrast
12. Gelfoam, coil, or plug embolization of the parenchymal tract can be performed to reduce bleeding
13. Recurrence of PVS within 6 mo after angioplasty should consider stent placement

Portal Venous Thrombosis (PVT) (Kessel D, Robertson I. Interventional Radiology: A Survival Guide. Elsevier; 2016; Am J Transplant 2013;13(9):2384–94; Cold Spring Harb Perspect Med 2014;4(5). pii: a015602; Transplantation 1997;63(2):250–5; AJR Am J Roentgenol 1995;165(5):1145–9; Transplantation 1994;57(2):228–31; AJR Am J Roentgenol 1986;147(4):657–63; J Gastroenterol Hepatol 2013;28(1):76–83; Am J Surg 1991;161(1):76–83; Liver Transpl 2006;12:330–51; AJR Am J Roentgenol 2004;183(6):1577–84; HPB (Oxford) 2004;6(2):69–75; World J Hepatol 2016;8(1):36–57; Transplant Proc 1997;29:2853–5; Liver Transpl 2001;7:75–81)
- Portal vein thrombosis occurs in about 1–2% of cases
- US: Thrombosis of the portal vein is characterized by no flow

- Access to the portal vein can be achieved via transhepatic, transjugular, or less commonly transplenic access
- Endovascular stenting of the portal vein can be performed in the setting of extrinsic compression, stenosis, or occlusion of the portal vein
- Portal venous stent placement provides rapid decompression of varices and palliation of symptoms with little morbidity to the patient helping to improve their quality of life and prognosis
- Stent placement should be considered when surgery is contraindicated, life expectancy is short, or other conservative methods of treatment have been exhausted

Technical Procedure (Kandarpa K. *Handbook of Interventional Radiologic Procedures*. Lippincott Williams & Wilkins; 2011; Kessel D, Robertson I. *Interventional Radiology: A Survival Guide*. Elsevier; 2016)

1. **Access:** Transhepatic or transjugular access into the portal vein
2. **Portogram:** Evaluate the extent of the thrombus
3. **TPA:** Administer at 0.5 mg/h (eg, 5–10 mg of TPA diluted in 500 mL NS, infused 25–50 mL)
4. **Venography:** Performed in 12–24 h, thrombolytic infusion is continued for a maximum of 36–48 h

IVC/Hepatic Vein Stenosis (Kandarpa K. *Handbook of Interventional Radiologic Procedures*. Lippincott Williams & Wilkins; 2011; *Am J Transplant* 2013;13(9):2384–94; *Cold Spring Harb Perspect Med* 2014;4(5). pii: a015602; *Transplantation* 1997;63(2):250–5; *AJR Am J Roentgenol* 1995;165(5):1145–9; *Transplantation* 1994;57(2):228–31; *AJR Am J Roentgenol* 1986;147(4):657–63; *J Gastroenterol Hepatol* 2013;28:18–25; *Am J Surg* 1991;161(1):76–83; *Liver Transpl* 2006;12:330–51; *AJR Am J Roentgenol* 2004;183(6):1577–84; *HPB (Oxford)* 2004;6(2):69–75; *World J Hepatol* 2016;8(1):36–57; *Transplant Proc* 1997;29:2853–5; *Liver Transpl* 2001;7:75–81; *Transplant Proc* 2006;38:2111–6) *Transpl Int* 2011;24:949–57; *Radiographics* 2003;23:1093–114; *Ann Ital Chir* 2001;72(2):187–05; *Semin Intervent Radiol* 2004;21(4):221–33; *J Vasc Interv Radiol* 1990;1:17–22; *AJR Am J Roentgenol* 2011;196(3 Suppl):WS15–25 Quiz S35–8; *Radiology* 2005;236:352–9; *AJR Am J Roentgenol* 1999;173:15–19; *Radiographics* 2001;21(5):1085–102)

- Complications of the IVC and the hepatic vein have a low combined incidence (<1%)
- **Clinical presentation:** Lower limb edema, hepatomegaly, ascites, pleural effusions, Budd-Chiari syndrome, liver and renal failure to hypotension → allograft loss and multiorgan failure
- Factors that may predispose to acute stenosis: Size discrepancy between the donor and recipient vessels or suprahepatic IVC kinking from organ rotation
- Delayed stenosis occurs from fibrosis, chronic thrombus, or neointimal hyperplasia
- Caval interposition anastomoses either the femoral or jugular approach may be used
- "Piggy-back" anastomosis, the jugular approach gives more direct access to the hepatic veins
- When using a jugular approach, liver biopsies can also be obtained
- IVC lesions are easily treated with balloon angioplasty, recurrence due to elastic recoil can be treated with stenting
- Stenoses involving the origins of the hepatic veins after a piggy-back anastomosis are more difficult to treat
- Anastomotic stenosis may be easily dilated from the jugular or femoral approach
- Recurrence of anastomotic stenosis can be treated with stent placement → extend the stent from the largest of the hepatic vein branches across the anastomosis with the IVC, crossing the origins of other hepatic vein branches

Technical Procedure

Venous Outflow Interventions

Anastomotic IVC stenosis or occlusion (Kessel D, Robertson I. *Interventional Radiology: A Survival Guide*. Elsevier; 2016; *Radiographics* 2003;23:1093–114; *Ann Ital Chir* 2001;72(2):187–205; *Semin Intervent Radiol* 2004;21(4):221–33; *J Vasc Interv Radiol* 1990;1:17–22; *AJR Am J Roentgenol* 2011;196(3 Suppl):WS15–25 Quiz S35–8)

1. **Access:** Obtain venous access with a micropuncture set. Use right common femoral access over the transjugular approach if the IVC stenosis is close to the cavoatrial junction. Insert a long vascular sheath with a side arm allowing continuous flushing
2. **Cavogram:** Performed via a coaxial pigtail catheter in both anteroposterior (AP) and lateral projections
3. **Pressure gradient measurements** are obtained (the gold standard for diagnosing IVC stenosis) >5 mmHg is abnormal
4. Once the stenotic lesion is traversed therapeutic IV heparin is administered
5. If thrombus burden is significant, mechanical and/or pharmaceutical thrombolysis over 12–48 h can be performed prior to angioplasty

6. **Angioplasty:** Starting with smaller caliber balloon, perform balloon dilatation serially increasing incrementally by 2 mm to 110% of the adjacent normal caval diameter
7. Monitor blood pressure when performing prolonged balloon inflation as it may drop significantly due to ↓ in venous return
8. Obtain postangioplasty pressures. Pressure gradient <5 mmHg is considered successful.
9. Consider stenting if there is immediate intraprocedural recoil or the cava has restenosed within 1–3 mo from a prior venoplasty
10. Catheters and guidewires are removed and hemostasis is achieved

Hepatic vein stenosis or occlusion (Kessel D, Robertson I. *Interventional Radiology: A Survival Guide.* Elsevier; 2016; *Radiographics* 2003;23:1093–14; *Ann Ital Chir* 2001;72(2):187–05; *Semin Intervent Radiol* 2004;21(4): 221–33; *J Vasc Interv Radiol* 1990;1:17–22; *AJR Am J Roentgenol* 2011;196(3 Suppl):WS15–25 Quiz S35–8)

1. **Access:** Right internal jugular vein using a micropuncture set and insert a vascular sheath with a side arm hooked to continuous flush
2. **Select:** The hepatic vein using a 5F catheter
   a. Stenosis is too tight to be crossed from the IVC → attempt transhepatic approach using a 22G Chiba needle
   b. After accessing the hepatic vein, pass a 0.018 in wire into the vein
   c. After crossing the stenosis, engage the wire with a snare inserted via jugular vein, and pulled through into the IVC. The procedure is continued via the transjugular approach to reduce the risk of capsular bleeding. However, some may perform the venoplasty from a transhepatic approach
3. Perform venography and pressure gradients
4. Once the stenotic lesion is traversed therapeutic IV heparin is administered
5. If significant thrombus is present, mechanical and possible pharmaceutical thrombolysis is performed over 12–48 h prior to angioplasty
6. **Venoplasty:** Starting with a small diameter balloon, perform balloon dilatation serially increasing incrementally by 2 mm to 110% of the adjacent normal venous diameter
7. **Venography and pressure measurements** are obtained. Successful if reduction of pressure gradient <5 mmHg
8. Consider stenting if there is immediate recoil or persistent gradient > 5 mmHg
9. The catheters and sheaths are removed and hemostasis is achieved

Biliary Complications (*Transplant Proc* 1997;29:2853–55; *Liver Transpl* 2001;7:75–81; *Transplant Proc* 2006;38:2111–6) *Transpl Int* 2011;24:949–57; *Radiographics* 2003;23:1093–114; *Ann Ital Chir* 2001;72(2):187–205; *Semin Intervent Radiol* 2004;21(4):221–33; *J Vasc Interv Radiol* 1990;1:17–22; *AJR Am J Roentgenol* 2011;196 (3 Suppl):WS15–25 Quiz S35–8; *Radiology* 2005;236:352–9; *AJR Am J Roentgenol* 1999;173:215–9; *Radiographics* 2001;21(5):1085–102)

- 25% of liver transplant recipients, usually within the first 3 mo after transplantation
- MR cholangiography → best noninvasive technique for evaluation of the biliary tree
- Obstruction is the most common biliary complication, usually stenosis at the anastomotic site
- Anastomotic strictures usually result from fibrotic proliferation with narrowing of the biliary lumen; less frequently, due to ischemia caused by hepatic artery thrombosis or stenosis
- Possible causes of nonanastomotic strictures include pretransplantation biliary diseases such as primary sclerosing cholangitis, biliary ischemia, and infection
- Various degrees of presentation, some with mild dilatation of the biliary tree with the absence of an actual mechanical obstruction or clinical and laboratory evidence of high-grade obstruction without visible dilatation of the biliary tree
- Some patients with clinical and biochemical evidence of biliary obstruction may have dilatation of both the donor and the recipient bile ducts
- Papillary dyskinesia or due to devascularization or denervation of the papilla of Vater during transplantation may result in diffuse ductal dilatation
- Ductal ischemia can lead to necrosis and its associated complications: Bile leak (fistula), ductal scarring with fibrosis (stenosis), and bile collection (biloma)
- Tx: Ductal stenosis with balloon dilatation. Ultimately, in most cases, retransplantation is necessary.
- Leaks most often occur at the T-tube site and rarely at the site of an anastomosis
- Bile can leak into the peritoneal cavity or form a perihepatic biloma. Tx: Stent placement and drainage of collections.

Postprocedure Management (Kandarpa K. *Handbook of Interventional Radiologic Procedures.* Lippincott Williams & Wilkins; 2011; Kessel D, Robertson I. *Interventional Radiology: A Survival Guide.* Elsevier; 2016)

- Routine postangiographic management for femoral access

- Transhepatic access
  - Bed rest at least 4 h, depends on the patient's anticoagulation status, size of transhepatic sheath
  - Access sites are checked within 12–24 h for bleeding or discharge (biliary or purulent)
  - Observe the patient for signs and symptoms of intra-abdominal bleeding, including increased abdominal girth
  - Obtain serial Hgb/Hct to monitor occult bleeding
  - Hydration depends on contrast volume and patient's volume status. In cases of severe IVC stenosis, patients may demonstrate postobstructive diuresis requiring adequate hydration
  - If stents were placed, patient should be started on anticoagulation (start with heparin, then Coumadin) and antiplatelet therapy (aspirin or clopidogrel) should continue for 6 mo postprocedure
  - Noninvasive imaging
    - Following arterial interventions baseline Doppler ultrasound is performed within 24–48 h and should be repeated at 1, 3, 6, and 12 mo, or as clinically indicated
    - Following embolization of pseudoaneurysms, Doppler ultrasound and/or CTA is performed within 24–48 h
    - Hepatic, IVC, or portal venous intervention → follow-up Doppler ultrasound and MR imaging should be obtained at 1 mo postprocedure

PERCUTANEOUS TRANSHEPATIC CHOLANGIOGRAM

Background (Kandarpa K. *Handbook of Interventional Radiologic Procedures.* Lippincott Williams & Wilkins; 2011; *J Gastrointest Surg* 2011;15(4):623–30; *J Vasc Interv Radiol* 2016;27(7):1056–69)
- **Procedure:** Percutaneous image-guided needle access into the biliary system with contrast injection to opacify the biliary tree
- Prior to the advances in noninvasive imaging (**MRCP, CT**) → cholangiograms were performed to visualize the biliary system to evaluate for pathology
- Now **percutaneous transhepatic cholangiography (PTC)** used as the first step in a number of percutaneous biliary interventions (biliary drain or stenting)
- 2 procedures used to evaluate the biliary anatomy: ERCP and PTC → ERCP is the first test of choice
- PTC is more invasive and painful than ERCP → PTC procedure involves puncturing the liver parenchyma → risk of hemoperitoneum and bile peritonitis
- PTC is now usually reserved for patients in whom ERCP is unsuccessful → biliary system cannot be cannulated or obstructing lesion prevents contrast material from opacifying the cephalic portions of the biliary system

Indications (Kandarpa K. *Handbook of Interventional Radiologic Procedures.* Lippincott Williams & Wilkins; 2011; *J Gastrointest Surg* 2011;15(4):623–30; *J Vasc Interv Radiol* 2016;27(7):1056–69)
- Evaluation of the biliary system after failed ERCP
- ERCP not feasible (eg, patients with gastrojejunostomy)
- Inaccessible papilla (eg, in ampullary carcinoma or duodenal obstruction from malignancy)
- Exclude extra hepatic bile duct obstruction, prior to biliary drainage procedure
- Demonstrate site of bile duct leak

Contraindications (Kandarpa K. *Handbook of Interventional Radiologic Procedures.* Lippincott Williams & Wilkins; 2011)
- Uncorrectable coagulation parameters (relative)

Anatomy
- **Intrahepatic biliary anatomy:** Bile canaliculi join to form segmental bile ducts → drain each liver segment. Segmental ducts unite to form sectional ducts:
  - Segments VI and VII drain into the right posterior duct (RPD)
  - Segments V and VIII drain into the right anterior duct (RAD)
  - Right posterior and anterior ducts joint to form the right hepatic duct (RHD)
  - Segmental bile ducts from II–IV unite to form the left hepatic duct (LHD)
- Left and right hepatic ducts join to form the common hepatic duct (CHD)
- Conventional intrahepatic anatomy is only present in 58–68% of the population
- Variations in the intrahepatic drainage anatomy is helpful for biliary drain decompression planning (Figure 13-7)
  A. Conventional (64%)
  B. Triple confluence with the right posterior, right anterior, and left hepatic ducts joining to form the common hepatic duct (14%)
  C. Right posterior duct drains into the left hepatic duct (12%)
  D. Right posterior duct drains directly into the common hepatic or cystic duct (8%)

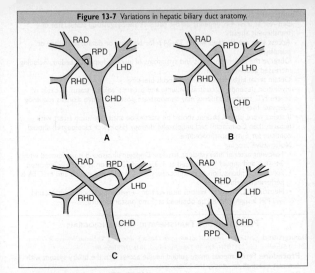

Figure 13-7 Variations in hepatic biliary duct anatomy.

Preprocedural Evaluation (Handbook of Interventional Radiologic Procedures. 2011: Lippincott Williams & Wilkins; Tech Vasc Interv Radiol 2006;9:69–76; J Vasc Interv Radiol 2010;21:611–30; J Gastrointest Surg 2011;15(4):623–30; J Vasc Interv Radiol 2016;27(7):1056–69; World J Gastroenterol 2007;13(29):3948–55; Indian J Palliat Care 2016;22(4):378–87; Asian Pac J Cancer Prev 2015;16(6):2543–6; Gut Liver 2014;8(5):526–35; World J Gastrointest Oncol 2016;8(6):498–508; J Vasc Interv Radiol 2010;21(6):789–95; Radiographics 2002;22(2):305–22; World J Gastroenterol 2007;13:3531–39; J Vasc Interv Radiol 2008;19(9):1328–35; J Vasc Interv Radiol 2003; 14(9 Pt 2):S243–6; Endoscopy 2009;41:323–8)

- Review cross-sectional imaging: Provides information about the pattern of biliary dilatation (uniform, segmental) and the level of obstruction, identify cause of obstruction
- Multiplanar MRI + MRCP → provides the best information about the cause and level of obstruction
- Coronal CT view → corresponds the AP fluoroscopy projection, helpful to better understand the anatomic background
- Informed consent
- Labs: PLT, INR

Equipment (Kandarpa K. Handbook of Interventional Radiologic Procedures. Lippincott Williams & Wilkins; 2011)
- 22G Chiba needle
- Connecting tube
- C-arm fluoroscopy
- Ultrasound machine
- Sedatives and analgesics

Procedure (Kandarpa K. Handbook of Interventional Radiologic Procedures. Lippincott Williams & Wilkins; 2011; Kessel D, Robertson I. Interventional Radiology: A Survival Guide. Elsevier; 2016)
1. **Preprocedural imaging:** Perform ultrasound to look for ductal dilatation before starting. Ultrasound guidance is almost always used for left lobe punctures but can be used to direct right-sided punctures as well.
2. **Access:** Locate the target.
   I. The duct is adjacent to the portal vein and artery. If duct is not dilated, use the portal vein as the target.
   II. Left-sided punctures are made from a subxiphoid approach (avoiding the pleural space) → target the segment 3 duct (anterior, superior to portal vein = safest)
   III. Right-sided punctures → If intercostal, approach above the rib to avoid blood vessels. If performing blind puncture target right flank below the 10th rib, mid-axillary line (avoid pleural space). Aim for segment 5, will help visualize most of the right lobe biliary ducts with contrast injection.

3. Inject local anesthetic (lidocaine) at the puncture site through the subcutaneous tissues and peritoneum
4. Puncture as peripherally as possible. Advance needle in the plane of the transducer in the trajectory of the targeted duct. For right-sided punctures, aim just cranial to the hilum of the liver while angulating the needle about 20° cranially and 20° ventrally.
5. The needle is advanced a few mm in the duct, the central stylet is removed and the connecting tube attached to the needle
6. *Cholangiogram:* Under fluoroscopy, gently inject contrast as the needle is withdrawn slowly
   I. Bile ducts → contrast tends to flow toward the hilum; obstructed ducts, the contrast often swirls as it dilutes
   II. Portal vein and hepatic artery → contrast flows toward the periphery of the liver
   III. Hepatic vein branches → contrast flows cranially toward the right atrium
   IV. Focal contrast with delayed clearance → parenchymal staining
7. Avoid overdistension of the bile ducts as it can cause bacteremia, sepsis, cholangitis
8. Left-sided ducts often do not fill after right duct contrast injection in supine patients → inject more contrast and carefully rotate the patient left side down

Procedural Imaging Findings (Kandarpa K. *Handbook of Interventional Radiologic Procedures.* Lippincott Williams & Wilkins; 2011)

- Filling defects seen on cholangiogram can be caused by:
  - Gallstones (smooth intraluminal filing defect)
  - Tumor (mural nodules or strictures)
  - Blood (extensive serpiginous intraluminal filling defect)
- Strictures are caused by tumor or sclerosing cholangitis
- Beading can be due to sclerosing cholangitis
- Dilated ducts are indicative of proximal duct blockage
- Displaced ducts can be secondary to an adjacent mass

Complications (Kandarpa K. *Handbook of Interventional Radiologic Procedures.* Lippincott Williams & Wilkins; 2011; *World J Gastroenterol* 2007;13(29):3948–55)

- Sepsis, cholangitis, bile leak, hemorrhage, or pneumothorax
- Reported rate 2%

PERCUTANEOUS BILIARY DRAIN PLACEMENT

Background (Kandarpa K. *Handbook of Interventional Radiologic Procedures.* Lippincott Williams & Wilkins; 2011; *Tech Vasc Interv Radiol* 2006;9:69–76; *J Vasc Interv Radiol* 2010;21:611–30; *J Gastrointest Surg* 2011;15(4):623–30; *J Vasc Interv Radiol* 2016;27(7):1056–69; *World J Gastroenterol* 2007;13(29):3948–55; *Indian J Palliat Care* 2016;22(4):378–87; *Asian Pac J Cancer Prev* 2015;16(6):2543–6; *Gut Liver* 2014;8(5):526–35; *World J Gastrointest Oncol* 2016;8(6):498–508; *J Vasc Interv Radiol* 2010;21(6):789–95; *Radiographics* 2002;22(2):305–22; *World J Gastroenterol* 2007;13:3531–9; *J Vasc Interv Radiol* 2008;19(9):1328–35; *J Vasc Interv Radiol* 2003; 14(9 Pt 2):S243–6)

- **Procedure:** Percutaneous placement of a drain within the biliary system for treatment of biliary obstruction (benign or malignant)
- Malignant causes of biliary obstruction include carcinoma of pancreas, cholangiocarcinoma, and metastatic disease
- Benign biliary obstruction: **Anastomotic strictures** after surgical bile duct repair or liver transplantation, **strictures secondary to intraoperative injury** (most commonly during laparoscopic cholecystectomy), **postoperative inflammatory strictures**, infections, sclerosing cholangitis
- Relief of obstruction → **improvement in pain, jaundice, and reduced occurrence of cholangitis**
- Biliary drainage is beneficial in **improving the liver function** prior to surgery or neoadjuvant chemotherapy
- Endoscopic treatment is the optimal initial management for benign biliary strictures
- Endoscopy is not possible for patients with high biliary strictures, bilioenteric anastomosis, tight low biliary strictures → percutaneous approach can be attempted
- Classified into external and internal/external percutaneous biliary drains
  - **External:**
    - *Straight drain:* Temporary, last resort → when unable to traverse the stricture into a large enough duct to form a pigtail, can dislodge easily
    - *Pigtail drain:* More secure than a straight catheter, but cannot cross the obstruction; however, able to access a large enough central duct to form a pigtail

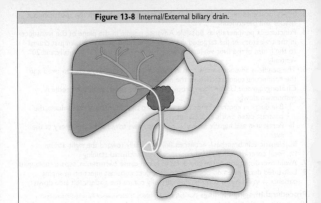

Figure 13-8 Internal/External biliary drain.

- **Internal/External:** Placed across the stricture, bile can be drained externally to a bag or internally to the duodenum. More secure, contains multiple side holes over the length of the catheter → additional side holes can be made along the catheter to increase drainage from the intrahepatic biliary tree (Figure 13-8).

Indication (Kandarpa K. *Handbook of interventional radiologic procedures.* Lippincott Williams & Wilkins; 2011; Kessel D, Robertson I. *Interventional Radiology: A Survival Guide.* Elsevier; 2016)

- Cholangitis, treatment of acute biliary sepsis
- Pain, pruritus alleviation
- Dilate biliary strictures
- Decrease serum bilirubin before the initiation of chemotherapy
- Access biliary system prior to stent placement
- Biliary stricture dilatation

Contraindication (Kandarpa K. *Handbook of Interventional Radiologic Procedures.* Lippincott Williams & Wilkins; 2011; Kessel D, Robertson I. *Interventional Radiology: A Survival Guide.* Elsevier; 2016)

Relative
- Coagulopathy/bleeding diathesis
- Ascites (can perform paracentesis prior to the procedure)

Pre-evaluation (Kandarpa K. *Handbook of Interventional Radiologic Procedures.* Lippincott Williams & Wilkins; 2016; Kessel D, Robertson I. *Interventional Radiology: A Survival Guide.* Elsevier; 2016)

- Informed consent
- Labs: PLT, INR, LFT (particularly bilirubin levels to establish baseline)
- Review cross-sectional imaging (CT, MR): Provides information and potential level of obstruction
  - Proximal obstruction: Primary biliary confluence may be blocked +/− secondary confluence → PTBD is preferred
  - Distal obstruction: Beyond the confluence, distal to the cystic duct insertion → ERCP is preferred method of drainage
- Select the appropriate target duct for biliary drainage → duct should drain at least 1/6th liver parenchyma
- Distal obstruction and primary confluence is patent, single drain should suffice
- **Anatomical variations:** If the right anterior or posterior ducts drain to the left main duct → left lobe drainage may be sufficient for palliation
- If the tumor is mainly involving the left ducts, then draining the right may be the best approach
- Hilar mass lesions require biductal biliary drainage (right and left biliary systems)
- Evaluate for atrophy or portal vein involvement → PTBD of the bile ducts within this lobe will not improve liver function due to the lack of functioning hepatic parenchyma
- If ascites, perform paracentesis prior to procedure (Ascites increases the risk of bleeding from the liver capsule and makes advancing stiff drainage catheters more difficult as the liver moves away from catheter)
- Antibiotic prophylaxis for biliary drainage → incidence of infectious complication after biliary drainage procedures 24–46%

- Most common isolates include Enterococcus species, as well as yeast, gram-negative aerobic bacilli, and *Streptococcus viridans*
- Risk factors for bacterial colonization: Periprocedural fever, previous biliary instrumentation, and bilioenteric anastomosis
- First-choice antibiotic agent: No consensus
- Common antibiotic choices:
  - 1-g ceftriaxone IV
  - 1.5–3 g ampicillin/sulbactam IV
  - 1-g cefotetan IV plus 4-g mezlocillin IV
  - 2-g ampicillin IV plus 1.5-mg/kg gentamicin IV
  (if penicillin-allergic, can use vancomycin or clindamycin and aminoglycoside)

Equipment
As for cholangiography, plus:
- Co-axial percutaneous access kit
- Dilators
- Guidewires: Stiff 0.018-in platinum-tipped wire, heavy duty 0.035-in 3-mm J wire, curved stiff hydrophilic wire, Amplatz wire
- Catheters: Variety used depending on what is needed to cross stricture—straight catheter, angled Kumpe, Cobra, Berenstein
- Drains: Pigtail, internal/external drain
- Peel-away sheath
- Sutures or catheter-retention device

Procedure (Kessel D, Robertson I. *Interventional Radiology: A Survival Guide.* Elsevier; 2016)
1. **Give antibiotics, sedation, and analgesia**
2. **Perform a cholangiogram:** Use a co-axial set → allows for conversion to a 0.035-in wire if a suitable duct is accessed. Identify area of obstruction.
3. **Choose the optimal duct for drainage:** Choose a dilated duct with a straight approach to the site of obstruction that can be accessed
4. **Puncture the duct:** Using fluoroscopic and/or ultrasound guidance access the duct at a point where it is large enough to accommodate the catheters/drains. Peripheral puncture will result in fewer complications.
5. **Confirm intraduct position:** Free back flow of bile indicates that you are in the duct. Gentle injection of contrast may be utilized. Advance the guidewire into the duct.
6. **2-stick technique:** If the initial access needle placement is suboptimal, use the initial needle access to opacify the biliary system, using this to aim/puncture an optimal duct with a second needle
7. **Exchange the 0.018-in wire for the 0.035-in J wire:** Using the co-axial set
8. **Dilate a tract into the duct:** Depending on the size of the catheter, use 5F or 6F dilators
9. **Introduce the catheter and wire to cross the stricture:** A variety of catheters and wires can used in various combinations
10. **As warranted, take a sample of bile:** For microbiology ± cytology
11. **Cross the stricture:** May need to use a curved hydrophilic wire
12. **Confirm intraluminal position:** Always ensure that you are either back in the bile duct or through to the duodenum
13. **Exchange for the heavy-duty J wire or Amplatz super-stiff wire:** An angled approach will need a stronger support wire
14. **Position the drain catheter:** Side holes along the internal/external drains should be on each side of the obstruction but not into the liver parenchyma as this can lead to leakage of bile. The locking pigtail should be distal to the point of obstruction → helps to maintain catheter position within the biliary tree
15. **Confirm free drainage**
16. **Fix the drainage catheter to the skin**

Postprocedure Management (Kandarpa K. *Handbook of Interventional Radiologic Procedures.* Lippincott Williams & Wilkins; 2011)
- Pain control, especially if intercostal space approach was used
- Pain decreases over 24–48 h
- Monitor vital signs q30 min for 1 h, then q1h for 4 h, then q6h for 24 h, then q shift (monitoring for sepsis)
- Check CBC and cultures (blood and bile) as needed
- Check liver function tests q daily for 2–3 d, then q2–3d, bilirubin should demonstrate a downward trend
- Catheters may be flushed with up to 10-cc saline every 8 h to prevent occlusion

- Record the output q8–12 h in the hospital, q daily at home
- Exchange every 2–3 mo or earlier as warranted
- Assess for drainage by clamping the drain 24–48 h prior to removing the biliary drainage catheter
- Wait at least 6–8 wk for the tract to mature prior to any removal

Major Complications (*World J Gastroenterol* 2007;13(29):3948–55)

Higher complication rates associated with patients with coagulopathies, cholangitis, stones, malignant obstruction, or proximal obstruction

- Sepsis
- Hemorrhage
- Localized inflammatory/infectious (abscess, peritonitis, cholecystitis, pancreatitis)
- Biliary peritonitis
- Pleural complications (pneumothorax, effusion, fistula)
- Death

Troubleshooting (Kandarpa K. *Handbook of Interventional Radiologic Procedures.* Lippincott Williams & Wilkins; 2011; Kessel D, Robertson I. *Interventional Radiology: A Survival Guide.* Elsevier; 2016)

- Bile leak around the catheter: May indicate occluded or dislodged catheter
  - Obtain KUB: Check to see if the side holes extend beyond the liver (dislodged/retracted)
  - If there is still significant biliary dilatation, additional side holes can be added to the drain to facilitate increased drainage or upsize the drain
  - Exchange drain if occluded
- Hemobilia
  - Confirm that the side holes of catheter have not migrated back to lie across a portal or hepatic vein
  - If so, advance the catheter
  - Sudden onset or hemobilia occurring 1–2 wk after the procedure is usually due to arterial injury → active extravasation or pseudoaneurysm → embolization
- Bile peritonitis
  - Drain the intraperitoneal bile collection
- Cellulitis or infection at the catheter site
  - Check the catheter for misplaced side holes. Infected of cloudy bile can look like "pus" around the catheter.
  - Apply antibiotics to skin around catheter daily
  - Remove/replace sutures
- Obstruction of the catheter, sluggish drainage
  - Perform cholangiogram
  - If catheter is occluded, exchange for a new catheter
- Dislodgement or removal of catheter
  - Evaluate in a time sensitive manner → if the tube is completely removed, the tract will close within hours unless it is chronic

Percutaneous Biliary Stent Placement (Tech Vasc Interv Radiol 2006;9:69–76; Radiology 1990;177: 793–7; Gastrointest Endosc 2010;72(5):915–23; Gastrointest Endosc 1993;39:43–9; Radiographics 1993;13:1249–63)

- **Procedure:** Placement of a metallic or plastic stent across a stenosed or obstructed CBD, in the setting of obstruction (benign and malignant diseases) to develop a communication between the biliary tree and the bowel allowing physiologic bile flow
- Usually a staged procedure after a week of initial biliary decompression when there is decreased risk of cholangitis/sepsis
- Types of stent include: Metallic (covered/uncovered) or plastic
- Placement of stent type is determined by the etiology of the obstruction (Figure 13-9)

Metallic Stent	Plastic Stent
Stainless steel or nitinol mesh, embedded into the biliary wall → decreased risk of migration	Increased risk of migration
Larger lumen, longer patency	Easily occluded with sludge because of their small diameter (12F endoscopy, 14F percutaneous)
Cannot be easily removed/exchanged	Easily exchanged/removed
Reserved for patients with inoperable malignant biliary obstruction and a life expectancy <12 mo	Usually used in treatment of benign strictures
Endoscope or percutaneous delivery	Usually via endoscope delivery system
More expensive	Least expensive

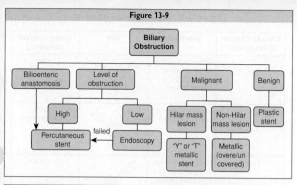

Figure 13-9

Biliary Obstruction
- Bilioenteric anastomosis
- Level of obstruction
  - High
  - Low
    - Endoscopy → (failed) → Percutaneous stent
- Malignant
  - Hilar mass lesion
    - "Y" or "T" metallic stent
  - Non-Hilar mass lesion
    - Metallic (overe/un covered)
- Benign
  - Plastic stent

Percutaneous stent

Covered Stent	Uncovered Stent
Exhibit longer patency durations and lower occlusion rates, reduce the length of hospital stay and decrease the need for periodic stent exchange	Lower shortening rate, and deployment is easier compared with covered stents
Prevent tumor ingrowth and avoid re-intervention	Tumor ingrowth via the metal mesh
Stent migration, occlusion of side-branches (cystic or pancreatic ducts → cholecystitis and pancreatitis)	Less expensive

- Benign strictures, plastic stenting is used because they are removable
- Malignant strictures, metallic stenting is used (higher patency, larger lumen); however, cannot be removed easily (lasts only 12 mo)
- Endoscopic treatment is the optimal initial management for benign biliary strictures
- Endoscopy is not possible for patients with high biliary strictures, bilioenteric anastomosis, tight low biliary strictures; therefore, percutaneous stenting can be attempted
- Percutaneous biliary stenting can be provided as a palliative procedure for inoperable malignant biliary obstruction
- Required number and configuration of stents depend on the degree of biliary obstruction
- Hilar mass lesions require biductal biliary drainage (right and left biliary systems) via 2 stents placement in Y-configuration. If CBD cannot be accessed from the left, T-configuration stenting can be performed (Figure 13-10).

- **Bismuth–Corlette classification system**: Provides anatomic description of the tumor location and longitudinal extension in the biliary tree (Figure 13-11)
- Need 2–3 cm of stent above the obstruction for good palliation

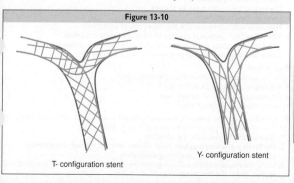

Figure 13-10

T- configuration stent

Y- configuration stent

Figure 13-11 Bismuth-Corlette Classification.

Bismuth-Corlette Classification	Description	Site	Stents to threat completely
Type I	Tumor involves the common hepatic duct distal to the biliary confluence	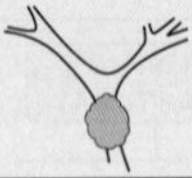	1 stent
Type II	Tumor involves the biliary confluence	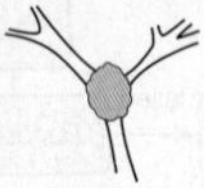	2 stents Y-configuration
Type III	Tumor involves the biliary confluence + right or left hepatic duct	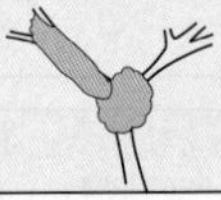	3+ stents
Type IV	Multifocal or extending to the bifurcation of the right and left hepatic ducts	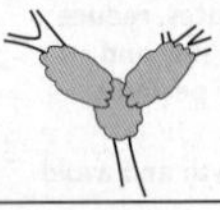	3+ stents

BISMUTH–CORLETTE CLASSIFICATION

Indications (Kandarpa K. *Handbook of Interventional Radiologic Procedures*. Lippincott Williams & Wilkins; 2011; Kessel D, Robertson I. *Interventional Radiology: A Survival Guide*. Elsevier; 2016; Radiology 1996;201(1): 167–72; J Vasc Interv Radiol 2014;25(12):1912–20; J Vasc Interv Radiol 2003;14(11):1409–16; Radiology 1990;177:793–7; Gastrointest Endosc 2010;72(5):915–23)

- Symptomatic **palliation for malignant obstruction** in patients who are not candidates for surgical intervention
- Altered/postsurgical anatomy that is **not able to be reached endoscopically**
- **High bile duct obstruction**, cannot be stented endoscopically

Contraindications (Kandarpa K. *Handbook of Interventional Radiologic Procedures*. Lippincott Williams & Wilkins; 2011; Kessel D, Robertson I. *Interventional Radiology: A Survival Guide*. Elsevier; 2016; Radiology 1996;201(1):167–72; J Vasc Interv Radiol 2014;25(12):1912–20; J Vasc Interv Radiol 2003;14(11):1409–16; Radiology 1990;177:793–7; Gastrointest Endosc 2010;72(5):915–23)

- Asymptomatic patients
- Presence of noncorrectable bleeding disorder
- Hemodynamic instability
- Cholangitis (biliary drain can be placed)
- Surgically resectable mass
- Hemobilia with intraductal clot (increased risk of occlusion)
- Worsening liver function in the face of adequate external drainage
- <30-d life expectancy and patient is stable with an external catheter
- Visible infection involving the percutaneous tract or entry site

Equipment
- As for percutaneous biliary drain placement, plus:
- Appropriate sheath size and length
- Angioplasty balloons of various sizes
- Biliary stents of various sizes

Procedure (Kandarpa K. *Handbook of Interventional Radiologic Procedures*. Lippincott Williams & Wilkins; 2011; Kessel D, Robertson I. *Interventional Radiology: A Survival Guide*. Elsevier; 2016)

1. Give antibiotics, sedation, and analgesia
2. **Perform a cholangiogram:** Inject diluted contrast through the external/internal biliary catheter confirming positioning
3. Using fluoroscopy, insert a 035-in guidewire through the drain with the distal end looped within the duodenum

4. **Exchange:** Typically, a percutaneous biliary drainage catheter is already in place. Cut the biliary catheter, releasing the pigtail and exchange the biliary drain over the guidewire for a sheath.
5. Define the length of the stenosis, the ductal diameter above the stenosis, and the proximal and distal landing sites.
6. **Choose the stent length** (at least 1 cm of stent expanded above and below the stenosis) → longer stent for rapidly growing tumors. Eg intrahepatic ducts (7–10 mm), CBD (10–12 mm)
7. **Deploy the stent,** then check position and flow with gentle injections through the sheath in at least 2 projections
8. Proximal portion of the stent should be placed below the first ductal bifurcation
9. Lower end of the stent may be kept above the ampulla to ↓ reflux and secondary cholangitis; however, the ampulla can be easily obstructed. If the tumor is invasive, rapidly growing or close to the ampulla → stent across the ampulla
   Intrahepatic bifurcation tumors → T- or Y-configuration stents
10. **Balloon dilatation** can be performed over the guidewire to further expand the stent if necessary (Figure 13-12)

Figure 13-12 Balloon dilatation of the stent.

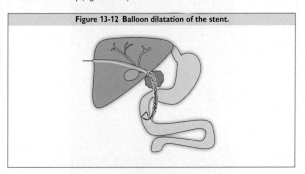

Figure 13-13 Stent placement in the region of the mass.

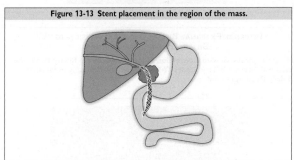

Postprocedure Management (Kessel D, Robertson I. *Interventional Radiology: A Survival Guide.* Elsevier; 2016)
- Pain control
- Monitor vitals
- Obtain labs, LFTS, CBC, lipase/amylase if concern for pancreatitis
- Follow-up cholangiogram, clinical evaluation

Major Complications (*Radiographics* 2002;22(2):305–22; *J Vasc Interv Radiol* 2008;19(9):1328–35)
Complications associated with biliary access
- Hemorrhage (peritoneal, subcapsular, hemobilia)
- Arterial injury (pseudoaneurysm, AVF, arterial-biliary fistula) → presents as delayed bleeding

- Balloon-induced duct rupture or bleeding → early presentation bleeding
- Bile leak/biliary peritonitis
- Cholangitis → occurred less frequently with EPTBD than with ERBD and IPTBD

Complications related to the biliary stent
- Stent migration
- Stent malfunction (intraluminal debris, stones, blood, tumor ingrowth)
- Stent occlusion (perform a new PBD, recanalize, or replace the stent)
- Cholangitis (tx w/abx)
- Duct occlusion → cholecystitis, pancreatitis

CHOLANGIOGRAM AT THE LEVEL OF THE **CBD** DEMONSTRATED BILIARY DILATATION WITH EXTRINSIC COMPRESSION OF THE COMMON HEPATIC DUCT BY A MASS

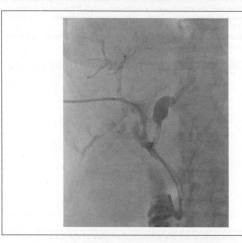

INTERNAL/EXTERNAL BILIARY DRAIN CONVERSION TO "Y"
BILIARY STENT CONFIGURATION

Fluoroscopically Guided Conversion of Internal–External Biliary Drains for Bilateral Internal Biliary Stents "Y-Configuration" Resulting in Internal Biliary Decompression

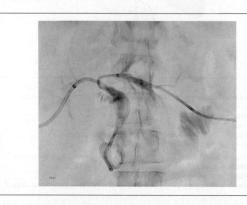

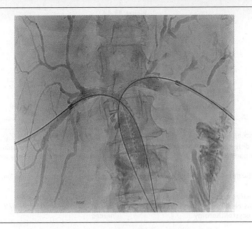

PERCUTANEOUS CHOLECYSTOSTOMY

BACKGROUND (Archives of Surgery 1999;134(7):727–32; HPB (Oxford) 2009;11(3):183–93; N Engl J Med 1994;330:403–8; Am J Surg 1983;146:719–22; AJR Am J Roentgenol 1997;168:1247–51)

- **Procedure:** Percutaneous catheter placement in the gallbladder lumen under imaging guidance for the treatment of acute cholecystitis
- **Diagnostic criteria of acute cholecystitis:** Clinical signs and symptoms, leukocytosis, and at least 1 ultrasonographic criteria including gallbladder stones/sludge, ultrasonographic Murphy sign, gallbladder wall thickening > 3 mm, pericholecystic fluid collection, and/or gallbladder distension
- Cholecystectomy is the definitive treatment for patients with acute cholecystitis and carries only a 0.8% risk of mortality for in low-risk cases and 18% in high-risk cases (Kandarpa K. Handbook of Interventional Radiologic Procedures. Lippincott Williams & Wilkins; 2011; Kessel D, Robertson I. Interventional Radiology: A Survival Guide. Elsevier; 2016)
- Percutaneous cholecystostomy (PC) is the treatment of choice for high-risk cases (calculus or acalculous cholecystitis)
- PC is used to decompress the gallbladder for managing cholecystitis definitively or as a temporizing measure until interval cholecystectomy is performed
- Acalculous cholecystitis → PC can be curative, cholecystectomy may not be needed

Indications (Kandarpa K. Handbook of Interventional Radiologic Procedures. Lippincott Williams & Wilkins; 2011; Kessel D, Robertson I. Interventional Radiology: A Survival Guide. Elsevier; 2016; Kaufman J, Lee M. Vascular and Interventional Radiology: The Requisites. Elsevier; 2016; Archiv Surg 1999;134(7):727–32)

- Cholecystitis in a patient who is critically ill/poor surgical candidate
- Unexplained sepsis in an ICU patient, other sources have been excluded (ICU patients → acalculous cholecystitis is a frequent and often underdiagnosed cause of sepsis)
- Access to the biliary tree after failed PBD
- Dissolution/removal of stones
- Divert bile from bile duct defect

Contraindications (Kandarpa K. Handbook of Interventional Radiologic Procedures. Lippincott Williams & Wilkins; 2011; Kessel D, Robertson I. Interventional Radiology: A Survival Guide. Elsevier; 2016; Kaufman J, Lee M. Vascular and Interventional Radiology: The Requisites. Elsevier; 2016; Archiv Surg 1999;134(7):727–32)

- **Absolute:** None
- **Relative:** Coagulopathy or antiplatelet/anticoagulant medication, ascites, gallbladder malignancy w/potential seeding

Preprocedure Evaluation (AJR Am J Roentgenol 1997;168:1247–51; J Vasc Interv Radiol 2010;21(6): 789–95; Hepatogastroenterology 2010;57(97):12–7; Hepatogastroenterology 2010;57(97):12–7)

- Informed consent
- Repeat the ultrasound imaging to confirm the anatomy and plan the approach
- Transhepatic or transperitoneal approach to percutaneous cholecystostomy (Figure 13-14)

Figure 13-14

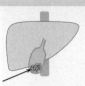

Transperitoneal

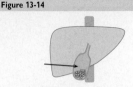

Transhepatic

Transhepatic	Transperitoneal
Bleeding can be tamponaded by the liver parenchyma	Technically more difficult → gallbladder more mobile near the fundus, may make it difficult to puncture
Gallbladder less mobile, closer to bare area	Transverse colon can overlie the fundus of the gallbladder
Increased risk of hemorrhage if large tracks required for percutaneous cholecystolithotomy	Large tracts can be dilated for percutaneous cholecystolithotomy if needed

Technique (Kandarpa K. *Handbook of Interventional Radiologic Procedures.* Lippincott Williams & Wilkins, 2011)
1. Perform sterile skin preparation—drape the patient and ultrasound transducer
2. Inject lidocaine into the skin and along the trajectory of the proposed tract to the liver or gallbladder
3. Puncture the gallbladder under ultrasound guidance
   - **Seldinger technique:** Perform tract dilatation and catheter placement under fluoroscopy
   - If the tract is going directly through the peritoneal cavity into a distended gallbladder, consider using a 6F or 8F catheter → no dilatation over wire, eliminate bile spill into peritoneum
   - Direct gallbladder entry can also be made with a "single exchange" technique by puncturing with a 5F sheathed needle, guidewire placed, then catheter
   - If dilatating or exchanging catheters, remove 10–20 mL of bile after original puncture to decrease intracholecystic pressure and minimize bile spill
4. **Fluoroscopy** → inject 3–5 mL of contrast through the first needle to enter the gallbladder → rough outline of the gallbladder to confirm that the needle is in the gallbladder lumen, not necrotic and leaking
5. Avoid diagnostic injections to prevent potential leaks and sepsis
6. Insert the wire, coil the wire 3 or 4 times in the gallbladder lumen
7. If necessary, dilate carefully. Be careful not to push the gallbladder away.
8. Insert an 8–10F locking pigtail catheter over the wire with the metal stiffener inside until the gallbladder lumen is reached, slowly pushing the catheter off the metal stiffener and wire thereafter
9. Secure the catheter to the skin
10. Send bile sample for Gram stain and culture
11. Do a limited low-volume contrast injection to confirm tube position, as warranted. If the procedure has been done at the bedside, a portable radiograph is recommended
12. Leave the catheter to gravity drainage, not bulb suction (increased chance of side hole catheter occlusion if suction is used)

Complications (*AJR Am J Roentgenol* 1997;168:1247–51; *J Vasc Interv Radiol* 2010;21(6):789–95; *Hepatogastroenterology* 2010;57(97):12–7; *Hepatogastroenterology* 2010;57(97):12–7)
- Bile leak with peritonitis → Drain any fluid collections outside the gallbladder, reestablish gallbladder access if lost
- Hemorrhage within gallbladder → due to rapid decompression, drain to gravity
- Bleeding from the transhepatic tract
- Sepsis
- Catheter dislodgement
- Vasovagal reaction

Postprocedure Management (Kaufman J, Lee M. *Vascular and Interventional Radiology: The Requisites.* Elsevier; 2016)
- Most patients improve within 72 h
- Irrigate the catheter 2–3×/d as warranted to decrease catheter occlusion

- Catheters must stay in place for a minimum of 2–4 wk before removal → mature track develops between the gallbladder and skin surface
- Premature removal → bile contamination of the peritoneal cavity
- Prior to removal, perform cholecystocholangiogram to confirm patency of the cystic duct and to exclude the presence of gallstones in the cystic duct, gallbladder, or bile duct
- If stones are present in the gallbladder, patient may need cholecystectomy or percutaneous cholecystolithotomy (if poor surgical candidate)
- Obstructive stone in the cystic duct → catheter should not be removed until the stone is either surgically or percutaneously removed
- Lastly, if there is a stone in the common bile duct, the patient will require ERCP and stone removal, or the stone can be removed percutaneously
- Technique for cholecystocholangiogram:
  - Remove the catheter over the guidewire. Use a Kumpe catheter or a 5F dilator over the guidewire into the opening of the percutaneous track
  - Inject contrast into the percutaneous track
  - Mature tract → contrast material will outline the track all the way to the gallbladder
  - Immature tract → contrast material will spill into the peritoneal cavity. Reinsert the catheter over the guidewire into the gallbladder
- Perform procedure at weekly intervals until the track is mature

ADDITIONAL RESOURCES

1. Behrens G, Ferral H. Transjugular liver biopsy. *Semin Interv Radiol* 2012;29(02). Thieme Medical Publishers.
2. Timothy C, Jeffrey MC, Jason S, et al. Optimizing needle direction during transjugular liver biopsy provides superior biopsy specimens. *Cardiovasc Intervent Radiol* 2014;37(6):1540–5.
3. Echenagusia M, Rodriguez-Rosales G, Simo G, et al. Expanded PTFE-covered stent-grafts in the treatment of transjugular intrahepatic portosystemic shunt (TIPS) stenoses and occlusions. *Abdom Imaging* 2005;30(6):750–4.
4. Inal M, Akgul E, Aksungur E, et al. Percutaneous placement of biliary metallic stents in patients with malignant hilar obstruction: Unilobar versus bilobar drainage. *J Vasc Interv Radiol* 2003;14(11):1409–16.
5. Johnson D, Kaplan J, Jensen A, et al. Adequacy of transjugular liver biopsy compared with percutaneous liver biopsy for staging fibrosis. *J Vasc Interv Radiol* 2017; 28(2):S205.
6. Kaassis M, Boyer J, Dumas R, et al. Plastic or metal stents for malignant stricture of the common bile duct? Results of a randomized prospective study. *Gastrointest Endoscopy* 2003;57(2):178–82.
7. Kim T, Yang H, Lee CK, et al. Vascular plug assisted retrograde transvenous obliteration (PARTO) for gastric varix bleeding patients in the emergent clinical setting. *Yonsei Med J* 2016;57(4):973–9.
8. Kiyosue H, Mori H, Matsumoto S, et al. Transcatheter obliteration of gastric varices: Part 2. Strategy and techniques based on hemodynamic features. *RadioGraphics* 2003;23:921–37.
9. Krokidis M, Orgera G, Rossi M, et al. Interventional radiology in the management of benign biliary stenoses, biliary leaks and fistulas: a pictorial review. *Insights Imaging* 2013;4(1):77–84.
10. Lammer J, Hausegger KA, Fluckiger F, et al. Common bile duct obstruction due to malignancy: treatment with plastic versus metal stents. *Radiology* 1996; 201(1):167–72.
11. Lee SJ, Kim MD, Lee MS, et al. Comparison of the efficacy of covered versus uncovered metallic stents in treating inoperable malignant common bile duct obstruction: a randomized trial. *J Vasc Interv Radiol* 2014;25(12):1912–20.
12. McNaughton DA, Abu-Yousef MM. Doppler US of the liver made simple *Radiographics* 2011;31(1):161–88.
13. Tsetis D, Krokidis M, Negru D, et al. Malignant biliary obstruction: the current role of interventional radiology. *Ann Gastroenterol* 2016;29(1):33–6.

GASTROINTESTINAL INTERVENTIONS

Background

- Interventional radiology is instrumental in the treatment of common gastrointestinal pathologies utilizing both intravascular and percutaneous methods.
- These methods often decrease morbidity and postprocedure recovery compared to surgical approaches.
- Intervention should be performed when appropriate after multidisciplinary consultation including gastroenterology and surgery, with complete discussion of treatment options, risks, and benefits of the procedure and goals of care.
- Most gastrointestinal procedures are considered "high risk" for bleeding—Recent INR (<1.5) and platelet (>50,000/µL) serology is required to reduce intraprocedure and postprocedure hemorrhage.
- Some gastrointestinal procedures may require antibiotic prophylaxis and will be listed as such in each of the following subsections.
- Interventions requiring arterial access are frequently performed from a common femoral arterial puncture.
- Preprocedure imaging of the gastrointestinal system should be performed to plan the approach and to identify variant anatomy.
  - CT—Best to evaluate the vascular and intestinal anatomy and surrounding structures. Both oral and intravascular contrast can be helpful to evaluate pathology/anatomy and may be necessary in the workup of common interventional procedures involving the gastrointestinal system. Specific indications will be discussed in this chapter.
  - Ultrasound—Infrequently utilized for evaluation of the alimentary tract due to artifact from bowel gas.
  - MR—More time consuming and expensive. Preprocedural MR is infrequently necessary for gastrointestinal intervention.

NONVASCULAR ESOPHAGEAL INTERVENTIONS

Background

- While gastroenterology/endoscopy services manage most esophageal diseases, some esophageal pathology is within the scope of interventional radiology.
- Fluoroscopic-guided intervention is a reasonable alternative when upper endoscopy is unavailable or when the patient is a high-risk surgical candidate.
- Interventional radiology may be consulted in the treatment of esophageal strictures, esophageal varices, and foreign-body removal.

Esophageal Strictures (*Image-Guided Interventions E-Book Expert Radiology Series.* Elsevier Health Sciences; 2013; *J Vasc Interv Radiol* 2006;17:831–5; *Abrams' Angiography: Interventional Radiology.* LWW; 2013; *Am J Gastroenterol* 2008;103:570–4)

- Etiology
  - Benign strictures
    - Fibrotic changes secondary to esophagitis, exposure to gastric acid or medications (NSAIDs), congenital and acquired esophageal motility disorders (achalasia) or after treatment of congenital anatomic abnormalities (esophageal atresia, tracheoesophageal fistula)
  - Malignant strictures
    - Primary squamous cell carcinoma and adenocarcinoma of the esophagus
- Patient Presentation:
  - Dysphagia (most common symptom), weight loss, regurgitation, aspiration, chest pain, and abdominal pain
- Initial Evaluation:
  - History and physical examination
  - Esophagram may be performed to determine the site and severity of the stricture
    - A water-soluble contrast agent should be used if there is any suspicion of perforation
  - If a malignant stricture is suspected, upper endoscopy and biopsy should be performed before image-guided intervention
  - CT, PET-CT, and endoscopic ultrasound can be obtained for staging of malignancy

Workup for Esophageal Balloon Dilation and Stent Placement (Image-Guided Interventions E-Book Expert Radiology Series. Elsevier Health Sciences; 2013; J Vasc Interv Radiol 2006;17:831–5; Abrams' Angiography: Interventional Radiology. LWW; 2013; Am J Gastroenterol 2008;103:570–4; Am J Roentgenol 2009;193:W278–82)

- Balloon dilation of the esophagus can be performed via both endoscopic and fluoroscopic guidance; coordination of care should be discussed with the gastroenterologist
- Indications:
  - To relieve symptoms of dysphagia from benign esophageal stricture
  - To palliate nonoperable malignant esophageal disease resulting in intrinsic obstruction, extrinsic compression, tracheoesophageal fistula, and perforation
  - To cover an anastomotic leak from prior surgery
  - To facilitate PO intake to nourish patients before undergoing surgical intervention or chemoradiation
- Contraindications:
  - Balloon dilation before stent placement should not be performed in the setting of known fistulas or perforation, which may worsen the area of weakness
  - A recent history of radiation therapy may increase the risk of hemorrhage and perforation
  - Existing tracheal compression from an esophageal mass may be aggravated by stent placement
- If the decision is made to proceed with intervention, all oral intake should be stopped the day prior to the procedure
- Blood work including complete blood count and coagulation studies must be obtained
- Previously obtained imaging, including esophagram and chest CT, should be reviewed prior to intervention

Balloon Dilation and Stent Placement Technique (J Vasc Interv Radiol 2006;17:831–5; Abrams' Angiography: Interventional Radiology. LWW; 2013; Am J Gastroenterol 2008;103:570–4; Am J Roentgenol 2009;193:W278–82; RadioGraphics 2003;23:89–105; Handbook of interventional radiologic procedures. Lippincott Williams & Wilkins; 2011; J Vasc Interv Radiol 2005;16:1705–9; J Vasc Interv Radiol 2001;12:283–97)

- The patient is placed on the fluoroscopy table in the left lateral decubitus position
- An esophagram is performed using water-soluble or iso-osmolar contrast to confirm the location and extent of the stricture
  - Contrast should be used carefully to prevent aspiration and the associated risks of pulmonary edema
- Anatomic landmarks are identified, such as vertebral body level, to recall the area of stricture
  - The patient's skin can be marked to identify the area of stricture
- Lidocaine spray can be used to anesthetize the pharynx before catheterization and conscious sedation is administered
- A 0.035-in Bentson guidewire or a stiff Amplatz wire (180 or 260 cm in length) is advanced from the oral cavity through the esophagus and gastroesophageal junction to the stomach or duodenum
- Wire advancement can be more easily achieved with the guidance of a 5F or 6F angiographic catheter or a sizing catheter that allow for simultaneous injection of contrast and measurement of stricture length
- Wire and catheter should be seen coiling within the stomach for secure access
- Once access is achieved, the sizing catheter can be exchanged for a balloon catheter over the stiff wire, which is advanced to the level of stenosis
  - A variety of balloon catheters exist that can be used for esophageal dilation
  - Balloon size for esophageal dilation ranges from 15–20 mm
  - Balloon diameter and length should be selected based on severity and length of the stricture
  - Start with a smaller diameter balloon and increase with subsequent dilations. Maximum balloon diameter should be the same as the normal adjacent esophageal lumen
- Balloon Inflation:
  - The balloon should be centered at the area of stricture that is predetermined with the contrast esophagram
  - Inflation should occur under continuous fluoroscopy so that the balloon can be readjusted if migration occurs
  - Resolution of the stenotic waist represents successful dilation
  - Repeat dilations can be performed until the waist is eliminated
  - The balloon should remain inflated for approximately one minute per dilation

- If blood is identified on the balloon between dilations or if the patient is experiencing pain despite sedation efforts, the procedure should be terminated
- Stent Selection and Deployment:
  - Plastic stents are less often utilized due to more frequently report postprocedure complications compared to metallic stents
  - Self-expanding metallic stents (more common) and balloon expandable stents can be placed
  - Both covered (for malignant stricture) and uncovered (for benign stricture) metallic stents can be utilized depending on the indication
    - Covered stents are less susceptible to tumor ingrowth
    - Uncovered stents are less prone to migration
  - Balloon dilation to 10–15 mm before stent placement can facilitate easier positioning and deployment
  - Positioning before deployment should ensure that more of the stent is placed above the area of stricture or tumor to reduce the chances of migration
  - The stent should cover at least 2 cm of normal esophagus both above and below the site of the stricture
  - Stent diameter should be selected based on maximum lumen possible for passage of food
  - Long strictures may require multiple overlapping stents. If more than one stent is required, the overlap length should be at least 1/3 of the entire stent length

Balloon Dilation and Stent Placement Technical Notes *(Abrams' Angiography: Interventional Radiology. LWW; 2013; Handbook of interventional radiologic procedures. Lippincott Williams & Wilkins; 2011)*

- Stents should not be placed across the upper esophageal sphincter, which may result in patient discomfort and aspiration
  - Typical anatomic landmark for the upper esophageal sphincter is the C5–C6 vertebral level
- Use of atropine may be helpful in decreasing vagal tone and controlling secretions
- Temporary retrievable stents can be placed before radiation therapy for malignant strictures to reduce complications that occur with placement of permanent stents
- Dilation for benign strictures can be repeated intermittently (for example, weekly) for optimal result
- If the inciting agent is known (such as caustic ingestion), dilation should be performed at least three weeks after initial injury. If dilation is performed sooner, there is an increased risk of perforation
- Stent placement for benign strictures is less likely to be successful compared to malignant strictures due to tissue hyperplasia and progressive restenosis
- Stent retrieval can be performed if complications occur or if the stent was placed only for a temporary purpose
  - Retrievable stents are equipped with drawstrings that can engage by a hooked catheter for removal

Complications of Balloon Dilation and Stent Placement *(RadioGraphics 2003;23: 89–105; Handbook of Interventional Radiologic Procedures. Lippincott Williams & Wilkins; 2011; Am J Roentgenol 1997;169:1281–4; Am J Roentgenol 2012;198:453–9)*

- Complications of esophageal intervention include stent migration, perforation, aspiration, hemorrhage, pain, the sensation of foreign-body ingestion, tumor ingrowth/outgrowth, gastric reflux, fistula formation, sepsis secondary to mediastinitis, pressure necrosis, and mucosal ulceration
- If the stent has migrated into the stomach, it can be left alone as long as the patient remains asymptomatic. Retrieval may be necessary in the setting of pain or obstruction

Postprocedure Care *(Image-Guided Interventions E-Book Expert Radiology Series. Elsevier Health Sciences; 2013; J Vasc Interv Radiol 2006; RadioGraphics 2003;23:89–105)*

- Postprocedure esophagram should be performed to document patency and accurate stent placement both immediately after the procedure with water-soluble contrast and then 24 h after the procedure
- Outpatient treatment should include at least 4 h of postprocedure observation prior to discharge. Alternatively, inpatient observation for the 1st 24 h after the procedure can be considered on a case-by-case basis
- Oral food intake can be gradually initiated after the follow-up esophagram is performed and demonstrates appropriate passage across stricture/through stent
- Patients should be instructed to chew solid food extensively before swallowing to minimize the chances of obstruction

- Carbonated beverages have been described to help maintain stent patency and can be recommended to the patient
- If the stent extends beyond the distal esophageal sphincter, the patient can be counseled to sleep in a semiupright position to minimize gastric reflux
- Proton pump inhibitors should be used in patients who develop reflux after stent placement
- Outpatient follow-up should be frequent and routine to evaluate for recurrent dysphagia
- If dysphagia recurs, repeat esophagram should be performed to look for defects along the stent that suggest tumor ingrowth, luminal narrowing, delayed emptying of the stent, new fistula formation, or migration

Esophageal Varices (Handbook of Interventional Radiologic Procedures. Lippincott Williams & Wilkins; 2011)
- Treatment of esophageal varices also falls within the scope of the gastroenterologist including medical management, endoscopic sclerotherapy, or ligation
- The role of interventional radiology in the treatment of esophageal varices is further discussed in the Hepatobiliary Interventions Chapter:
  - Transjugular intrahepatic portosystemic shunt (TIPS) to decrease portal pressures and to reduce variceal flow
  - Transcatheter embolization/sclerosis of varices

Fluoroscopic-Guided Esophageal Foreign-Body Removal (Image-Guided Interventions E-Book Expert Radiology Series. Elsevier Health Sciences; 2013; J Vasc Interv Radiol 1998;9:95–103)
- The gastroenterology team most often performs foreign-body retrieval within the esophagus via rigid endoscopy
- If rigid endoscopy is unavailable, balloon catheter extraction with fluoroscopic guidance is an option
  - The foreign body is either pushed retrograde into the oropharynx or anterograde into the stomach if the object is safe to pass
  - Contraindications to fluoroscopic retrieval include esophageal edema with airway compression, perforation, and pneumomediastinum
  - In addition to previously mentioned complications related to esophageal interventions, foreign-body retrieval could lead to respiratory compromise from displacement of the object from the esophagus into the airway

---

NONVASCULAR LOWER INTESTINAL INTERVENTION

Background
- While gastroenterology/endoscopy services manage most intraluminal interventions, some procedures are within the scope of interventional radiology
- Fluoroscopy-guided intervention is a reasonable alternative when endoscopy is unavailable
- Interventional radiology may be consulted in the treatment of colorectal strictures and colonic fistulas

Colorectal Strictures
- Etiology of lower intestinal strictures:
  - Inflammatory bowel disease, ischemia, diverticulitis/infection, malignancy, and scarring from postsurgical anastomosis
- Both endoscopic and fluoroscopic-guided stent placement techniques have been described for treatment of colorectal strictures (J Vasc Interv Radiol 2010;21:1244–9)
- Indications for intervention (J Vasc Interv Radiol 2003;14:P272–P6):
  - Stricture resulting in acute large bowel obstruction, which is a medical and surgical emergency
  - Temporary stenting can be performed as a bridge to surgical resection or for palliative purposes
    - Allows time for proper presurgical medical management and tumor staging (in cases of malignant stricture)
    - Presurgical stent placement and decompression may decrease need for colostomy compared to primary emergent surgery in the treatment of malignant strictures (Dis Colon Rectum 2002;45:401–6)
- Contraindications for Intervention (Am J Gastroenterol 2008;103:570–4):
  - Bowel perforation resulting in peritonitis
  - Long-segment strictures, multiple strictures, or proximal strictures within the ascending colon or small bowel should not be attempted for stenting
  - Extension of malignant stricture with tumor involving the anal sphincter

- Preprocedure Work-up (*Handbook of Interventional Radiologic Procedures.* Lippincott Williams & Wilkins; 2011; *J Vasc Interv Radiol* 2003;14:P272–6):
  - Physical exam with evaluation for appropriateness of conscious sedation
  - Digital rectal examination prior to catheterization to evaluate for anal/low rectal invasion of tumor
  - Colonoscopy or barium enema to identify the location of stricture
  - Abdominal radiography and CT may be performed for evaluation of obstruction
  - Cleansing enema to clear stool
  - CBC, coagulation panel with correction of coagulopathy prior to intervention
  - IV hydration and nasogastric tube placement for bowel decompression in the setting of acute large bowel obstruction
- Fluoroscopy-guided stent placement technique (*Handbook of Interventional Radiologic Procedures.* Lippincott Williams & Wilkins; 2011; *J Vasc Interv Radiol* 2003;14:P272–6):
  - Patient positioning on the fluoroscopy table is based on operator preference but most often lateral decubitus
  - The angiographic catheter (6F) and guidewire (0.035 in) are placed through the anus beyond the level of the stricture with fluoroscopic guidance
  - Water-soluble contrast can be injected through the catheter to demonstrate the level and length of stricture
  - The guidewire is exchanged for a stiff 0.035-in wire such as an Amplatz
  - An uncovered or covered metallic expandable stent is then passed over the wire and deployed across the area of the stricture
    - Length of stent is dependent on the length of obstruction
      - Should extend 3–6 cm beyond the stricture on each side
    - Typically 20 or 24 mm in diameter
  - Contrast is again injected after stent deployment to evaluate patency and to check for perforation
- Postprocedural complications (*Gut Liver Gut Liver* 2010;4(Suppl 1):S9,S9–18):
  - Stent migration most common complication, including rectal expulsion
  - Stent obstruction usually due to tumor ingrowth/overgrowth or fecal impaction
  - Bowel perforation, sepsis, pain, and rectal hemorrhage (less common)
  - Unlike esophageal stenting, balloon dilation before colonic stent placement is typically not performed due to a risk of perforation
- Postprocedure Management (*Image-Guided Interventions E-Book Expert Radiology Series.* Elsevier Health Sciences; 2013; *Clin Endosc* 2014;47:415–19):
  - Serial physical examinations and abdominal radiographs should be performed every 24 h to document decompression
  - If there is clinical concern for repeat obstruction, water-soluble contrast enema can be repeated to document patency
  - Low residue diet is recommended to minimize chance of impaction
  - While the majority of patients demonstrate improvement of obstructive symptoms, some patients continue to be symptomatic either because of incomplete stent expansion or unrecognized more proximal strictures

Colonic Fistulas
- Similar to the treatment of colonic strictures, covered stents can be placed fluoroscopically to obstruct fistulous tracts (*Image-Guided Interventions E-Book Expert Radiology Series.* Elsevier Health Sciences; 2013; *Handbook of Interventional Radiologic Procedures.* Lippincott Williams & Wilkins; 2011)

UPPER GASTROINTESTINAL HEMORRHAGE

Background
- Upper gastrointestinal (GI) hemorrhage originates proximal to the Ligament of Treitz and is more common than lower GI bleeding (*Image-Guided Interventions E-Book Expert Radiology Series.* Elsevier Health Sciences; 2013)
- Causes include direct bleeding into the lumen (gastroduodenal ulcer, Mallory–Weiss tear, gastritis/duodenitis, vascular malformations, hemorrhagic tumor), transpapillary (hemobilia, transpancreatic duct) and variceal bleeding (*Image-Guided Interventions E-Book Expert Radiology Series.* Elsevier Health Sciences; 2013; *Baillieres Clin Gastroenterol* 1995;9:53–69; *Am J Roentgenol* 2015;205:753–63; *J Vasc Interv Radiol* 2009;20:461–6)
  - The following discussion will focus on nonvariceal upper GI bleeding. See Hepatobiliary Interventions for discussion of variceal hemorrhage.

- Patients present with hematemesis and/or melena (acute); hematochezia (massive acute upper GI bleed); chronic iron deficiency anemia (chronic) *(Image-Guided Interventions E-Book Expert Radiology Series. Elsevier Health Sciences; 2013; Bailieres Clin Gastroenterol 1995;9:53–69; Am J Roentgenol 2015;205:753–63; Gastrointest Endosc 2012;75:1132–8)*
- Majority of cases stop bleeding spontaneously (80%) and the minority recur (20–30%) *(J Vasc Interv Radiol 2009;20:461–6; Ann Intern Med 2003;139:843–57)*

Relevant Anatomy *(Semin Interv Radiol 2009;26:167–74)*
- The celiac axis originates from the abdominal aorta (level of the T12 vertebral body) and supplies the gastroesophageal junction to the distal duodenum
- Celiac artery (CA) branches include left gastric, splenic, and common hepatic arteries to supply the lesser curvature of the stomach, spleen, and liver, respectively
- The common hepatic artery gives off the gastroduodenal artery (GDA), which courses between the pancreas and the duodenum
- After the GDA take off, the common hepatic artery becomes the proper hepatic artery that divides into the right and left hepatic arteries
- The GDA gives rise to the superior pancreaticoduodenal arteries supplying the pancreatic head and duodenum through anastomoses with the inferior pancreaticoduodenal arteries that originate from the super mesenteric artery (SMA)
- The terminal branch of the GDA is the right gastroepiploic artery that supplies the greater curvature of the stomach and eventually anastomosis with the left gastroepiploic artery that arises from the splenic artery
- Pancreaticoduodenal arcade connects the GDA (and therefore the celiac axis) to the inferior pancreaticoduodenal artery and SMA *(Cardiovasc Intervent Radiol 2017; 40:465–9)*
- Extensive ring circulation exists between the right/left gastric, short gastric, right/left gastroepiploic arteries, and the pancreaticoduodenal arcades *(Image-Guided Interventions E-Book Expert Radiology Series. Elsevier Health Sciences; 2013; Bailieres Clin Gastroenterol 1995;9:53–69; Semin Interv Radiol 2009;26:167–74)*
- Common variant anatomy includes *(Image-Guided Interventions E-Book Expert Radiology Series. Elsevier Health Sciences)*:
  - Replaced or accessory right hepatic artery from the SMA
  - Replaced or accessory left hepatic artery from the left gastric artery
  - Left gastric, hepatic, or splenic arteries arising directly from the aorta
  - Common celiac and mesenteric trunk
  - Dorsal pancreatic or inferior phrenic arteries arising from the celiac trunk
  - GDA arising from the right or left hepatic artery
  - Arc of Buehler (vertically oriented arterial anastomosis between the celiac artery and SMA)

Initial Evaluation *(Gastrointest Endosc 2012;75:1132–8)*
- Assessment of hemodynamic stability and need for resuscitation with crystalloid IV fluids and need for blood transfusion
- Consider nasogastric tube placement and proton pump inhibitor therapy
- Emergent upper endoscopy is 1st line in unstable severe upper GI hemorrhage allowing for fast diagnosis and treatment
- Upper endoscopy is recommended within 24 h in hemodynamically stable patients Colonoscopy should be performed if upper endoscopy is negative to look for a lower GI source *(Handbook of Interventional Radiologic Procedures. Lippincott Williams & Wilkins; 2011)*
- Alternative diagnostic tests can be performed if upper/lower endoscopy is nondiagnostic in a hemodynamically stable patient including capsule endoscopy, radionuclide imaging (sensitivity 0.1–0.2 mL bleeding/min), CTA (0.3–0.5 mL/min), and catheter angiography (sensitivity 0.5–1.0 mL/min).

Indications for Catheter Directed Angiography (CDA) and Intervention
- Continued bleeding documented by radionuclide imaging (tagged RBC scan) or CTA indicates that CDA will likely be successful at diagnosis and treatment. Since the sensitivity of angiography is less than these noninvasive examinations (see above), if noninvasive imaging is negative, angiography will also likely be nondiagnostic and is usually not indicated *(Handbook of Interventional Radiologic Procedures. Lippincott Williams & Wilkins; 2011)*
- CDA should be considered if 1st-line endoscopy is negative, nondiagnostic (limited visualization due to continuous bleeding), or if initial endoscopic treatment fails, resulting in recurrent hemorrhage *(Bailieres Clin Gastroenterol 1995;9:53–69)*

Celiac Trunk Arterial Anatomy

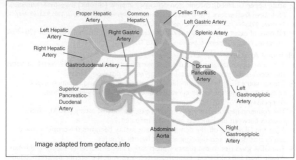

Image adapted from geoface.info

Celiac Trunk Arterial Anatomy

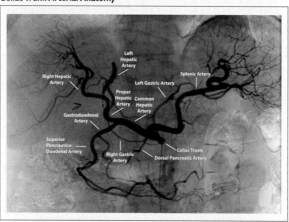

- CDA should be considered in appropriate patients with upper GI bleed prior to surgical intervention
- Angiography should be performed as soon as possible after/during hemorrhage to increase the likelihood of documenting active extravasation *(Image-Guided Interventions E-Book Expert Radiology Series. Elsevier Health Sciences; 2011; Baillieres Clin Gastroenterol 1995;9:53–69)*

Contraindications for Catheter Directed Angiography (CDA) and Intervention

- Absolute contraindications: None in the setting of emergency
- Relative contraindications: History of extensive upper GI surgery or radiation therapy, severe visceral atherosclerosis (increased risk of infarction), in addition to general risks of angiography (contrast allergy, renal failure, uncorrectable coagulopathy, etc.) *(Image-Guided Interventions E-Book Expert Radiology Series. Elsevier Health Sciences; 2011; Handbook of interventional radiologic procedures. Lippincott Williams & Wilkins; 2011)*
- Cardiovascular risk factors must be considered when intra-arterial vasopressor infusion is used for treatment of hemorrhage *(Baillieres Clin Gastroenterol 1995;9:53–69)*

Preprocedure Workup

- Thorough patient history and physical exam may help provide diagnostic information to identify the source of bleeding *(Handbook of Interventional Radiologic Procedures. Lippincott Williams & Wilkins; 2011)*

- Assess hemodynamic stability—Hemorrhagic shock (systolic BP <100 mmHg and HR >100) and hemoglobin/hematocrit drop that is nonresponsive to repeat transfusions are indicators of active bleeding (*Image-Guided Interventions E-Book Expert Radiology Series.* Elsevier Health Sciences; 2013). Hemodynamic stability suggesting absence of active bleeding can result in negative/nondiagnostic angiography (*Image-Guided Interventions E-Book Expert Radiology Series.* Elsevier Health Sciences; 2011; *Handbook of Interventional Radiologic Procedures.* Lippincott Williams & Wilkins; 2011; *Baillieres Clin Gastroenterol* 1995;9:53–69).
- Resuscitation efforts should not delay intravascular diagnosis and treatment and can be continued in the angiography suite
- Localization of hemorrhage with CTA before angiography has been advocated to provide anatomical information, decrease procedural time, contrast volume, and overall patient/operative exposure to radiation (*Radiol Bras* 2015;48:381–90; *Egypt. J Radiol Nucl Med* 2016;47:161–8)
- Evaluate coagulopathy; if possible, correct before the procedure

Procedural Technique

- Intra-arterial access is usually obtained via common femoral, brachial, or radial artery catheterization (*Baillieres Clin Gastroenterol* 1995;9:53–69). A sheath, typically 5F, must be used to maintain access.
- Primary visceral branch selection is dependent on the clinical suspicion of the most likely site of hemorrhage based on history, physical exam, and pre-angiography diagnostic testing (*Handbook of Interventional Radiologic Procedures.* Lippincott Williams & Wilkins; 2011; *J Vasc Interv Radiol* 2009;20:461–6)
- For suspected upper GI bleeds the CA and SMA are the most likely culprits and should be studied 1st
- From common femoral artery access, guidewire and catheter are advanced into the abdominal aorta superior to the expected location of the CA ostium above of the level of the T12 vertebral body
- The curve of the catheter is then manipulated to point anteriorly and the catheter is slowly pulled caudally until the catheter tip engages the celiac axis or SMA
- After a small volume test injection of contrast confirms successful CA or SMA catheterization, higher-volume diagnostic arteriography is performed (rate of 5–6 mL/s for 4–5 s) (*Radiology* 2010;255:278–88; *Abrams' Angiography: Interventional Radiology.* LWW; 2013)
- If contrast extravasation cannot be identified by injection of the main CA and SMA trunks, sequential subselective catheterization should be performed until the location of hemorrhage is identified
  - Even once the site of bleeding is located, angiographic documentation of all possible feeding arteries must be completed to avoid missing additional sites of hemorrhage (*World J Gastroenterol WJG* 2012;18:1191–201).
  - Imaging should be carried out into the venous phase with each contrast injection
- A variety of 5F, 0.038-in catheters can be used to access the celiac axis/SMA depending on operator preference and branch vessel anatomy as determined on preprocedure CTA; commonly used visceral artery selecting catheters include Cobra, reverse curve Sos, and Simmons-shaped catheters
- Once the site of active hemorrhage is identified, subselection into smaller vessels may be necessary to minimize nontarget embolization
- Subselection into vessels smaller than the gastroduodenal artery is achieved with a 3F microcatheter/0.018-in microwire coaxial system passed through the 4F or 5F catheter and sheath (*Radiology* 2010;255:278–88; *World J Gastroenterol WJG* 2012;18:1191–201; *J Vasc Interv Radiol* 2013;24:422–31).
- Before embolization, stable catheter position should be documented via test injection of contrast (*Image-Guided Interventions E-Book Expert Radiology Series.* Elsevier Health Sciences; 2011)
- Choice of embolization agent used is dependent on the pathology being treated, catheter position and operator preference (see below) (*Image-Guided Interventions E-Book Expert Radiology Series.* Elsevier Health Sciences; 2011)
- Embolization coils, pushable or detachable, are the most commonly used embolic agent in the setting of GI bleed
- Standard 0.035-in metallic embolization coils are deployed through a 4F to 5F catheter and can be used for larger selected arteries. Smaller microcoils are deployed through appropriately sized microcatheters (*Baillieres Clin Gastroenterol* 1995;9:53–69)

- When a patient is volume depleted, coils may be slightly oversized to avoid recanalization after the intravascular volume has been restored (*Image-Guided Interventions E-Book Expert Radiology Series*. Elsevier Health Sciences; 2011)
- Polyvinyl alcohol (PVA) particles ranging from 300–500 μm or N-Butyl-2-Cyanoacrylate (NBCA) glue can be used when hemorrhage originates from small vessels that cannot be subselectively catheterized (*J Vasc Interv Radiol* 2013;24:422–31)
- Nonradiopaque particles should be mixed with contrast (50%) and injected under continuous fluoroscopy to minimize reflux of particles into nontarget vessels (*Image-Guided Interventions E-Book Expert Radiology Series*. Elsevier Health Sciences; 2011)
- Use of particulate embolic material in the treatment of GI bleed can increase the risk of infarction
- Temporary occlusion can be achieved with gelatin sponge material (Gelfoam); however, also results in more distal arterial occlusion and increases the risk of ischemia
- Ethanol should be avoided as it may migrate to the capillaries and result in tissue necrosis (*Image-Guided Interventions E-Book Expert Radiology Series*. Elsevier Health Sciences; 2011)
- Postembolization angiography should then be performed to document hemostasis and collateral vasculature to the site of bleeding
- Access closure after catheter and sheath removal can be achieved by manual compression or use of a closure device
- Intraprocedural monitoring of blood pressure, electrocardiography, pulse oximetry, capnography, and body temperature is essential in hemorrhaging patients (*Handbook of Interventional Radiologic Procedures*. Lippincott Williams & Wilkins; 2011; *J Vasc Interv Radiol* 2009;20:461–6)

Identifying Site of Hemorrhage
- Contrast extravasation into the bowel lumen is the only direct angiographic sign of hemorrhage
- Indirect signs that suggest the location of bleeding include vessel irregularity or spasm, the presence of true or false aneurysms, shunting, and neovascularity (*Image-Guided Interventions E-Book Expert Radiology Series*. Elsevier Health Sciences; 2011)
- If endoscopy precedes endovascular intervention, the endoscopist can place several metallic clips at the site of bleeding as a target for embolization

Selection of Embolic Agent
- **Diffuse bleeding (gastritis, duodenitis):** When multiple vessels are likely contributing to hemorrhage consider use of a Gelfoam slurry or PVA particles
  - Blood flow will carry Gelfoam and PVA particles to more downstream arterial branches and result in distal embolization to the perfused vascular territory
  - Use of larger PVA particles can decrease chances of ischemia and necrosis
  - Local infusion of vasopressin (0.1–0.4 units/min), a vasoconstricting agent, can be considered as an alternative treatment. However, vasopressin has become less favorable due to frequent rebleeding after the infusion is stopped and cardiovascular complications (*Image-Guided Interventions E-Book Expert Radiology Series*. Elsevier Health Sciences; 2011; *Baillieres Clin Gastroenterol* 1995;9:53–69; *J Vasc Interv Radiol* 2003;14:535–43)
- **Gastroduodenal artery hemorrhage or single large eroded artery (peptic ulcer):** Use coils to embolize both distal (to avoid reconstitution of flow from collaterals beyond the site of bleeding) and proximal to the site of hemorrhage
- **Hemobilia:** The bleeding vessel should be embolized both distally and proximally to the source of arterial bleeding, most often with coils
- **Coagulopathy:** NBCA glue can be considered in irreversible coagulopathy since this material does not rely on thrombus formation like coils and PVA particles (*J Vasc Interv Radiol* 2013;24:422–31)
- **True visceral aneurysms:** Can be treated with coiling of aneurysm sac, stent graft exclusion, stent-assisted sac coiling, or with distal and proximal coils if the involved vessel can be safely sacrificed
- Hemorrhagic complications of pancreatitis will be discussed in the Pancreatic Interventions section of this chapter

Technical Notes
- If the site of bleeding has already been documented by endoscopy, active hemorrhage does not need to be documented during angiography and embolization of the

target vessel can be performed if there is adequate collateral circulation to prevent ischemia
- If there is active bleeding, the bleeding point must be occluded both proximally and distally
- Collateral supply to the point of bleeding may be revealed after embolization and therefore postembolization angiography is necessary for documentation of successful hemostasis and for evaluation of any residual bleeding from collaterals (Image-Guided Interventions E-Book Expert Radiology Series. Elsevier Health Sciences; 2011)
- Antiperistaltic agents (glucagon or hyoscine butylbromide) can be used during the procedure to minimize artifact from bowel motion (Image-Guided Interventions E-Book Expert Radiology Series. Elsevier Health Sciences; 2011)

Provocative Angiography for Occult Gastrointestinal Hemorrhage (Cardiovasc Intervent Radiol 2006;30:1042–6; J Vasc Interv Radiol 2001;30:477–83)

- Provocative angiography (PA) can be employed in situations when noninvasive imaging, endoscopy, and conventional angiography fail to localize the site of hemorrhage
- PA entails the incremental addition of locally administered intra-arterial medication to promote hemorrhage; success rate ranges from 29–80% (Cardiovasc Intervent Radiol 2007;30:1042–6)
- Commonly used pharmacologic agents including anticoagulants (both systemic and intra-arterial heparin), vasodilators (intra-arterial nitroglycerine, verapamil, papaverine), and thrombolytics (intra-arterial tPA)
- Once the site of hemorrhage is identified, routine embolization can be performed
- Although rare, the most severe complication of PA is massive uncontrollable hemorrhage and care must be taken to procure blood products prior to the procedure, in addition to frequent intraprocedural patient monitoring. Use of vasopressin and heparin reversal agents may be necessary in the setting of uncontrolled bleeding after PA.

Complications

- General complications of angiography (contrast allergy, worsening of renal failure, puncture site hematoma or hemorrhage, vessel dissection and rupture, etc.) (J Vasc Interv Radiol 2006;17:831–5; J Vasc Interv Radiol 2010;21:283–97)
- Critical ischemia of the stomach and duodenum is a rare complication of embolization due to rich collateral vasculature within the celiac axis; however, ischemia may result in strictures, ulcerations and necrosis (World J Gastroenterol WJG 2012;18:1191–201)
  - Ischemic complications are increased in patients with limited collateral vasculature from prior surgery/radiation or advanced atherosclerotic disease
  - Surgical resection may be required in the setting of bowel infarction
  - Chronic ischemia-related bowel strictures might be amendable to balloon dilation therapies that are typically performed endoscopically
- Nontarget embolization occurs when embolic material passes into vasculature that is unintended for occlusion
  - Most commonly, nontarget embolization results from excessive pressure when injecting particles or from dislodgement of the catheter from the intended vessel during embolic deployment
  - Removal of the embolic material with suction or retrieval with a snare may be considered if a critical organ is affected
- Coil erosion through vessels or bowel wall, a rare complication, can result in massive recurrent hemorrhage

Postprocedural Care

- Patient follow-up is instrumental for early detection and repeat treatment of recurrent hemorrhage and management of postprocedure complications
- Risk of rebleeding is variable based on patient anatomy, location of hemorrhage, and viability of vascular collaterals
- Frequent monitoring of vital signs and postprocedural hemoglobin/hematocrit for documentation of stability and evaluation of recurrent hemorrhage
- Postprocedure immobility of the extremity distal to the puncture site (with femoral access), neurovascular checks, and frequent inspection of the puncture site for hematoma formation should be compulsory (Handbook of Interventional Radiologic Procedures. Lippincott Williams & Wilkins; 2011)
- Consistent tracking of nasogastric tube and bloody stool output

LOWER INTESTINAL HEMORRHAGE

Background
- Lower-intestinal hemorrhage originates distal to the Ligament of Treitz and is less common than upper GI bleeds (20% of all cases of intestinal hemorrhage) (*Image-Guided Interventions E-Book Expert Radiology Series. Elsevier Health Sciences; 2013; Gastroenterol Clin North Am 2005;34:643–64; Gastrointest Endosc 1999;49:228–38*)
- Etiology includes diverticular disease (most common, up to 55% of cases), vascular disease (angiodysplasia, AVM, ischemia, radiation-induced), inflammatory disease (infectious or inflammatory bowel disease), and neoplasia (*World J Gastroenterol WJG 2012;18:1191–201; Gastrointest Endosc 1999;49:228–38*)
- Hematochezia (passage of fresh blood per rectum) is the most common presentation and likely indicative of colonic or rectal hemorrhage (*Gastrointest Endosc 1999; 49:228–38*)
- Majority of cases, like upper GI hemorrhage, resolve spontaneously (*Image-Guided Interventions E-Book Expert Radiology Series. Elsevier Health Sciences; 2013; Gastroenterol Clin North Am 2005;34:643–64; Gastrointest Endosc 1999;49:228–38*)

Relevant Anatomy (*Semin Interv Radiol 2009;26:167–74*)
- The superior mesenteric artery (SMA) originates from the abdominal aorta (level of the L1–2 vertebral body) and supplies the distal duodenum to the distal transverse colon via the inferior pancreaticoduodenal, intestinal, ileocolic, right colic, and middle colic arteries
- The inferior mesenteric artery (IMA) originates from the abdominal aorta (L3–4 vertebral body level) and supplies the distal transverse colon to the distal rectum via the left colic and superior rectal arteries
- Distal branches of the IMA supply the upper rectum as the superior rectal or hemorrhoidal artery
- The lower rectum is supplied by middle and inferior rectal branches arising from the anterior division of the internal iliac arteries
- Common variant anatomy includes (*Image-Guided Interventions E-Book Expert Radiology Series. Elsevier Health Sciences; 2013*)
  - Middle colic artery arising from the dorsal pancreatic branch of the celiac artery. This variant can be identified by an absence in the perfusion territories of the SMA and IMA in the region of the distal transverse colon.
  - Arc of Buhler connecting the celiac trunk and the SMA
  - SMA and IMA communication through the marginal artery of Drummond and the Arc of Riolan
  - Collateral vascular supply to the IMA may arise from middle hemorrhoidal branches originating from the internal iliac arteries

Initial Evaluation (*Am J Gastroenterol 2016;111:459–74*)
- Assessment of hemodynamic stability and need for emergent resuscitation including IV fluids, blood transfusion, and correction of coagulopathy if applicable
- Initial evaluation should also include risk stratification for the appropriate level of care
- Colonoscopy is 1st line in the majority of cases of lower intestinal hemorrhage and should be performed in all hemodynamically stable symptomatic patients
- If the patient is hemodynamically unstable, surgical or interventional radiology consultation should be obtained after resuscitation is started
- High suspicion for upper GI hemorrhage in patients who present with hematochezia and hemodynamic instability should prompt a low threshold for nasogastric lavage and upper endoscopy
- CTA and tagged RBC scan can be obtained as noninvasive diagnostic tests if there is uncertainty whether there is active bleeding and the patient remains hemodynamically stable

Indication for Catheter-Directed Angiography (CDA) and Intervention
(*Am J Gastroenterol 2016;111:459–74*)
- Hemodynamically unstable patients with ongoing hemorrhage who cannot tolerate adequate bowel preparation or colonoscopy should be considered for diagnostic and therapeutic angiography (*Baillieres Clin Gastroenterol 1995;9:53–69*)
- Active hemorrhage is required for positive angiographic diagnosis in acute intestinal hemorrhage

Mesenteric Arterial Anatomy

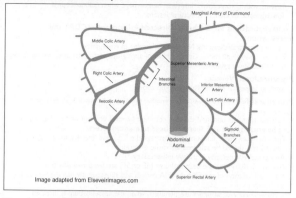

Mesenteric Arterial Anatomy

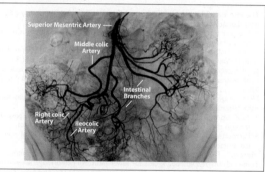

Mesenteric Arterial Anatomy

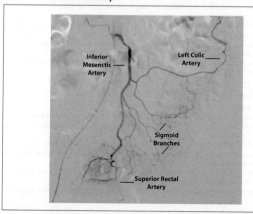

- Although most often beneficial in the acute setting, angiography can be helpful in patients with chronic lower intestinal hemorrhage when colonoscopy is nondiagnostic to identify structural lesions

Contraindications for Catheter-Directed Angiography (CDA) and Intervention
- Absolute contraindications: None in the setting of emergency
- Relative contraindications: General risks of angiography (contrast allergy, renal failure, uncorrectable coagulopathy, etc.)

Preprocedural Workup
- Same as upper GI hemorrhage workup above

Procedural Technique (Image-Guided Interventions E-Book Expert Radiology Series. Elsevier Health Sciences; 2013)
- Vascular access is obtained through common femoral, brachial, or radial artery catheterization and a 5F sheath is placed to maintain access
- For suspected lower intestinal hemorrhage the SMA and IMA are the most likely culprits and should be selected for catheterization
- Abdominal aortography is usually unnecessary
- Guidewire (0.035 in) and base catheter (4F or 5F) are fed proximally to the expected location of the SMA or IMA ostium and subsequently manipulated to point anteriorly
  - Reverse curved catheters are beneficial when the vessel ostium is directed caudally, while less curved catheters are beneficial when the ostium is directed at a right angle
- The wire and catheter are then slowly pulled caudally under fluoroscopy guidance until the catheter tip is lodged within the SMA and IMA ostium
  - Catheter tip should be advanced far enough into the vessel to prevent recoil back into the aorta
- Contrast injection should be performed to document successful SMA or IMA catheterization (rate of 5–6 mL/s for 4–5 s for the SMA and a rate of 3 mL/s for 4–5 seconds for the IMA) (Image-Guided Interventions E-Book Expert Radiology Series. Elsevier Health Sciences; 2013; Handbook of interventional radiologic procedures. Lippincott Williams & Wilkins; 2011)
- Hemorrhagic vessels are most likely in the periphery and will require subselective catheterization
  - Achieved with a 3F microcatheter/0.018-in microwire coaxial system passed through the 5F catheter and sheath (World J Gastroenterol WJG 2012;18:1191–201)
  - Microcatheter should be advanced as close as possible to the point of contrast extravasation to prevent embolization of a large segment of bowel
- Microcoils, PVA particles (300–500 microns), and NBCA glue are the most commonly utilized embolic agents for lower intestinal hemorrhage (Image-Guided Interventions E-Book Expert Radiology Series. Elsevier Health Sciences; 2013; J Vasc Interv Radiol 2013;24: 422–31)
- PVA particles and NBCA glue should be suspended in contrast material before injection for visualization
- Deployment of embolic material should be performed at or beyond the marginal artery but proximal to the terminal intramural arcades
- Postembolization angiography should be obtained to document hemostasis and collateral vasculature
- Access closure after catheter and sheath removal can be achieved with manual compression or use of a closure device

Identifying Site of Hemorrhage
- Refer to upper GI hemorrhage "Identifying Site of Hemorrhage" above

Technical Notes
- If prior imaging is available, the 1st targeted vessel should be selected based on the most likely suspected location of hemorrhage (World J Gastroenterol WJG 2012;18:1191–201)
- If the location of bleeding is suspected to be originating from the IMA or if the location is unknown, the IMA should be studied first to avoid overlap between the vascular and the urinary bladder as it fills with excreted contrast
- Imaging of the aorta is usually unnecessary but may be helpful if the ostium to the SMA and IMA is difficult to locate and cannulate
- Oblique projections may need to be obtained to identify the site of hemorrhage

Provocative Angiography for Occult Gastrointestinal Hemorrhage
- Refer to upper GI hemorrhage "Provocative Angiography for Occult Gastrointestinal Hemorrhage" above

Complications
- General complications of angiography (contrast allergy, worsening of renal failure, puncture site hematoma or hemorrhage, vessel dissection and rupture, etc.) (*Image-Guided Interventions E-Book Expert Radiology Series. Elsevier Health Sciences; 2013; Handbook of Interventional Radiologic Procedures. Lippincott Williams & Wilkins; 2011*)
- Bowel ischemia and infarction is the most severe complication related to embolization resulting in stricture, ulceration, necrosis, and bowel perforation (*J Vasc Interv Radiol 2014;25:10–9*)
  - Ischemic complications have been reported with a rate of 0–25% with minor changes, such as abdominal pain and asymptomatic mucosal changes, occurring more frequently than major complications such as infarction and stricture. Recent studies report rates in the lower end of this range (*Handbook of Interventional Radiologic Procedures. Lippincott Williams & Wilkins; 2011; J Vasc Interv Radiol 2014;25:10–19; J Vasc Interv Radiol 2001;12:1399–405; J Vasc Interv Radiol 2003;14:1503–9*)
- Complications related to lower intestinal embolization are more likely compared to the treatment of upper GI hemorrhage due to relatively fewer collateral vessels
- Recurrent bleeding after embolization has been reported with rates from 8.8–26% occurring more frequently in the small bowel compared to the colon (*Handbook of Interventional Radiologic Procedures. Lippincott Williams & Wilkins; 2011; J Vasc Interv Radiol 2014;25:10–9*)

Postprocedural Care
- Immediate postprocedure care of lower intestinal hemorrhage is similar to care for upper GI bleed including frequent monitoring of vital signs, stool output, serum hemoglobin, and hematocrit to evaluate the need for repeat intervention or blood transfusion
- Once cessation of hemorrhage is achieved, colonoscopy should be performed on a nonemergent basis to define the pathology and to evaluate the bowel for postembolization ischemic changes
- Hemorrhage from angiodysplasia and AVM is unlikely to resolve with intra-arterial treatment with a high rate of rebleeding. Surgical resection is the definitive treatment for these lesions (*Baillieres Clin Gastroenterol 1995;9:53–69*).

MESENTERIC ISCHEMIA

Acute Mesenteric Ischemia and Chromic Mesenteric Ischemia

Background
- Acute mesenteric ischemia (AMI) is a life-threatening emergency (*Image-Guided Interventions E-Book Expert Radiology Series. Elsevier Health Sciences; 2013*)
  - More common in elderly patients >50 y of age with multiple comorbidities
  - High mortality rates (52–93%) depending on etiology and time from symptom onset to treatment (*Handbook of Interventional Radiologic Procedures. Lippincott Williams & Wilkins; 2011; Radiol Oncol 2013;47:239–43*)
  - Etiology:
    - Arterial Embolus (most common cause)—Frequently in the setting of cardiac dysfunction such as arrhythmia, cardiomyopathy, recent myocardial infarction, or arterial intervention
    - Acute Arterial Thrombosis—Typically in setting of severe chronic atherosclerotic disease
    - Venous Thrombosis—Hypercoagulable state, dehydration, oral contraceptives, cirrhosis/portal hypertension, abdominal infection, pancreatitis, malignancy, trauma. Intestinal edema of the bowel wall leads to decreased arterial flow and tissue necrosis
    - Nonobstructive Mesenteric Ischemia (NOMI)—Bowel hypoperfusion due to vasoconstriction or vasospasm in the setting of severe illness (ARDS, cardiac shock, sepsis). NOMI can also result from substances that cause vasoconstriction such as cocaine, vasopressors, digitalis, and ergot
    - Aortic dissection—Extension of dissection into the mesenteric arteries
  - Patient Presentation: Rapid onset severe abdominal pain out of proportion to physical examination, fever, nausea, vomiting, diarrhea, and bloody stool
    - Peritoneal signs indicate progression from ischemia to infarction (*Handbook of Interventional Radiologic Procedures. Lippincott Williams & Wilkins; 2011*)

- Chronic Mesenteric Ischemia (CMI) (*J Vasc Interv Radiol* 2014;25:1515–22)
  - More common in elderly patients >50 y of age with multiple comorbidities
  - Etiology:
    - Severe atherosclerosis resulting in high-grade arterial stenosis or occlusion
      - SMA is most commonly involved in symptomatic patients
      - Celiac artery and IMA are less likely to be involved due to collateralization
      - Usually asymptomatic unless there is multivessel disease
    - Fibromuscular dysplasia, vasculitis, and median arcuate ligament syndrome are less common etiologies of CMI
  - Patient Presentation: Intermittent postprandial abdominal pain, weight loss, malabsorption, "fear of food"
  - CMI can progress to AMI if symptoms go undiagnosed and untreated

Relevant Anatomy
- See above for mesenteric anatomy

Indications for Endovascular Intervention (*Image-Guided Interventions E-Book Expert Radiology Series*. Elsevier Health Sciences; 2013; *J Vasc Surg* 2009;50(2):341–8.e1)
- AMI:
  - Surgery remains the standard of care for AMI in the setting of lactic acidosis and peritoneal signs (bowel infarction)
  - Endovascular treatment has become a more common alternative in patients who are poor surgical candidates and do not have signs of bowel infarction
  - Benefits of Endovascular Intervention:
    - Lower morbidity and mortality
    - Use of conscious sedation rather than general anesthesia
    - Avoidance of open surgery in high-risk patients
    - More targeted therapy without the need for bowel resection
- CMI:
  - Not all cases of severe mesenteric atherosclerotic disease require endovascular treatment or surgery
  - Revascularization should be considered in symptomatic patients and should be strongly considered in asymptomatic cases of chronic triple vessel mesenteric arterial occlusive disease (celiac, SMA, and IMA)
  - Mesenteric revascularization in asymptomatic chronic single vessel disease that is identified incidentally on CTA/MRA is controversial
- Endovascular therapy can act as a bridge or adjunct to definitive surgery in both cases of acute and chronic mesenteric ischemia and can be done sequentially in hybrid operating/endovascular suites

Contraindications to Intervention (*Handbook of Interventional Radiologic Procedures*. Lippincott Williams & Wilkins; 2011)
- No absolute contraindications to intervention in cases of acute mesenteric ischemia
- Relative contraindications include those general to angiography (contrast allergy, renal failure, uncorrectable coagulopathy, etc.)
- Symptomatic compression of the celiac artery by the median arcuate ligament is treated surgically and not with stent placement (stents can migrate and fracture at this location)
- Risk of distal embolization should be strongly considered in patients with severe atherosclerotic plaque, in which case surgical bypass may be of greater benefit than endovascular treatment
- Locally infused papaverine, an intra-arterial vasodilator that is frequently used for treatment, is contraindicated in complete heart block
- Absolute and relative contraindications to thrombolysis in other organ systems also apply to treatment of AMI including, but not limited to, active hemorrhage, trauma, recent surgery or CVA

Initial Evaluation (*Image-Guided Interventions E-Book Expert Radiology Series*. Elsevier Health Sciences; 2013; *Handbook of Interventional Radiologic Procedures*. Lippincott Williams & Wilkins; 2011; *World J Gastroenterol WJG* 2006;12:3243–7)
- History of Presenting Illness—Including onset, timing (postprandial vs. constant), duration, and nature of the abdominal pain
- Physical Examination—Evaluation for tenderness and peritoneal signs of guarding and rigidity
- Laboratory Evaluation—Evaluate lactic acid level, leukocytosis, fecal occult blood positive
- Imaging Evaluation:

- Angiography—Gold standard for diagnosis
- CTA—Most commonly utilized for rapid diagnosis due to direct demonstration of thrombosis, intramural or portal venous gas, or lack of bowel wall enhancement
- Abdominal radiograph—Nonspecific dilated loops of bowel (ileus)
- Ultrasound—Limited for evaluation of the mesenteric vessels distally but Doppler can detect stenosis or occlusion within the proximal vessels

Preprocedure Management (Image-Guided Interventions E-Book Expert Radiology Series. Elsevier Health Sciences; 2013; Handbook of Interventional Radiologic Procedures. Lippincott Williams & Wilkins; 2011)

- AMI:
  - Fluid resuscitation (mean arterial pressure >65), pain control, systemic heparinization if embolic or thrombotic disease is suspected, broad-spectrum IV antibiotics, no oral intake and possible need for nasogastric suction
- CMI:
  - Aspirin (81 or 325 mg PO) or clopidogrel (300 mg PO) the day of/before the procedure
- Continued monitoring of vital signs and fluid status
- Serial abdominal physical examination for development of peritoneal signs

Procedural Technique (Image-Guided Interventions E-Book Expert Radiology Series. Elsevier Health Sciences; 2013; Handbook of Interventional Radiologic Procedures. Lippincott Williams & Wilkins; 2011; J Vasc Interv Radiol 2002;13:P149–54)

- If the decision is made for the patient to undergo endovascular therapy, it must be initiated as soon as possible after presentation of symptoms to treat reversible ischemia before progression to bowel infarction
- Mesenteric angiography is performed with conscious sedation and appropriate intraprocedural cardiopulmonary monitoring
- Access can be obtained through the radial or brachial artery for ease of cannulation of the caudally oriented origin of the SMA. If femoral access is preferred, a reverse curved catheter/sheath can be used for cannulation
- Catheterization occurs through a vascular sheath with a 4F or 5F base catheter over a 0.35-in hydrophilic guidewire

Diagnostic Angiography (Handbook of Interventional Radiologic Procedures. Lippincott Williams & Wilkins; 2011; J Vasc Interv Radiol 2002;13:P149–54)

- AP and lateral projections with a pigtail catheter placed in the aorta are obtained to document origin of the mesenteric arteries, patency, and overall perfusion of the bowel
- Imaging should be carried out into the venous phase to document the mesenteric veins, especially if there is concern for venous thrombosis
- Celiac artery, SMA and IMA can then be subselected based on the area of concern
- Imaging Findings:
  - Arterial embolus/thrombus—SMA is most commonly involved with identification of an intraluminal filling defect and lack of flow distal to the origin. Most often clot is lodged at the middle colic artery bifurcation
  - NOMI—Vasospasm resulting in segmental or diffuse narrowing
  - Venous thrombus—Intraluminal filling defect in a mesenteric vein with evidence of venous congestion, prolonged mucosal opacification, and resulting arterial spasm

Therapeutic Intervention (Handbook of Interventional Radiologic Procedures. Lippincott Williams & Wilkins; 2011; J Vasc Interv Radiol 2002;13:P149–54)

- Endovascular Infusion of Vasodilators (Abrams' Angiography: Interventional Radiology. LWW; 2013; Handbook of Interventional Radiologic Procedures. Lippincott Williams & Wilkins; 2011)
  - Treatment for diffuse vasospasms
  - May be initiated by IR as an adjunct before emergent open surgery
  - Intra-arterial papaverine is the most commonly used vasodilator
  - A 45–60 mg bolus of papaverine is administered into the SMA followed by continuous infusion that is adjusted (30–60 mg/h) for at least 24 h based on the response
  - Catheter is flushed after 24 h of infusion with normal saline for 30 min
  - Diagnostic angiography is repeated to evaluate response
  - Catheter can be removed if vasospasm and symptoms resolve
  - Cycle is repeated every 24 h for a maximum of 5 d if vasospasms persist
- Endovascular Infusion of Thrombolytics (Handbook of Interventional Radiologic Procedures. Lippincott Williams & Wilkins; 2011; J Vasc Interv Radiol 2005;16:317–29)
  - Treatment for embolic and thrombotic disease
  - Tissue plasminogen activator (tPA) is the most common agent used

- Catheter is positioned intra-arterially upstream of or within the clot
- Bolus dose (20 mg) can be administered directly into the embolus/thrombus
- Alternatively, tPA can be given as an infusion with a rate of 1 mg/h
- Angiography should be frequently repeated (every 4–8 h) to reassess patency
- Anticoagulation with intra-arterial heparin and continuous IV heparin infusion is administered simultaneously throughout catheter-directed thrombolysis
- Surgery should be performed if symptoms persist after 4 h despite treatment or if the patient develops peritoneal signs suggestion of infarction
- Catheter-Directed Mechanical Thrombectomy/Aspiration Thrombectomy (Radiol Oncol 2013;47:239–43; Vasc Endovascular Surg 2017;51:91–4)
  - Treatment for embolic disease
  - Removal of clot without the need for local thrombolysis or surgery
  - Mechanical thrombectomy devices disrupt clot and facilitate aspiration through the catheter
- Angioplasty and Stenting (Image-Guided Interventions E-Book Expert Radiology Series. Elsevier Health Sciences; 2013; J Vasc Interv Radiol 2014;25:1515–22)
  - Treatment of atherosclerotic and thrombotic disease, less frequently embolic disease
  - Pressure transducers can be used to measure a trans-stenotic/lesional gradient to determine the potential benefit of angioplasty (significant gradient = >20 mmHg or 10% difference)
  - Balloon expandable or self-expanding stents can maintain clot between the stent and the vessel wall to prevent distal embolization

SMV and Portal Vein Thrombosis (Abrams' Angiography: Interventional Radiology. LWW; 2013)
- Initial treatment of SMV thrombosis involves medical management of the precipitating factors (anticoagulation, correcting fluid status, treating infection, etc)
- If medical management fails, thrombolysis or mechanical thrombectomy can be performed through transhepatic or transjugular access

Acute Mesenteric Ischemia due to Aortic Dissection
- Treatment is directed toward increasing perfusion to the mesenteric vascular bed(s). Surgical and endovascular techniques can be considered.

Complications (Image-Guided Interventions E-Book Expert Radiology Series. Elsevier Health Sciences; 2013; Abrams' Angiography: Interventional Radiology. LWW; 2013)
- General complications of angiography (contrast allergy, worsening of renal failure, puncture site hematoma or hemorrhage, vessel dissection and rupture, etc.)
- Hypotension with infusion of vasodilators especially if the catheter is dislodged from the SMA into the aorta
- Distal embolization after thrombolysis or angioplasty resulting in AMI
  - Look for delay in forward flow of contrast despite positive result after recanalization
  - Distal embolization can be treated with subsequent thrombolysis
- Reperfusion Injury
  - Ischemia–reperfusion facilitates formation of reactive oxygen species resulting in inflammation and tissue injury
  - Symptoms can include those of systemic inflammatory response or acute respiratory distress syndrome
  - Allopurinol (xanthine oxidase inhibitor) has shown to decrease intestinal cell injury and the severity of reperfusion damage (J Pediatr Surg 1992;27:968–73; J Vis Exp 2016;111. doi: 10.3791/53881.)

Postprocedure Care (Image-Guided Interventions E-Book Expert Radiology Series. Elsevier Health Sciences; 2013; Handbook of Interventional Radiologic Procedures. Lippincott Williams & Wilkins; 2011)
- Admission to the intensive care unit for cases of AMI
- Continuous monitoring of vitals, laboratory results (lactic acid, fibrinogen levels) and sequential abdominal physical examination
- Continued fluid resuscitation and therapeutic anticoagulation with IV heparin or an appropriate alternative
- IV antibiotics (especially in cases of venous ischemia leading to edema and mucosal barrier disruption) should be administered
  - Piperacillin/tazobactam (Zosyn) 3.375 g IV q6h
  - Alternatively, metronidazole and levofloxacin
- No oral intake or clear liquid diet for at least 12 h after intervention

- Follow-up Imaging:
  - Follow-up CTA should be performed 1 mo after the procedure even in asymptomatic patients
  - 6-mo follow-up CTA should also be performed after mesenteric stent placement to evaluate for early restenosis
    - Consider repeat intervention if there is >70% restenosis
- If a stent is placed, continue aspirin 81 mg or 325 mg daily for life and clopidogrel 75 mg for at least 30 d after treatment
- Medical management of comorbidities and risk factor modification for mesenteric ischemia (lipid lower medication, blood pressure control, glucose management)

PANCREATIC INTERVENTION

Background
- The role of interventional radiology primarily involves treatment of complications from pancreatitis, pancreatic cancer, and pancreatic transplantation
- Similar to other gastrointestinal procedures, close collaboration with gastroenterology and surgery should be maintained to establish goals of care and appropriate management

Complications of Pancreatitis (Image-Guided Interventions E-Book Expert Radiology Series. Elsevier Health Sciences; 2013; Pol Przegl Chir 2015;87:485–90; RadioGraphics 2005;25:S191–211)
- **Pseudoaneurysm**
  - Etiology:
    - A focal weakening of the arterial wall due to inflammatory erosion from surrounding proteolytic pancreatic enzymes
    - Splenic artery is most commonly involved
      - Gastroduodenal, pancreaticoduodenal, dorsal pancreatic, gastric and hepatic arteries are less frequently involved
    - Pseudoaneurysm rupture can occur within a pseudocyst, into the peritoneum, into the bowel (upper GI bleed) or the pancreatic duct (hemosuccus pancreaticus)
      - Overall mortality of 37% (J Vasc Interv Radiol 2007;18:591–96)
  - Patient Presentation: Abdominal pain, hypovolemic shock, hemodynamic instability. May be discovered incidentally on diagnostic imaging in asymptomatic patients.
  - Indication for Intervention:
    - Pseudoaneurysms (equivalent to a contained hemorrhage) must be treated in the setting of pancreatitis regardless of size
    - Transcatheter embolization is 1st-line treatment (lower morbidity and mortality compared to open surgery)
  - Contraindications:
    - No absolute contraindications in the case of emergency
    - Standard relative contraindications to angiography.
  - Endovascular Treatment Options:
    - Embolization
    - Stent graft placement
    - Percutaneous thrombin injection
  - Embolization Procedural Technique (RadioGraphics 2013;33:E71–96):
    - Femoral or radial arterial access is secured with a vascular sheath
    - A base catheter (4F or 5F) is positioned at the celiac artery and angiography is performed to determine the location of the pseudoaneurysm
    - Microcatheter/microwire system is used to cannulate the pseudoaneurysmal vessel
    - Detachable and pushable microcoils are deployed to occlude normal segments of the artery 1st distal and then proximal to the neck of the aneurysmal sac
    - Postembolization angiography should demonstrate vascular stasis, with no further filling of the pseudoaneurysm or contrast extravasation
  - Stent Graft Placement (Image-Guided Interventions E-Book Expert Radiology Series. Elsevier Health Sciences; 2013):
    - Covered stent placement to exclude the pseudoaneurysm while preserving flow through the involved vessel

- Less commonly performed compared to embolization
- Usually only placed in large caliber vessels (splenic, hepatic, SMA) where complete embolization might result in clinically significant downstream ischemia
- Difficult to manipulate larger catheters required for stent placement in smaller visceral arteries
- Care should be taken to avoid covering vital nonaneurysmal vessels
- Percutaneous Thrombin Procedural Technique (*Handbook of Interventional Radiologic Procedures. Lippincott Williams & Wilkins; 2011; RadioGraphics 2013;33:E71–96*):
  - Can be performed if embolization is unsuccessful due to inability to cannulate the celiac artery
  - Performed under ultrasound or contrast-enhanced CT guidance
  - Percutaneous access is obtained via a 22G needle with the tip positioned directly into the pseudoaneurysm lumen
  - Thrombin is injected serially in small volumes until thrombosis is achieved. Eg, 100 units (0.1 mL of a 1000:1 dilution in saline) are delivered slowly for a total of 500–4,000 IU
  - No linear relationship between the size of pseudoaneurysm and dose to achieve occlusion (*RadioGraphics 2013;33:E71–96*)
- Complications (*Image-Guided Interventions E-Book Expert Radiology Series. Elsevier Health Sciences; 2013*)
  - Rebleeding
  - Splenic infarction/atrophy after splenic artery embolization
  - Microcoil or stent migration
  - Clinical postembolization syndrome is a rare complication due to extensive vascular collateralization of involved arteries around the pancreas
- Special Notes (*Handbook of Interventional Radiologic Procedures. Lippincott Williams & Wilkins; 2011*):
  - Filling only the sac with coils rather than distal and proximal embolization may cause expansion of the pseudoaneurysm and rupture
  - With embolization, complete occlusion distally should be ensured before proximal coiling because direct access to that vessel is compromised/eliminated after embolization
- Postprocedure Care:
  - Routine post angiography care
  - Follow up cross-sectional imaging (CTA or MRA) is obtained 1 mo after the procedure to document pseudoaneurysm thrombosis and to evaluate for distal organ infarction
- **Venous Complications of Pancreatitis**
  - Portal vein thrombosis
  - Splenic vein thrombosis
  - SMV thrombosis (for management of Portal Vein and SMV Thrombosis see Mesenteric Ischemia section)
- **Percutaneous Drainage of a Pseudocyst** (*World J Gastroenterol 2008;14:4841–3; J Vasc Interv Radiol 2002;13:P106–8*)
  - Etiology:
    - Well-circumscribed collection containing proinflammatory pancreatic fluid and a fibrous pseudocapsule
    - May be associated with a pseudoaneurysm
    - May be superinfected or hemorrhagic even without an associated pseudoaneurysm
  - Treatment Options:
    - Percutaneous drainage catheter placement (Interventional Radiology)— Preferred for an infected pseudocyst with an immature wall
    - Endoscopic drainage or cystogastrostomy tube placement (Gastroenterology)— Preferred for a chronic pseudocyst with a mature wall
    - Surgical removal (Surgery)—Reserved for complicated cases of pancreatitis with evidence of necrosis
  - Percutaneous Drainage Catheter Placement:
    - Indication for Intervention:
      - Pseudocysts >6 cm in diameter that persist over 6 w or in symptomatic patients (abdominal pain, obstruction)
    - Contraindications for Intervention:
      - Standard contraindications to percutaneous drainage catheter placement
    - Procedural Technique:
      - See technique for percutaneous drainage catheter placement described in Body Interventions chapter

- Safe catheter placement includes avoiding injury to surrounding structures such as colon or peripancreatic blood vessels
- Common Approaches: Via the anterior abdominal wall for drainage of pseudocysts located at the pancreatic head and body. Through left flank and anterior pararenal space for pseudocysts located at the pancreatic tail.
  - Complications:
    - Risk of pseudocyst recurrence after catheter removal
    - Catheter obstruction due to thick, viscous pseudocyst contents resulting in inadequate drainage
    - Pancreatic-percutaneous fistula formation
- **Percutaneous Treatment of Pancreatic Duct Strictures** (*J Vasc Interv Radiol* 2001;12:104–10)
  - An infrequent option for failed endoscopic treatment in the setting of proximal pancreatic duct stricture
  - Procedural techniques include percutaneous access into the pancreatic duct, dilation, and drainage catheter placement. Due to the rarity of the procedure, discussion of these techniques is beyond the scope of this guide

Complications of Pancreatic Cancer

- Biliary obstruction is the most common complication of a pancreatic head mass
- If pancreatic cancer is suspected and imaging is nondiagnostic, percutaneous needle aspiration for cytological and microbiological evaluation can be performed

Vascular Complications of Pancreatic Transplantation (*Abrams' Angiography: Interventional Radiology*, LWW; 2013)

- Vascular complications of pancreatic transplantation, like any solid organ transplant, include thrombosis, anastomotic stenosis, and pseudoaneurysm formation
- The pancreatic allograft is usually placed in the pelvis
  - The most common surgical technique results in anastomosis of the transplanted pancreas to the recipient iliac vasculature ("Y-graft" procedure)
- Patient Presentation:
  - Worsening or new insulin dependence, pancreatitis
  - Gastrointestinal or intra-abdominal hemorrhage in the setting of ruptured pseudoaneurysm
- Diagnostic Imaging Workup:
  - Contrast-enhanced MRA or CTA
  - Limited role of ultrasound due to overlying bowel gas, variable surgical anatomy, and concomitant complexity of imaging in patients with pancreatitis
- Endovascular Treatment:
  - Infrequently performed and reported due to the rarity of pancreatic transplantation and associated complications
  - Similar techniques to other locations in the body/solid organ transplantation:
    - Arterial stenosis → balloon angioplasty and stent placement
    - Arterial thrombosis → thrombolysis
    - Active hemorrhage → embolization
- Postprocedural Care and Followup:
  - Dependent on the type of intervention performed

GASTROINTESTINAL FEEDING INTERVENTION

Fluoroscopic-Guided Nasogastric/Nasojejunal Tube Placement

Background (*Gastroenterology* 2011;141:742–65)
- Depending on indication, tube placement locations include nasogastric, nasoduodenal, or nasojejunal
  - If for feeding placement, nasojejunal tubes have less risk of aspiration due to less gastric residuals
- Can be placed by three primary methods:
  - Blind placement bedside with subsequent KUB to confirm position
  - Fluoroscopic placement
  - Endoscopic placement

Clinical and Preprocedural Workup (*J Vasc Interv Radiol* 2012;23:727–36; *Essential Clinical Procedures: Expert Consult*, Elsevier Health Sciences; 2013)
- Classified as low risk bleeding procedures. Anticoagulant and antiplatelet therapy typically can be continued.

- Clinical history is important to assess for contraindications prior to placement, as listed below

Indications (*Interventional Critical Care: A Manual for Advanced Care Practitioners.* Springer; 2016)
- Therapeutic
  - Short-term feeding in patients who are malnourished or at risk for aspiration (neurologic conditions, unconscious/vented or sedated)
  - Medication delivery
  - Gastric decompression (removing water, blood, ingested substances, or air)
- Diagnostic
  - Evaluate for upper gastrointestinal bleeding
  - Administer enteric contrast

Contraindications (*J Vasc Interv Radiol* 2012;23:727–36; *Laryngoscope* 2014;124:916–20)
- Acute trauma or surgery to the skull base or face
- Risk of bleeding (esophageal varices or severe coagulation abnormality)
- Esophageal perforation or risk of esophageal perforation such as alkaline ingestion
- Moderate to severe esophageal stricture
- Tracheoesophageal fistula

Type of Nasogastric Tubes (*Interventional Critical Care: A Manual for Advanced Care Practitioners.* Springer; 2016)
- Levin tube:
  - Single lumen. For medication and nutrition
    - Sizes from 3–18F (for nasogastric tubes do not place larger than 18F due to increased risk of trauma)
- Salem sump tube:
  - Double lumen tube: a larger lumen for gastric decompression (fluid and air) or medication delivery and a smaller lumen for air vent

Procedural Technique (*Gastroenterology* 2011;141:742–65; *Interventional Critical Care: A Manual for Advanced Care Practitioners.* Springer; 2016; *Interventional Radiology: A Survival Guide.* Elsevier Health Sciences; 2016)
- **Position patient** with neck flexed (decreases chance of tracheal placement)
- **Local anesthetic spray** to the back of the throat can be administered for comfort
- **Assess length** from bridge of the nose to earlobe to xiphoid process
- **Lubricate** and insert the nasogastric tube in the nasal cavity
- **If patient awake** ask to take sips of water to facilitate placement into esophagus
- **Confirm fluoroscopic placement** by following the tube to the stomach or duodenum. Once in the expected location of the stomach, **contrast injection can identify the gastric outlet**
- **Turn patient in right lateral decubitus position to facilitate advancement through the pylorus**
- **Secure in position** with tape

Troubleshooting (*Gut* 2003;52:vii1–12)
- **If difficult postpyloric placement,** an angled angiographic catheter with torquable hydrophilic guidewire can be used to gain access and then a feeding tube is placed over the wire. IV metoclopramide can facilitate forward movement.

Complications (*Gastroenterology* 2011;141:742–65; *Interventional Critical Care: A Manual for Advanced Care Practitioners.* Springer; 2016)
- Incorrect placement: Airways or mouth
- Gastric wall damage and hemorrhage
- Nasal mucosal damage
- Aspiration pneumonia
- Sinusitis
- Chronic use may lead to esophageal stricture

Postprocedural Care (*Interventional Critical Care: A Manual for Advanced Care Practitioners.* Springer; 2016; *Interventional Radiology Procedures in Biopsy and Drainage.* Springer London; 2011)
- Ensure tube is working by using a large syringe to inject air with simultaneous auscultation
- Maintain patency by daily flushing with normal saline
- Assess nasal cavity and nasopharynx for ulceration or tissue necrosis
- Do not keep in place for long term (more than 4–6 w)

PERCUTANEOUS GASTROINTESTINAL TUBE PLACEMENT

Percutaneous Gastrostomy
Types of Percutaneous Gastrostomy Tubes (*Gut* 2003;52:vii1–12; *Clin Radiol* 2003;58:398–405)
- Radiologically inserted gastrostomy (RIG)

- Per-oral image-guided gastrostomy (PIG) or pull gastrostomy
  - PIG has an equally successful rate to RIG and lower rates of re-intervention (*Am J Roentgenol* 1997;169:1281–4)
  - Contraindicated in patients with nasopharyngeal cancer
  - Larger caliber than RIG tubes, 14F–20F vs. 12F–16F, which are less likely to clog
  - PIG approach can allow the placement of a larger primary tube when compared with some RIG tubes
- Note that image-guided percutaneous gastrostomy tubes are placed by radiologists and include Radiologically inserted gastrostomy (RIG) and Per-oral image-guided gastrostomy (PIG). This is differentiated from percutaneous endoscopic gastrostomy (PEG), which is performed endoscopically.

Background (*Interventional Radiology Procedures in Biopsy and Drainage.* Springer London; 2011)
- For patients who have normal absorption and motility but inadequate or absent oral intake
- For patients who need long-term nutrition (more than 4–6 w)

Clinical and Preprocedural Workup (*Handbook of Interventional Radiologic Procedures.* Lippincott Williams & Wilkins; 2011; *Gastroenterology* 2011;141:742–65; *J Vasc Interv Radiol* 2012;23:727–36; *Essential Clinical Procedures: Expert Consult.* Elsevier Health Sciences; 2013; *Gut* 2003;52:vii1–12)
- **Imaging evaluation:**
  - CT may be performed to assess the percutaneous access route and evaluate for contraindications
  - At the time of the procedure, ultrasound can be used to identify the left lobe of the liver
  - Administration of ~200 mL dilute barium 12 h before the procedure can outline colon. Otherwise, can use colonic gas to identify colon or if little colonic gas then retrograde air per rectum can be injected before the procedure.
- **Laboratory workup:** Check INR, PTT, Platelets
  - **If low-risk bleeding procedure (ie,** placement of percutaneous tube through a present mature stoma)
    - No need to hold anticoagulant or antiplatelet therapy
  - **If moderate-risk bleeding procedure (ie,** initial percutaneous placement)
    - Preprocedure laboratory goal: INR <1.5 and Platelet >50000
    - Medications:
      - Clopidogrel: Withhold for 5 d before the procedure
      - Aspirin: Do not withhold
      - Low-molecular-weight heparin (therapeutic dose): Withhold 1 dose before the procedure
- **NPO:** 8–12 h prior to procedure
- **NG tube placement prior to procedure:** For access to insufflate air into stomach → brings stomach close to the anterior abdominal wall. If difficult NG tube placement bedside then perform fluoroscopic-guided NG tube placement during the procedure.
- **Antibiotic prophylaxis** in patients undergoing per-oral image-guided gastrostomy (PIG) due to oral flora. Recommend penicillin-based prophylaxis such as cefazolin or per local/regional antibiotic susceptibility guidelines.
- **Indications** (*J Vasc Interv Radiol* 2012;23:727–36; *World J Gastroenterol WJG* 2014;20:7739–51; *Semin Interv Radiol* 2004;21:181–9)
- Patients with inadequate or absent oral intake
  - Due to dysphagia or risk of aspiration
    - Neurological (stroke, brain injury, neuromuscular disorders, cerebral palsy)
    - Neurocognitive disorders (dementia)
  - Due to obstructive lesions
    - Esophageal cancer, head and neck cancer, or mediastinal cancer
  - Due to head/neck trauma or surgery
- Diversion of feeding from esophageal leaks due to recent surgery or trauma
- Palliative decompression
  - Proximal small bowel or gastric outlet obstruction (however, cannot be used for feeding)
  - Advanced abdominal malignancies causing chronic obstruction/ileus
  - Gastroparesis (diabetic gastropathy, scleroderma) or other bowel dysmotility disorders
- Intestinal access for biliary procedures (eg, patients with Roux-en-Y anastomosis)

Contraindications *(Handbook of Interventional Radiologic Procedures. Lippincott Williams & Wilkins; 2011; Gastroenterology 2011;141:742–65; J Vasc Interv Radiol 2012;23:727–36; Semin Interv Radiol 2004;21:181–9; Vascular and Interventional Radiology: The Requisites. 2nd ed. Elsevier Health Sciences; 2013)*

- Absolute Contraindications
  - Uncorrectable coagulopathy (INR >1.5, PTT >50 s, platelets <50000/mm³)
  - Massive ascites (perform preprocedural paracentesis)
  - Hemodynamically unstable
  - Sepsis, peritonitis, abdominal wall infection at selected site of placement
  - Peritoneal carcinomatosis
- Relative Contraindications
  - Technically challenging
    - Colonic or liver interposition between the stomach and anterior abdominal wall
    - Previous gastric surgery makes difficult access and requires advanced techniques and/or CT guidance
    - Ascites
    - Large hiatal hernia
- Considerations
  - Patients with portal hypertension and varices have a potential for massive hemorrhage
  - Immunosuppression associated with higher rates of pericatheter leakage
  - Possible increased risk of ascending meningitis in patients with ventriculoperitoneal shunts
  - Inflammatory, neoplastic, or infectious involvement of the gastric wall (may result in poor wound healing and tract formation)

Radiologically Inserted Gastrostomy (RIG) Procedural Technique *(Handbook of Interventional Radiologic Procedures. Lippincott Williams & Wilkins; 2011; Gastroenterology 2011;141:742–65; Clin Radiol 2003;58:398–405)*

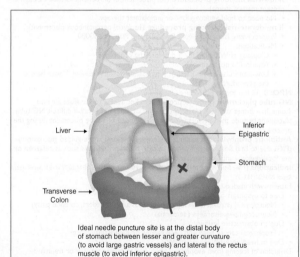

Ideal needle puncture site is at the distal body of stomach between lesser and greater curvature (to avoid large gastric vessels) and lateral to the rectus muscle (to avoid inferior epigastric).

1) **Preoperative medications:** Glucagon (0.5–1.0 mg) or butylscopolamine (20 mg) IV may be administered to diminish gastric peristalsis
2) **Sedation:** Local anesthesia with moderate sedation
3) **Prep and drape:** Epigastrium and left subcostal area with sterile technique. Localize liver edge and transverse colon.
4) **Insufflate** stomach with air via NG tube

5) **Entry site:** Left upper quadrant → Distal body of stomach between lesser and greater curvature (to avoid large gastric vessels) and lateral to the rectus muscle (to avoid inferior epigastric)
   a. **+/− Gastropexy:** Need for T fasteners debated
      i. **With Gastropexy:** Consider in patients with poor wound healing and impaired ability to form a mature tract (chronic steroids) or at high risk for peritoneal leakage (ascites). Perform with needle preloaded with a T-fastener anchor system. Confirm intragastric positioning and insert stylet through the needle to advance anchor into the stomach and remove needle and stylet leaving the anchor suture. Secure anchor suture to bring the anterior gastric wall to the abdominal wall. In total, insert of 2–4 gastric T-fasteners.
   b. **Without gastropexy:**
      i. Maintain air distention of the stomach to maintain placement adjacent to the anterior abdominal wall
6) **Puncture stomach:**
   a. → Aim needle toward pylorus → Facilitates future G to GJ tube conversion
7) **Confirm needle position:** With injection of contrast outlining gastric rugal folds. With the Seldinger needle tip in the stomach, insert a stiff 0.035-in guidewire to gain access and coil within the stomach
8) **Dilate the tract:** Using push dilators or balloon catheter
9) **Place gastrostomy tube:** Over the wire, potentially through a peel-away sheath
10) **Confirm placement:** Inject contrast to confirm proper position
11) **Secure:** With sutures or retaining devices

Per-Oral Image-Guided Gastrostomy (PIG/pull gastrostomy) Procedural Technique (*Handbook of Interventional Radiologic Procedures.* Lippincott Williams & Wilkins; 2011; *Gut* 2003;52:vii1–12)

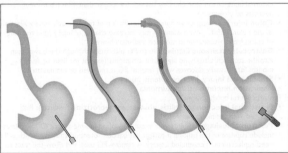

A) Needle access to the stomach. B) Retrograde passage of a guidewire through the esophagus. C) Gastrostomy tube is pulled down over the wire. D) Gastrostomy tube is pulled out through the needle puncture site and internal fixation collar affixed against the gastric mucosa.

- Similar to RIG procedure, however, no need for gastropexy
1) Inflate stomach via NG tube
2) Percutaneously puncture stomach
   a. Direct needle toward the gastroesophageal junction to facilitate cannulation of the esophagus
3) Insert guidewire, then place a 4F–5F sheath through the gastrostomy tract
4) Then perform retrograde catheterization of the esophagus with a hydrophilic guidewire and a 4F or 5F angiographic catheter and advance the guidewire out of the mouth.
5) A snare included in pull-gastrostomy kit will tighten onto the wire
6) Warn the patient and pull the gastrostomy tube down the esophagus to the stomach adjacent to the anterior gastric wall
7) Remove the wire and affix the internal fixation collar against the gastric mucosa

Troubleshooting (*Handbook of Interventional Radiologic Procedures.* Lippincott Williams & Wilkins; 2011; *Gut* 2003;52:vii1–12; *WJG* 2014;20:8505–24)

- **If abnormal anatomy or difficult access,** CT guidance can be used
- **If tenting of gastric wall on attempted puncture,** try a short stabbing motion to puncture the thick muscular gastric wall.

- RIG
  - Due to thick muscular wall of the stomach, use caution when using the dilator as this step may push the stomach away and possibly lead to displacement out of the stomach into the peritoneum. **If difficulty dilating the gastrostomy tract,** make sure the stomach is insufflated adequately. If T-fasteners are in place, additional traction on these will also pull the gastric wall anteriorly.
- PIG
  - **If unable to catheterize the esophagus retrograde,** place an antegrade wire through the nasogastric tube and snare the wire
  - **If access is lost after tract dilation,** reaccessing is extremely difficult and the procedure will have to be performed at a later date. Treat the patient with supportive care, due to the gastric leakage.
  - **If gastrostomy tube falls out**
    - **For an immature tract,** they usually close within 24–48 h. However, sometimes access can be reobtained by using a Kumpe catheter and guidewire. If tract is closed, the procedure will have to be performed again.
    - **For a mature tract,** a Foley catheter can be used to maintain access until tube replacement. Thereafter, access can be reobtained by a Kumpe catheter and hydrophilic guidewire and a new gastrostomy tube can be placed.

Complications (WJG 2014;20:7739–51; Radiology 1995;197:699–704)
- Procedure-related 30-d mortality under 0.5% (Am J Roentgenol 2012;198:453–9)
  - Surgical and endoscopically placed gastrostomies carry higher mortality and complication rates (Gut Liver Gut Liver 2010;4(Suppl 1):S9–S18)
- Procedural complications
  - **Pneumoperitoneum:** Benign and self-limiting, resolves in 24–72 h. 50% of patients.
  - **Bleeding:** From the puncture either from the stomach (due to puncture of the gastroepiploic artery or its branches) or from the abdominal wall → tightening the external bumper can stop bleeding but not for longer than 48 h (to prevent necrosis or ulceration)
  - **Colon injury:** Prevent by adequate air insufflation of the stomach and localization of the colon. Pitfall → overdistention may increase chance of injury (due to lifting of colon from overdistended stomach and small bowel)
  - **Gastrocolocutaneous fistula:** Due to PG placement through the bowel then into the stomach. Usually, no significant symptoms (except for ileus or fever) → months later usually discover when original PG is removed or manipulated.
  - **Small bowel injury, liver or splenic injury**
  - **Aspiration pneumonitis/pneumonia**
- Postprocedural complications
  - **Peristomal infection (cellulitis, abscess, or necrotizing fasciitis):** Risk reduced with antibiotic prophylaxis
  - **Peristomal leakage:** Patients with impaired wound healing at risk. Other causes include rupture of the balloon if patient has balloon retention catheter which will need replacement. If continued leakage → remove PG tube and allow the tract to mature/close for a couple days and replace with a new PG tube (only if mature tract and enough time passed for stomach to be scarred to abdominal wall). Do not replace with larger tube → enlarges the tract and worsens leakage.
  - **Pressure ulcers:** Reduce excessive traction to reduce risk
  - **Leak of gastric contents into peritoneum:** Most serious complication. Treat with holding tube feeds and surgical management.
  - **Peptic ulcers:** Seen in approximately 15% of patients. Treat with medical management with PPIs.
  - **Gastric outlet obstruction:** Caused by obstruction of the pylorus or duodenum by part of the PG tube
  - **Ileus or gastroparesis:** Postprocedural ileus is common, managed conservatively
  - **PG tube dislodgement:** Usually in patients with dementia or combative patients. Prevent with an abdominal binder.
  - **PG tube clogged:** Common especially with thick feeds, medications, and bulking agent administration. Prevent with adequate and frequent flushing with warm water (not saline → can crystalize and further clog). Dwell catheter solutions also include carbonated beverage such as cola. In addition, flushing catheter with a smaller 1 cc syringe (Medallion) provides more pressure.
  - **Post PG diarrhea:** Common, in about 10–20% of patients. Majority of the time due to diet → treat with diet modification (dilute solutions, lactose-free and low-fat diets).
  - **Tumor implantation at PG site:** Uncommon. Reduce risk by PG placement after removal of primary cancer. Poor prognosis.

- **Buried bumper syndrome:** Internal bumper becomes dislodged along the PG tract. Due to excess tension between the internal and external bumpers leading to necrosis/ulceration at the bumper site. Usually presents around ~2–4 mo. Can be fatal.

Postprocedural Care (Handbook of Interventional Radiologic Procedures. Lippincott Williams & Wilkins; 2011; Gut 2003;52:vii1–12; Clin Radiol 2003;58:398–405; World J Gastroenterol 2014;WJG 20:7739–51)
- Watch for signs for peritonitis with serial abdominal examinations
- Fast for 6 h postprocedurally. If this is tolerated, can administer 25–50 mL of water through the tube for a total of 6 h. If this is also tolerated, feeding can start the next day.
- Gastrostomy tube care
  - "Fresh" tubes which have not had a chance to form a tract yet, should not be manipulated if possible to reduce the risk of leaking gastric contents into the peritoneum and causing peritonitis
  - PEG tube tract starts to mature after 7–10 d → matures in usually in 1–3 w. However, malnourished or immunocompromised patients can take up to a month.
  - Remove T-fasteners after the gastropexy has started to form, ranges per operator from 2 d to 2 w
- Replace water in the balloon every 7–10 d
- Routine changes of the gastrostomy tube not usually performed and are replaced when malfunctioning
- Tube exchanges should not be performed on immature stomal tracts to reduce risk of leaking of gastric contents and peritonitis

Percutaneous Gastrojejunostomy
Indications (Handbook of Interventional Radiologic Procedures. Lippincott Williams & Wilkins; 2011; Clin Radiol 2003;58:398–405)
- Risk of gastroesophageal reflux or aspiration
- Feeding for patients with gastric outlet obstruction

Types (Handbook of Interventional Radiologic Procedures. Lippincott Williams & Wilkins; 2011)
- Single lumen
- Double lumen
  - One lumen in the jejunum and the other in the stomach. The second gastric lumen can be used for decompression or medication administration.

Procedural Technique (Handbook of Interventional Radiologic Procedures. Lippincott Williams & Wilkins; 2011)
- **Initial feeding tube placement (primary percutaneous gastrojejunostomy)**
  - Direct needle puncture toward pylorus.
  - Use angled catheter and guidewire to obtain access into the jejunum
  - Dilate entry site and place peel-away sheath
  - Insert PGJ tube
  - Confirm position
  - Secure catheter
- **Conversion of gastrostomy tube to a gastrojejunostomy tube**
  - Can be performed after successful placement of a percutaneous gastrostomy
    - If gastropexy was previously done, conversion can be attempted at any time; otherwise, waiting 1–3 w after gastrostomy tube placement for tract maturation is recommended
  - Can be difficult if angle of primarily placed PG tube is towards the fundus → attempt to redirect with rigid sheath or cannula but if unsuccessful perform a new puncture directed towards the pylorus
- Position PGJ beyond ligament of Treitz and gastric tube in the stomach lumen

Complications (Gastroenterology 2011;141:742–65)
- Same as for percutaneous gastrostomy (above)
- Prevent dumping syndrome with an elemental diet and slow pump infusion

Percutaneous Jejunostomy
Background (Gastroenterology 2011;141:742–65)
- In patients where the stomach needs to be bypassed

Indications (Handbook of Interventional Radiologic Procedures. Lippincott Williams & Wilkins; 2011; Gastroenterology 2011;141:742–65)
- Prior gastric surgery such as gastrectomy
- Abnormal gastric position
- Obstruction of duodenum or proximal jejunum
- Chronic aspiration

Procedural Technique (Handbook of Interventional Radiologic Procedures. Lippincott Williams & Wilkins; 2011; Gastroenterology 2011;141:742–65; Radiology 1998;209:747–54; Hepatology 57:1651–3)
- More technically challenging to puncture the jejunum

- Use angled catheter with a guidewire or long nasoenteric balloon catheter to enter the nostril and go down to the level of the jejunum
- Then dilate the jejunum with saline, air, or balloon inflation
- Subsequently, puncture the distended jejunum under CT, fluoroscopy, or ultrasound
- Confirm position of the needle
- Insert T-fastener to secure the jejunum to the anterior abdominal wall
- Insert guidewire into the jejunum and advance to secure access
- Perform serial dilatation to the feeding tube size
- Insert feeding tube over the guidewire and remove the guidewire

Complications (Gastroenterology 2011;141:742–65)
- Same as for percutaneous gastrostomy (above)
- Prevent dumping syndrome with an elemental diet and slow pump infusion

Percutaneous Cecostomy

Indications (Handbook of Interventional Radiologic Procedures. Lippincott Williams & Wilkins; 2011; J Vasc Interv Radiol 2012;23:727–36)
- Decompression or diversion
  - Fecal incontinence (especially neurologic causes such as cerebral palsy, meningomyelocele, or spinal cord injury)
  - Chronic colonic pseudo-obstruction (Ogilvie syndrome) or chronic colonic obstruction
  - Chronic refractory constipation
  - Cecal volvulus
- Antegrade medication delivery
  - Chronic obstruction due to neurogenic colon

Procedural Technique (Handbook of Interventional Radiologic Procedures. Lippincott Williams & Wilkins; 2011)
- Anterior intraperitoneal approach
- Distend cecum with air with rectal Foley catheter if needed
- Perform single wall puncture via fluoroscopy
- Confirm needle position
- Insert T-fasteners
- Proceed with guidewire to facilitate dilation

Complications (Handbook of Interventional Radiologic Procedures. Lippincott Williams & Wilkins; 2011)
- Rare

REFRACTORY ASCITES

Background (Hepatology 2013;57:1651–3; J Hepatol 2010;53(3):397–417; Semin Interv Radiol 2012;29: 129–34; Ann Surg 2004;239:883–91; Am J Transplant 2005;5:1886–92)
- According to American Association for the Study of Liver Diseases (AASLD) and European Association for the Study of the Liver (EASL) guidelines, refractory ascites is defined as ascites unresponsive to medical therapy (sodium-restricted diet and high-dose diuretic treatment [400 mg/d of spironolactone and 160 mg/ furosemide]) or has rapid recurrence after therapeutic paracentesis.
- Around 60% of patients with compensated cirrhosis develop ascites within 10 y during their disease course. Of these patients, refractory ascites occurs in less than 10%. After the development of refractory ascites, the 1-y mortality rate has been estimated around 50%. Due to the high mortality rates, patients with refractory ascites should be considered for liver transplantation; after liver transplant, the 2-y survival rates are around 85%.

Management of Refractory Ascites (Hepatology 2013;57:1651–3; J Hepatol 2010;53(3):397–417; Semin Interv Radiol 2012;29:129–34; Ann Surg 2004;239:883–91; Am J Transplant 2005;5:1886–92)
- 1st line: Large-volume paracentesis + Albumin (generally 6–8 g albumin per liter of fluid removed after 5 L)
- 2nd or 3rd line: TIPS vs. Peritoneovenous shunts (PVS)
  - Consider in patients requiring frequent paracentesis more than every 2–3 w or not agreeable to frequent paracentesis
  - EASL and AASLD guidelines, peritoneovenous shunts have almost completely been replaced by the TIPS procedure because of its reduced morbidity and reduced interference with anticipated liver transplantation. However, there is much debate on this and some authors and emerging research demonstrate that PVS can serve as a bridge to liver transplantation. In the appropriate patient population, PVS can improve the quality life with faster treatment of ascites when compared to TIPS
  - Meta-analysis with 5 RCTs have shown mixed results in respect to survival, when comparing TIPs vs. PVS (J Vasc Interv Radiol 2006;17:831–5)

- PVS showed better early control of ascites after shunting (73% vs. 46% after 1 mo) (Ann Surg 2004; 239:883–91)
- TIPS showed better long-term efficacy (1–5) of ascites control after shunting (85% vs. 40% after 3 y) (Ann Surg 2004;239:883–91)
- Shunt occlusion occurs in both TIPS and PVS or also known as a Denver shunt, with median shunt primary patency of 4.4 and 4 mo for TIPS versus PVS. However, the assisted shunt patency is better with TIPS (31.1 months vs. 13.1 mo) (Ann Surg 2004;239:883–91). Notably, TIPS primary patency is improved with the use of more commonly used covered stent grafts.
- Pleurx Catheter
  - Within the recent years, studies have found that the Pleurx catheter is effective management for patients with malignant ascites.
  - There are relatively high patency rates of ~85%. (J Vasc Interv Radiol 2008;19:S1723–31) with low reported complication rates including peritonitis (1–11%), catheter occlusion (2.5–37%), and catheter leakage (2–11%). (J Pain Symptom Manage 2009;38:341–9) (J Vasc Interv Radiol 2008;19:S1723–31).
  - Studies have also found in patients with malignant ascites, although there is a more expensive initial procedural cost. Overall, it may be less costly if a need for repeated paracentesis >9–10 times. (Am J Roentgenol 2015;205(5):1126–34).

	Large Volume Paracentesis	TIPS	Denver Shunt	Pleurx Catheter
Patient considerations	Better for: – Patients who are well controlled with repeated large volume paracentesis – Require relatively infrequent paracentesis or are agreeable to repeat paracentesis with higher frequency	Better for: – Patients with longer estimated life-span – Loculated ascites – Cirrhotic patients with history of SBP – History of variceal bleed or large varices – Budd Chiari (treats hepatic venous outflow obstruction)	Better for: – Patients who need faster ascites control with shorter estimated life-span (<3 mo ie, MELD score >18) – Patients unable to tolerate TIPS procedure due to portal vein thrombosis, prior hepatic resection, or HCC in a critical location – Patients with good functioning status able to perform maintenance of the shunt – Able to tolerate increased intravascular volume with sufficient cardiac function – Good success rates in chylous ascites (J Vasc Interv Radiol 2014;25:S127)	Better for: – Patients not well controlled with repeated paracentesis – Patients able to perform catheter maintenance – For malignant and non-malignant ascites (although most studies in patients with malignant ascites
Pros	– Low-risk procedure – No risk of device-related complications	– Better long-term ascites control – Nutrient retention – Preserves transplant candidacy	– Immediate ascites control – Nutrient retention – Reversible – Improvement of renal function and thereby lower rates of hepatorenal syndrome (Am J Transplant 2005;5:1886–92)	– Immediate ascites control – Reversible – Decreased hospital/clinic visits – High Patency rates of ~85% (J Vasc Interv Radio 2008;19:S1723–31)

| Cons | – Frequent procedures
– Loss of nutrients | – Difficult to reverse
– Hepatic encephalopathy 30–50% of the patients. (J Vasc Interv Radiol 2014;25:S127)
– Shunt thrombosis and stenosis (less frequent with covered stents)
– Liver failure | – High maintenance
– Does not control variceal bleeding
– Not for loculated ascites
– Higher rates of shunt occlusion vs. TIPS
– Infection, sepsis, DIC | – Loss of nutrients
– Peritonitis (1–11%), catheter occlusion (2.5–37%) and catheter leakage (2–11%) |

PERITONEOVENOUS SHUNTING

Background (Am J Transplant 2005;5:1886–92)
- Initially created by Harry Leveen in 1974, as a subcutaneous catheter continuously shunting protein-rich ascitic fluid into the central venous system via a 1-way pressure activated valve
- Subsequently modified by Denver Biomedical and has replaced the Leveen shunt with the Denver shunt
- Now the applications of peritoneovenous shunting have expanded to include not only shunting ascites but also pleural effusions

Relevant Anatomy

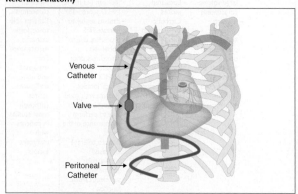

Venous Catheter

Valve

Peritoneal Catheter

Clinical and Preprocedural Workup (Semin Interv Radiol 2012;29:129–34)
- **Patient selection:**
  - Can be placed for patients of all ages, even neonates
  - Need to choose patients with good functional status who are able to perform necessary maintenance to maintain patency of the shunt. Patients also need to have good cardiorespiratory function to tolerate the increased venous return after device placement.
  - One of the advantages of this procedure over TIPS in the management of refractory ascites is that it is easily reversible
  - In patients with cirrhosis and variceal bleeding, PVS is less appropriate, as does not control variceal bleeding
  - Studies have reported improved renal function and liver function after PVS placement
- **Imaging evaluation:**
  - Ultrasound prior to the procedure to ensure that the ascites is without loculation and there is an adequate amount to access for paracentesis
  - Also, ultrasound the venous access site to determine patency
- **Laboratory workup:** Check INR, PTT, Platelets, WBC

- Patients should be without concern for active infection, fever, leukocytosis
- **Moderate-risk bleeding procedure**
  - Preprocedure laboratory goal: INR: <1.5 and Platelet: >50000
- **Antibiotic prophylaxis:** Broad spectrum antibiotics are administered at the start of the procedure and continued for 7–10 d after the procedure

Indications (Handbook of Interventional Radiologic Procedures. Lippincott Williams & Wilkins; 2011; Semin Interv Radiol 2012;29:129–34; J Vasc Interv Radiol; 2014;25:S127; J Vasc Surg Venous Lymphat Disord 2017:5:538–46; J Vasc Interv Radiol 2013;24:1073–4)
- Recurrent refractory ascites (cirrhotic or malignant)
  - Especially in patients with a shorter estimated life-span (<3 mo, ie MELD score >18), in need of faster ascites control
  - Patients unable to tolerate TIPS procedure due to portal vein thrombosis, prior hepatic resection, or HCC in a critical location
- Recurrent chylous ascites

Contraindications (Semin Interv Radiol 2012;29:129–34)
- Sepsis
- Uncorrectable coagulopathy
- Loculated ascites
- Morbid obesity (shunt valve must be placed against a firm structure such as the rib or sternum)

Components (Semin Interv Radiol 2012;29:129–34; Ann Surg 1974;180:580–90)
- **Compressible pump chamber:** Manual pump implanted in the subcutaneous tissues over lower ribs. Function to prevent occlusion by flushing fluid through the shunt (avoids build-up of proteinaceous debris) and maintain patency as well as determine patency when malfunctioning.
- **Silicone miter valves:** One-way valves to direct ascitic or pleural fluid to the venous system. Opens when pressure is 3 cmH$_2$O above CVP.
  - **Double valve:** More common
    - 1st valve: Opens when pressure is 3 cmH$_2$O above CVP
    - 2nd valve: Prevents reflux of fluid or blood during manual compression
  - **Single valve**
    - Higher flow rates and better in patients with viscous ascitic or pleural fluid and in patients with large amounts of ascites
- **Radiopaque Catheters:**
  - **Fenestrated peritoneal or pleural catheter:**
    - 15.5F
  - **Venous catheter:**
    - **15.5F:** For internal jugular, subclavian or peritoneosaphenous placement → double valve (flow rate 25–40 mL/min) or single valve (flow rate 40–55 mL/min)
    - **11.5F:** For subclavian placement → double valve (flow rate 20–30 mL/min) or single valve (flow rate 30–40 mL/min)

Procedural Technique (Semin Interv Radiol 2012;29:129–34; Eur Radiol 2002;12:1188–92)
1. **Side choice:** Standard surgical field preparation and draping from the neck to the pelvis on the side of the body with the most fluid
2. **Anesthesia:** Typically local with moderate conscious IV sedation
   a. Local anesthesia at the peritoneal/pleural access site, venous access site, and subcutaneous tunnel
3. **Prime shunt:** Immerse in normal saline and compress pump valve to remove air
4. **Plan placement:**
   a. **Compressible valve**
      i. Over noncompressible lower rib
   b. **Peritoneal or pleural space placement**
   c. **Venous placement**
      i. Internal jugular vein: 11.5F or 15.5F
      ii. Subclavian vein: 11.5F preferable
      iii. Saphenous vein: 15.5F
5. **Gain peritoneal or pleural fluid access:** Under ultrasound guidance
   a. **Pre-drain fluid:** Either partially drain to have abdomen lax for procedure or completely drain and replace with 4 L of normal saline ("less risk of DIC") → primes the shunt system to start continuous low flow after placement
6. **Make skin incision to create subcutaneous pocket** and insert compressible valve over a noncompressible rib
7. **Tunnel peritoneal/pleural catheter end** to the peritoneal/pleural access site using a hemostat

8. **Gain central venous access:** Under ultrasound guidance
   a. If IJ access, place as close to the clavicle as possible
   b. Secure access with 5F outer transitional catheter with a 0.035-in guidewire advanced to the level of the IVC
9. **Tunnel central venous end** to the venous access site using a hemostat
10. **Prime pump valve** again by compressing to initiate flow then stop flow with hemostat at the venous limb
11. Measure distance to the right atrium and cut catheter to appropriate length
12. Insert shunt catheter through a 12F or 16F peel-away sheath in the central venous end and a 16F peel-away sheath in the peritoneal/pleural end
13. Suture compressible valve

Complications (Semin Interv Radiol 2012;29:129–34; Eur Radiol 2002;12:1188–92; Arch Surg 1982;117:924–8; J Gastroenterol Hepatol 2007;22:2161–6; J Pediatr Surg 2011;46:315–9; Arch Surg 1982;117: 631–5; Cardiovasc Intervent Radiol 2011;34:980–8; J Vasc Interv Radiol 2015;26:S39)

- Shunt occlusion:
  - If chamber does not refill → then peritoneal/pleural (lower) tubing blocked
  - If chamber is hard → then venous (upper) tubing is blocked or blood clot in the chamber
- Catheter fracture
- Infection
- Ascitic fluid leakage
- Disseminated intravascular coagulopathy (DIC)
- Catheter-related venous thrombosis
- Pulmonary edema
- Pneumoperitoneum/pneumothorax

Postprocedural Care
- **Manual pumping to prevent clogging of the system:** Recommended twice a day (20 times each session) in supine position
  - **Special attention for single-valve systems:** Must compress venous end of shunt during manual pumping to prevent blood reflux into chamber which would cause occlusion

---

ADDITIONAL RESOURCES

1. Anderson GS, Levine MS, Rubesin SE, et al. Esophageal stents: Findings on esophagography in 46 patients. Am J Roentgenol 2006;187:1274–9.
2. Davies RP, Kew J, & West GP. Percutaneous jejunostomy using CT fluoroscopy. Am J Roentgenol 2001;176:808–10.
3. LaBerge J. Interventional Radiology Essentials. Lippincott Williams & Wilkins; 2000.
4. Schrag SP, Sharma R, Jaik NP, et al. Complications related to percutaneous endoscopic gastrostomy (PEG) tubes. A comprehensive clinical review. J Gastrointestin Liver Dis 2007;16:407–18.
5. Courtney A, Nemcek AA Jr, Rosenberg S, et al. Prospective evaluation of the PleurX catheter when used to treat recurrent ascites associated with malignancy. J Vasc Interv Radiol 2008;9(12):1723–31.
6. Fleming ND, Alvarez-Secord A, Von Gruenigen V, et al. Indwelling catheters for the management of refractory malignant ascites: A systematic literature overview and retrospective chart review. J Pain Symptom Manage 2009;38:341–49.
7. Bohn KA & Ray CE Jr. Repeat large-volume paracentesis versus tunneled peritoneal catheter placement for malignant ascites: A cost-minimization study. Am J Roentgenol 2015;205(5):1126–34.
8. Lungren MP, Matthew P, Kim CY, et al. Tunneled peritoneal drainage catheter placement for refractory ascites: Single-center experience in 188 patients. J Vasc Interv Radiol 2013; 24(9)9:1303–8.
9. Tapping CR, Ling L & Razack A. PleurX drain use in the management of malignant ascites: Safety, complications, long-term patency and factors predictive of success. Br j radiol 2012; 85(1013):623–28.

Background

• Pediatric interventional radiology is a continually evolving and growing subspecialty. Although interventional radiology procedures have been performed on children for decades, historically by "adult" trained interventional radiologist or pediatric radiologists, the number of pediatric interventional radiology fellowship training programs has steadily increased over the last 10 years as has the Peds IR workforce (Pediatr Radiol 2017;47:651–6). Types of diseases and response to pathology are distinctly different in children and such requires a certain level of expertise. In this chapter, specific clinical and technical considerations for pediatrics will be discussed. In addition, procedures commonly seen in pediatrics that have not been discussed elsewhere, including pediatric GI procedures and treatment for vascular malformations and varicoceles, will be described.

Clinical Considerations in Pediatrics

• **Periprocedure and Intraprocedure Care:**
  • Consent/Assent: Informed consent is obtained from the patient's parent or guardian, preferably a minimum of a few hours in advance and not immediately before the procedure. It may be better to not explain the procedure in front of a young patient as this might increase anxiety. An older child or adolescent should give assent, meaning they agree to the procedure.
  • Child life specialists: Utilize child life specialist before, and even during the procedure. These specialists have appropriate age-level training to help children cope with the procedure and can provide distraction and support during a nonsedate procedure, such as joint injections or gastrojejunostomy (GJ) replacements.
  • NPO guidelines for sedation/anesthesia: 2 h for clear liquids, 4 h for breast milk, 6 h for formula/milk, 8 h for solid foods
  • Coagulation studies: Abnormal platelets and coagulation factors are common in the neonatal period. Even if these studies are normal, platelets and factor function may be abnormal. For procedures with moderate or high risk of bleeding in neonates, considerer obtaining a type and cross with blood products on hold or in the procedure room. Be cognizant of blood loss and waste during procedures as the total blood volume in a term neonate (3 kg) is only about 250 mL.

Artery/Patient Weight	10–20 kg	20–50 kg	>50 kg
Aorta	5–10 for 8–15	10–20 for 20–40	20–25 for 25–50
Celiac	2–3 for 10–20	3–5 for 15–30	5–8 for 30–60
Splenic	2–3 for 10–15	3–5 for 15–20	5–8 for 20–50
Hepatic	2–3 for 5–10	3–5 for 10–20	5–8 for 15–25
Superior mesenteric	2–3 for 10–15	3–5 for 15–30	5–8 for 30–50
Inferior mesenteric	*	1–3 for 6–9	2–3 for 10–15
Renal	2–4 for 3–5	3–5 for 6–9	5–8 for 10–15
Subclavian	2–3 for 4–6	3–4 for 6–15	5–8 for 15–25
Common Carotid	2–3 for 3–5	4–6 for 5–10	6–8 for 10–15
Internal Carotid	1–2 for 3–5	2–4 for 5–8	4–5 for 6–10
Vertebral	*	2–5 for 4–6	4–7 for 6–9
Pulmonary	5–8 for 8–15	10–15 for 15–30	15–20 for 25–40

*Hand injection is recommended. In patients under 10 kg, hand injection is recommended for arteriography procedures. Minimum frame rate of 4 frames/s for arterial phase is suggested.

(Reprinted from Springer: Heran MK, Marshalleck F, Temple M, et al. Joint quality improvement guidelines for pediatric arterial access and arteriography: from the Societies of Interventional Radiology and Pediatric Radiology. Pediatr Radiol 2010;40(2):237–50. Copyright © Springer-Verlag 2009, with permission.)

• Radiation exposure: In pediatrics, radiation safety is of the utmost importance since children are most susceptible to the negative effects of radiation exposure. Always attempt to use low-dose pediatric protocols for fluoroscopy and CT-guided procedures. Intermittent fluoroscopy with a low frame rate should be utilized (1–4 frames/s). Last image hold, rather than overhead exposures, should be used when possible to minimize addition radiation exposure. Limit digital subtraction imaging since it contributes a large amount to the overall exposure during a procedure. Magnification should be avoided if possible. If desired, digital zoom can be employed instead. Use filters and collimation to decrease field of

view, and hence, skin entry and overall patient dose. Routine shielding is not recommended. When possible, utilize imaging modalities that do not emit ionizing radiation (ie, ultrasound, MRI).
- Body temperature: Due to increased surface area to volume ratio, infants and children decrease in body temperature more rapidly than adults. You should consider utilizing warm blankets or warmed air (bear hugger) during procedures lasting longer than 30 min. Also, keep room temperature higher, especially with neonates and infants.
- Contrast amount: Attempt to limit dose to 4–5 mL/kg. Must plan out runs as to optimize images and decrease need to repeat injection. Suggested contrast injection rate (mL/s) and total volume (mL) for commonly evaluated arteries are listed in the table below *(Pediatr Radiol 2010;40:237–50)*
- Medication dosing: Pediatric medications are prescribed in a weight based manor, usually with a maximum dose:
  - Antibiotics:
    Cefazolin 50 mg/kg IV, max 2 g
    Cefoxitin 40 mg/kg IV, max 2 g
    Ceftriaxone 50 mg/kg IV, max 2 g
    Clindamycin 10 mg/kg IV, max 900 mg
    Piperacillin/Tazobactam infant—80 mg/kg IV; children and adolescent—100 mg/kg IV, max 3.375 g
  - Analgesia:
    Acetaminophen 15 mg/kg PO
    Fentanyl 1 μg/kg IV
    Morphine 0.05 mg/kg IV
    Local:
    1% Lidocaine—max 0.4 mL/kg
    0.5% Bupivacaine—max 0.4 mL/kg
  - Sedatives:
    Ketamine 1 mg/kg IV
    Midazolam 0.05 mg/kg IV
  - Cardiac/vascular:
    Heparin bolus 100 μ/kg, max 5000 units (suggested for angiography in patients under 10 kg)
    Nitroglycerin 1–3 μg/kg intra-arterially for vasospasm
    Epinephrine:
    Anaphylaxis 0.01 mg/kg IM (1 mg/mL), max 0.5 mg
    Cardiac arrest 0.01 mg/kg IV (0.1 mg/mL), max 1 mg
  - Reversal agents:
    Flumazenil 10 mg/kg IV, may repeat 1–3 min × 4
    Naloxone 5 μg/kg IV (partial), 0.1 mg/kg (full)
  - Other:
    Diphenhydramine 1 mg/kg IV, max 50 mg
- Vital signs: Normal ranges for pulse, BP, and respiratory rate vary depending on patient age. Estimates are summarized below.

Age	Weight (kg)	HR	RR	SBP
Newborn	3.5	80–200	30–60	>60
6 mo	7.5	80–180	24–29	>65
1 y	10	60–150	22–30	>72
3 y	14	60–150	22–30	>76
5 y	18	60–115	20–24	>80
10 y	30–32	60–100	16–22	>90
12 y	40	60–100	16–22	>90
14 y	45	60–100	14–20	>90

- Fluid volume: Administering saline flushes and running fluids through a sheath can significantly increase the patient's fluid volume. Be cognizant of amount of fluid being given during the procedure. Consider utilizing 3 or 5 mL syringes instead of the 10–20 mL syringes used for adults.
- Maintenance fluid guidelines: For the 1st 10 kg = 4 mL/kg/h; 2nd 10 kg (11–20 kg) = 2 mL/kg/h; and >20 kg = 1 mL/kg/h. Eg, 26-kg child: (10 kg × 4) + (10 kg × 2) + (6 kg × 1) = 40 + 20 + 6 = 66 mL/h

- **Anesthesia, Sedation, and Analgesia**
  - IR procedures in pediatric patients frequently require general anesthesia or deep sedation, whereas the same procedure in an adult might require mild or moderate sedation, or even no sedation with only local anesthetic
  - Many pediatric hospitals and facilities that provide pediatric IR services have sedation teams that are certified in providing deep sedation. Deep sedation must be administered by a physician, nurse anesthetist, or anesthetist assistant that have been properly trained and credentialed. The sedation provider should be experienced with positive pressure mask ventilation and endotracheal intubation
  - Careful screening of patients, including a thorough review of medical history and review of systems, is necessary to identify patients who are high risk for sedation and may require anesthesia instead. Some "red flags" for sedation include: History of apnea, infants less than 1 mo old, respiratory compromise, uncontrolled GERD or vomiting, craniofacial abnormality, or cardiac disease. Also, if the procedure is very painful, long in duration, high risk, or if complete immobilization is required, general anesthesia should be utilized (*Pediatric Interventional Radiology: Handbook of Vascular and Non-Vascular Interventional.* Springer; 2014)
  - Patients must be continuously monitored during sedation, including EKG, pulse oximetry, capnography, and BP
- **"Pediatric" Equipment and Devices**
  - Most of the equipment we use in pediatric IR is off label and not FDA approved for children. This is primarily related to the ethics involved in pediatric medical trials.
  - Angiography unit with procedure specific low dose pediatric protocols. You do not need a textbook crystal clear image to perform a joint injection or exchange a GJ tube. Start out on the lowest dose and frame rate and increase these as needed (ie, 120-kg football player).
  - Ultrasound machine with a high-frequency linear probe (12–18 MHz) and a hockey stick probe (12–14 MHz), which has a smaller footprint and allows for in plane needle guidance
  - Recommend **latex free**. Many children with chronic illnesses (ie, myelomeningocele) develop an allergy to latex. Latex gloves, equipment, or bandages are not allowed at our institution
  - Suggested devices for pediatric procedures (*Tech Vasc Interventional Radiol* 2011;14:2–7):
    Arterial introducer sheaths: 3F–4F
    Aortography in infant: 4F multisidehole straight
    Cerebral angiography: 4F angled glide catheter
    Visceral angiography: 4F Sos Omni
    Biopsy devices: 16G & 18G core Temno or BioPince
    Transjugular liver biopsy: Pediatric kit
    Vascular access or FNA: 21G, 4 cm echo tip
    PICC: 1.9F single lumen, 2.6F dual lumen
    PICC exchange: 0.010, 0.014, & 0.018 hydrophilic guidewires
    IVC Filter placement: Retrievable Denali, Celect, or Option
    DVT thrombolysis: AngioJet with 6F Solent Omni and Proxi catheter
    Abscess drainage/nephrostomy tube: 6F and 8 F, 15 cm, and 25 cm Dawson Mueller locking pigtail
    Chest tube: 8.5F nonlocking Merit medical
    Enteric tubes: Low-profile gastrostomy 12F, 0.8 stoma length, Low-profile gastrojejunostomy 14F, 1.0 cm stoma length, 15 cm length

Diagnosis and Treatment of Vascular Anomalies

- **According to ISSVA classification, Vascular Anomalies should be divided into two categories: Vascular Tumors & Vascular Anomalies**
- **Vascular tumors**
  - Infantile Hemangioma (Fig. 15-1)
    - Most common tumor of infancy, 20% are multiple
    - Skin is most common location ("raspberry spot")
    - Liver is 2nd most common location (Fig. 15-2)
      - 3 types: Focal, multiple, and diffuse
    - Usually appear 2–4 w after birth
    - Three phases (*Pediatric Interventional Radiology: Handbook of Vascular and Non-Vascular Interventional.* Springer; 2014):
      - "Proliferative"—up to 9–12 mo of age, hypervascular, rapid growth, high flow
      - "Involuting"—over 5–7 y, reduced vascularity, gradual size reduction
      - "Involuted"—after 5–9 y of age, residual fibrofatty tissue

Figure 15-1

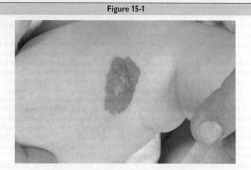

Figure 15-2

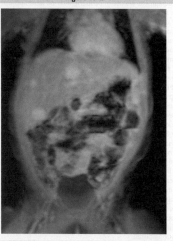

- 50/70/90 rule: 50% resolve by age 5, 70% resolve by age 7, 90% resolve by age 9
- Usually no intervention or treatment needed, but embolization may be indicated with infantile hepatic hemangiomas causing high-output heart failure
- Medical therapies include propranolol and steroids
- Surgical resection is an option for large cutaneous lesions for cosmetics
- Can be mistaken for AVM due to high flow, but associated mass makes the distinction
- Can be mistaken for VM or LM of exam if deeper in subcutaneous tissue due to "bluish" skin discoloration
- GLUT1 positive on histochemical staining
- Congenital Hemangioma (Fig. 15-3)
  - Rare, fully developed at birth, GLUT1 negative
  - 3 different proposed varieties:
    - RICH—"Rapidly involuting": Large protuberant mass, usually regress by 12 mo, may cause high output heart failure early in life and require embolization
    - NICH—"Noninvoluting": Slightly raised area of bluish discoloration, telangiectasias, and pale halo, persists through life, surgical resection is an option
    - PICH—"Partially Involuting": Intermediate clinical characteristics with partial regression

Figure 15-3

PEDIATRIC 15-5

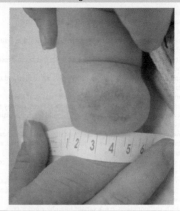

- Kaposiform Hemangioendothelioma (Fig. 15-4)
  - Aggressive, locally invasive, violaceous protuberant mass, commonly on shoulder, trunk or thigh
  - Kasabach–Merritt Phenomenon
    - Consumptive coagulopathy with severe thrombocytopenia
    - Medical therapy options include vincristine and sirolimus
    - Platelet transfusion not routinely recommended
    - Catheter embolization could be performed as an adjunct to medical therapy in severe cases, but only temporary increase in platelets

Figure 15-4

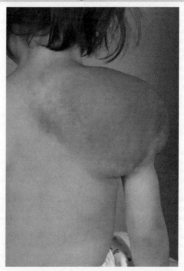

- **Vascular Malformations Classifications**
  - **Low flow**
    - Venous malformation (VM)
      - Most common vascular malformation treated by IR
      - Most are sporadic and unifocal
      - Composed of abnormal dilated venous channels with thin walls lined by endothelial cells
      - Congenital lesions that may be evident at birth, but often present in early childhood due to pain and swelling
      - Most commonly in soft tissues, but can involve all tissues and cross multiple tissue planes (muscle, bone)
      - Most common locations are extremities and head and neck
      - Variable appearance clinically: Dilated superficial veins, spongy focal lesion, complex venous channels crossing through multiple tissue planes, or diffuse extremity involvement
      - Most have bluish discoloration of the overlying skin, are soft and near completely compressible, refill with blood after compression, enlarge with dependent position or Valsalva
      - Variable communication with normal veins, will enlarge with compression of outflow veins
      - Acute pain can be caused by focal thrombosis within the VM, chronic intermittent pain is usually due to blood pooling and swelling, but also with muscle or joint involvement
      - *Glomuvenous malformations* are a variant lined by glomus cells, usually clinical diagnosis. Less amenable to traditional sclerotherapy options
      - *"Blue rubber bleb nevus syndrome"* is a disease of multiple VMs in the skin, subcutaneous tissues and GI track. Anemia is common due to chronic GI bleeding, often requiring treatment with iron and even blood transfusions
      - *"Hepatic hemangiomas"* and *"vertebral hemangiomas"* in adults are actually venous malformations
    - Lymphatic malformation (LM)
      - Cysts that contain lymphatic fluid and are lined by endothelial cells
      - Macrocystic (>1 cm), microcystic (<1 cm), or mixed types
      - Formerly called "cystic hygroma" or "lymphangioma"—inaccurate terminology that should not be used
      - Usually noted at birth, but can present later due to rapid growth related to superinfection, hemorrhage, or illness. Can also be diagnosed on prenatal imaging
      - Usually unifocal, but can have diffuse involvement of subcutaneous tissues
      - Most commonly involve subcutaneous soft tissue, but can involve any tissue, including bone
      - Most commonly located in head/neck and axillary regions
    - Capillary malformation (CM)
      - Most common vascular malformation
      - Cutaneous, flat, pink or red lesions
      - Present at birth
      - Most common seen in head and neck
      - Also called "Port-wine stains"
      - Can be associated with syndromes: Sturge–Weber, Klippel–Trenaunay
      - Can be treated with pulsed laser by plastics or dermatology, no role for IR
    - Combined (ie, CLM, VLM, etc.)
  - **High flow**
    - Arteriovenous malformation (AVM)
      - Complex network of abnormal vessels (nidus) between feeding arteries and veins without intervening capillary bed
      - Congenital, but usually dormant through childhood, can exhibit rapid growth during puberty, pregnancy or after trauma
      - Commonly "observed" in childhood with annual clinical follow-up
      - Commonly involve extremities, truck, and viscera and can be localized or extensive *(Pediatric Interventional Radiology: Handbook of Vascular and Non-Vascular Interventional. Springer; 2014)*
      - Can involve soft tissues and bone
      - May present as a pink skin lesion at birth and be mistaken for a CM *(Pediatric Interventional Radiology: Handbook of Vascular and Non-Vascular Interventional. Springer; 2014)*
      - Overgrowth and warmth of affected limb occurs due to local hypervascularity
      - Skin ulceration can occur due to venous congestion

- Can result in a steal phenomenon with ischemia to affected limb and rarely high output heart failure
- Clinically divided into 4 stages (Schobinger staging)
  - Stage 1: Quiescent—warm, vascular stain
  - Stage 2: Expansive—warmer, bruits/thrills, enlarging
  - Stage 3: Destructive—ulcers, bleeding, pain, bone lysis
  - Stage 4: Cardiac failure
- Arteriovenous fistula (AVF)
  - Simpler form with direct artery to vein connection with no intervening capillaries or nidus (Fig. 15-5)
  - Includes pulmonary "AVM" and Vein of Galen Malformation
  - Often acquired (ie, trauma, iatrogenic)

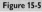

Figure 15-5

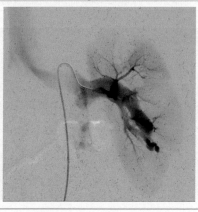

- **Syndromes Associated with Vascular Malformations**
  - Klippel–Trenaunay (CLVM): Evident at birth, sporadic, triad—(1) CM, (2) VM/varicosities, (3) regional growth disturbance, usually single lower extremity, soft tissue, and bone hypertrophy—may require surgical correction, pain usually related to venous congestion and thrombophlebitis, complications include recurrent LM infections/cellulitis, hemorrhage, and PE
  - Parkes Weber (CLAVF): Evident at birth, sporadic high flow vascular malformations composed of macro and micro AV fistulae, usually affect the extremities, associated with RASA-1 mutation, vascular skin stain ("pseudo CM") and overgrowth with prominent veins, LMs can occur as well (*Pediatric Interventional Radiology: Handbook of Vascular and Non-Vascular Interventional.* Springer; 2014)
  - Hereditary hemorrhagic telangiectasia (HHT):
    - Also called Osler–Weber–Rendu
    - Rare, autosomal dominant disorder
    - Multiple AVMs, often with the lungs, liver, and brain
    - Of all people with pulmonary AVMs, the majority will have HHT
    - Brain AVMs may cause headaches or seizure
    - May be asymptomatic until complicated by hemorrhage (stroke, hemoptysis)
    - Severe shunting can cause high output heart failure or hypoxia/cyanosis (pulmonary AVM)
    - Telangiectasias ("spider veins") seen on skin and mucous membranes
  - CLOVES syndrome: Acronym for **C**ongenital, **L**ipomatous, **O**vergrowth, **V**ascular malformations, **E**pidermal nevi, **S**pinal/skeletal anomalies; extremely rare overgrowth syndrome, somatic mutation in the PIK3CA gene
- **Imaging of Vascular Anomalies**
  - Most vascular anomalies can be diagnosed clinically and do not require imaging (ie, hemangiomas, capillary malformations)
  - If imaging is indicated, MRI and/or Ultrasound can be performed

- Ultrasound findings *(Semin Roentgenol 2012;47(2):106–17; Tech Vasc Interv Radiol 2011;14(1):22–31)*:
  - Infantile hemangioma: Circumscribed mass lesion, usually echogenic, but variable. High vessel density, hypervascular lesion with high flow during proliferative phase
  - Venous malformation: Often multiple hypoechoic and anechoic channels but can also be ill-defined solid echogenic lesions *(Semin Roentgenol 2012;47(2):106–17)*, compressible, occasional hyperechoic clots. May augment on spectral waveform imaging, may see monophasic slow flow on color Doppler, but often no flow noted.
  - Lymphatic malformation: Usually multispatial with numerous anechoic cysts, can be macrocysts (>1 cm) or microcysts (<1 cm), or "mixed" type (Fig. 15-6). If purely microcystic, often difficult to distinguish individual cysts. Can have echogenic debris from internal hemorrhage or infection. On Doppler, no internal blood flow, but can see flow in septations.
  - Arteriovenous malformation/fistula: Cluster of vessels without discrete mass, color Doppler shows arterial and venous waveforms, arterialization of draining veins

Figure 15-6

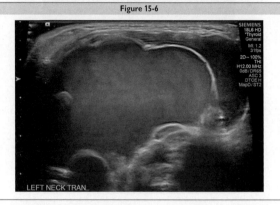

- MRI findings *(Semin Roentgenol 2012;47(2):106–17; Tech Vasc Interv Radiol 2011;14(1):22–31)*:
  - Infantile hemangioma: High signal on T2W, iso-signal on T1W, "flow void" artifact, intense diffuse postcontrast enhancement
  - Venous malformation: T1W intermediate signal, often heterogeneous, high signal on T2W FS, irregular patchy enhancement on early postcontrast imaging, diffuse enhancement if small or delayed postcontrast imaging (Fig. 15-7)
  - Lymphatic malformation: Low T1, high T2 signal, no internal postcontrast enhancement, septal enhancement (Fig. 15-8)
  - Arteriovenous malformation: Serpiginous flow voids, no associated soft tissue mass, MR angiogram may be helpful, as is dynamic postcontrast imaging (aka TWIST, TRICKS), to evaluate arterial component and identify the characteristic early draining vein(s). Feeding arteries are usually enlarged and outflow veins are enlarged and tortuous (Fig. 15-9)

- **Sclerotherapy for Venous Malformations**
  - Indications: Pain, joint involvement, disfigurement
  - If indicated, should be performed early in life since smaller lesions require fewer treatments. Risk of anesthesia in infants should also be considered.
  - Although sclerotherapy is the initial treatment of choice, other treatment options include: Surgical resection, laser photocoagulation, or a combination of these. No treatment option will consistently cure these lesions.
  - Anesthesia is typically required
  - When visible, ultrasound guidance should be utilized for needle access
  - 20G or 22G angiocatheters or other micropuncture needles can be utilized. Free back flow of blood should be noted after needle access.
  - After confirmed needle access and securement of the needle, dilute contrast should be injected slowly under fluoroscopy or digital subtraction imaging to evaluate for any extravasation and to look for brisk venous outflow (Fig. 15-10)
  - After contrast and blood are allowed to backflow through the access needle, the lesion is injected with an opacified sclerosant

Figure 15-7

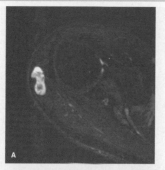

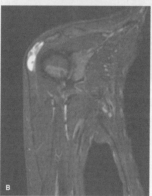

Figure 15-8

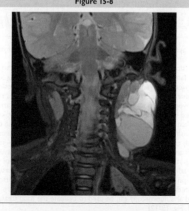

Figure 15-9

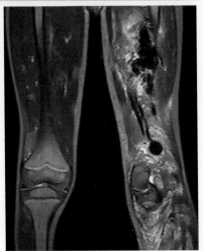

Figure 15-10

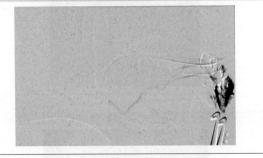

- Sclerosant options: 1% or 3% sodium tetradecyl sulfate (STS), dehydrated ethanol, bleomycin, or polidocanol
- Agent selection takes into account the side-affect, risk profile, location of the lesion, and familiarity and comfort of the operator. Consider using STS as 1st line, with bleomycin reserved for very superficial or orbit or tongue lesions (less inflammation). Ethanol has also been shown to be efficacious but carries risks of tachycardia, tachypnea, pulmonary hypertension, and cardiopulmonary arrest, and should only be used by experienced operators. STS can be mixed with lipiodol and air to create a foam that will allow for better stasis and contact with the endothelial cells lining the malformation (2 mL STS + 1 mL lipiodol + 2 mL air). Bleomycin can be diluted with contrast and sterile saline in the pharmacy (1 U/mL—max 0.5 U/kg, 15 U total) and chemotherapy precautions need to be taken *(Tech Vasc Interv Radiol 2011;14(1):22–31)*. Bleomycin carried the risk of hyperpigmentation of the skin and use of any adhesive material on the skin should be avoided. No cases of bleomycin associated pulmonary fibrosis have been reported with sclerotherapy doses.
- Multiple needle access sites are usually needed to cover the entire lesion. Ultrasound and fluoroscopy can be used to evaluate the total treatment area (Fig. 15-11, Fig. 15-12)

Figure 15-11

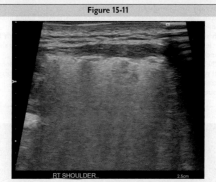

RT SHOULDER   2.5cm

Figure 15-12

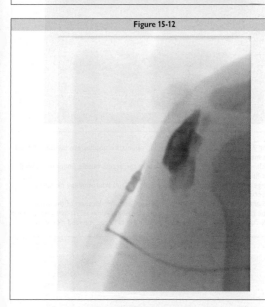

- Unless otherwise indicated (airway compression, unusual amount of pain), patients are discharged home same day. Pain medication is sometimes indicated. A pediatric pain scale should be utilized, especially in younger children (ie, Faces Pain Scale)
- Needles are removed and light manual pressure held until hemostasis is achieved
- Complications: Skin blistering and ulceration, nerve injury, hemoglobinuria, oliguria, DVT, hyperpigmentation (bleomycin)
- Goals of treatment: Pain resolution/improvement, shrinkage of the lesion (usually multiple treatments needed 6–8 w apart), rarely preoperative fibrosis to improve surgical outcome (less bleeding, improved safety and visibility)
- Usually outpatient same day procedure, may need admission if near airway or extensive lesion. Rarely need pain medication other than OTC options
- Patients are re-evaluated 4–6 w after the procedure and the decision to pursue addition treatments is made, usually at 6–8-w intervals

- **Sclerotherapy for Lymphatic Malformations**
  - Indications: Macrocystic disease, reduce size of mass, prevent future infection and spontaneous internal hemorrhage
  - As with venous malformations, intervention should be performed early in life since smaller lesions require fewer treatments. Risk of anesthesia in infants should also be considered.
  - Sclerotherapy is the initial treatment of choice. Other treatment options include: Surgical resection, medical therapy (sirolimus), or a combination of these. No single treatment option will consistently cure these lesions.
  - Ultrasound guidance should be utilized for needle access (Fig. 15-13)

Figure 15-13

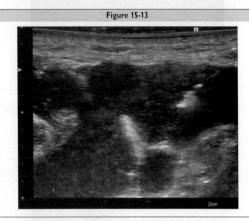

- 20G or 22G angiocatheters or other micropuncture needles can be utilized. Fluid within macrocysts should be aspirated.
- The sclerosant of choice is injected thought the access needle under ultrasound and/or fluoroscopic guidance (Fig. 15-14)
- For large macrocysts, consider drain placement and sclerotherapy performed on 3 consecutive d (*Pediatric Radiology* 2012;42:1080–8)
- Sclerosant choice again depends on operator comfort, location of the lesion and subtype (macro verses microcystic). Consider doxycycline as 1st-line agent, diluted in 50% contrast for a concentration of 10 mg/mL. Recommended max dose is

Figure 15-14

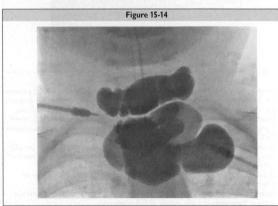

300 mg for patients <12 mo and 1200 mg in patients >12 mo (*Pediatric Radiology* *2012;42:1080–8*). Other agents that can be considered include OK-432 (0.1 mg in 10 mL saline, max 0.2 mg), bleomycin, STS, alcohol, or a combination of these (*Tech Vasc Interv Radiol 2011;14(1):22–31*). Consider bleomycin as first choice for microcystic disease or lesions near the airway or within the orbit or tongue (*Intervent Radiol 2014;37:1476–81*).

- Complications: Nerve injury, skin breakdown or ulceration, compartment syndrome (rare) (*Tech Vasc Interv Radiol 2011;14(1):22–31*)
- Usually performed as a nonurgent outpatient procedure, and unless the treated lesion is in a precarious location (orbit, tongue, next to airway), most patients are discharged home on the same day
- Patients are re-evaluated 4–6 w after the procedure and the decision to pursue addition treatments is made, usually at 6–8-w intervals (Fig. 15-15)

Figure 15-15

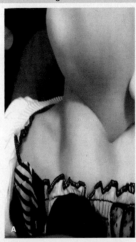

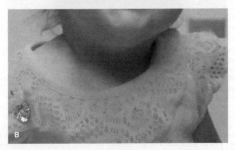

- **Embolization for the Treatment of AVM**
  - Most AVMs will eventually require treatment due to symptoms
  - Embolic treatment of AVMs carries significant risk and requires extensive experience and knowledge of the natural history of the lesion
  - Simple AVFs can be cured with embolization. More complex AVMs often require multiple embolization treatments, at 6–8-w interval, which will allow for symptom control, but will *not* cure the AVM (*Pediatric Interventional Radiology: Handbook of Vascular and Non-Vascular Interventional. Springer; 2014*)

- Conventional angiography is the gold standard to fully assess AVMs, but is not needed until treatment in eminently indicated
- Stage 3 and 4 lesions, and some stage 2 lesions, should be treated
- Diagnostic angiography should be performed for pretreatment planning, but can be done in conjunction with 1st embolization procedure
- General anesthesia is needed for pain management and paralysis during these lengthy procedures
- For lower extremity lesion, the "up and over" technique is preferred with contralateral common femoral artery access
- Ultrasound guidance and micropuncture technique should be used and a 4F or 5F sheath placed based on diagnostic catheter size and microcatheter compatibility
- Should perform "global" angiography of the entire limb affected with power injection and digital subtraction at a fast frame rate in multiple projections (Fig. 15-16). Also done at the start of subsequent treatment sessions. A "working" projection can then be identified. Consider use of road map technology to aid with subsequent selective catheterization (Pediatric Interventional Radiology: Handbook of Vascular and Non-Vascular Interventional. Springer; 2014; Tech Vasc Interv Radiol 2011;14(1):22–31).

Figure 15-16

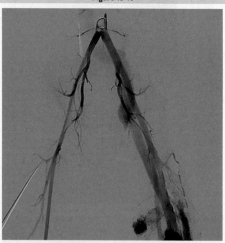

- The 4F or 5F diagnostic/guiding catheter should be advanced into the origin of a large feeding vessel, taking care not to impede flow (Fig. 15-17)
- If spasm occurs, consider administration of nitroglycerin
- AVMs can be treated by transarterial or transvenous approaches, or via direct access to the nidus. Combinations of these techniques are also used (Tech Vasc Interv Radiol 2011;14(1):22–31)
- For transarterial approach, a microcatheter and guidewire should be advanced through the diagnostic/guide catheter to the distal feeding artery near the nidus. Pre-embolization DSA, usually via had injection, must always be performed to evaluate for any opacification of nontarget arterial branches that should be spared, assess rate of antegrade flow, and monitor for reflux. Postembolic contrast is also performed to evaluate result and/or need for further embolization.
- For transvenous technique, a large draining vein is accessed in a retrograde fashion using ultrasound guidance with a small gauge needle (21G). Embolic agent may then be administered retrograde into the nidus while occluding venous outflow. (Tech Vasc Interv Radiol 2011;14(1):22–31)
- Direct access of a large nidus can also be performed with ultrasound-guided access and embolic agent administered directly into the nidus. Venous outflow must be occluded as well to prevent embolic agent for extending into the outflow vein and possibly into pulmonary artery circulation.

Figure 15-17

PEDIATRIC 15-15

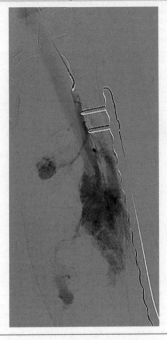

- Embolic agents
  - As with sclerosant use in low flow vascular malformation treatment, the specific embolic agent for AVM treatment will depend on the comfort level and experience of the operator, the location of the lesion, and the complexity of the AVM (# of feeding vessel, size and number of the nidi, flow rate through the lesion, and number and size of draining veins)
  - Embolic options include: Liquid (ethanol), semi-liquid (Onyx, NBCA glue), and solid (particles, gelfoam, coils). Combinations of techniques and agents can be used.
  - Ethanol: Steep learning curve for use, should be injected through a microcatheter in a distal feeding artery at a rate and volume determined during prior contrast injection, does not need opacification, can be repeated as needed, 0.2–2 mL per injection, waiting a minimum of 5–10 min between injections, most effective at endothelial destruction but can cause life-threatening hemodynamic changes (tachycardia, tachypnea, and hypertension)
  - n-Butyl-2-cyanoacrylate (NBCA) glue: Diluted and opacified with ethiodol, concentration will depend on flow rate and complexity of the nidus, with goal being to fill the nidus. If not dilute enough, it can plug up the feeding artery. If too dilute, it can traverse the nidus and enter to venous system with associated complications. For most AVMs, ratios of 1:3 (25%) or 1:4 (20%) are utilized. Dextrose 5% is used to flush the catheter before glue injection. Glue is injected slowly (~1 min) under imaging guidance, after which the microcatheter should be immediately retracted. Risk of "gluing" the catheter into the vessel.
  - Onyx (ethylene vinyl alcohol copolymer): Cohesive (nonadhesive) agent with more predictable flow behavior than glue, commonly used in brain AVMs (*Tech Vasc Interv Radiol* 2011;14(1):22–31)
  - Particles: Large particles can be used for preoperative devascularization, but use is not recommended for large shunts due to risk of extension into the pulmonary circulation

- Coils/plugs: Not recommended for most AVMs since occlusion of the feeding artery will limit future access ("burning bridges") and the nidus will recruit new feeding vessels; may be used to occlude distal feeding artery in simple AVFs (Fig. 15-18) or pulmonary AVM, or used in transvenous or direct nidus access to help fill the nidus and draining vein which will decrease the flow rate and allow for better penetration with a liquid embolic

Figure 15-18

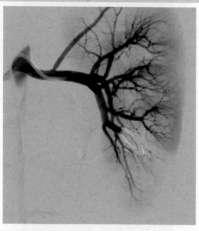

- Most patients are admitted postprocedure for at least 24 h to monitor for complications, usually related to nontarget embolization or embolic agent utilized. Swelling is common and may last up to 1 w. Skin ulceration can be managed in conjunction with plastic surgery. Aggressive hydration (2 times maintenance) is essential when ethanol is used due to hemoglobinuria. Bedrest is indicated for 6 h postfemoral sheath removal and peripheral pulses evaluated with vitals (Pediatric Interventional Radiology: Handbook of Vascular and Non-Vascular Interventional. Springer; 2014)
- Patients are discharged when tolerating fluids, pain is controlled by oral analgesics, and urine is normal in color and volume. Rigorous activity is avoided for at least 2 w (Pediatric Interventional Radiology: Handbook of Vascular and Non-Vascular Interventional. Springer; 2014)

Treatment of Scrotal Varicoceles
- **Definition** (J Ultrasound 2014;17(3):185–93)
  - Abnormal dilatation of the veins of the pampiniform venous plexus
- **Epidemiology** (J Ultrasound 2014;17(3):185–93; Urology 2007;70(2):362–5)
  - Incidence in adolescents/adults is between 10–20%
    - 6% of 10-y olds, 15% of patients >13 y
- **Pathophysiology** (J Ultrasound 2014;17(3):185–93; In: Coley B., ed. Caffey's Pediatric Diagnostic Imaging. Philadelphia, PA: Elsevier; 2013:126)
  - Scrotal varices formed due to increased venous pressure in the veins that drain the testicles
    - Continuous or intermittent reflux of venous blood into the pampiniform plexus → increased venous pressure with bulging of the veins and venous stasis → progressive dilatation and stagnation lead to hyalinization and weakening of the venous walls
      - Reflux of blood is usually due incompetent valves in either the main spermatic vein or a side branch (Fig. 15-19)
  - If unilateral, 99% are left sided
    - Bilateral varicoceles are common
    - Isolated right varicocele should prompt further workup for intraabdominal tumor or other etiology
      - The right spermatic vein enters directly into the IVC at an oblique angle, which results in less pressure and less back up of blood

Figure 15-19

PEDIATRIC 15-17

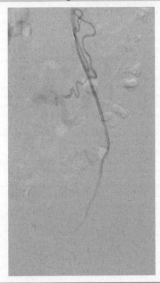

- Isolated right varicocele may be due extrinsic compression or narrowing of either the proximal IVC or right spermatic vein
- **Clinical Presentation** (*J Ultrasound* 2014;17(3):185–93; *J Vasc Intervent Radiol* 2012;23(2):206–10; *Ann Surg* 1988;207(2):223–7)
  - Often presents with "achy" pain or discomfort
  - Infertility:
    - Engorgement of venous blood around testicles leads to an increase in the temperature of the seminiferous tubules, which leads to issues with sperm quality
    - Impossible to predict which adolescent patients with varicoceles are at risk for infertility. Early treatment, even in asymptomatic individuals, may lead to increased testicular volume and increased sperm counts.
- **Diagnosis** (*Image-Guided interventions*. Philadelphia, PA: Saunders/Elsevier; 2014:79; *RadioGraphics* 2005;25(5):1197–14)
  - Most commonly found on physical exam of symptomatic patients. Palpation likened to feeling a "bag of worms"
    - Grading system of Dubin and Amelar:
      - Grade 0 = Not palpable.
      - Grade 1 = Palpable only with the patient standing and performing a Valsalva maneuver
      - Grade 2 = Palpable without Valsalva
      - Grade 3 = Visible
  - Imaging:
    - Tortuous, tubular, anechoic structures surrounding the testicles, representing dilated veins. Usually seen superior, lateral, and/or posterior to the testis. Blood flow on color Doppler imaging.
- **Indication for Treatment** (*Image-Guided interventions*. Philadelphia, PA: Saunders/Elsevier; 2014)
  - Primary indications include: Subfertility/infertility in adult men, testicular atrophy in adolescent or pediatric patients, or pain
- **Contraindications to Treatment** (*Image-Guided interventions*. Philadelphia, PA: Saunders/Elsevier; 2014)
  - Absolute:
    - Severe allergy to contrast

- Relative:
  - Coagulopathy requiring correction
- **Treatment** (*J Vasc Intervent Radiol* 2012;23(2):206–10; *Image-Guided Interventions.* Philadelphia, PA: Saunders/Elsevier; 2014; Treating Urogenital Vascular Conditions. In: *Interventional Radiology: A Survival Guide.* Elsevier; 2017:40)
  - Endovascular technique:
    - Initial venous access is obtained from either a femoral or jugular venous approach
      - Jugular has the added benefit of allowing for easier access of either the left or right spermatic veins from a single puncture
    - After obtaining venous access, a 7F–8F sheath is inserted
    - If the right groin is accessed, a modified Cobra catheter can be used to selectively catheterize the left renal vein and orifice of the left spermatic vein
    - For right-sided varicoceles, a nontapered 7F Simmons-1 guide catheter is used to select the origin of the right internal spermatic vein, commonly just below the right renal vein, anteriorly
    - If right internal jugular is accessed, a gently curved catheter can be used to either select the right or left spermatic vein
  - Left spermatic vein embolization:
    - The left renal vein is selected using the catheter and small injection of contrast is used to look for reflex into the spermatic vein (Fig. 15-20)

Figure 15-20

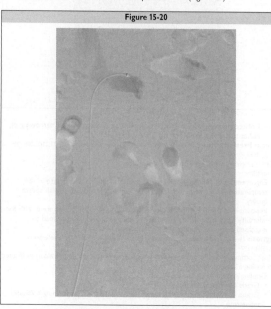

- Next the spermatic vein is selected using either the catheter or a hydrophilic wire. After this, between 10–20 mL of contrast material is injected to perform a selective venogram while the patient performed a Valsalva maneuver (Fig. 15-21)
  - Collimated fluoroscopic images are taken with the focus being from the veins orifice to the pubic symphysis to limit radiation dose to the testicles
- A variety of material can be used to occlude the vein: Embolization coils, microcoils, tissue adhesives, plugs, and sclerosant agents
- When using coils, a 5F nontapered straight catheter is used coaxially through the guide catheter to better control coil placement.
- When using coils or plugs, the vein is packed from the distal portion, just above the pubic symphysis, to its origin with the end point being complete occlusion (Fig. 15-22)

Figure 15-21

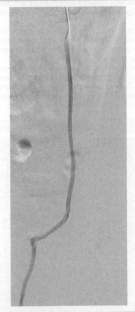

Figure 15-22

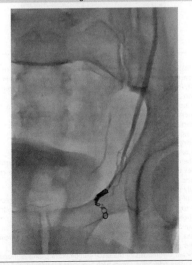

- Intermittent contrast injection is used to confirm placement and to check for the presence of large collateral veins that may also need embolized
- Must select large enough coils so that they pack well and will not become dislodged
- If a sclerosing agent is used, an occlusion balloon catheter is positioned just above the superior pubic ramus. After distal balloon occlusion, contrast is injected into the vein to approximate the amount of sclerosing agent needed. The balloon deflated before injection of the agent.
- Alternatively, coils may be packed within the distal spermatic vein to both estimates the required volume of agent need and to prevent reflux of the agent into the testicle. Coils are placed at the level of the pubic symphysis. The agent is then injected slowly, allowing for greater control. Intermittent contrast injection is performed to confirm occlusion (Fig. 15-23).

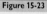

Figure 15-23

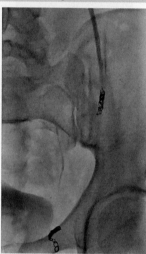

- Traditionally, only the sclerosing agent is injected into the vein to allow for occlusion. However, newer methods include injection of an agent, such as boiling contrast, followed by intermittent introduction of gelatin pledgets to aid in occlusion
  - After confirmation of occlusion, the catheters and sheath are removed
- Right spermatic vein embolization:
  - Technique is similar to the left, once the right spermatic vein is accessed
  - May require use of a microcatheter using a coaxial method
- Pitfalls during treatment:
  - No reflux of contrast into the spermatic vein
    - May be due to a competent valve near the origin of the spermatic vein
    - Implies that reflux maybe from a side branch rather than the renal vein
  - Spermatic vein spasm:
    - Usually self-limiting
    - A small dose of nitroglycerin, such as 100 µg, can be given directly into the vein. Wait approximately a minute and repeat the venogram after administration.
- Complications:
  - Less than 5% of cases.
    - Nausea, groin hematoma, reaction to contrast, and femoral vein thrombosis are the more common complications
    - Significant thrombosis of the distal pampiniform plexus is more common when using sclerosing agents with a reported incidence of 1–4%

- Recurrence rate between 4–11%, which is less than traditional surgery
- Retreatment using catheter-directed embolization is more difficult in patients who previously underwent the procedure verses those who had the traditional surgical approach
- **Postprocedure Care** (*Image-Guided Interventions*. Philadelphia, PA: Saunders/Elsevier; 2014)
  - Patients are observed for 4–6 h postprocedure
    - Maintenance intravenous fluids until the patient can tolerate PO
    - Pain control with NSAIDs
    - Rest is encouraged for the remainder of the day, then restoration of normal activity
  - Heavy lifting and sports may be resumed in 2 w
- **Long Term Follow-up**
  - None required unless symptomatic or recurrence

Pediatric Gastrointestinal (GI) Procedures

- **Overview** (*J Vasc Intervent Radiol* 2014;25(12):1983–91)
  - The vast majority of GI procedures covered in the adult chapter can be, and are, performed in the pediatric population with the most common being procedures for gastroenteric access to provide a route for feeding or decompression
- **Gastroenteric Access** (*Techn Vasc Intervent Radiol* 2010;13(4):222–8; *Image-Guided Interventions*. Philadelphia, PA: Saunders/Elsevier; 2014:133; *J Vasc Intervent Radiol* 2011;22(8):1089–106; *Pediatr Neurosurg* 2006;42(2):95–9; *Pediatric Radiology* 1998;28(7):521–3; *Arch Dis Child* 2009;94(9):668–73)
  - Background:
    - Most pediatric patients requiring gastroenteric access have neurodevelopmental or metabolic disorders
    - Proper nutrition is an extremely important aspect of a child's growth and development
    - Oral feeding may not be possible due to safety or adequacy concerns
      - Short-term nutrition supplementation can be provided via nasogastric (NG) or nasojejunal (NJ) tubes, usually no longer than 3 mo
      - Long-term nutritional requirements may require a gastrostomy or gastrojejunostomy tube
  - Indications:
    - Any child who will require frequent, long-term feeding support
      - Common diagnoses requiring long-term gastroenteric access
        - Neurologic impairment (congenital and acquired)
        - Gastrointestinal issues (severe reflux, dysmotility, malabsorption)
        - Chronic medical conditions (cardiac disease, end-stage renal failure, cystic fibrosis, high metabolic states)
    - More general indications include: Failure to thrive, recurrent aspiration, inadequate caloric intake, reflux, swallowing dysfunction, special dietary requirements, or medications
    - Achieving a specific weight may be a prerequisite to undergo certain surgeries (ie, cardiac, transplant)
  - Contraindications:
    - Absolute:
      - Uncorrectable, severe coagulopathy
      - Abnormal anatomy preventing the procedure from being done safely, which may require surgical approach or assistance with endoscopy
      - Unrepaired congenital diaphragmatic hernia or anterior abdominal wall defect
      - Severe intestinal obstruction (unless placed purposely for decompression)
    - Relative:
      - Coagulopathy requiring correction
      - Clinically unstable
      - Recent VP shunt placement
        - Increased risk of shunt infection (recommend waiting >1 mo)
  - Special considerations:
    - Gastrostomy (G) vs. gastrojejunostomy (GJ)
      - Any patient with gastroesophageal reflux and a severe condition requiring gastroenteric access will likely not tolerate G-tube feeding
      - Children with significant comorbidities often do better with a GJ
      - G feeds are usually boluses and require shorter feeding hours
      - GJ feeds are usually continuous at a lower rate with longer feeding hours
      - If G feeds are ideal in a patient with comorbidities and reflux, anti-reflux surgery (ie, Nissen) can be combined with the gastrostomy in an attempt to increase tolerance
      - Often a G-tube will be the initial feeding tube placed, but it can be converted to a GJ in the future (after 4–6 w)

- Social aspects:
  - Need for gastroenteric access and tube feeds can be psychologically and emotionally very difficult for patients and caregivers. Food and meals are a large part of many cultures and it can be difficult for a caregiver to accept their child's inability to participate.
  - A multidisciplinary approach is recommended to assess the needs of the child
  - Caregiver education and ability to perform feeding tube maintenance is also a necessary skill
- **Procedure** (*J Vasc Intervent Radiol* 2014;25(12):1983–91; *Techn Vasc Intervent Radiol* 2010;13(4):222–8; *Image-Guided Interventions.* Philadelphia, PA: Saunders/Elsevier 2014:133; *J Vasc Intervent Radiol* 2011;22(8): 1089–106; *Interventional radiology: A survival guide.* Elsevier; 2017:42; *Cochrane Database Syst Rev* 2006:(4): CD005571; *Radiology* 1996;201(3):691–95)
  - Technical aspects independent of technique:
    - Pediatric fasting guidelines are followed
      - Avoiding long fasting periods
      - Maintain hydration and euglycemia using IV hydration or clear fluids with dextrose
  - Antibiotic prophylaxis
    - Patients undergoing gastroenteric access are often at risk for infection due to poor nutrition, immunocompromised status, or significant comorbidities
    - Antegrade technique for access has a reported incidence of 5.4–30% stoma infection, probably related to contamination by oral flora. Therefore, patients undergoing antegrade technique should receive antibiotic prophylaxis.
    - Prophylaxis with the retrograde technique is controversial, but many proceduralists will give a single preprocedure prophylactic dose
  - 0.2–0.5 mg of Glucagon IV can be given to achieve gastric atony and pyloric constriction
  - In both techniques, the lower margins of the spleen and liver can be identified using ultrasound and marked on the skin
  - If the location of the colon is a concern, it can be filled with dilute barium, either given by mouth hours before the procedure or by enema immediately before
  - G-tube size recommendations:
    - Weight based: <10 kg = 10F; 10–25 kg = 12F, >25 kg =14F
    - Varies depending on institution
  - Retrograde Technique—G-tube:
    - Widely used method because it can be performed without general anesthesia and has a low incidence of major complications
    - Can be used in patients with esophageal stricture, esophageal atresia, or oropharyngeal abnormalities
      - In patients with esophageal atresia, the retrograde method has been described after gastric distension through puncturing the stomach with a 22G needle under ultrasound guidance
    - While the patient is in the supine position, a nasogastric (NG) tube is placed
    - Air is then pumped into the stomach, through the NG, until it is sufficiently distended
    - The site of access is then chosen using a combination of fluoroscopy and ultrasound
      - The ideal target it at the mid to distal gastric body, equidistant from the lesser and greater curvatures, to minimize the risk of arterial injury
      - Generally lateral to the rectus muscle and 2 cm from the lower costal margin is a good location. But better to go through the rectus muscle than too close to the pylorus
    - Once the site of puncture is chosen, local anesthesia is administered, and an 18G needle preloaded with a pediatric retention suture is used to puncture the air distended stomach under intermittent fluoroscopy
      - The needle is also connected to a contrast filled syringe through a T connector so a small amount of contrast can be injected once the puncture is complete to confirm intraluminal gastric location
      - Angling the initial puncture toward the pylorus may be useful if there is a possibility of future G to GJ conversion (Fig. 15-24)
    - A small nick in the skin is made along the needle tract to allow for easier passage of the dilators and eventually the tube
    - The retention suture is deployed by advancing a 0.035-in guide wire
      - The retention suture thread is secured

Figure 15-24

PEDIATRIC

15-23

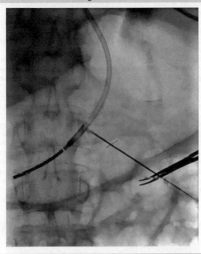

- The needle is removed and the tract dilated to accommodate the intended tube size
  - The tract must be larger than the tube itself. Some studies suggest 2F beyond the size of the chosen tube is ideal. Alternatively, a peel away sheath can be utilized.
- The G-tube is then inserted into the stomach over the wire using intermittent fluoroscopy guidance
- There are multiple types of tubes, anything from a standard pigtail catheter secured to the skin to a button G tube with a retention balloon can be used
- If a pigtail catheter is initially used, eventual conversion to a "button" low profile G tube is ideal as they are easier to use for the caretakers
- Antegrade or "Pull" Technique—G-tube:
  - Requires a specific tube designed for the procedure that is significantly longer than the retrograde type
    - Tapered distal end that acts as a dilator with the proximal end functioning as an internal fixator
    - Distal tapered end has a looped wire attached
  - Much like the retrograde technique, an NG is passed into the stomach
  - Adjacent to the NG, a goose-neck type snare catheter is passed per orally into the stomach
    - Once in the stomach, the snare is opened under fluoroscopy
  - The stomach is insufflated and the site of access chosen
  - After selecting an appropriate site, local anesthesia is administered and the stomach punctured with an 18G needle attached to a syringe of contrast
    - The tip of the needle is aimed toward the center of the snare within the stomach
  - After stomach puncture, a small nick is made in the skin with a scalpel to facilitate passage of the feeding tube
  - Once gastric location is confirmed, a looped wire is passed through the needle into the stomach. Length of the looped wire is key since it will need to span the entire length of the thorax and mouth while maintaining percutaneous access into the stomach.
  - The looped wire is then snared by the goose-neck snare catheter from above
  - The oral catheter, with the looped wired entering through the stomach firmly snared, is pulled up slowly through the esophagus and out the mouth
  - The special G-tube with the loop attached at the distal, tapered end is then safely and securely attached to the looped wire coming from the gastrostomy needle

- Next, using gentle traction from below and intermittent fluoroscopy, the looped wire with the G-tube attached is slowly pulled down through the esophagus, into the stomach, and out the puncture site
- The tube is pulled until resistance is felt, indicating the end of the tube with the internal fixation portion has been reached
- The catheter often also comes with an external fixator that is attached after placement to help hold it in place
- The long, "dilator" portion of the tube is cut and the hub is attached to allow for medication administration and feeding. Some catheters have premeasured markings on where to cut the excess off. If not, it can be cut approximately 10–15 cm from the stomach.

- **GJ Tube:**
  - A retrograde G-tube can be converted to a GJ tube once the tract has matured (~6 w)
    - Performed with fluoroscopic guidance utilizing a guidewire and angled guide catheter to cross the pylorus and access the proximal small bowel
    - Alternatively, the GJ tube can be "stiffened" with a guidewire, advanced through the gastrostomy, and across the pylorus to access the proximal small bowel. This works best with smaller children and a favorable stoma trajectory.
    - GJ conversions and exchanges are routinely performed without sedation, with the aid of child life specialists. Parents may be allowed to come in for the procedure at the discretion of the proceduralist.
    - Contrast should be injected following placement to confirm tip position (Fig. 15-25)

Figure 15-25

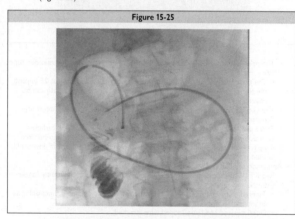

- After tube is in position, the retention balloon can then be inflated with sterile water (recommended) or dilute contrast. If an "adjustable" stoma length GJ is utilized, contrast should also be injected via the Gastrostomy port to confirm balloon position
- There is some controversy as to if, and when, to perform "routine" GJ exchanges. Many pediatric IRs do perform routine exchanges between 3–6 mo, prior to tube malfunction, clogging, or balloon failure/dislodgement
- If a primary GJ is to be placed, the technique is similar to that of a retrograde G-tube
  - If colonic visualization is required, keep barium to a minimum as to not obscure portions of the small bowel
  - Glucagon should not be given as to make passage of a catheter through the pylorus easier
  - Once the stomach is punctured, using intermittent fluoroscopy, a long 0.035-in, floppy tip wire is advanced to deploy the retention anchor and maintain access
  - While maintaining the wire in the stomach, the needle is removed and an angled catheter is advanced into the stomach over the wire

- With the wire still in the catheter, under fluoroscopic guidance, the catheter is manipulated to gain access into the duodenum, and catheter and wire are then advanced to the level of the duodenojejunal junction (DJJ)
  - The catheter is then removed while maintaining wire access, and the GJ tube is advanced over the wire into the proximal small bowel
- Complications:
  - Published rates of complications are limited in pediatric literature but range from 0.39–9%.
  - Potential complications:
    - Accidental organ puncture (liver, colon, etc.)
    - Retention suture breaks (if a functioning retention suture is required, it can be placed directly adjacent to the tube)
    - Inadvertent peritoneal placement, which usually occurs during dilation. Fluoroscopy during dilation or use of a stiffer wire will help minimize this risk
    - Pneumoperitoneum (large pneumoperitoneum may require needle decompression)
- **Postprocedural care** (*Techn Vasc Intervent Radiol* 2010;13(4):222–8; *Image-Guided Interventions.* Philadelphia, PA: Saunders/Elsevier; 2014:133)
  - Patients are usually monitored as an inpatient for up to 3 d
  - Patients are usually kept NPO for 12–24 h postprocedure with the G tube to gravity drainage
    - IV hydration with isotonic fluid containing glucose is used to maintain euglycemia.
    - After 12 h, if bowel sounds are present, the NG is clamped and the diet advanced to clear liquids through the G-tube
      - Advanced gradually over the next 48 h to full feeds (consider nutrition consult)
      - If tolerating feeds, NG is removed
  - Glucose level is checked if glucagon was given due to risk of rebound hypoglycemia
  - Pain control:
    - Morphine IV may be required initially
    - Afterward, acetaminophen 15 mg/kg PO or rectally is usually sufficient
  - If barium was given for colon visualization, consider a stool softener
  - The retention anchor suture can be cut approximately 14 d post procedure.
  - It takes the tract around 6 w to mature, but once mature, if a generic pigtail catheter was used, it is replaced with a more traditional, low-profile tube
- **Long-term followup** (*Image-Guided Interventions.* Philadelphia, PA: Saunders/Elsevier 2014:133; *Pediatr Radiol* 2008;38(9):963–70)
  - A feeding tube requires a commitment to ongoing maintenance by the caregiver and constant reevaluation of the child's nutritional status and needs, including: ability to feed orally, presence of reflux, safety with different food consistencies, further need for a G/GJ tube, and potential need to convert a G into a GJ
  - Children usually show weight gain in the 1st 6 mo
  - If a pigtail catheter is used initially, it is in both the patient's and caregiver's best interest to convert to a button tube as quickly as possible (6 w).
  - If conversion from a G to a GJ tube is necessary, often a tube placed in IR is easier to convert than one placed surgically or using endoscopy
- **Cecostomy placement** (*Pediatric Interventional Radiology: Handbook of Vascular and Non-Vascular Interventional.* Springer; 2014)
  - **Indications**
    - Chronic constipation, colonic dysmotility, and associated fecal incontinence not responding to medical management
    - Commonly in utilized in patients with spina bifida or cerebral palsy
    - Allows for anterograde bowel irrigation instead of enemas, improving patient quality of life with better control of bowel movements and less incontinence
    - Multidisciplinary decision (GI, surgery, dieticians, IR)
    - Performed less frequently with the advent of appendicocecostomy (Malone Procedure), which creates a surgical route for bowel irrigation
  - **Preprocedure**
    - Clears liquid diet for 2 d prior
    - Bowel prep the day prior (similar to colonoscopy prep, vary by institution)
  - **Procedure**
    - Usually GA or sedation required
    - Prophylactic antibiotic needed (cefoxitin)
    - Ultrasound can be utilized to map out the liver margin and urinary bladder

- The colon is insufflated with air
- Cecum is localized under fluoroscopy
- An 18G needle is advanced into the cecum and contrast injected to confirm placement
- Anchor sutures can then be deployed through this needle access
- A stiff guidewire is then advanced through the needle and needle removed
- The tract is then dilated over the guidewire, and an 8F locking pigtail catheter of choice is placed
- The catheter is secured with suture and sterilely dressed
- **Postprocedural care**
  - Overnight admission for observation (fever, diffuse abdominal pain)
  - Advance diet as tolerated
  - Normal saline flushed started after 24 h
  - Retention sutured can be cut at 14 d
  - At 6–8 w, the catheter is exchanged for a low-profile cecostomy tube (commonly a Chait Percutaneous Cecostomy Catheter—Cook Medical)
  - Cecostomy tubes should be replaced as needed when malfunction or dislodgement occurs, and at a minimum, annually

GYNECOLOGIC INTERVENTIONS

UTERINE ARTERY EMBOLIZATION

Uterine Fibroid Embolization

Patient Selection

- **Indications**
  Symptomatic fibroid disease: Menorrhagia, dysmenorrhea, pelvic pain, urinary frequency, hydronephrosis
- **Contraindications**
  Absolute: Pregnancy, active PID, prior pelvic radiation, suspected uterine/endometrial/cervical cancer
  Relative: Fibroids that may respond best to hysterectomy/myomectomy → intracavitary and <3 cm, subserosal and large/pedunculated, total uterine size >24 w, location within the cervix or broad ligament

Preprocedural Management

- **Endometrial Biopsy (to r/o malignancy)**
  - Warranted in ALL postmenopausal patients
  - Consider in premenopausal patients with irregular menses (more frequent than q21d and/or lasting longer than 10 d)
- **Rx**
  - Gonadotropin-releasing meds → often used in treatment of fibroids; constrict uterine artery; should be stopped for 3 mo prior to procedure
  - Antipyrexial + Antiemetic + Opioid → to prevent postembolization syndrome: Regimen varies by institution, but typically ketorolac + ondansetron + hydromorphone before and during the procedure
- **Imaging of Fibroids**
  - **Goal: Document treatable fibroid(s), exclude alternative pathology**
  - US is a reasonable imaging option, but pelvic MR has added information (extrauterine pathology, enhancement characteristics) (*J Vasc Interv Radiol* 2002;13:1149–53)
  - Predictors of best response: Submucosal > intramural > subserosal location, smaller fibroids, avid enhancement
  - Pedunculated subserosal fibroids show less shrinkage post UAE, and thus, less symptom relief (*J Vasc Interv Radiol* 2008;19:662–7)
  - Cervical fibroids have robust vascularity (possibly alternative or collateral) and have low success rates with UAE (*J Vasc Interv Radiol* 2012;23:236–40)
  - **High T2 signal on MR predicts good response to therapy**

Equipment

- Angio suite w/: roadmapping capability, available pulsed fluoro rate of ≤15/s
- 4F or 5 F catheter for internal iliac a. selection
- 0.025 or 0.028-in microcatheter with microwire for uterine a. (UA) selection
- **Embolic Material**
  - Targeting precapillary level: 500–900 μM beads (*Cardiovasc Intervent Radiol* 2010;33:943–8; *Abdom Imaging* 2004;29:128–31)
  - **Goal = preserve cervicovaginal + ovarian arteries** → These are <500 μM
  - Infibroid centripetal arteries are <500 μM, but perifibroid plexus arteries are 500–100 μM → this allows for selective embo with calibrated microspheres
  - Spherical PVA or TAGM → RCTs have shown better fibroid infarction and long term clinical outcomes with TAGM as compared to conventional spherical PVA
  - No RCT data on new embolics: PVA hydrogel or Polyzene F-coated hydrogel

Technique

- **Access Options**
  - Femoral a. access → steps detailed below
  - Radial a. access
    - **Benefit:** Avoid postprocedural lower-extremity immobilization
    - **Limitation:** Longer distance to target vessel, may exceed catheter length in tall patients
    - **Technique:** Anterior division of each internal iliac artery can be accessed with an MPA (in contrast to steps below)
- *Bilateral UAE is required* regardless of fibroid location → to prevent formation of new collaterals

GYNECOLOGIC INTERVENTIONS & PREGNANCY

Procedure

1. Obtain arterial access + place 5F sheath
2. Position pigtail flush catheter in the infrarenal abdominal aorta
3. Perform DSA + generate roadmap
4. Advance Bentson through the catheter + position system over the iliac bifurcation
5. Advance Bentson into the external iliac artery
6. Remove flush catheter and advance a uterine catheter or MPA. Puff contrast and advance the catheter to the origin of the uterine artery. Perform DSA as needed to define anatomy.
7. Position the image intensifier to optimize visualization of the UA origin
8. Advance the microcatheter into the horizontal segment of the uterine artery
9. Perform power injected DSA to check for collaterals to ovary (3 cc/s for 9 cc)
10. Mix embolic. Embolize under fluoro
11. Flush and remove microcatheter
12. Push uterine catheter into the aorta with wire. Form Waltman loop. Get Bentson down the ipsilateral internal iliac and pull uterine catheter down
13. Repeat embolization on ipsilateral side
14. Close

Technical Notes

- Optimized view of UA origin conventionally achieved with **10° of ipsilateral oblique**, but in reality varies with anatomy
- UA anatomic variants:
  - Origin from the anterior division of the internal iliac a. as 2nd or 3rd branch in 51% of pts → best imaged in contralateral anterior oblique
  - Origin from a trifurcation of the internal iliac a. in 40% → best imaged in ipsilateral anterior oblique
  - Origin from the ipsilateral ovarian a. in 1% of pts
- UA Selection: 4F or 5F catheter may be used to access the UA, but if causes spasm should be retracted to the internal iliac a. and a microcath advanced coaxially to the UA
  - For nontortuous UA: Advance catheter to **major medial turn of the vessel** and place in proximal portion of the transverse segment beyond origin of any side branches
  - For tortuous UA: Advance to just proximal to the first severely angulated segment to avoid spasm
- *If suspicion for collateral supply to ovaries based on run,* may use 700–900 μM beads instead of 500–700 μM as a precaution
- Embolization endpoint = Subtotal occlusion (5 beat stasis)
  - TAGM → Embolize until UA forward flow slows to sluggish, with occlusion of fibroid feeding distal branches and patent UAs ("pruned tree" appearance)
  - All other spherical embolics (ie, PVA) → embolize to stasis/near stasis
  - Always wait a few minutes after apparent endpoint to ensure no early recanalization
- Postembolization intraarterial administration of 1% lidocaine → associated with lower pain scores, no change in analgesic requirements, and moderate to severe vasospasm (*J Vasc Interv Radiol* 2001;12:1065–9)
- *Collateral branches off the ovarian artery typically also feed fibroids* → if large caliber (≥IMA diameter), may also warrant treatment (700–900 μM beads)

Postprocedure Management

Overnight Admission for:

1. **Pain Control**
   - 1000 mg acetaminophen IV 1× in PACU
   - Ibuprofen 600 mg PO q6h + PCA while inpatient
2. **PRN Antiemetic**
3. **IV Fluids**

Typical return to work time = 1 w

- **Postembolization Syndrome** (*Semin Intervent Radiol* 2013;30:354–63)
  - Expected postprocedural syndrome of pain, nausea/vomiting, malaise/fever, and low-grade fever related to iatrogenic infarction
  - Pain usually peaks at 8–12 h

- Systemic symptoms usually peak at 2–3 d
- Etiology: Thought to be related to infarction of nontarget, normal myometrium → ischemia induces acidosis, anaerobic metabolism, accumulation of lactate and adenosine which induce pain via chemoreceptors
- **"Rule of 3 d"** → starts w/ in 3 d, resolves within 3 d; if meets these criteria, no blood cultures required
- Higher risk with larger tumors

Complications
- **Fibroid Passage**
  - Incidence: 2.5% (Obstet Gynecol 2002;100:873–80)
  - Symptoms: Pain, bleeding, infection
  - Occurs only in submucosal fibroids
  - Occurs 3 mo–3 y after UAE
  - Requires pelvic exam and MR evaluation
  - Treatment: NSAIDs/oral narcotics, PO/IV abx, sometimes D&C
- **Severe Infection** → Requires abx or surgical intervention in 1.2% (J Vasc Interv Radiol 2004;15:1415–21)
- **Access Site Injuries** → Artery or nerve; 0.1% of cases
- **Premature menopause:** Incidence = 7.3%; risk is higher in pts over 45 y.o.; likely 2' nontarget embolization of the ovarian arteries via tubal branches (Obstet Gynecol 2005;106:1309–18)
- **DVT/PE:**
  - Incidence = 1 in 200 pts (Obstet Gynecol 2001;98:29–34), decreasing compression of pelvic veins as fibroids shrink → allows clot to migrate
  - Ppx w/ SCDs for all pts, consider LMWH for high risk patients
- **Pregnancy Complications**
  - RCT compared reproductive outcomes following myomectomy vs. UFE (Cardiovasc Intervent Radiol 2008;31:73–85) @ 2 y: UFE less likely to become pregnant (RR 0.45), less likely to deliver full term (RR 0.64), and more likely to miscarry (RR 2.7); however still had 50% chance of getting pregnant
  - Systematic review reveals no increased odds of preterm delivery, malpresentation, or IUGR, but increased risk of miscarriage (OR 2.8), C-section (OR 2.1), and postpartum hemorrhage (OR 6.4) with UFE vs. myomectomy

Follow-Up
Protocol: F/U MR + Clinic Visit @ 6 mo
- Fibroids decrease in volume by 40–60% → shrinkage may not yet be seen with shorter interval imaging f/u

Outcomes (Cochrane Database Syst Rev 2014;(12):CD005073; Obstet Gynecol 2005;106:933-9)
- Largest registry is SIR's **FIBROID registry** (2729 pts)
  - 87% w/ improvement in symptom scores 1 y posttreatment
  - 85% of pts satisfied with outcome 3 y posttreatment
  - 9.8% hysterectomy, 2.9% myomectomy, 1.8% repeat UAE at 3 y followup
- RCTs comparing UFE vs. Surgery
  - **EMMY Trial** (multicenter): UFE vs. Hysterectomy
    - Shorter hospital stays with UFE vs. hysterectomy
    - At 2 y: Similar symptom control, health related QoL, and pt satisfaction; but 24% of UAE pts had undergone subsequent hysterectomy
    - At 5 y: Similar symptom control, plus an additional 4% of UAE pts had undergone subsequent hysterectomy
  - **REST Trial** (multicenter): UFE vs. Hysterectomy or Myomectomy
    - No difference in complication rates
    - Higher reintervention rate among UFE pts (20% by 32 mo, 32% by 5 y)
    - At 5 y: Symptoms and health related quality of life similar in both groups

Other Applications of Uterine Artery Embolization

Postpartum Hemorrhage
- Embolic material: Foam or glue

Adenomyosis
- Embolic material: 300–500 μM beads (targeting capillary level; higher risk of ovarian embo/premature ovarian failure than in UFE) typically followed by 500–700 μm beads
- Outcomes → ~50% of patients achieve durable relief of symptoms and avoid need for surgical reintervention (Semin Intervent Radiol 2008;25:387–93)

Ovarian Vein Embolization for Pelvic Congestion Syndrome

Patient Selection
- Indications
  - Pelvic pain, dyspareunia, menstrual abnormalities, vulvar/lower extremity varices PLUS **gonadal vein diameter of 10 mm** or greater PLUS **reflux and stasis** of the ovarian veins during diagnostic angiography
  - Note: **Low PPV for dilated vessels alone!** → Present in 50% of multiparous women
  - Typically, symptomatic worsening with: Upright positioning, toward the end of the day, with sexual arousal, during menstruation
- Etiology
  - Incompetent valves at ovarian v. orifices (incidence: **L >> R**) → reflux into ovarian v. and sometimes even iliac v.
- Epidemiology
  - Increased incidence with: Prior pregnancy, tubal ligation, IUD, nutcracker syndrome

Preprocedural Management
- Dx of exclusion after complete GYN workup and attempted medical management, sometimes including ex lap
- CT or MR → documenting dilation of ovarian veins to 10 mm (5 mm = normal)

Equipment (Cardiovasc Intervent Radiol 2015;38:806–20)
- Microcath system for selection
- 4F or 5F sheath for embolic delivery
- Sclerosant or embolic: ie, 3% sodium tetradecyl sulfate diluted to 2% with contrast, polidocanol; ie, Gelfoam
- Coils or plugs: Oversizing important to prevent nontarget embo of renal v. or pulmonary a., esp. bc these veins are usually incompetent → 1–2 mm oversizing is recommended for each vein; corresponds to 20–30% oversizing for ovarian v. and 15–20% oversizing for iliac v. (J Vasc Interv Radiol 2018; 29:45–53)

Technique—Ovarian Vein Embolization
1 Obtain venous access—IJ or femoral
2 Place 7F sheath
3 Select L renal v. with 7F guidecath: Diagnostic run as detailed below
4 Advance 5F hydrophilic catheter coaxially over guide wire into L ovarian v. to the level of the pelvis
5 Perform ovarian venogram
6 Mix sclerosant and/or embolic (varies by institution) and inject
7 Wait 3–5 min—then occlude main L ovarian v. with coils or plugs
8 Repeat on R—origin (usually) directly from IVC
9 Close

Technical Notes
- Access
  - IJ or CFV → Recurved cath and long curve guide cath or sheath for CFV access
- Note: L ovarian v. targeted 1st bc more easily accessed and more commonly affected than R
- L renal venogram → + dx when reflux into L ovarian vein is documented, plus:
  - Dilated to 10 mm
  - Shows stasis (~10 min) → then generally drains to contralateral normal ovarian v. or hypogastric v.
- Staged Treatment Approach
  - 1st Treatment Session: Sclerosis of parauterine venous plexus + coil/plug ovarian veins
  - 2nd Treatment Session (PRN based on symptoms): Coil/plug internal iliac veins → typically 3–6 w later

Postprocedural Management
- Pain/pressure → may increase for days to weeks postprocedure, self-limiting
- Potential complications
  - Iliac or renal v. thrombosis
  - PE

Followup
- Clinic visits: Typically 3–4 mo post, then 12 mo post
- Long-term symptom relief → achieved in 82–94% of pts (Cardiovasc Intervent Radiol 2007;30:655–61; Cardiovasc Intervent Radiol 2007;36:1006–14; Cardiovasc Intervent Radiol 2013;36:1006–14)

Fallopian Tube Recanalization (Curr Opin Obstet Gynecol 2004;16:221–9; Radiographics 2000;20:1759–68)

Preprocedural Management
- Epidemiology
  - 30% of cases of female subfertility are tubal in origin
  - Tubal origin infertility is often a consequence of PID or endometriosis
- Pt Selection
  - Pts w/ distal disease (ie, fimbrial) better treated with surgery or IVF
  - Pts with proximal tubal obstruction (PTO) may be candidates for fluoroscopic or endoscopic intervention → may be due to fibrosis, debris, adhesions
- Indication: **Female subfertility** + HSG with **bilateral PTO**
- Contraindications: Active pregnancy, active PID, abnormal recent pap
- ABX: 100 mg doxycycline PO BID for 5 d, starting 2 d preprocedure

Equipment
- Speculum
- Transcervical catheter (ie, 12F transcervical cannula w/ 5F inner)
- 1:2 dilution of iodinated contrast in normal saline
- 40 cm angled tip 4F or 5F cath for selective salpingography
- 0.018 or 0.035 hydrophilic angled tip guidewire for traversing obstructed tube ± 3F microcath for column strength

Technique—Fallopian Tube Recanalization

Cervical Cannulation
1 Insert speculum into vagina to achieve visualization of the cervix
2 Swab and cannulate cervix with occlusive catheter—seal with endocervical balloon
3 Inject 30% water soluble contrast to opacify uterine cavity—proceed if fallopian tubes do not opacify normally

Selective Salpingography
4 Advance 5F curved cath over a guidewire to the cornua
5 Gently inject contrast—proceed if reveals PTO

Fallopian Tube Recanalization
6 Advance 3F tapered catheter over a 0.015 guidewire coaxially through 5F system to cross the tubal obstruction
Repeat 4–6 for contralateral side PRN
Repeat selective salpingography

*** **Troubleshooting:** 0.016 floppy tipped tapered guidewire or 0.035 angled tip hydrophilic guidewire can be used as 2nd line to cross most obstructions
- Endpoint = Patent tube with free intraperitoneal contrast spillage, or patent proximal tube unmasking distal blockage @ fimbriae (needs surgery)

IR and Special Considerations in Pregnancy (J Vasc Interv Radiol 2012;23:19–32)

Dose Limits/Limiting Dose
- Threshold dose for effects to fetus: >100–200 mGy
- Nonemergent fluoroscopic procedures are contraindicated during pregnancy
  - Early Pregnancy → Risk for fetal genetic mutation
  - Late Pregnancy → Risk for fetal mental retardation or leukemia
- Emergent cases
- Close collaboration with medical physicist and OB required
- Minimize fetal exposure by:
  - Minimizing pulse rate
  - Minimizing patient distance from detector
  - Maximizing patient distance from X-ray tube
  - Excluding fetus from beam if possible
  - Collimating
  - Neck or upper extremity access if possible (vs. groin)
  - Maximizing kVP/minimizing mA
- If pt and fetus survive acute scenario, formal fetal dose calculation is warranted → to guide possible recommendation for termination

Iodinated Contrast
- Risks of iodinated contrast to fetus have not been fully studied → however, no reports in literature of adverse effects
- ACOG and ACR positions: Iodinated contrast is safe in pregnancy (J Vasc Interv Radiol 2012;23:19–32)
  - Theoretical risk of hypothyroidism in neonates exposed to iodinated contrast in utero → recommended thyroid function panel in first few days of life

TRAUMATIC LIVER INJURIES

Background

- The liver is the 2nd most commonly injured organ in blunt abdominal trauma after the spleen with an incidence of 15–20% (*Surg Clin North Am* 1975;55:387–07)
- Dual blood supply of liver lends to frequent hepatic vascular injury which may present as intraperitoneal hemorrhage (hemoperitoneum), hepatic laceration, subcapsular hematoma, intraparenchymal hematoma, arteriovenous fistula (AVF), pseudoaneurysm (PSA), hemobilia, or thrombosis (*Handbook of Interventional Radiology Procedures*. 2011: Lippincott Williams & Wilkins)
- Clinically significant hemorrhage from traumatic liver injuries can occur from hepatic arterial or hepatic venous injury (*Handbook of Interventional Radiologic Procedures*. 2011: Lippincott Williams & Wilkins)
- Hepatic venous injury (hepatic veins or IVC) carries high mortality (*Handbook of Interventional Radiological Procedures*. 2011: Lippincott Williams & Wilkins)
- Hepatic arterial injury is more common and can be treated with embolization in select patients (*Handbook of Interventional Radiologic Procedures*. 2011: Lippincott Williams & Wilkins)
- Can rarely present with retroperitoneal hemorrhage (hemoretroperitoneum) if bare area of liver is injured (*AJR Am J Roentgenol* 1993;160(5):1019–22)
- American Association for the Surgery of Trauma (AAST) grading system used for liver injures (grades I–VI) (table included)
- High-grade injuries associated with significant mortality (>50%) (*J Trauma* 1995;38(3):323–4)

Workup

- Depends on hemodynamic status of the patient
- If the patient is hemodynamically unstable (SBP <90 and HR >120 without adequate response to fluid resuscitation) then the patient should go straight to surgery
- If hemodynamically stable then patient should undergo multidetector contrast-enhanced CT (MD-CECT) of the chest, abdomen, and pelvis (CAP) (*J Trauma Acute Care Surg* 2012;73:S288–93)

Imaging

- MD-CECT is the initial modality of choice, and the AAST grading system based on MD-CECT findings (Table 17-1)
- Laceration appears as linear or branching hypodensities, and are graded based on the depth of the laceration and percentage of hepatic lobe involvement
- Subcapsular hematomas appear as crescentic hemorrhage collection between the liver capsule and parenchyma. Graded based on percentage of surface area of liver involved
- Intraparenchymal hematoma is ill-defined hypodensity within hepatic parenchyma. Graded based on size (*J Trauma* 1995;38(3):323–4)
- It is important to look for active extravasation of contrast material which indicates on-going active hemorrhage. It appears as ill-defined areas of dense extraluminal contrast and will increase in size and density on delayed imaging
- PSA has a similar appearance but is more defined and will typically remain stable in size and density on delayed images (*Radiology* 2007;243(1):88–95)

Table 17-1 Classification of traumatic liver injuries. Adapted from AAST, 1994 revision (*J Trauma* 1995;38(3):323–4)

Grade	Injury	Description
I	Hematoma	Subcapsular, <10% of surface area
	Laceration	Capsular tear, <1 cm parenchymal depth
II	Hematoma	Subcapsular, 10–50% of surface area Intraparenchymal, <10 cm diameter
	Laceration	1–3 cm parenchymal depth, and <10 cm length
III	Hematoma	Subcapsular, >50% of surface area or expanding Intraparenchymal, >10 cm or expanding
	Laceration	>3 cm parenchymal depth
IV	Laceration	Parenchymal disruption involving 25–75% of hepatic lobe or involving 1–3 segments
V	Laceration	Parenchymal disruption involving >75% of hepatic lobe or >3 segments
	Vascular	Juxtahepatic venous injury
VI	Vascular	Hepatic avulsion

Treatment

- Depends on hemodynamic status of patient and grade of injury
- Hemodynamically unstable patients typically require emergent surgical intervention (exploratory laparotomy)
- Hemodynamically stable patients with low-grade injuries (grades I–III) are typically managed conservatively, with or without angioembolization (*J Trauma Acute Care Surg* 2012; 73:S288–93)
- Specific indications for angiographic evaluation and angioembolization listed below

Indications for Angioembolization (*Handbook of Interventional Radiologic Procedures.* 2011: Lippincott Williams & Wilkins)

- Stable patients with high-grade injury (≥grade III)
- Focal contrast extravasation and clinical evidence on ongoing hemorrhage
- Persistent hemobilia suggesting arterio-biliary fistula
- Following exploratory laparotomy and surgical packing in patients with severe liver injury in order to definitively treat ongoing hemorrhage and reduce risk of delayed hemorrhage
- Persistent or ongoing hemorrhage despite initial surgical intervention

Procedure Technique

- Arterial access gained via the common femoral or radial artery using a micropuncture needle, and subsequent placement of a vascular sheath (usually 5F)
- The celiac artery and SMA are selected using a curved or reverse curve catheter such as a Cobra or SOS catheter
- Ideally assessment should include both SMA and celiac arteries, to assess for variant anatomy such as replaced or accessory hepatic arteries. Angiograms should be carried out through venous phase to document portal vein patency. Assessment depends on condition of patient
- If need for emergent hemostasis, full angiographic assessment may be carried out after initial emergent hemostasis is achieved.
- When performing common or proper hepatic angiogram meticulous evaluation of DSA images is required to identify sites of active extravasation which may appear as areas of contrast blush on angiogram (*Handbook of Interventional Radiologic Procedures.* 2011: Lippincott Williams & Wilkins)
- It is important to identify the cystic artery as to avoid nontarget embolization of the gallbladder (*J Vasc Interv Radiol* 1993;4(3):359–65)
- If multiple areas of extravasation are present, nonselective embolization can be performed using gelfoam slurry or large particles (>500 microns) into the left, right, or proper hepatic artery. Embolization should be performed with catheter distal to cystic artery
- If a single area of extravasation identified, then subselective catheterization of the injured branch is performed using a coaxial microcatheter. Embolization can be performed using either gelfoam, coils, or particles dependent on location and severity of the injury
- If an arteriovenous, arterioportal, or arteriobiliary fistula is discovered, the feeding artery should be separated from the draining vein or biliary duct via coil embolization (*Handbook of Interventional Radiologic Procedures.* 2011: Lippincott Williams & Wilkins)

Expected Outcomes/Results

- Technical success rate ranging from 88–100% (*Clin Radiol* 2014;69(12):e505–e11)
- Postcoiling angiogram should demonstrate cessation of contrast blush
- The success rate is dependent on the injury grade, with higher-grade injuries having a higher rate of re-bleeding after embolization

Complications

- It is important to differentiate trauma related complications from procedural-related complications (*Handbook of Interventional Radiologic Procedures.* 2011: Lippincott Williams & Wilkins)
- Known complications of traumatic liver injuries unrelated to angioembolization include hemobilia, bile peritonitis, bilious ascites, hemoperitoneum, abdominal compartment syndrome, hepatic abscess, and delayed hemorrhage (*J Trauma Acute Care Surg* 2012;73:S288–93)
- Complications related to angioembolization include nontarget embolization of the gallbladder leading to gallbladder necrosis. Liver infarction and necrosis is rare given dual blood supply of liver but can occur. It is important to evaluate the patency of the portal venous system prior to embolization as compromise of the portal venous system is a risk factor for liver necrosis (*Clin Radiol* 2014;69(12):e505–e11)
- Postembolization syndrome and iatrogenic vascular injury including but not limited to arterial access hematoma, PSA formation, and dissection

Background

- The spleen is the most commonly injured solid organ in blunt abdominal trauma (Malays J Med Sci 2011;18:60–7)
- Historically traumatic splenic injuries were treated with splenectomy or observation (Handbook of Interventional Radiologic Procedures. 2011: Lippincott Williams & Wilkins)
- Recently, nonoperative management has become the standard of care for hemodynamically stable patients (Br J Surg 2010;97(11):1696–03)
- The goal of nonoperative therapy is to preserve splenic function as the spleen plays a vital role in immune function, especially in the defense against encapsulated organisms (J Trauma Acute Care Surg 2012;72(1):229–34)
- Splenic embolization continues to gain acceptance and has had an increasing role in the past 2 decades in treating patients with traumatic splenic injuries (Handbook of Interventional Radiologic Procedures. 2011: Lippincott Williams & Wilkins)
- It is currently an effective treatment in select patients with splenic injury
  - In fact, 1 study showed that trauma centers with the highest rates of splenic embolization had the highest rates of splenic salvage (J Trauma Acute Care Surg 2013;75(1):69–5)
- The spleen is a very vascular organ with abundant collateral circulation from pancreatic, gastroduodenal, and gastric branches which allow distal perfusion to the spleen in the setting of proximal embolization of the splenic artery (Semin Intervent Radiol 2010;27(1):14–28)
- AAST grading system used for splenic injuries based on MD-CECT findings (grades I–V) (Semin Intervent Radiol 2010;27(1):14–28) (Table 17-1)

Workup

- See workup in "Hepatic Trauma"

Imaging

- MD-CECT is the modality of choice. AAST grading system based on CT findings (Semin Intervent Radiol 2010;27(1):14–28; Radiology 2012;265:678–93) (Table 17-2)

Table 17-2 Classification of traumatic splenic injuries. Adapted from AAST, 1994 version (J Trauma 1995;38(3):323–4)

Grade	Injury	Description
I	Hematoma	Subcapsular, <10% of surface area
	Laceration	Capsular tear, <1 cm parenchymal depth
II	Hematoma	Subcapsular, 10–50% surface area Intraparenchymal, <5 cm diameter
	Laceration	1–3 cm parenchymal depth, and not involving a trabecular vessel
III	Hematoma	Subcapsular, >50% surface area or expanding Intraparenchymal, ≥5 cm or expanding Ruptured subcapsular or intraparenchymal
	Laceration	>3 cm or involvement of trabecular vessels
IV	Laceration	Involvement of segmental or hilar vessels producing >25% devascularization or the spleen
V	Laceration	Completely shattered spleen
	Vascular	Hilar vascular injury leading to devascularization of the spleen

- Splenic injury commonly associated with hemoperitoneum (Semin Intervent Radiol 2010;27(1):14–28; Radiology 2012;265:678–93)
- Injuries range from lacerations, hematomas (intraparenchymal or subcapsular), PSA, AVF, shattered spleen, and hilar injury leading to devascularization (Semin Intervent Radiol 2010;27(1):14–28; Radiology 2012;265:678–93)
- Lacerations appear as linear or branching hypodensities and are graded based on size and involvement of hilar vessels which may lead to devascularization of the spleen (Semin Intervent Radiol 2010;27(1):14–28; Radiology 2012;265:678–93)
- Subcapsular hematomas are crescentic hemorrhagic collections between the spleen and capsule. They are graded based on surface area coverage of the spleen by the hematoma (Semin Intervent Radiol 2010;27(1):14–28; Radiology 2012;265:678–93)
- Intraparenchymal hematomas are round ill-defined intraparenchymal hypodensities and are graded based on size (Semin Intervent Radiol 2010;27(1):14–28; Radiology 2012;265:678–93)
- Injury to the hilar vessels is considered a grade-V injury and is associated with a high rate of mortality (Semin Intervent Radiol 2010;27(1):14–28; Radiology 2012;265:678–93)

- A shattered spleen is also considered a grade V injury (Semin Intervent Radiol 2010;27(1): 14–28; Radiology 2012;265:678–93)
- It is important to look for active extravasation on MD-CECT which indicates ongoing active hemorrhage. It appears as ill-defined areas of dense extraluminal contrast and will increase in size and density on delayed imaging (Radiology 2007;243(1):88–95)
- Splenic trauma can also lead to contained vascular injury such as PSA and AVF (Can J Surj 2008;51(6):464–72)

Treatment

- Depends on hemodynamic stability of patient. Patients with hemodynamic instability are usually treated surgically while stable patients are treated conservatively with observation or embolization (J Trauma Acute Care Surg 2012;73:S294–00)
- Stable patients with low-grade injuries (I–III) typically treated with observation with or without angioembolization (J Trauma Acute Care Surg 2012;73:S294–00)
- Historically splenic injuries were treated with splenectomy or observation (J Trauma Acute Care Surg 2012;73:S294–00)
- There was a reported high rate of infection and sepsis after splenectomy, therefore there has been an increasing role for splenic salvaging therapy, namely angioembolization (J Trauma Acute Care Surg 2012;73:S294–00)
- The goal being to avoid splenectomy and preserve viable splenic function (J Trauma Acute Care Surg 2012;73:S294–00)

Indications for Angioembolization

- Contrast blush on MD-CECT in stable patients with ≥ grade III injury Contrast blush in grades I–III injuries is controversial (Am Surg 2013;79(10):1089–92)
- Hemodynamically stable patients with high-grade injuries (≥ grade III) (J Trauma Acute Care Surg 2012;73:S294–00)
- Presence of AVF or PSA on MD-CECT which indicates ineffective embolization or observational management (Can J Surj 2008;51(6):464–72)
- Delayed bleeding following conservative management (Semin Intervent Radiol 2012;29(2): 147–49)

Procedure Technique

- 1st access is gained via the femoral or radial artery using a micropuncture technique, and the transitional dilator is exchanged for a 5F vascular sheath over a 0.035 wire
- Then the celiac axis is selected using a wire and a curved or reverse curved selective catheter such as a Cobra or SOS (Diagn Interv Imaging 2014;95(9):825–31)
- A celiac angiogram is performed through the portal venous phase with particular attention to not only the splenic but left gastric artery as it is an important collateral feeder vessel to the spleen and typically the 1st vessel arising off of the celiac trunk (Diagn Interv Imaging 2014;95(9):825–31)
- The catheter is then advance into the splenic artery, and meticulous evaluation of DSA angiographic images is required to evaluate for active extravasation indicated by contrast blush (Semin Intervent Radiol 2012;29(2):147–49)
- If no contrast blush is identified the decision must be made by both the interventional radiologist and the trauma surgeon whether to observe the patient or embolize the splenic artery. This depends on the status of the patient (Semin Intervent Radiol 2012;29(2):147–49)
- If an intraparenchymal blush is identified, embolization can be performed using either a proximal or a more distal selective approach which is at the discretion of the operator
- It is controversial which technique is superior
- Numerous studies have shown a lower rate of infarction and postembolization syndrome for proximal embolization as opposed to distal (Diagn Interv Imaging 2014;95(9): 825–31)
- Typically, proximal embolization is desired for active ongoing hemorrhage in order to rapidly control hemorrhage (Diagn Interv Imaging 2014;95(9):825–31)
- Proximal embolization temporarily decreases the vascularization pressure within the spleen which controls further hemorrhage and allows vascular injuries to heal (Can J Surj 2008;51(6):464–72)
- Proximal embolization is performed by coil embolization of the main splenic artery
  - Care should be taken to embolize distal to the origin of the dorsal pancreatic artery to preserve collateral supply to the spleen through collateral vessels, namely the short gastric and gastroepiploic arteries (Diagn Interv Imaging 2014;95(9): 825–31)
  - Coils should be sized 20–25% larger than the vessel diameter as vessels are typically vasoconstricted in the setting of hemorrhage (Can J Surj 2008;51(6):464–72)

- Distal embolization is typically favored for extraparenchymal hemorrhage, AVF, and PSA (Semin Intervent Radiol 2012;29(2):147–49)
- Distal embolization is performed using a coaxial microcatheter system to access the distal injured vessel and embolization is performed using microcoils (Diagn Interv Imaging 2014;95(9):825–31)

Expected Outcomes/Results
- Splenic embolization is effective in achieving hemostasis in over 90% of cases of splenic injury (Can J Surg 2008;51(6):464–72)
- Proximal embolization of the main splenic artery is successful in avoiding splenectomy in 90–95% of cases (Can J Surg 2008;51(6):464–72)
- Most studies have shown little difference in outcomes of proximal versus distal embolization (J Trauma 2004;56(3):542–47)
- A postcoiling angiogram should demonstrate cessation of contrast blush

Complications
- Rebleeding is the most common complication which is typically defined as major (requiring splenectomy) or minor (not requiring splenectomy)
- Infarction is a common complication, especially for distal embolization
  - The clinical significance of an incidentally found peripheral infarction on imaging in an asymptomatic patient is debatable (Semin Intervent Radiol 2012;29(2):147–49)
- Development of an abscess is another complication which was described in 4% of patients in a large multi-institutional series

---

BRONCHIAL ARTERY EMBOLIZATION

Background
- 1st reported in 1973 as a therapeutic option for massive hemoptysis by Remy et al. (Intervent Radiol 2012;29:155–60)
- In the vast majority of cases (>90%), the bronchial arteries are the culprit for massive hemoptysis (Intervent Radiol 2012;29:155–60)
- Bronchial artery embolization (BAE) is a minimally invasive alternative to surgery, and aims to preserve pulmonary function (Arch Surg 1998;133:862–66)

Indications
- Massive hemoptysis is defined as >300 mL in 24 h or 100 mL daily for at least 3 d. Minor bleeding with hemodynamic instability is also an indication (J Vasc Interv Radiol 2014; 25:221–28)
- Conditions related to massive hemoptysis include cystic fibrosis, bronchiectasis, neoplasm, infections such as TB and aspergillosis, pulmonary fibrosis, AVF, aneurysms etc (Intervent Radiol 2012;29:155–60)

Contraindications
- No absolute contraindications
- Relative contraindications to angiography in general include uncorrectable coagulopathy, renal insufficiency, and serious contrast allergy
- Congenital pulmonary artery stenosis (CPAS) is a relative contraindication as these patients may rely heavily on bronchial artery circulation for pulmonary parenchymal perfusion (Semin Intervent Radiol 2008;25:310–18)
- Care must be taken when performing BAE on patients with a major radiculomedullary branch (ie, artery of Adamkiewicz) arising from the target bronchial artery as there is a risk of spinal cord infarction in these patients (The Practice of Interventional Radiology: With Online Cases and Videos. Philadelphia, PA: Elsevier; 2012:443–70)

Imaging and Anatomic Considerations
- The bronchial arteries are branches directly arising from the thoracic aorta providing blood supply to the airways
- Bronchial artery anatomy is highly variable
  - The most common pattern is 2 bronchial arteries on the left and 1 on the right
  - The right bronchial artery typically arises from a common intercostobronchial trunk
  - Cauldwell patterns of orthotopic bronchial artery branching (Figure 17-1) (Radiographics 2002;22:1395–09)
    - Type I: 41%
    - Type II: 21%
    - Type III: 21%
    - Type IV: 10%

Figure 17-1 The 4 most common branching patterns of bronchial artery anatomy. Type I: Single right intercostobronchial trunk (ICBT) and 2 paired left bronchial arteries. Type II: Single right ICBT and a single left bronchial artery. Type III: Paired right bronchial arteries with one arising from ICBT and paired left bronchial arteries. Type IV: Paired right bronchial arteries with one arising from an ICBT and a single left bronchial artery. (Reprinted from Sopko DR, Smith TP. Bronchial artery embolization for hemoptysis. *Semin Intervent Radiol* 2011;28(1):48–62. Copyright © Georg Thieme Verlag KG, with permission.)

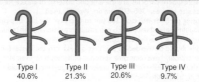

| Type I | Type II | Type III | Type IV |
| 40.6% | 21.3% | 20.6% | 9.7% |

- Bronchial arteries typically arise from the thoracic aorta at the T5–T6 vertebral body level. The right bronchial artery typically arises from the posterolateral aspect of the thoracic and the left from the anterolateral aspect.
  - Another helpful landmark is the left mainstem bronchus on frontal projection (*Eur Radiol* 2007;17(8):1943–53)
- CT angiogram (CTA) is the study of choice for evaluating bronchial artery anatomy prior to embolization
  - CTA is extremely helpful for guiding catheter placement during the procedure
  - CTA can also help avoid unnecessary catheterization (*Eur Radiol* 2007;17(8):1943–53)
- Unlike abdominal sources of bleeding, angiographically visible active extravasation from bronchial arteries is extremely rare
- On CTA culprit bronchial arteries will appear as abnormally dilated tortuous vessels
- The role of bronchoscopy is controversial. Historically, bronchoscopy had a major role in diagnosis and localization of hemoptysis
  - However, recent data suggests bronchoscopy may have a limited role in hemoptysis due to low detection rates as excessive blood in the airways often obscures the bronchial tree (*J Vasc Interv Radiol* 2014;25:221–28)

Preprocedural Workup (*Handbook of Interventional Radiologic Procedures.* 2011: Lippincott Williams & Wilkins)
- Important to obtain a detailed history and thorough physical examination
- Evaluation of airway and respiratory status is important as patient may need to be intubated, and the procedure scheduled with general anesthesia
- Labs including CBC, BMP, PT/INR should be obtained prior to procedure
  - Platelets be >50,000 and INR >1.5
- Also, be sure to check creatine and GFR
- Make sure patient does not have serious contrast allergy

Procedure Technique
- Arterial access gained via the common femoral artery using a 4F or 5F sheath
- Next, a thoracic aortogram may be performed using a pigtail catheter if CTA is not available. The aortogram should be carefully reviewed to determine the site and origin of the vessel(s) most amenable to embolization
- The pigtail catheter is exchanged for the catheter of choice to select the target bronchial artery(ies). The Mickelson catheter is a popular choice
- The target vessel is then selected with the catheter using the T5–T6 vertebral body levels as well as the left mainstem bronchus as landmarks
  - Target vessel abnormalities include aneurysm/pseudoaneurysm, active extravasation (rarely), or most commonly enlargement and tortuosity (*Handbook of Interventional Radiologic Procedures.* 2011: Lippincott Williams & Wilkins)
- A DSA bronchial artery angiogram is performed
  - Important to evaluate for presence of the anterior spinal artery (ASA) as it arises from the right intercostobronchial trunk in 5–10% of cases
    - Anterior spinal artery is a small caliber longitudinal vessel that receives supply from up to eight anterior segmental medullary arteries that have classic hairpin configuration, the most prominent of these is the so-called Artery of Adamkiewicz which typically arises from an intercostal branch between the T9 and T12 level
    - Nontarget embolization of the anterior spinal artery can result in cord ischemia and rarely paraplegia (*Intervent Radiol* 2012;29:155–60)
- Once the vessel is selected a coaxial wire/microcatheter is used to gain more distal access

- Then a DSA angiogram of the bronchial arteries is performed through the microcatheter
  - Confirm that microcatheter is in proper location and distal enough in the bronchial artery to avoid reflux of particles into the thoracic aorta
  - Catheter must be distal to origin of ASA if present to avoid cord ischemia
- Once microcatheter is properly positioned then particles can be delivered through the microcatheter
  - PVA or microsphere particles are the embolic material of choice for BAE
    - Particles size between 300–500 μm are typically used
    - Avoid using particles less than 300 μm to decrease the risk of passage into bronchopulmonary shunts which can result in pulmonary infarction (*Handbook of Interventional Radiologic Procedures.* 2011: Lippincott Williams & Wilkins)
  - Use of coils should be avoided to preserve access into the vessel for future BAE as patients typically have recurrent episodes of hemoptysis even after BAE
  - Particles should be delivered slowly under fluoro guidance to avoid reflux and nontarget embolization
  - Embolization should be performed to near stasis
- A postembolization DSA angiogram should be performed
- Catheter and sheath are then removed and hemostasis secured

Postprocedural Care
- Must perform a comprehensive neurologic exam to evaluate for nontarget embolization of anterior spinal artery
- Continue to treat underlying cause of hemoptysis
- If intubated may need to be monitored in ICU

Results
- Technical success rate >90% (*The Practice of Interventional Radiology: With Online Cases and Videos.* Philadelphia, PA: Elsevier; 2012:443–70)
- Clinical success defined as ability to control massive hemoptysis, up to 98% (*Intervent Radiol* 2012;29:155–60)
- High recurrence rates of hemoptysis (2–27% at 1 mo and 10–52% at 46 mo) as there is rapid recruitment of collateral vessels
- Therefore, repeat BAE is common (*Handbook of Interventional Radiologic Procedures.* 2011: Lippincott Williams & Wilkins)

Complications
- Most feared complication is transverse myelitis/paralysis secondary to nontarget embolization of the anterior spinal artery via a medullary branch (1.4–6.5%) (*Intervent Radiol* 2012;29:155–60; *Radiographics.* 2002;22:1395–1409)
- Other complications include chest pain (24–91%), dysphagia secondary to embolization of esophageal branches (0.7–18%), catheter related vascular injury such as bronchial artery dissection, contrast nephropathy, and access site complications (*Radiology* 1990;175(2):401–05)
- Delayed complications include risk of bronchial necrosis and pulmonary infarction (higher risk if significant bronchopulmonary shunting) (*AJR Am J Roentgenol* 1983;141(3): 535–37; *Presse Med* 1983;12(33):2056–57)

EXTREMITY TRAUMA

Background
- Vascular injury in the extremities is most commonly seen in the setting of penetrating trauma such as gunshot wounds and stab wounds
- However, vascular injury can also result from blunt trauma in cases of crush injuries, degloving injuries, joint dislocations, and lacerations (*Semin Intervent Radiol* 2006;23(3):270–78)

Workup
- History and physical exam is key in triaging and diagnosing vascular injury
  - 1st, the extremity should be examined to identify the entry and exit wounds in cases of penetrating trauma as to estimate the trajectory of the projectile in the body. In addition, one should search for lacerations, abrasions, superficial hematomas, and other signs of extremity trauma
  - Next, a detailed neurovascular exam should be performed
    - Predictive findings for extremity trauma have been described as either hard or soft findings. The presence of hard signs has a 95% positive predictive value for vascular injury whereas the presence of soft signs has a 30% positive predictive value for vascular injury

- Hard signs: Loss of distal pulses, expanding or pulsatile hematoma, thrill or bruit, active hemorrhage, and critical limb ischemia
- Soft signs: Nonexpanding hematoma, nonpulsatile bleeding, pallor or change in skin color, neurologic deficit, and unexplained hypotension
- In stable patients CTA is commonly used to diagnose vascular injury and ascertain the need for intravascular or surgical intervention
  - Imaging findings of vascular injury in the extremities includes pseudoaneurysm, arteriovenous fistula, active extravasation, spasm, occlusion, intimal flap or stenosis (*Radiographics* 2005;25:S133–S42)

Indications for Angiography
- Blunt trauma:
  - Angiography indicated if pulse deficit persists after orthopedic reduction
  - Joint dislocations as well as severely displaced fractures associated with vascular injury
- Penetrating trauma:
  - If hard signs of vascular injury exist, angiography is warranted (*Handbook of Interventional Radiologic Procedures*. 2011: Lippincott Williams & Wilkins)
  - If the path of a high-velocity missile (ie, bullet) comes in close proximity to a major vessel, angiography should be performed even in the absence of hard signs
    - The energy of the missile within the tissue causes pressure changes and shock wave injury centimeters from the projectile tract which can cause significant vascular injury such as pseudoaneurysm, AV fistula, thrombosis, intimal flap, intramural hematoma, or vasospasm (*Radiographics* 2005;25:S133–S42)

Procedure Technique
- 1st a nonselective arteriogram should be performed of either the thoracic aortic arch for upper extremity trauma or abdominal aorta/common iliac artery for lower-extremity trauma
- Then, a more selective angiogram should be performed in multiple obliquities at the site of injury (*Radiographics* 2005;25:270–78)
  - Contrast injection should be proximal to the site of injury to evaluate for collateral blood flow (*Handbook of Interventional Radiologic Procedures*. 2011: Lippincott Williams & Wilkins)
- Treatment strategy depends on the type of vascular injury as well as the location of the vessel(s) involved
  - In larger vessels such as the popliteal artery, superficial femoral artery, subclavian, etc. stent grafts are typically utilized for injuries such as PSA, active extravasation, AVFs, or dissection (*Handbook of Interventional Radiologic Procedures*. 2011: Lippincott Williams & Wilkins)
  - In smaller arteries as well as distal muscular branches coil embolization is typically employed to achieve hemostasis. When using coil embolization, it is important to confirm adequate collateral blood flow and distal circulation (*J Trauma Acute Care Surg* 2014;77(6):920–25)
  - Treating AVFs can be difficult. It is important to cut off the arterial inflow to the fistula. In smaller vessels coiling distally and proximally to the fistula is typically an effective strategy. Care must to taken to avoid coil migration into the venous system (*Handbook of Interventional Radiologic Procedures*. 2011: Lippincott Williams & Wilkins)

PELVIC TRAUMA

Background
- Pelvic trauma is seen in both high speed blunt trauma as well as in penetrating trauma
- Pelvic fractures occur in approximately 3–9% of blunt trauma patients (*Ann Surg* 2001; 233(6):843–50)
- Pelvic fractures are commonly associated with arterial hemorrhage leading to hypovolemic shock
- Retroperitoneal hemorrhage occurs in 13–44% of pelvic fractures (*Ann Surg* 1990; 211(2):109–23)
- Pelvic trauma with hemorrhagic shock is associated with high mortality rate (as high as 30–50% in some studies) (*Injury* 2014;45(4):738–41; *Handbook of Interventional Radiologic Procedures*. 2011: Lippincott Williams & Wilkins)

Workup and Initial Management
- Initial management includes resuscitation with pRBCs and IV crystalloids
- Patients typically undergo pelvic x-ray initially followed by Panscan including CT head, C-spine, chest, abdomen, and pelvis

- Management options include placement of a pelvic binder initially followed by external fixation of pelvic fractures and packing ± angioembolization
- Angioembolization in the setting of hemorrhagic shock secondary to pelvic fractures should not be delayed for operative external fixation
- Patients with penetrating trauma injuries typically undergo exploratory laparotomy

Indication for Angioembolizations

- Hemorrhagic shock refractory to initial fluid resuscitation in a patient with pelvic fractures or retroperitoneal hemorrhage and no evidence of intraperitoneal hemorrhage
- Hemorrhagic shock secondary to pelvic fractures requiring more than 4U of pRBCs in 24 h or 6U in 48 h
- Pelvic hematoma with active extravasation seen on CE-CT in a patient with hemodynamic instability
- Patients with penetrating injuries who have a large expanding pelvic hematoma discovered during laparotomy *(Handbook of Interventional Radiologic Procedures. 2011: Lippincott Williams & Wilkins; J Trauma Acute Care Surg 2014; 76(2):374–79)*

Contraindications

- All contraindications are relative as pelvic angioembolization is typically performed in the setting of life threatening hemorrhagic shock

Anatomy and Imaging Findings

- On CE-CT present as pelvic and/or retroperitoneal hematoma
- Arterial injury on CE-CT or diagnostic angiogram can present as occlusion, stenosis, spasm, intimal tear, pseudoaneurysm, arteriovenous fistula, or active extravasation *(Semin Intervent Radiol. 2006;23(3):270–78)*
- The majority of the blood supply to the pelvis comes from the internal iliac artery and its branches. There is an extensive network of collateral blood supply in the pelvis
- The most commonly injured vessels in pelvic trauma are the internal iliac arteries and its branches (Figure 17-2)
- Injury to the external iliac arteries and its branches are uncommon *(Semin Intervent Radiol. 2006;23(3):270–78)*

Procedure and Technique

- 1st, the common femoral artery contralateral to the most severe pelvic injury/fracture is accessed, and a 5F vascular sheath is placed
- The technique will depend on the stability of the patient
  - If the patient is unstable and emergent embolization is needed, then rapid selection of the internal iliac artery on the ipsilateral side of the most severe injury and nonselective embolization of the posterior branch with gelfoam is warranted. Occlusion of the posterior branch with an Amplatzer device can also be performed *(Injury 2014;45(4):738–41)*
- Once stabilized an abdominopelvic aortogram should be performed using a pigtail catheter as there is high association with retroperitoneal arterial and solid organ injury
- The internal iliac artery contralateral to the access site should be selected. An internal iliac arteriogram is performed and careful evaluation for active extravasation/arterial injury is sought. Multiple projections may need to be obtained to clearly delineate the vessels involved
- The internal iliac artery ipsilateral to the access site should be selected afterward, and an internal iliac arteriogram performed *(Semin Intervent Radiol 2004;21(1):23–35)*
- Different techniques for embolization can be used depending on the type of injury
  - If only a single focus of hemorrhage is identified involving a distal branch of the internal iliac artery then subselective embolization can be performed using a microcatheter for selection and gelfoam or coils for embolization
  - If multiple foci of hemorrhage are identified then more proximal embolization of the posterior branch of the internal iliac artery can be performed using gelfoam slurry
    - Care should be taken to avoid reflux into the anterior division of the internal iliac artery or external iliac artery
- Because of the extensive collateral supply in the pelvis, normal collateral vessels may need to be coiled in order to achieve hemostasis *(Handbook of Interventional Radiologic Procedures. 2011: Lippincott Williams & Wilkins)*

Results

- Technical success rate approaching 100%, and clinical success rate of 95% *(J Trauma 2002;53(2):303–08)*
- Results are dependent on time to embolization. Rapid embolization is associated with improved outcomes *(Injury 2014;45(4):738–41)*

Complications

- Recurrent hemorrhage in 5.8–7.5% of embolization cases *(Am Surg 2000;66(9):858–62)*
- Reported cases of ischemic necrosis of the rectum or gluteal muscles and peripheral nerve damage. This is seen more commonly when smaller particles or embolic materials are used which causes occlusion at the capillary level *(Cardiovasc Intervent Radiol 1997; 20(1):50–3)*
- Distal lower-extremity ischemia secondary to nontarget embolization is a potential risk. This is why it is important to avoid reflux of embolic material *(AJR Am J Roentgenol 1979;133(5):859–64)*
- Impotence is also a potential risk *(J Trauma 2004;56(4):734–41)*

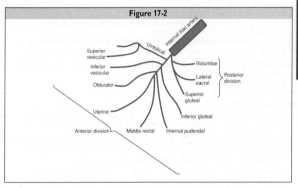

Figure 17-2

THORACIC DUCT EMBOLIZATION

Background

- Chylous leaks are a result of leakage of lymphatic fluid from the thoracic duct or its tributaries
- It results in chylous ascites, chylothorax, chylopericardium, or postoperative chylous leaks
- Divided into traumatic and nontraumatic causes
  - Traumatic causes include blunt/penetrating trauma as well as iatrogenic causes
  - Nontraumatic causes include idiopathic, malignant, congenital, systemic, lymph vessel disease, and infectious
- The most common cause is iatrogenic after thoracic or abdominal surgeries, particularly after esophagectomy
- Thoracic duct embolization is a minimally invasive procedure to treat chylous leaks above the diaphragm, and is an alternative to surgery *(Semin Intervent Radiol 2011;28(1):63–74)*

Anatomic Considerations

- The thoracic duct carries 1–2 L of lymphatic fluid, the majority of which comes from intestinal and hepatic lymphatic ducts *(J Clin Invest 1953;32(7):637–49)*
  - Varies depending on diet of patient (increased in patients with fatty diets, particularly triglycerides)
  - Elevated in conditions that raise hepatic sinusoidal pressure such as cirrhosis and right heart failure *(N Engl J Med 1960;263:471–74)*
- The thoracic duct drains all the lymph from the body with the exception of drainage from the right hemithorax, right head, right neck, and right arm
- It is the largest lymph vessel measuring approximately 45 cm in length
- The thoracic duct originates in the upper abdomen (cisterna chyli at the T12 level) and enters the thoracic cavity through the aortic hiatus coursing between the aorta and azygos vein (aorta on the left and azygos on the right)
- It courses just anterior to the surface of the vertebral bodies in the thoracic cavity and empties into the venous system near the confluence of the left internal jugular and subclavian veins *(Surg Oncol Clin N Am 2007;16(1):1–16)*

- Many anatomic variations of the thoracic duct exist (*Der Ductus Thoracicus der Japane. In Das Lymphgefässssystem der Japaner.* Tokyo: Kenkyusha; 1953)
- The cisternal chyli is typically located in the retrocrural location between the T12–L2 levels just to the right of the aorta
  - Formed by confluence of intestinal trunk/lumbar lymphatic trunks, and receives chyle from intestines (*AJR Am J Roentgenol* 2000;175(5):1462)

Indications for Lymphangiogram and Potential Embolization

- High-volume chylothorax (>1000 mL/d)
  - High mortality due to electrolyte abnormalities, dehydration, immune comprise, respiratory distress, and nutritional depletion
- Chylopericardium
- Failure of conservative management
  - Conservative management includes chest tube placement, total parenteral nutrition (TPN), and limiting fat intake
  - Conservative management is typically successful in lower volume chylothoraces (<500 mL/d) (*Handbook of Interventional Radiologic Procedures.* 2011: Lippincott Williams & Wilkins)

Contraindications (*Handbook of Interventional Radiologic Procedures.* 2011: Lippincott Williams & Wilkins)

- Uncorrectable coagulopathy
- Severe contrast allergy
- Pseudochylous effusion

Preprocedural Workup

- History and physical should be performed to assess for thoracic duct injury. Also, an assessment of the airway should be performed prior to moderate conscious sedation (*Handbook of Interventional Radiologic Procedures.* 2011: Lippincott Williams & Wilkins)
- Laboratory analysis of the pleural or pericardial fluid should be performed prior to the procedure to confirm chylous effusion
  - Chylous fluid will have elevated triglycerides and lymphocytes
  - Presence of chylomicrons in the fluid is diagnostic for chyle unless the fluid contains blood (*Chest* 2007;133(6):1436–41)
- Preprocedural MRI (heavily T2 weighted) can be obtained to delineate thoracic duct anatomy (*Eur Radiol* 2013;23:702–11)
- Prophylactic periprocedural antibiotics should be administered
  - Typically, 1 g of IV cefazolin is used (*Handbook of Interventional Radiologic Procedures.* 2011: Lippincott Williams & Wilkins)

Procedure Technique

- 1st, lymphangiography is performed using either the traditional pedal technique or intranodal technique (*J Vasc Interv Radiol* 2012;23(5):613–16)
  - Pedal technique: Methylene blue is injected into either the 1st or 2nd toe webspace. The methylene blue is taken up by the lymphatics in the foot and blue streaks appear under the skin. Cutdown is performed and a lymph vessel is cannulated with a 30G catheter, and ethiodol is injected. Serial fluoroscopic images are obtained every 15–20 min until the cisterna chyli is opacified (*J Med Imaging Radiat Oncol* 2010;54(1):43–6).
  - Nodal technique: The hilum of the bilateral inguinal lymph nodes is accessed under ultrasound guidance with a 25G spinal needle. Then ethiodol (up to 6 mL) is injected each lymph node using the needles using a balloon insufflator maintaining a pressure of around 1–2 mmHg. Serial fluoroscopic images are obtained until the cisterna chyli is opacified. Then 20 mL of saline is injected through the same needles to allow better and more rapid opacification of the cisterna chyli and thoracic duct.
    - Takes much less time, smaller puncture site, and increased technical success when compared to the pedal technique
- Next, the cisterna chyli or target lymphatic channel is accessed using transabdominal right paramedian percutaneous approach with a 22G Chiba needle under fluoroscopic guidance. A super stiff 0.018 wire is advanced through the needle into the thoracic duct.
- A 3F 65-cm microcatheter is then advanced over the wire into the thoracic duct. DSA lymphangiogram is performed by injecting water-soluble contrast via the microcatheter with a 1 cc syringe. Careful evaluation for contrast extravasation or ductal obstruction should be performed.
- The catheter is then advanced to the level of ductal injury and embolization is performed
  - Embolization is performed with a combination of coils and n-butyl cyanoacrylate (NBCA) glue just upstream to the leak/ductal injury

- The coils provide a scaffold for the glue
- Prior to glue injection, the catheter should be flushed with 0.2 mL of D5W solution to avoid polymerization of the glue within the catheter
- The glue is typically diluted 1:1 in lipiodol although other concentrations may be used
- Perform type II embolization if thoracic duct unsuccessfully cannulated
  - If the thoracic duct is unsuccessfully cannulated, the cisternal chyli and retroperitoneal lymphatics can be macerated using multiple passes with a 22G needle to divert chyle into the retroperitoneum, thus allowing the thoracic duct to heal (Semin Intervent Radiol 2011;28(1):63–74; Handbook of Interventional Radiologic Procedures. 2011: Lippincott Williams & Wilkins)

Postprocedural Care (Handbook of Interventional Radiologic Procedures. 2011: Lippincott Williams & Wilkins)
- Outpatients are typically monitored overnight
- Postprocedural pain is minimal
- Chest tube output should be monitored. Output should significantly decrease after the embolization
- Continue dietary restriction of fatty intake
- Serial chest x-rays can be obtained to assess for treatment response

Results
- In largest series, overall intent-to-treat success rate for traumatic chylous leak was 71%
- The success rate is directly associated with the ability to select the thoracic duct/cisternal chyli with the microcatheter
- Clinical success rate improved when combination of glue and coils used (91%) vs. coils alone (84%) (J Thorac Cardiovasc Surg 2010;139(3):584–90)

Complications
- Immediate complications:
  - 2 reported cases of pulmonary embolism with glue (1 symptomatic and the other asymptomatic) (J Thorac Cardiovasc Surg 2010;139(3):584–90; Chest 2013;143:158–63)
  - Theoretical risk of bowel or vessel injury, although no reported cases
- Long-term complications include lower-extremity edema, chronic diarrhea, breast swelling, and abdominal swelling (J Vasc Interv Radiol 2012;23(1):76–9)

APPROACH TO THE TRAUMA PATIENT

Background
Trauma is the leading cause of death in USA for both men and women under the age of 45 and is the 4th most common cause of overall mortality for all ages (http://www.cdc.gov/injury/wisqars. Published 2007. Accessed January 10, 2017)
- Divided into blunt and penetrating injuries
  - Penetrating injuries further divided into gunshot wounds and stab wounds
- More severe injuries associated with multisystem trauma
  - Must assess patients' hemodynamic status in order to properly triage. Hemodynamically unstable patients typically require surgical intervention, whereas stable patients can be managed nonsurgically (World J Emerg Surg 2013;8:14)

Initial Assessment and Resuscitation (Advanced Trauma Life Support Program for Physicians. 9th ed. Chicago, IL: 2012)
- Primary survey (ABCDE)
  - Airway, breathing, circulation, disability, and exposure
  - Must fully expose patient by removing clothing
  - Assess gross mental status using Glasgow Coma Scale (GCS)
- Resuscitation:
  - Placement of large bore IVs, cardiac monitoring, and oxygen
  - Endotracheal intubation in patients with altered mental status and those unable to protect their airways
  - Resuscitation with blood transfusion and crystalloid IV fluids in the setting of hypovolemic shock
  - Cervical stabilization for suspected C-spine injuries
- Secondary Survey
  - After initial survey and resuscitation phase
  - Involves conducting a thorough head to toe examination

- Requires careful inspection of exposed patient for deformities, abrasions, bruises, hemorrhage
- Abdominal exam requires careful palpation of all 4 quadrants, although abdominal exam is typically unreliable in alcohol or drug intoxication as well as in multisystem trauma
- At this point history should be obtained
  - May need to piece together history from multiple sources including witnesses, emergency responders, family members, etc.
  - Important to ascertain mechanism of injury, use of seatbelt or helmet, airbag deployment, vital signs, treatments administered in the field, and change in mental status
  - AMPLE pneumoninic for history: Allergies, medications, past medical history, last meal, and events leading up to the injury

Labs

- Type and screen, CBC, ABG, BMP or CMP, EKG, UA, toxicology screen (others may be necessary depending on the mechanism of injury as well info gathered from the H&P)
- LFTs and lipase if suspect solid abdominal organ injury

Imaging Modalities

- Hemodynamically unstable patients undergo chest x-ray, pelvic x-ray, and focused assessment with sonography for trauma (FAST) prior to surgery (ACR appropriateness criteria: https://acsearch.acr.org/docs/69409/Narrative/)
  - FAST exam is used to screen for intraperitoneal and retroperitoneal free fluid and/or hemoperitoneum
    - 4 standard views are obtained (transverse subxiphoid, longitudinal view of the right upper quadrant, longitudinal view of the left upper quadrant, as well as transverse and longitudinal views of the suprapubic region) (Radiographics 2008;28: 255–44)
    - Minimum amount of free fluid detected is approximately 200 cc (Radiographics 2008; 28:255–44)
  - After stabilized, patients may require additional x-rays of extremities if there is obvious deformity or concern for fracture
  - Diagnostic peritoneal lavage has been largely replaced by FAST exam
- Hemodynamically stable patients should undergo noncontrast CT head and cervical spine followed by contrast-enhanced CT (CE-CT) of the chest, abdomen, and pelvis using IV contrast (100–150 mL of low or iso-osmolar contrast) in the portal venous phase (65–80 s after the start of contrast administration) (Radiology 2012;265:678–93)
  - If patient has hematuria or if there is high clinical suspicion for renal collecting system/ureteral injury 5-min delayed postcontrast imaging should be performed to evaluate for contrast extravasation suggesting a urine leak (AJR Am J Roentgenol 2006; 187(5):1296–02)
  - In cases of pelvic fractures, hematuria, suspected bladder, or ureteral injury a CT cystogram should be performed by administering 300–500 cc of dilute contrast via Foley catheter into the bladder. Contrast extravasation suggests bladder injury (AJR Am J Roentgenol 2006;187(5):1296–02)

Imaging Findings in Trauma

- Hemoperitoneum:
  - CT is more accurate than US when evaluating for hemoperitoneum as well localizing the source of bleeding (Radiology 1983;148(1):187–92)
  - On CT hemoperitoneum has an attenuation of 30–45 HU (Radiology 1983;148(1):187–92)
  - On US hemoperitoneum is hard to discern from simple free intraperitoneal fluid as the identification of internal echoes is operator and machine dependent
  - Hemoperitoneum like free fluid tends to accumulate in dependent sites in the abdomen such as Morrison's pouch and the pouch of Douglas (rectovesicle pouch in males) (Radiology 1983;148(1):187–92)
  - Clotted blood located adjacent to the site of injury tends to be slightly hyperdense (40–75 HU) compared to nonclotted blood hence the term sentinel clot sign (AJR Am J Roentgenol 1989;153(4):747–9)
    - This is helpful in localizing the source of bleeding when the source is not obvious
- Active extravasation:
  - Refers to IV administered extravascular contrast material on CT (Radiology 2012; 265:678–93)
  - Indicates ongoing active hemorrhage and may be an indication for angioembolization

Treatment

- Hemodynamically unstable patients who do not respond to initial resuscitation typically go straight to surgery after initial workup (*J Trauma Acute Care Surg* 2012;73:S294–00; *J Trauma Acute Care Surg* 2012;73:S288–93)
  - Penetrating trauma has a lower threshold for surgical intervention as the rate of solid organ injury is very high
- Hemodynamically stable patients undergo CE-CT and are typically managed conservatively with observation and angioembolization when indicated (*J Trauma Acute Care Surg* 2012;73:S294–00; *J Trauma Acute Care Surg* 2012;73:S288–93)
- Angiography allows simultaneous diagnosis and treatment of solid organ injury
- Angioembolization aims to achieve hemostasis and organ salvage in a minimally invasive manner
- There is a 90% success rate of angioembolization for blunt and penetrating solid organ trauma, for both intraperitoneal and retroperitoneal injuries (*World J Surg* 2000; 24(5):539–45)

Indication for Angioembolization

- Angioembolization is appropriate for hemodynamically stable patients with contrast extravasation on CE-CT scan or high-grade injury to a solid organ
  - Angioembolization is a minimally invasive technique that aims to control arterial hemorrhage using controlled occlusion of vessels using various techniques such as particles, coils, gelfoam, Amplatzer plugs, etc.
- Indications for angioembolization are likely to broaden in the very near future

Technique (*Semin Intervent Radiol* 2010;27(1):14–28)

- The technique depends on the location, severity, and type of injury. Specific techniques are described later for each individual section.
- No matter what the injury is, arterial access is typically obtained using the common femoral, brachial, or radial artery
  - If there is extremity or pelvic injury, the side opposite of the injury should be accessed
- Larger vessels typically require coils for embolization whereas smaller vessels can be embolized with particles or gelfoam
- End organs without abundant collateral blood supply should be embolized using a superselective distal approach (ie, the kidneys) to avoid large areas of infarction/necrosis
- Organs with dual vascular supply (ie, the liver) or organs with extensive collateral blood supply (ie, the pelvis) can tolerate large areas of embolization
- Need for emergent hemostasis in unstable patients with multiple areas of extravasation/vascular injury can be treated with nonselective approach using a temporary embolic agent such as gelfoam
- Treatment of pseudoaneurysms (PSA) can be achieved by either packing the PSA densely or by using a sandwich technique where embolization is performed distal and proximal to the vascular injury in order to prevent collateral filling of the injured vessel
- Organs with extensive collateral supply, such as the spleen, can tolerate proximal embolization
- Stents and stent grafts can be used to control bleeding while maintaining luminal patency when larger conduit vessels such as the aorta, iliac, femoral, subclavian, and renal arteries are involved

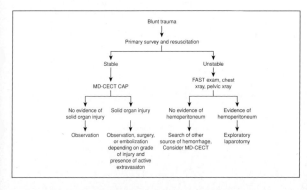

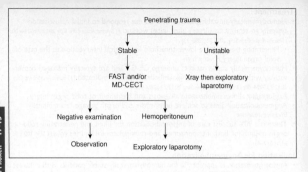

Outline

- Major anatomy of the head and neck
- Ischemic stroke
- Cerebral aneurysms
- Carotid artery atherosclerotic disease
- Epistaxis
- Spinal angiography
- Intracranial atherosclerotic disease
- Brain arteriovenous malformations
- Intracranial arteriovenous fistulae
- Complications specific to neurointerventional procedures

Major Anatomy of the Head and Neck

- **Arteries of the Neck and Head**

  Aorta

  Most common aortic variations (Q Bull Northwest Univ Evanst Ill Med Sch 1957;31(2):136–43)

    Bovine Arch (see Fig. 18-1, bottom right panel)—The brachiocephalic (also called innominate) and left common carotid arteries share a common origin from the aortic arch (27%)

    Direct origin of the left vertebral artery from the aortic arch proximal to the left subclavian artery origin (2.5%)

    Aberrant origin of the right subclavian artery distal to the left subclavian artery (<1%)

  Type 1, 2, 3 arch (J Neurointerventional Surg 2014;6(3):219–24)

    Defined by the location of the origin of the brachiocephalic artery (Fig. 18-1)

    The aorta elongates with age, making type 2 and 3 arches more common in the elderly population

    Type of arch affects choice of diagnostic and/or base catheter; type 3 arches can make interventional procedures more difficult

> **Figure 18-1 Top left:** Type I aortic arch; Brachiocephalic artery originates from top of aortic arch **Top right:** Type II aortic arch; Brachiocephalic artery originates below the top of the aortic arch **Bottom left:** Type III aortic arch; Brachiocephalic artery originates below the inferior aspect of the aorta at the level of the aortic arch **Bottom right:** Bovine arch; solid arrow point to common origin of left subclavian and left common carotid artery **A:** Descending aorta; **B:** Left subclavian artery; **C:** Left vertebral artery; **D:** Left common carotid artery; **E:** Brachiocephalic artery (also called innominate artery); **F:** Right common carotid artery; **G:** Right vertebral artery; **H:** Right subclavian artery; **I:** Ascending aorta.

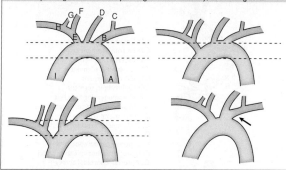

Innominate/Brachiocephalic Artery—1st branch of the aorta, bifurcates into the right subclavian artery, which gives off the right vertebral artery, and the right common carotid artery, which bifurcates into the

  Right Internal Carotid Artery

  Right External Carotid Artery

Left Common Carotid Artery—2nd branch of the aorta, bifurcates into the

  Left Internal Carotid Artery

  Left External Carotid Artery

Left Subclavian Artery—3rd branch of the aorta, which gives off the Left Vertebral Artery

External carotid artery branches—Mnemonic for remembering the order of branches: "SALFOPS Max"

Superior thyroid
Ascending pharyngeal
Lingual
Facial
Occipital
Posterior auricular
Superficial temporal
Maxillary artery (aka internal maxillary artery)

Internal carotid artery—Divided into 7 sections (see Fig. 18-2)

1st major branch is in the cavernous segment, the meningohypophyseal trunk (MHT), which divides into the

Dorsal meningeal artery
Inferior hypophyseal artery
Tentorial artery (of Bernasconi and Cassinari)

The internal carotid artery becomes intradural at the clinoid segment

The outer dural ring separates the cavernous and clinoid segments
The inner dural ring separates the clinoid and ophthalmic segments

Branches of the "supra-clinoid" ICA; mnemonic for order of branches is "OSPAMA"

Ophthalmic artery
Superior hypophyseal artery
Posterior communicating artery
Anterior choroidal artery
Middle cerebral artery
Anterior cerebral artery

- **Main venous drainage from the brain**

Superior sagittal sinus from cortical veins over cerebral convexities
Straight sinus formed by the Vein of Galen and Inferior Sagittal Sinus, Vein of Galen from Internal Cerebral + Basal vein of Rosenthal
Superior sagittal sinus and straight sinus join to form the confluence of sinuses/ torcula Herophili

---

Figure 18-2 Segments of the internal carotid artery and branches.

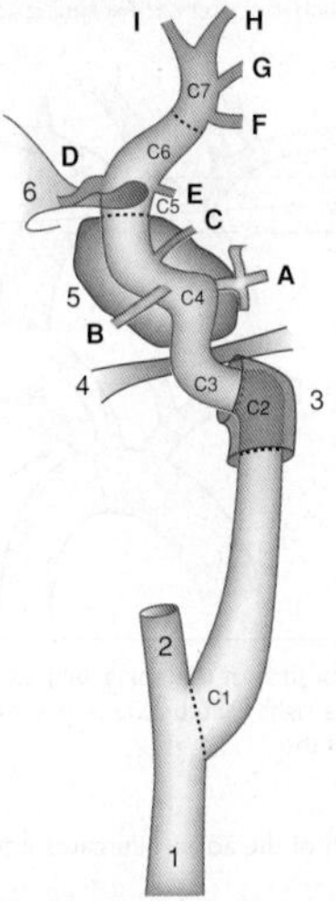

C1: Cervical segment
C2: Petrous segment
C3: Lacerum segment
C4: Cavernous segment
C5: Clinoid segment
C6: Ophthalmic segment
C7: Communicating segment
A: Meningohypophyseal trunk
B: Inferolateral trunk
C: McConnell's capsular arteries
D: Ophthalmic artery
E: Superior hypophyseal artery
F: Posterior communicating artery
G: Anterior choroidal artery
H: Middle cerebral artery
I: Anterior cerebral artery
1: Common carotid artery
2: External carotid artery
3: Carotid canal
4: Petrolingual ligament
5: Cavernous sinus
6: Anterior clinoid process

Figure 18-3 Anterior circulation anatomy, Right internal carotid artery injection, AP **A:** Right internal carotid artery (ICA) **B:** Right middle cerebral artery (MCA) **C:** Right lenticulostriate penetrating arteries **D:** Right anterior cerebral artery (ACA) **E:** Anterior communicating artery (ACommA) **F:** Left ACA.

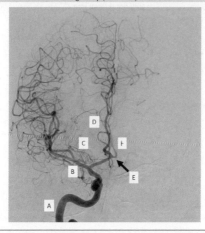

Figure 18-4 Anterior circulation anatomy, Right internal carotid artery injection, lateral **A:** ICA **B:** Meningohypophyseal trunk (MHT) **C:** Ophthalmic artery (OA) **D:** Posterior communicating artery (PCommA) **E:** Anterior choroidal artery (AChA) **F:** MCA branches **G:** ACA **H:** Callosomarginal artery **I:** Pericallosal artery.

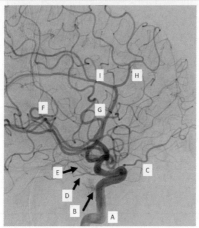

- From the confluence, a transverse sinus, formed by dura at the edge of the tentorium, drains laterally on both sides, each joins the superior petrosal sinus to form the sigmoid sinus
- The sigmoid sinus drains inferolaterally and joins the inferior petrosal sinus to become the jugular bulb, thus forming the origin of the internal jugular vein

Figure 18-5 Posterior circulation anatomy, Right vertebral artery injection, AP **A:** Right vertebral artery (VA) **B:** Right posterior inferior cerebellar artery (PICA) **C:** Right anterior inferior cerebellar artery (AICA) originating from the distal right VA **D:** Basilar artery (BA) **E:** Left AICA originating from the BA **F:** Right superior cerebellar artery (SCA) **G:** Right posterior cerebral artery.

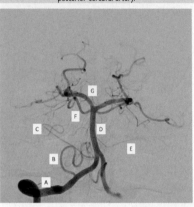

Figure 18-6 External carotid artery anatomy, right external carotid artery injection, lateral **A:** External carotid artery **B:** Superior thyroid artery **C:** Ascending pharyngeal artery **D:** Lingual artery **E:** Facial artery **F:** Occipital artery **G:** Posterior auricular artery **H:** Superficial temporal artery **I:** Maxillary artery **J:** Middle meningeal artery.

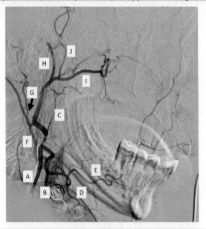

The internal jugular vein exits the skull via the jugular foramen and drains inferiorly to join the subclavian vein to form the brachiocephalic or innominate vein

The left and right innominate veins join to form the superior vena cava

- **Dangerous ECA-ICA anastomoses** (Cardiovasc Intervent Radiol 1991;14(6):325–33; AJNR Am J Neuroradiol 2009;30(8):1459–68)

  Taken into consideration when embolizing through ECA branches; embolic material can flow into ICA branches and cause blindness or stroke

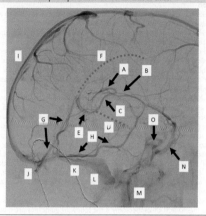

Figure 18-7 Cerebral venous anatomy, right internal carotid artery injection (venous phase), lateral **A:** Thalamostriate vein **B:** Caudate vein **C:** Internal cerebral vein **D:** Basal vein of Rosenthal (represented by dashed line) **E:** Vein of Galen **F:** Inferior sagittal sinus (represented by dashed line) **G:** Straight sinus **H:** Vein of Labbe **I:** Superior sagittal sinus **J:** Confluence of sinuses **K:** Straight sinus **L:** Sigmoid sinus **M:** Internal jugular vein **N:** Sphenoparietal sinus **O:** Cavernous sinus.

Most common is arterial supply to the retina from the middle meningeal artery, a branch of the internal maxillary artery

Prior to embolization of the middle meningeal artery, a DSA run must be obtained to look for a retinal blush

Less common, distal IMA to ophthalmic artery anastomoses

Ascending pharyngeal anastomoses with the cavernous ICA

Occipital artery anastomoses with the vertebral artery

- **Cranial nerve supply by ECA branches to cranial nerves VII, IX–XII**
  (Cardiovasc Intervent Radiol 1991;14(6):325–33)

  Particularly important when embolizing with polyvinyl alcohol particles; cranial nerve palsies can occur

  Supply to geniculate ganglion (VII) via facial arcade from petrous branch of the MMA and stylomastoid branch of the posterior auricular artery

  Neuromeningeal trunk of the ascending pharyngeal artery supplies parts of cranial nerves IX–XII

Ischemic Stroke

- **Background**

  Ischemic stroke accounts for 87% of strokes in the United States; intracerebral hemorrhage accounts for 10% and subarachnoid hemorrhage 3%

  5th leading cause of death *(National Center for Health Statistics Data Brief No 293. Hyattsville, MD: National Center for Health Statistics; 2017)*; one of the leading causes of disability

  Caused by poor perfusion or blockage of an intracerebral vessel due to:

  Intrinsic atherosclerotic disease

  Thrombus formation in the vessels that supply the brain (eg, from a ruptured atherosclerotic plaque or a vessel dissection) and subsequent embolization to the brain

  Embolus from heart, either due to thrombus formation in the left heart (often from atrial fibrillation and subsequent stagnant blood), or a "paradoxical embolus" from the right heart that crosses to the left heart via a patent foramen ovale

  Hypoperfusion, either due to systemic dysfunction or due to critical stenosis of a vessel supplying the brain combined with absent collateral flow from an incomplete circle of Willis

  Small vessel ischemic disease

  Lipohyalinosis due to chronic hypertension, amyloid deposition due to amyloid angiopathy, and endothelial dysfunction due to hyperglycemia

- **Presentation**

  Ischemia in the brain causes predictable neurological deficits based on the location

  Hemiplegia, hemineglect (sensory, spatial, and visual), aphasia are common

  After large vessel occlusion, there is a "core infarct," which represents unsalvageable brain tissue, and an "ischemic penumbra" of oligemia which causes neurological dysfunction but is still salvageable with restoration of blood flow

- **Evaluation**

  Patients evaluated in field by EMS and taken to nearest hospital able to administer IV tissue plasminogen activator (tPA, alteplase)

  STAT CT Head without contrast is obtained to rule out hemorrhage and IV tPA is administered if certain criteria are met

  > Some cities are equipped with mobile stroke units with CT scanners in the vehicle that are dispatched to evaluate suspected stroke patients

  Concurrent to the evaluation and administration of IV tPA, patients are also evaluated for emergent mechanical thrombectomy, but this evaluation should not delay the administration of IV tPA

  Based on 2018 AHA/ASA guidelines, mechanical thrombectomy is the standard of care and should be performed on all AIS patients if certain criteria are met

  (2018 Guidelines for the Early Management of Patients With Acute Ischemic Stroke: A Guideline for Healthcare Professionals From the American Heart Association/American Stroke Association. *Stroke.* January 2018. doi:10.1161/STR.0000000000000158)

  Most centers evaluate a stroke patient within 6 h of symptom onset for mechanical thrombectomy with a noncontrast CT Head to estimate core infarct size using the ASPECT score (see below) and a CT angiogram of the head and neck to identify site of occlusion; if evaluating for mechanical thrombectomy after 6 h, advanced imaging must be performed (either an MRI DWI ± MR perfusion, or a CT perfusion scan)

  If groin puncture can be initiated within 6 h of symptom onset, patients should undergo mechanical thrombectomy if the following guidelines are met:

  > Prestroke modified Rankin score of 0 or 1
  >
  > Causative occlusion of the ICA or proximal MCA
  >
  > Age ≥18 y
  >
  > NIHSS score of ≥6
  >
  > ASPECTS of ≥6

  If groin puncture can be initiated within 16 h (level I recommendation) or 24 h (level IIa recommendation) from last known well, patients should undergo mechanical thrombectomy if guidelines from the DAWN (*N Engl J Med* 2018;378(1):11–21) or DEFUSE 3 (*N Engl J Med* 2018;378(8):708–18) trial are met:

  > For DAWN, same criteria as above, except core infarct must be measured with either an MRI DWI sequence or a CT perfusion study and patient must fit into one of these 3 categories
  >
  > > <80 y old + NIHSS ≥20, core <51 cc
  > >
  > > <80 y old + NIHSS 10–20, core <31 cc
  > >
  > > ≥80 y old + NIHSS ≥10, then core <21 cc
  >
  > For DEFUSE III, an MR or CT perfusion study must be performed, and the following criteria must be met
  >
  > > Baseline mRS 0–2
  > >
  > > NIHSS ≥6
  > >
  > > Occlusion of ICA or MCA-M1
  > >
  > > Initial infarct size of <70 mL, and a
  > >
  > > Ratio of the volume of ischemic tissue on perfusion imaging to infarct volume of 1.8 or more

Modified Rankin Scale (mRS)	
0	No symptoms
1	No significant disability despite symptoms; able to perform all usual duties and activities
2	Slight disability; unable to perform all previous activities but able to look after own affairs without assistance
3	Moderate disability; requires some help, but able to walk without assistance
4	Moderately severe disability; unable to walk without assistance and unable to attend to own bodily needs without assistance
5	Severe disability; bedridden, incontinent, and requires constant nursing care and attention

(Modified Rankin Scale: Used to quantify degree of disability in stroke patients (*Scott Med J* 1957;2(4):127–36; *Stroke* 1988;19(12):1497–500.))

National Institute of Health Stroke Scale (NIHSS)	
0	No stroke
1–4	Minor stroke
5–15	Moderate stroke
16–20	Moderate to severe stroke
21–42	Severe stroke

National Institute of Health Stroke Scale (NIHSS): 0–42 point score based on level of consciousness, motor and sensory function, language, neglect, gaze, vision, ataxia (*Stroke* 1989;20(7):864–70;1994;25(11):2220–6).

ASPECT Score: Alberta Stroke Program Early CT Score
(*Lancet* 2000;355(9216):1670–4)

CT Head without contrast is evaluated for presence of grey–white differentiation in 10 different areas of the MCA distribution; 1 point is given for presence of grey–white differentiation (10 is a normal scan)

- Caudate
- Putamen
- Internal capsule
- Insular cortex
- M1: "Anterior MCA cortex," corresponding to frontal operculum
- M2: "MCA cortex lateral to insular ribbon" corresponding to anterior temporal lobe
- M3: "Posterior MCA cortex" corresponding to posterior temporal lobe
- M4: "Anterior MCA territory immediately superior to M1"
- M5: "Lateral MCA territory immediately superior to M2"
- M6: "Posterior MCA territory immediately superior to M3"

(Reprinted from Barber PA, Demchuk AM, Zhang J, et al. Validity and reliability of a quantitative computed tomography score in predicting outcome of hyperacute stroke before thrombolytic therapy. ASPECTS Study Group. Alberta Stroke Programme Early CT Score. *Lancet* 2000;355(9216):1670–4. Copyright © 2000 Elsevier, with permission.)

- **Treatment**
  Intra-arterial thrombectomy with a stent-retriever is 1st line based on the 2018 AHA/ASA AIS treatment recommendations (2018 Guidelines for the Early Management of Patients With Acute Ischemic Stroke: A Guideline for Healthcare Professionals From the American Heart Association/American Stroke Association. *Stroke*. January 2018. doi:10.1161/STR.0000000000000158)
    1st-pass using an aspiration catheter may be equally effective, but further trials are needed
    Intra-arterial thrombolysis may also be effective for carefully selected patients <6 h from symptom onset, but there is no medication approved by the FDA for IA thrombolysis available
      The only medication to show a benefit was pro-urokinase, which is not available in the US; tPA is used off-label in select cases, including for rescue therapy if mechanical thrombectomy is unsuccessful
  The technical goal of the thrombectomy procedure should be reperfusion to a modified Thrombolysis in Cerebral Infarction (mTICI) 2b/3 angiographic result to maximize the probability of a good functional clinical outcome

Modified Treatment in Cerebral Infarction (mTICI) Perfusion Score	
(*Stroke* 2013;44(9):2650–63)	
0	No perfusion
1	Flow beyond occlusion without distal branch reperfusion
2a	Reperfusion of less than half of the downstream target arterial territory
2b	Reperfusion of more than half, yet incomplete, in the downstream target arterial territory
3	Complete reperfusion of the downstream target arterial territory, including distal branches with slow flow

Patients may undergo general anesthesia or conscious sedation for the procedure
  Conscious sedation preferred if there is a delay to undergo general anesthesia (eg, anesthesiologist not immediate available)
  Efforts should be made not to drop blood pressure during induction

Procedure Basics for Mechanical Thrombectomy
  Groin puncture, Seldinger technique to place an 8F sheath
  6F base or guide catheter or balloon base or guide catheter navigated over a 5F or 6F "select" catheter over a glidewire into the proximal

cervical internal carotid artery, and the select catheter and glidewire are removed

A DSA run is obtained confirming the site of vessel occlusion. A road map is made from the run.

A microcatheter is advanced over a microwire past the occlusion, the microwire is removed, and a small amount of contrast is pushed through the microcatheter to ensure it is distal to the site of occlusion

Next, the stent-retriever is advanced through the microcatheter. Once the distal tines are pushed through the microcatheter, the stent retriever is held in place and the microcatheter is pulled back to completely unsheathe the stent retriever.

After allowing the stent retriever to integrate into the clot for several minutes, it is carefully withdrawn and removed from the base catheter; the thrombus is wiped from the stent and an injection is obtained through the base catheter to confirm recanalization of the occluded vessel

Next, the base catheter is withdrawn into the sheath and a run is obtained of the common femoral artery to ensure no vessel injury

If IV tPA was administered prior to the stroke intervention, many interventionalists will choose to leave the sheath in place for 12–24 h due to risk of a femoral hematoma; others will remove the sheath immediately following the intervention and close the arteriotomy using a collagen plug-based closure device (eg, AngioSeal)

Postintervention care

Following intervention, the patient is managed in an ICU setting; a neuro- or stroke-specific unit is recommended by the AHA/ASA. Strict blood pressure <180/105 mmHg is recommended, while some practitioners use a lower maximum allowable systolic blood pressure of 160 mmHg

While the sheath is in place, patients must lie with the head of bed flat or nearly flat (<15°), to reduce risk of injury to the common femoral artery injury and leg ischemia. Hourly neurovascular checks are performed by the ICU nurse

- **Evidence for Treatment with Mechanical Thrombectomy**

1980s, case series of intra-arterial thrombolysis for basilar artery occlusion published, suggesting superiority over no treatment (AJNR Am J Neuroradiol 1983;4(3):401–4)

IV tPA approved by FDA for acute ischemic stroke in 1996, but poor efficacy on proximal large vessel occlusion and only approved for <3 h from onset initially (now up to 4.5 h in select patients)

PROACT I: IA recombinant pro-urokinase (r-pUK) vs. IA saline for MCA occlusion <6 h stopped early due to IV tPA being approved, but analysis of 43 patients already treated showed benefit (Stroke 1998;29(1):4–11)

PROACT II published in 1999: IA r-pUK vs. IV heparin for MCA occlusion <6 h. 186 pts, improved clinical outcomes by 15% (NNT 7). Ultimately r-pUK not approved by FDA, but study established that IA therapy can be safe and effective, launching the era of endovascular therapy (JAMA 1999;282(21):2003–11)

MERCI device already in use for retrieval of coils, single arm study of 153 pts showed MERCI opened 48% of intracranial vessels with low rate of ICH, but overall mortality still high at 42%. Approved by FDA for thrombectomy in 2004 under a special device clearance path (510-K) that only had to show equivalence to a current device (Stroke 2005;36(7):1432–8)

3 RCTs of medical therapy vs. endovascular therapy published in 2013 failed to show efficacy of endovascular therapy (IMS-III, SYNTHESIS, MR-RESCUE), but flawed in many ways (use of MERCI device, poor patient selection, IA tPA frequently used) (N Engl J Med 2013;368(10):893–903; N Engl J Med 2013;368(10):904–13; N Engl J Med 2013;368(10):914–23)

In 2015, 5 independent randomized control trials were published demonstrating efficacy for endovascular therapy over medical therapy alone with newer devices and improved patient selection (MR CLEAN, EXTEND-IA, ESCAPE, SWIFT PRIME, REVESCAT) (N Engl J Med 2015;372(1):11–20; N Engl J Med 2015;372(11):1009–18; N Engl J Med 2015;372(11):1019–30; N Engl J Med 2015;372(24):2285–95; N Engl J Med 2015;372(24):2296–306)

After endovascular treatment, 30–71% were independent at 90 d vs. 19–40% with medical treatment alone

Absolute increase in functional independence by 13–31% at 90 d after endovascular therapy vs. medical therapy alone

In 2018, 2 RCTs published that show overwhelming benefit for intervention greater than 6 h, up to 16 or 24 h, in carefully selected patients (DAWN, DEFUSE 3) (N Engl J Med 2018;378(1):11–21; N Engl J Med 2018;378(8):708–18)

In these 2 studies, functional independence was 90 d was 45–49% in the thrombectomy group as compared with 13–17% in the control group

Mortality at 90 d was equivalent in DAWN, 19% in thrombectomy group vs. 18% medical group, and in DEFUSE, there was a significant difference in mortality, 17% in the thrombectomy group vs. 45% in the medical group

Intervention does not increase overall risk:

The risk of symptomatic brain hemorrhage was 2–8% with endovascular treatment vs. 2–6% with medical therapy alone

The risk of death at 3 mo was 9–21% after endovascular treatment and 12–22% after medical therapy alone

Risk of any major adverse event at 90 d is 31–47% with endovascular treatment vs. 36–42% with medical therapy

- **Imaging in Stroke Using an Illustrative Case Example (Figures 18-8, 18-9, and 18-10):**

Figure 18-8 Left: Noncontrast CT head in a patient with AIS; loss of grey–white differentiation in the insula; ASPECTS 9. **Right:** Coronal MIP reconstruction of CT angiogram head/neck demonstrating occlusion of the left M1 segment.

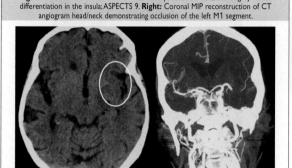

Cerebral Aneurysm
- **Background**

Defined as an abnormal outpouching of an intracranial artery

May be saccular ("berry"), fusiform (dissecting or dolichoectatic), or mycotic (infectious)

Saccular aneurysms are likely caused by combination of hereditary and acquired factors; outpouching forms at a weakness in the artery wall

Unruptured aneurysms present in 2–3% of general population (N Engl J Med 2007;357(18):1821–8; Lancet Neurol 2011;10(7):626–36)

Annual incidence of subarachnoid hemorrhage (SAH) 10 per 100,000, or about 30-40,000 per year in the United States (Stroke 1998;29(1):251–6)

Risk factors for intracranial aneurysm rupture (Stroke 2013;44(9):2414–21):

Hypertension, cigarette smoking, posterior circulation aneurysm, anterior communicating artery aneurysm, larger aneurysm size, family history of intracranial aneurysm

Conditions predisposing one to intracranial aneurysm:

Polycystic kidney disease, Ehlers–Danlos syndrome, Marfan syndrome, fibromuscular dysplasia, or Moyamoya syndrome

- **Presentation**

Unruptured aneurysms

Usually asymptomatic; found incidentally on neuroimaging obtained for other reason

Rarely, cranial nerve palsy, such as oculomotor nerve palsy from a posterior communicating artery aneurysm

If very large, may cause headache or seizures due to brain edema

Ruptured aneurysms

High initial mortality, about 30% mortality within the 1st 48 h (Stroke 1994;25(7):1342–7)

Symptoms in patients who make it to the hospital: Classically a thunderclap headache ("worst headache of life"), also may be asymptomatic, may present with a mild headache, nausea/emesis, obtundation, or coma

Up to 40% report a recent severe headache (sentinel headache) within the preceding month

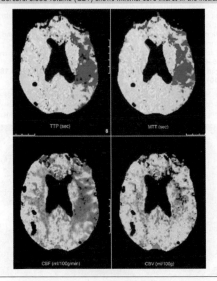

Figure 18-9 CT perfusion maps. Time to peak (TTP), mean transit time (MTT), and cerebral blood flow (CBF) demonstrate large perfusion deficit in the left MCA distribution. Cerebral blood volume (CBV) shows minimal core infarct in the insula.

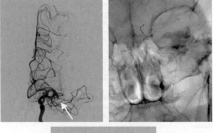
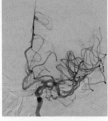

Figure 18-10 Left: DSA run shows left MCA M1 cut off (*white arrow*). Middle: Stent retriever deployed in M1 segment. Right: After withdrawal of stent retriever, full perfusion in left MCA distribution.

- **Diagnosis**
  Noncontrast head CT scan is performed if there is clinical suspicion, eg, severe
  headache; sensitivity 90–100% if performed within the 1st 6 h of onset
  If the CT scan is negative for acute blood but there is a high clinical suspicion, a
  lumbar puncture must be performed
  MRI brain T2 and FLAIR sequences also highly sensitive for blood products, but if
  negative with high clinical suspicion, an LP must still be performed so MRI
  generally not recommended
  Lumbar puncture
    Classical findings associated with SAH: High opening pressure and elevated red
    blood cell count that does not decrease from tube 1–4
    Drop in RBC count from tube 1–4 may be seen in both traumatic taps and SAH,
    so not the most reliable indicator
    Xanthochromia is the most sensitive indicator; detectable 2 h to several weeks
    after aneurysm rupture
    If CT Head and LP are negative, no further testing is required
    If SAH recognized on CT Head or LP, vascular imaging is performed
      CT angiogram head often obtained initially; may not detect aneurysms less than
      3 mm
      If CT angiogram negative, diagnostic digital subtraction angiography (DSA) is
      performed
      If DSA negative for aneurysm, a repeat angiogram must be performed 4–14 d
      afterward; up to 20% of repeat angiograms will identify an aneurysm
- **Grading Scales**

Hunt Hess scale (Lancet 1974;304(7872):81–4)	
Grade I	Asymptomatic, or minimal headache (HA) and slight nuchal rigidity
Grade II	Moderate to severe HA, nuchal rigidity, no neurological deficit other than cranial nerve palsy
Grade III	Drowsiness, confusion, or mild focal deficit
Grade IV	Stupor, moderate–severe hemiparesis
Grade V	Deep coma, decerebrate rigidity, moribund appearance

(Reprinted from Teasdale G, Jennett B. Assessment of coma and impaired consciousness. A practical scale.
Lancet 1974;2(7872):81–4. Copyright © 1974 Elsevier, with permission.)

World Federation of Neurosurgical Societies (WFNS) scale (J Neurosurg 1968;28(1):14–20)	
Grade I	Glasgow Coma Scale (GCS) 15, no motor deficit
Grade II	GCS 13–14 without deficit
Grade III	GCS 13–14 with focal neurological deficit (eg, hemiparesis, aphasia)
Grade IV	GCS 7–12, with or without deficit
Grade V	GCS <7, with or without deficit

Modified Fischer Scale (J Neurol Neurosurg Psychiatry 1988;51(11):1457)		
Modified Fischer Scale	Criteria	Incidence of Symptomatic Vasospasm (%)
Grade 0	No SAH, no intraventricular hemorrhage (IVH)	0
Grade 1	Thin focal or diffuse SAH, no IVH	24
Grade 2	Thin focal or diffuse SAH, IVH present	33
Grade 3	Thick focal or diffuse SAH, no IVH	33
Grade 4	Thick focal or diffuse SAH, IVH present	40

(Reproduced from Teasdale GM, Drake CG, Hunt W, et al. A universal subarachnoid hemorrhage scale:
report of a committee of the World Federation of Neurosurgical Societies. *J Neurol Neurosurg Psychiatry*
1988;51(11):1457, with permission from BMJ Publishing Group Ltd.)

Glasgow Coma Scale (Neurosurgery 2006;59(1):21–7; discussion 21–7) (sum of 3 factors, score 3–15)			
Points	Eye Opening Response	Verbal Response	Motor Response
6			Obeys commands
5		Oriented	Purposeful movement

4	Spontaneous	Confused, able to answer questions	Withdraws from pain
3	Open to voice	Inappropriate words	Flexion to pain
2	Open to pain	Incomprehensible speech	Extension to pain
1	No response	No response	No response

(From Frontera JA, Claassen J, Schmidt JM, et al. Prediction of symptomatic vasospasm after subarachnoid hemorrhage: the modified fisher scale. *Neurosurgery* 2006;59(1):21–7; discussion 21–7. Reproduced by permission of the Congress of Neurological Surgeons.)

- **Treatment**
  Surgical: Only treatment option until the invention of the detachable coil
    Craniotomy for clip embolization
      A metallic clip is placed across the neck of the aneurysm
    Trap and bypass: For very large or fusiform aneurysms
      Vessel sacrifice proximal to the aneurysm and an arterial bypass to the vessel distal to the aneurysm
    For blister aneurysms, wrapping the vessel with Gore-Tex is an option
  Endovascular coiling
    Guglielmi detachable coil (GDC) invented 1990, FDA approved 1995 for surgically high risk aneurysms
      Platinum coils with shape memory, advanced through a microcatheter into an aneurysm where the shape reforms
      Electrolytic detachment allows precise placement with a pusher wire then the ability to detach and remove the pusher wire
      Many variations of platinum coils are now on the market with different size, shape, texture qualities using mechanical and electrolytic detachment devices
    Adjunct devices to platinum coils for wide-necked aneurysms
      Aneurysms with a dome to neck ratio of <2:1 can be difficult to coil due to coil herniation into the parent vessel
      "Balloon remodeling" technique utilizes a balloon catheter inflated in the parent vessel lumen while the coil is advanced into the aneurysm lumen
      Stent-assisted coiling; a nitinol stent is deployed in the parent vessel and then the coils are deployed into the aneurysm lumen. Requires dual antiplatelet therapy, so not ideal for patient with SAH
  Flow Diverting Stent
    Intracranial stent with 30–35% metal surface area coverage (vs. approximately 10% for other stents), placed in the parent vessel across the aneurysm neck which directs blood flow past the aneurysm, resulting in gradual thrombosis of the aneurysm over days to months
    Due to gradual thrombosis and need for antiplatelet therapy, not generally used to treat ruptured aneurysms; may be some utility for ruptured blister aneurysms which are not amenable to clip or coil embolization
    FDA approval for Pipeline Embolization Device achieved in 2011 based on the results of the PUFS trial (see below "Landmark Trials"). The PITA trial was the initial multicenter prospective trial demonstrating safety and efficacy of the device.
    A 2nd generation, easier to deploy flow diverter, the Pipeline Flex, was approved by the FDA in 2015. Procedure related morbidity and mortality rates have dropped from 5.6% with the 1st generation to 1.9% with the 2nd generation device (*J Neurosurg* 2018:1–7)
  Clip vs. coil
    The decision to treat with open clipping or endovascular coiling is made on a case-by-case basis, depending on aneurysm and patient characteristics
    For ruptured aneurysms, if the aneurysm is judged to be amenable to both clipping and coiling, coiling should be considered per AHA/ASA guidelines (also see ISAT below in "Landmark Trials")
    For elective treatment of intracranial aneurysms, the aneurysm and patient characteristics must be weighed with the technical expertise of the performing surgeon/interventionalist
    In general, clipping has a higher perioperative risk of complication than coiling, but coiled aneurysms have a higher rate of recanalization, increased rate of delayed rupture, and higher retreatment rate
  When to Treat
    Ruptured aneurysms must be treated due to the high risk of rerupture; 3–4% in the initial 24 h, and 50% in the 1st 30 d from historical studies. Rerupture is associated with high mortality

Unruptured aneurysms in a patient that has had a subarachnoid hemorrhage should be treated; these are at higher risk of rupture than aneurysms of equivalent size in patients that have not had SAH

Incidentally discovered aneurysms are treated on a case-by-case basis; studies have tried to predict which aneurysms will rupture (see ISUIA II, UCAS, SUAVe below under "Landmark Trials") with imperfect results

In general, unruptured intracranial (and intradural) aneurysms will be treated if
- Patient with a life expectancy over 5 y
- Aneurysm is 7 mm or greater
- There is presence of a daughter sac/bleb
- Aneurysm arises from the posterior circulation
- Growth of aneurysm over serial scans

Aneurysms less than 7 mm in the anterior circulation can be monitored with serial scans in a patient willing to accept the small risk of aneurysmal rupture

- **Complications of Endovascular Coiling**

Intraprocedural complications include cerebral thromboembolism, aneurysm perforation, coil migration, parent vessel injuries, retroperitoneal hematoma, limb ischemia

Published morbidity and mortality rates for endovascular coiling vary widely, morbidity ranging from 1.4–14.4%, clinically significant or permanent morbidity 0.27–7.7%, and mortality from 0–1.7% (AJNR Am J Neuroradiol 2005;26(3):506–14; AJNR Am J Neuroradiol 2008;29(1):63–8; AJNR Am J Neuroradiol 2009;30(1):79–84)

- **Landmark Trials**

International subarachnoid aneurysm trial (ISAT) (Lancet Lond Engl 2005;366(9488):809–17; Lancet Neurol 2009;8(5):427–33): Outcome of clipping vs. coiling ruptured aneurysms. 1994–2002; 2143 patients enrolled

Stopped early at interim analysis due to better outcomes with coiling

23.5% of patients treated with coil embolization were dead or dependent at 1 y vs. 30.9% of the clipping group

5 y, however, the proportion of independent patients were equivalent, 83% of patients in the coiling group vs. 82% in the clipping group

There was still a mortality benefit, 11% of the coil group was dead at 5 y vs. 14% of the clipping group

Critiques of ISAT:

9559 patients enrolled initially, most excluded due to lack of "clinical equipoise," introducing selection bias

Negatives for coiling: Lower complete aneurysm obliteration rate (82% vs. 66%), retreatment rate higher (8.8% vs. 0.9% in the latter group), higher rebleeding rate (0.6% vs. 0.3%) (Neurosurgery 2010;66(5):961–2)

International Study of Unruptured Intracranial Aneurysms (ISUIA) II (Lancet Lond Engl 2003;362(9378):103–10):

4060 patients—1692 did not have aneurysm repair, 1917 had open surgery, and 451 had endovascular procedures

5-y cumulative rupture rates for patients without prior SAH with aneurysms located in anterior circulation were 0%, 2.6%, 14.5%, and 40% for aneurysms less than 7 mm, 7–12 mm, 13–24 mm, and 25 mm or greater, respectively, compared with rates of 2.5%, 14.5%, 18.4%, and 50%, respectively, for the same size categories involving the posterior circulation (including posterior communicating artery aneurysms)

The 0% rupture rate of anterior circulation aneurysms under 7 mm despite a majority of ruptured cerebral aneurysms measuring <7 mm is likely explained by the fact that aneurysms are acquired lesions, and the risk of rupture is highest when the aneurysm grows

Unruptured Cerebral Aneurysm Study (UCAS) (N Engl J Med 2012;366(26):2474–82):

5720 patients with newly identified unruptured intracranial aneurysms 3 mm or larger, followed over 11,660 aneurysm-y, ruptures were documented in 111 patients, with an annual rate of rupture of 0.95%

Yearly rate of rupture per aneurysm: 3–4 mm is 0.36%, 5–6 mm is 0.50%, 7–9 mm is 1.69%, 10–24 mm is 4.37%, 25 mm or larger is 33.4%

Aneurysms of the posterior and anterior communicating arteries were more likely to rupture than in the MCA

Aneurysms with a daughter sac were more likely to rupture

Small unruptured intracranial aneurysm verification study (SUAVe) (Stroke 2010;41(9):1969–77):

Followed 446 pts with unruptured aneurysms <5 mm

Overall annual risk of rupture was 0.54%, 0.34% for single unruptured aneurysms, 0.95% for multiple aneurysms

Pipeline embolization device for the intracranial treatment of aneurysms (PITA) trial *(AJNR Am J Neuroradiol 2011;32(1):34–40)*:

31 unruptured intracranial aneurysms with either a wide neck (>4 mm), unfavorable dome/neck ratios (<1.5) or failed previous therapy were enrolled

Complete aneurysm occlusion noted in 28 (93.3%) of 30 patients who underwent a followup angiogram at 180 d. 2 patients (6.45%) experienced periprocedural ischemic strokes

Pipeline for uncoilable or failed aneurysms (PUFS) trial *(Radiology 2013;267(3): 858–68; Neurosurgery 2017;80(1):40–8)*:

109 complex ICA aneurysms in 107 patients treated

Occlusion rate of 73.6% at 6 mo, 86.8% at 1 y, 93.4% at 3 y, and 95.2% at 5 y

5.7% of aneurysms required retreatment

5.6% procedure-related morbidity and mortality rate

96.3% of patients at the 5-y followup were independent (mRS <3)

No delayed neurological death or hemorrhagic or ischemic cerebrovascular events reports beyond 6 mo

No recanalization of previously occluded aneurysms

Carotid Artery Atherosclerotic Disease

- **Definition**

  Atherosclerotic plaque formation and subsequent internal carotid artery stenosis, usually within the 1st 2 cm of the common carotid artery bifurcation

  Considered symptomatic if ipsilateral stroke, TIA, or amaurosis fugax (transient monocular blindness)

  Moderate stenosis 50–69%, high-grade stenosis 70–99%

- **Pathophysiology**

  Atherosclerotic plaque formation with subsequent inflammation and oxidative stress

  Plaque ulceration, rupture, thrombosis, and hemorrhage can occur

  Emboli destination: MCA > ACA > ophthalmic artery

- **Clinical Manifestation**

  Can cause ipsilateral TIA due to hypoperfusion or stroke due to embolus

  Hypoperfusion produces stereotyped TIAs

  Embolus causes vessel occlusion with subsequent neurological manifestations

  Carotid bruit may be heard, but this is a poor predictor or degree of carotid stenosis or stroke risk

- **Evaluation of carotid artery stenosis**

  Screening not recommended for asymptomatic patients without risk factors *(Stroke 2011;42(8):e420–63)*

  Carotid Artery Duplex Ultrasonography often used as 1st-line screening test in patient with risk factors (PVD, CAD, atherosclerotic aortic aneurysm, HTN, HLD, tobacco smoking, strong family history) and patients with carotid bruit *(Radiology 2004;232(2):431–9)*

  Carotid US has sensitivity of 0.89 (95% CI 0.85–0.92) and a specificity of 0.84 (95% CI 0.77–0.89) to detect 70–99% carotid stenosis versus conventional angiography *(Lancet Lond Engl 2006;367(9521):1503–12)*

Diagnosis and stratification of ICA stenosis on carotid artery duplex ultrasound *(Radiology 2003;229(2):340–6)*				
ICA stenosis %	**ICA PSV cm/s**	**ICA EDV cm/s**	**PSV ratio (ICA/CCA)**	**B-mode imaging characteristics**
<50%	<125	<40	<2.0	Plaque or intimal thickening is visible
50–69%	125–230	40–100	2.0–4.0	Plaque is visible
>70%	>230	>100	>4.0	Visible plaque and luminal narrowing
Near occlusion	Variable	Variable	Variable	Markedly narrowed lumen
Total occlusion	Undetectable	Undetectable	Not applicable	No flow identified

(From Grant EG, Benson CB, Moneta GL, et al. Carotid artery stenosis: gray-scale and Doppler US diagnosis–Society of Radiologists in Ultrasound Consensus Conference. *Radiology* 2003;229(2):340–6. DOI:10.1148/radiol.2292030516. Copyright © 2003 Radiological Society of North America, with permission.)

MR Angiography

The sensitivities of both time-of-flight or contrast-enhanced MRA technique for the identification of carotid artery occlusion or severe stenosis were similar and ranged from 91–99%, while specificities ranged from 88–99% (Stroke 2008;39(8):2237–48)

CT Angiography

CTA compared with intra-arterial cerebral angiography for the diagnosis of 70–99% carotid stenosis had a sensitivity of 0.77 (95% CI 0.68–0.84) and a specificity of 0.95 (95% CI 0.91–0.97)

Catheter Angiography

Gold standard, but generally not indicated prior to treatment due to accuracy of noninvasive imaging

Indicated if multiple studies are ordered and there is disagreement

- **Indications for treatment and choosing a treatment modality**

For asymptomatic carotid artery stenosis <60%, medical management and continued surveillance is recommended

Based on the results of the ACAS trial, asymptomatic patients with >60% stenosis should undergo carotid endarterectomy (CEA)

Asymptomatic Carotid Atherosclerosis Study (ACAS) (JAMA 1995;273(18):1421–8):

Established CEA as standard of care in patients with asymptomatic carotid stenosis >60% over contemporary medical management alone

1987–1993, 1662 patients with asymptomatic carotid artery stenosis of 60% or greater reduction in diameter were randomized to medical management versus CEA

5-y aggregate risk of ipsilateral stroke/periop stroke or death was 5.1% for CEA vs. 11% for medical management only

Relative risk reduction 0.53%

Less effective in women

Medical management has improved and smoking rates have declined since ACAS, so may be less benefit with CEA

For symptomatic patients, multiple clinical trials have demonstrated benefit of intervention + medical therapy over contemporary medical management alone

North American Symptomatic Carotid Endarterectomy Trial (NASCET)
(N Engl J Med 1991;325(7):445–53):

Established CEA as standard of care in patients with symptomatic carotid stenosis >70% over medical management (ASA)

662 symptomatic patients with carotid stenosis >70% randomized between 1988–1991 to CEA vs. aggressive medical management

2-y risk of any ipsilateral stroke 26% (medical) vs. 9% (CEA)

Major or fatal ipsilateral stroke 13.1% (medical) vs. 2.5% (CEA)

CEA "highly beneficial" in patients with recent hemispheric stroke, retinal TIA, or nondisabling strokes and ipsilateral high-grade stenosis

Carotid artery stenting (CAS) developed as an alternative to CEA; initially only available in clinical trials

Stenting vs. Endarterectomy for Treatment of Carotid-Artery Stenosis (CREST) (N Engl J Med 2010;363(1):11–23):

Established CAS as an alternative to CEA in subgroup of high risk patients; led to FDA approval of carotid stents

2502 patients randomized to CEA vs. CAS in asymptomatic and symptomatic patients

Asymptomatic patient eligible if stenosis >60% on angiography, >70% on US, or >80% on CTA or MRA if US 50–69%

Symptomatic patients eligible if stenosis >50% on angiography, >70% on US, or >70% on CTA or MRA if US 50–69%

4-y rate of stroke or death was 6.4% with CAS and 4.7% with CEA. Symptomatic patients 8.0% CAS, 6.4% CEA, asymptomatic patients 4.5% CAS, 2.7% CEA

Higher risk of periprocedural stroke with stenting (4.1% vs. 2.3%)

Higher risk of periprocedural MI with CEA (2.3% vs. 1.1%)

After 30 d, incidence of ipsilateral stroke similar between CAS (2.0%) and CEA (2.4%)

>70 y: Favored surgery over stenting due to higher risk of primary end-points (stroke, MI, death)

Stenting favored younger patients

After 10 y, no difference in ipsilateral stroke or death; CAS 11.8% and CEA 9.9% (N Engl J Med 2016;374(11):1021–31)

Stenting and Angioplasty with Protection in Patients at High Risk for Endarterectomy (SAPPHIRE) Trial (N Engl J Med 2004;351(15):1493–501):

Established noninferiority of stenting symptomatic and asymptomatic high-grade stenosis in patients at high surgical risk

334 patients with increased surgical risk who had either symptomatic stenosis of 50% or greater or asymptomatic stenosis of 80% or greater.

Criteria for high risk (at least 1): clinically significant cardiac disease (CHF, abnormal stress test, or need for open heart surgery), severe pulmonary disease, contralateral carotid occlusion, contralateral laryngeal nerve palsy, previous radical neck dissection or radiation therapy to neck, recurrent stenosis after a CEA, age >80

Primary endpoints death, stroke, or MI at 30 d, and death or ipsilateral stroke at 1 y

12.2% primary endpoint in CAS, 20.1% for CEA (significant for noninferiority)

At 1 y, carotid revascularization repeated in 0.6% s/p CAS and 4.3% CEA

At 3 y, primary end point 24.6% for CAS and 26.2% for CEA (N Engl J Med 2008;358(15):1572–9)

Randomized trial of stent vs. surgery for asymptomatic carotid stenosis trial (ACT I) (N Engl J Med 2016;374(11):1011–20)

Established noninferiority of stenting asymptomatic high-grade stenosis without high risk

1453 patients enrolled CAS vs. CEA for asymptomatic carotid stenosis who were not considered to be at high risk for surgery

Primary endpoints death, stroke, or MI at 30 d, and ipsilateral stroke at 1 y

Primary endpoint 3.8% for CAS and 3.4% in CEA. Stroke or death in 30 d was 2.9% in CAS and 1.7% in CEA. Cumulative 5-y rate of stroke-free survival 93.1% in stenting group and 94.7% in endarterectomy group

• Treatment

Carotid Endarterectomy (CEA)

Preoperative

Imaging examined to identify if surgically accessible lesion with attention to the angle of the jaw; most carotid lesions at the level of the C3/4 interspace are accessible

Patients placed on ASA 81 mg prior to procedure

Operation

EEG neuromonitoring during the procedure to identify intraprocedural ischemia during temporary occlusion

Carotid artery bifurcation exposed and dissected from the surrounding tissue

Heparin bolus administered

Temporary occlusion of ICA then CCA then ECA (ensures any embolic material is directed away from the brain)

Arteriotomy along distal CCA and proximal ICA over the plaque

Plaque and intimal layer removed, debris irrigated away

Arteriotomy sutured with interrupted or running suture

Temporary clips removed in reverse order (ECA then CCA then ICA)

Closure with meticulous hemostasis; heparin may be partially or totally reversed with protamine if needed

Postoperative

Observation overnight

Close BP monitoring to prevent BP spikes with frequent neurovascular and neurological exams

ASA 81 mg is continued postoperatively; often indefinitely

A baseline carotid duplex ultrasound is obtained to track for restenosis

Complications

Cerebral infarct due to ischemia or embolus

Neck hematoma with subsequent respiratory compromise

Laryngeal nerve palsy

Esophageal perforation (rare)

Postoperative ipsilateral intracerebral hemorrhage

Delayed restenosis

Carotid Artery Stenting (CAS)

Preoperative

CAS most appropriate for symptomatic patients with high-grade stenosis and one of the following:

High surgical risk due to cardiac or pulmonary disease

Contralateral carotid artery occlusion or isolated ipsilateral anterior circulation

Contralateral laryngeal nerve palsy

Previous radical neck dissection or radiation

Restenosis after prior CEA

Patient is started on aspirin 81 mg and Plavix 75 mg at least 5 d prior, or loaded with aspirin 650 mg and Plavix 600 mg prior to the procedure

In addition to basic endovascular preop management (see separate chapter), a detailed neurological exam must be personally obtained by the interventionalist

Procedure

Generally performed under conscious sedation monitored by an anesthesia team with arterial BP monitoring unless patient is unable to tolerate; neurological exams may be performed during the procedure if embolus suspected

Atropine should be drawn up and ready to give in the event of prolonged bradycardia/asystole with manipulation of the carotid body

Groin access obtained with placement of a long (80–90 cm) 6F sheath

Patient heparinized after access; bolus + drip vs. intermittent bolus dosing; ACT should be monitored approximately every 20 min and maintained approximately double the patient's baseline ACT

Guide/base catheter navigated to the mid-distal common carotid artery and a DSA run is performed; measurements obtained of the percent stenosis, diameter of the CCA proximal to the lesion, diameter of the ICA distal to the lesion, and length of the lesion

Stent length should be at least several mm longer than the lesion

Stent diameter determined by CCA diameter; tapered stent may be used

Note is also made of the lesion location in reference to the vertebral bodies; if there is movement or loss of a roadmap, the stent can still be deployed in the correct location

An embolic protection device (EPD) with a diameter equivalent to the diameter of the mid-distal ICA is navigated past the lesion and deployed; care is taken not to allow the EPD to scrape along the ICA to avoid intimal injury

Balloon angioplasty may be required prior to or after stent deployment; a balloon should never be sized greater than the diameter of the normal parent vessel or of the stent; poststent angioplasty increases the risk of vessel dissection

The stent is navigated over the EPD wire and carefully deployed covering the entire lesion

The lesion is considered treated if there is less than 50% residual stenosis; some interventionalists aim for a lower percent residual stenosis

The EPD is recaptured and removed after stent and angioplasty if necessary

The heparin drip or intermittent boluses should be stopped after EPD removal; partial reversal with protamine is optional

The sheath is removed and the common femoral arteriotomy is closed with a device and manual pressure or pressure alone

Postoperative

Observation overnight

Close BP monitoring to prevent BP spikes with frequent neurovascular and neurological exams

A baseline carotid duplex US is obtained

Plavix continued for minimum 6 w to 6 mo to allow for neointimal growth in the stent; aspirin 81 mg usually continued indefinitely

Complications

Ischemic stroke from embolus

Vessel dissection

Intracerebral hemorrhage

Postoperative ipsilateral intracerebral hemorrhage

Delayed restenosis

Epistaxis

- **Background**

Uncontrolled epistaxis often idiopathic, but may be also be caused by tumors, postradiation changes, trauma *(AJR Am J Roentgenol 2000;174(3):845–51)*

Treatment can involve embolization of external carotid artery branches

- **Evaluation**

Initial evaluation by ENT physicians to determine if bleeding site is from the anterior or posterior nasal mucosa

Anterior bleeding can usually be controlled by chemical or electrical cautery along with nasal packing

Endoscopic evaluation of the posterior nasal mucosa with electrocautery may control the bleeding source, but if unable to visualize or control the bleeding, transarterial embolization may be required

CTA of the head/neck may provide evidence of the source, but contrast extravasation is often not seen

CTA head/neck is useful in uncontrolled bleeding caused by postradiation changes as there is often associated vasculopathy with steno-occlusive disease of the CCA, ICA, and ECA

- **Treatment**
  Due to massive blood loss prior to intervention, the presence of an anesthesia team is useful to provide general anesthesia or provide conscious sedation

  Groin access is obtained with 6F sheath in the common femoral artery

  A 6F guide catheter is navigated into the ECA on the side of the epistaxis and a DSA run is obtained to identify contrast pooling or distal vessel damage

  Embolization may be accomplished with polyvinyl alcohol particles, Embospheres, embolic glues such as nBCA or Onyx, Gelfoam, platinum coils, or a combination of these

  Particles are often used because they can be carried to the small arterioles adjacent to the mucosa, rather than just occluding the vessel proximally and potentially allowing collateral blood flow to continue to perfuse the injured mucosa

  Use of embolic glues can cause mucosal necrosis due to permanent loss of perfusion

Spinal Angiography
  A full diagnostic spinal angiogram involves DSA runs of the:

  Vertebral arteries

  Common carotid arteries

  Subclavian arteries (including thyrocervical and costocervical trunks and internal thoracic arteries)

  Paired intercostal arteries

  Paired lumbar arteries

  External iliac and internal iliac arteries

  Diagnostic spinal angiography is most commonly performed due to suspicion for dural arteriovenous fistula (AVF)

  A preangiography gadolinium bolus spinal MRA is useful to localize the dural AVF so a more focused spinal angiogram may be performed

Spinal AVF Classification (*J Neurosurg* 1994;81(2):221–9)	
Type I	AV fistula between radicular artery and intradural medullary vein
Type II	Intramedullary glomus malformations
Type III	Extensive juvenile malformations, often extending into paraspinous structures
Type IV	Intradural perimedullary AV fistulas
Type IV, subtype a	Simple extramedullary fistula fed by single arterial branch
Type IV, subtype b	Intermediate-sized fistulas with multiple arterial feeders
Type IV, subtype c	Giant multipediculated fistulas

(From Barrow DL, Colohan AR, Dawson R. Intradural perimedullary arteriovenous fistulas (type IV spinal cord arteriovenous malformations). *J Neurosurg* 1994;81(2):221–9. DOI: 10.3171/jns.1994.81.2.0221. Reprinted by permission of American Association of Neurological Surgeons.)

  Preoperative embolization of spine metastases is the most common spinal interventional procedures

  Embolization with PVA particles, embolic glue, or coils can reduce blood loss during resection of spinal metastases

  Renal cell, thyroid, and melanoma mets tend to be hypervascular and resection can result in massive blood loss; preoperative embolization can result in significantly less blood loss

Intracranial Atherosclerotic Disease
- **Definition**
  Atherosclerotic plaque formation in an intracranial vessel with subsequent stenosis

  Generally discovered incidentally or upon workup of stroke

  Most common intracranial locations are the distal ICA, proximal MCA, and mid-basilar artery

- **Treatment**
  Prior to 2011, balloon-expandable intracranial stents were used in patients with TIA or stroke caused by intracranial atherosclerotic disease (ICAD) to prevent further strokes

  Due to negative clinical trial results vs. medical therapy (see below, "SAMMPRIS" and "VISSIT"), only a select few patients benefit from intervention for ICAD

  Medical therapy consists of antiplatelets, statins, BP lowering medication, and lifestyle modification

  The Wingspan stent mounted on a Gateway balloon (Stryker Neurovascular), Fremont, CA is the only device available in US, and is approved under a humanitarian device exemption (HDE) for patients meeting all of the following requirements:

  Age between 22–80

2 or more strokes despite aggressive medical management

Most recent stroke occurred more than 7 d prior to the procedure

70–99% stenosis due to atherosclerosis of the intracranial artery related to the recurrent strokes

Have made a good recovery from prior strokes, with a pretreatment modified Rankin score of 3 or less

Stenting vs. aggressive medical therapy for intracranial arterial stenosis (SAMMPRIS) (N Engl J Med 2011;365(11):993–1003; Lancet Lond Engl 2014;383(9914):333–41):

Patients eligible if recent TIA or stroke attributed to 70–99% stenosis of a major intracranial artery

Assigned to aggressive medical management or aggressive medical management plus percutaneous transluminal angioplasty and stenting (PTAS) with the Wingspan stent

Primary endpoint stroke or death within 30 d, or stroke after revascularization for the qualifying lesion during the follow-up period, or stroke in the territory of the qualifying artery beyond 30 d

Enrollment stopped after 451 patients randomized, 30-d stroke or death in the PTAS group 14.7%, and 5.8% in the medical management group. 1-y rates of primary endpoint 20% in PTAS group vs. 12.2% in medical management group

During a median followup of 32.4 mo, 15% of patients in the medical group and 23% of patients in the stenting group had a primary endpoint event. Beyond 30 d, 10% of patients in each group had a primary endpoint event

The early benefit of aggressive medical management over stenting with the Wingspan stent for high-risk patients with intracranial stenosis persists over extended followup

Effect of a balloon-expandable intracranial stent vs. medical therapy on risk of stroke in patients with symptomatic intracranial stenosis (VISSIT) (JAMA 2015;313(12):1240–8):

Vitesse Intracranial Stent Study for Ischemic Stroke Therapy

112 patients randomized to receive the balloon expandable stent and medical management vs. medical management alone

Halted early due to publication of SAMMPRIS trial

Primary endpoint stroke in the same territory within 12 mo or TIA >10 min between 2 d and 12 mo after treatment; stroke, death, or ICH within 30 d or TIA >10 min between 2 and 30 d

30-d stroke, death, ICH, or TIA >10 min 24.1% in stent group vs. 9.4% in medical group

1-y stroke or TIA >10 min 36.2% in stent group vs. 15.1% in medical group

Brain Arteriovenous Malformation (AVM)
- ### Background
  Rare (0.1% of population)

  Presenting symptoms

  ICH (41–79%), especially in children

  Seizure (11–33%)

  Headache

  Focal neuro deficit (rare)

  The overall annual hemorrhage rate is 3.0% (95% CI 2.7–3.4%) (J Neurosurg 2013;118(2):437–3)

  2.2% (95% CI 1.7–2.7%) for unruptured AVMs

  4.5% (95% CI 3.7–5.5%) for ruptured AVMs

  Increased risk of hemorrhage

  Prior hemorrhage (HR 3.2, 95% CI 2.1–4.3)

  Deep AVM location (HR 2.4, 95% CI 1.4–3.4)

  Exclusively deep venous drainage (HR 2.4, 95% CI 1.1–3.8)

  Associated aneurysms (HR 1.8, 95% CI 1.6–2.0)

  Trend toward increase hemorrhage risk:

  Any deep venous drainage (HR 1.3, 95% CI 0.9–1.75)

  Female sex (HR 1.4, 95% CI 0.6–2.1)

  Not significantly associated with rupture risk

  Small AVM size

  Older patient age

  Estimation of lifetime rupture risk:

  105—Patient age

- ### Treatment
  #### Surgical Excision
  Longest history

  Highest rates of cure (95%)

  Spetzler–Martin grade affects surgical risk

Stereotactic radiosurgery (*J Neurol Neurosurg Psychiatry* 2000;68(5):563–70)

Complete cure is considerably higher with smaller lesions; an overall 80% obliteration rate by 3 y occurs with lesions that are 3 cm or smaller

Larger lesions have reported obliteration rates of 30–70% at 3 y

Still risk of rupture during latency period (estimated to be equivalent to untreated AVM)

Complication rate 8–10% (CN deficit, seizures, radiation necrosis)

Endovascular therapies

Not considered curative alone

Partial embolization can increase pedicle pressure and risk of hemorrhage

Used as adjunct, preoperatively or before radiosurgery to reduce volume of treatment area

Most useful for deep or high flow feeding vessels

Embolic materials include n-BCA (n-Butyl Cyanoacrylate) and Onyx

Smallest microcatheters (flow-directed microcatheters) are used

Risk of treatment (*JAMA* 2011;306(18):2011–9)

Overall, 5.1–7.4% risk of permanent neurologic complication or death

Decision to treat unruptured brain AVMs unclear

A Randomized Trial of Unruptured Brain Arteriovenous malformations (ARUBA) attempted to answer this question for unruptured AVMs (*Lancet Lond Engl* 2014; 383(9917):614–21)

Compared interventions (any modality alone or in combination) vs. medical management in heterogeneous group of unruptured AVMs

Halted after 223 patients enrolled over 7 y, due to stroke or death of 29% in interventional arm vs. 10% in medical arm over a 33-mo mean followup

Limited by selection bias: Of 726 eligible patients, 323 refused enrollment, 177 treated outside of randomization, and 223 randomized

Higher than average treatment complications: many high-grade lesions (10% grade 4, 25% grade 3), 1/3rd of patients treated with embolization alone, only 15% microsurgical treatment

Very short-term followup minimizes lifetime risks

Due to heterogenous AVM grades, heterogenous treatment modalities, and short followup, the results are not generalizable to specific patients (*Stroke* 2014;45(9):2808–10)

More favorable results in case series of surgical treatment for unruptured AVMs (*Stroke* 2017;48(1):136–44):

Of 977 AVM patients, 155 ARUBA-eligible patients had microsurgical resection (71.6% surgery only and 25.2% with preoperative embolization)

Mean follow-up was 36.1 mo. Complete obliteration was achieved in 94.2% after initial surgery and 98.1% on final angiography

Early disabling deficits and permanent disabling deficits occurred in 12.3% and 4.5%, respectively, whereas any permanent neurological deficit (modified Rankin Scale score ≥1) occurred in 16.1%

Among ubAVM of Spetzler–Martin grades 1 and 2, complete obliteration occurred in 99.2%, with early disabling deficits and permanent disabling deficits occurring in 9.3% and 3.4%, respectively

Major bleeding was the only significant predictor of early disabling deficits on multivariate analysis ($P < 0.001$)

Spetzler–Martin Grade for Brain AVMs (*J Neurosurg* 1986;65(4):476–3)
Higher Grade Corresponds to a Higher Surgical Risk. From 0% with SM Grade 1–31% with SM Grade 5

Score of 1–6 based on sum of 3 attributes:

Size of nidus

small (<3 cm) = 1

medium (3–6 cm) = 2

large (>6 cm) = 3

Eloquence of adjacent brain*

noneloquent = 0

eloquent = 1

Venous drainage

superficial veins only = 0

deep veins = 1

*Eloquent brain: Sensorimotor, language, visual cortex, hypothalamus, thalamus, brain stem, cerebellar nuclei, or regions immediately adjacent to these structures

Noneloquent brain: Frontal lobe, temporal lobe, cerebellar hemispheres

(From Spetzler RF, Martin NA. A proposed grading system for arteriovenous malformations. *J Neurosurg* 1986;65(4): 476–83. DOI:10.3171/jns.1986.65.4.0476. Reprinted by permission of American Association of Neurological Surgeons.)

Intracranial Arteriovenous Fistulae

- **Background**

  Direct connection between artery and vein without intervening capillaries

  May present with intracranial hemorrhage, intracranial hypertension, seizures, focal neurological deficit, high output cardiac failure, or myelopathy

  Carotid-cavernous fistula represent a special case of intracranial AVF and often present with unilateral chemosis from superior ophthalmic vein hypertension/congestion

  2 main classifications of intracranial dural arteriovenous fistulae

Borden (J Neurosurg 1995;82(2):166–79)	Cognard (Radiology 1995;194(3):671–80)
Type I: 1 or more meningeal arteries drain directly into dural venous sinus or meningeal dural vein; anterograde flow	Type I: Fistula flow confined to sinus, anterograde flow
	Type IIa: Fistula flow confined to sinus, retrograde flow into sinus but not into cortical veins
Type II: 1 or more meningeal arteries drain directly into dural venous sinus; retrograde flow into subarachnoid veins	Type IIb: Fistula drains into sinus with reflux into cortical veins, anterograde flow
	Type IIa+b: Fistula drains into sinus with reflux into cortical veins, retrograde flow
Type III: 1 or more meningeal arteries drain directly into subarachnoid veins located at or on the wall of dural sinus	Type III: Fistula drains directly into cortical veins
	Type IV: Fistula drains directly into cortical veins with venous ectasia
	Type V: Fistula with spinal perimedullary venous drainage

(From Borden JA, Wu JK, Shucart WA. A proposed classification for spinal and cranial dural arteriovenous fistulous malformations and implications for treatment. J Neurosurg 1995;82(2):166–179. DOI: 10.3171/jns.1995.82.2.0166. Reprinted by permission of American Association of Neurological Surgeons; Cognard C, Gobin YP, Pierot L, et al. Cerebral dural arteriovenous fistulas: clinical and angiographic correlation with a revised classification of venous drainage. Radiology 1995;194(3):671–80. DOI: 10.1148/radiology.194.3.7862961)

Cognard Type I and IIa: 0% risk of intracranial hemorrhage

Cognard Type IIb and IIa+b have about a 10% change of hemorrhage

Cognard Type III: 40% intracranial hemorrhage rate

Cognard Type IV: 65% intracranial hemorrhage rate

Cognard Type V: 40% hemorrhage rate; 50% with myelopathy

Barrow Classification of Caroticocavernous Fistulae (J Neurosurg 1985;62(2):248–56)	
Type A (Direct)	Direct connection between the intracavernous internal carotid artery (ICA) and the cavernous sinus
Type B (Indirect)	Dural fistula between the meningeal branches of the intracavernous ICA and the cavernous sinus
Type C (Indirect)	Dural fistula between the meningeal branches of the external carotid artery (ECA) and the cavernous sinus
Type D (Indirect)	Dural fistula between meningeal branches of both the ICA and ECA and the cavernous sinus

(From Barrow DL, Spector RH, Braun IF, et al. Classification and treatment of spontaneous carotid-cavernous sinus fistulas. J Neurosurg 1985;62(2):248–56. DOI:10.3171/jns.1985.62.2.0248. Reprinted by permission of American Association of Neurological Surgeons.)

- **Treatment**

  Observation may be warranted for Cognard type I and IIa fistulae as these have a 0% intracranial hemorrhage risk, especially in the elderly population, however progression is often noted on serial scans

  Successful treatment requires occlusion of the fistulous point where the artery meets the vein

  Treatment options include surgical and endovascular occlusion; location of the fistula is the primary determinant when deciding how to treat

  Dural AVFs adjacent to the superior sagittal sinus (SSS) can be difficult to access endovascularly and are easily treated surgically by performing a craniotomy and placing a clip at the fistulous location

  Tentorial dural AVFs are also often treated surgically

  Access to the fistulous location endovascularly can be reached transarterially or transvenously

  Dural AVFs at the torcula can be particularly difficult to treat because:

  The venous side cannot be embolized

There are frequently feeding arteries from bilateral ECA and vertebral distributions

Surgical treatment generally has an unacceptably high risk due to massive hemorrhage encountered during exposure

Transverse-sigmoid junction dural AVFs can be occluded by a combination of transarterial embolization (using a liquid embolic such as Onyx) and transvenous embolization of the transverse sigmoid junction (using coils) if there is a patent contralateral transverse sinus

Direct carotid-cavernous fistula can be treated by coiling off the cavernous sinus either transarterially (by passing the microwire/microcatheter through the fistula) or transvenously through the inferior petrosal sinus

Complications Specific to Neurointerventional Procedures

It is important to personally perform a comprehensive neurological exam on the patient prior to any procedure, this will allow the interventionalist to detect subtle changes during and after the procedure that may signal a complication

- **Intracranial hemorrhage**

  Intracranial vessel perforation with subsequent subarachnoid hemorrhage can occur during any procedure requiring microwire/microcatheter manipulation within the cerebral vasculature

    Vast majority of these procedures are done under general endotracheal intubation with muscle paralysis to prevent movement while navigating the intracranial vessels (acute ischemic stroke intervention is an exception)

  During certain high-risk procedures when small, distal branches must be navigated, such as navigating to a distal AVM feeder, mycotic aneurysm, or pial AV fistula, it is good practice to have a fast-acting embolic glue (eg, n-BCA glue) open and mixed on the back table

  In the event of vessel perforation, the vessel can be immediately sealed to reduce size hemorrhage

  Vessel perforation can be suspected if there is a sudden jump of the wire or microcatheter, when the wire or catheter is seen outside a vessel on a roadmap image, or when there are signs of elevated intracranial pressure such sudden bradycardia and hypertension

  When coiling an aneurysm, always have the 1st coil open and on the back table before attempting to access the aneurysm with the microwire and microcatheter

  If there is perforation of the aneurysm, do not pull back on the wire/catheter

  If the wire perforates aneurysm, advance the microcatheter past the wall of the aneurysm and remove the wire; if the microcatheter perforates the aneurysm, leave it in place

  Quickly advance the open coil into the microcatheter, deploying some loops out of the aneurysm, and pulling back through the perforation and deploying the rest inside the aneurysm

  If this procedure is practiced, often there is minimal subarachnoid hemorrhage

  Forceful microcatheter injections in small, delicate intracranial vessels can also cause vessel perforation, particularly during a stroke intervention when there is already breakdown of the blood–brain barrier

  An examination of the pupils should be performed if a hemorrhage is suspected; signs of herniation warrant an immediate neurosurgical consult for possible external ventriculostomy drain placement or emergent hemicraniectomy

  Mannitol 1 g/kg should be administered to reduce brain swelling and protamine should be administered to reverse heparinization

- **Retroperitoneal hematoma**

  Potentially life-threatening complication that must be identified as soon as possible and treated

  Arteriotomy should be made over the lower 3rd of the femoral head, and below the inguinal ligament; this is identified prior to groin puncture by placing a radiopaque marker, eg, a hemostat, over the CFA in the groin to identify the correct location. Ultrasonography may also be used to obtain access.

  A retroperitoneal hematoma may or may not be accompanied by a groin hematoma, so visual inspection may not identify a hemorrhage into the retroperitoneal space

  Often the patient will complain of achy pain in the lower quadrant

  A deep, firm hematoma can be palpated, particularly when compared to the contra-lateral groin

  At times, the only sign of a retroperitoneal hemorrhage is hypotension and tachycardia

Direct firm pressure should be held over the arteriotomy site, but this may be ineffective in stopping retroperitoneal hemorrhage as the presence of a retroperitoneal hematoma suggests an arteriotomy proximal to the inguinal ligament in a noncompressible location

If a retroperitoneal hematoma is suspected, a STAT CT angiogram of the iliofemoral vessels should be obtained unless there is presence of hemorrhagic shock in which case vascular surgery should be consulted for emergent operative repair

Use of a larger bore sheath, antiplatelet medication, supratherapeutic heparinization, and obesity increase the risk of developing a symptomatic hematoma

- **Ischemic infarct**

  Common during neurointerventional procedures; usually these are small and caused by tiny emboli from:

  Thrombi due to stagnation of blood in catheters

  Small particulate matter picked up by catheters and wires while on the back table if inadequately wiped prior to reintroduction

  Air bubbles from poor technique

  Symptomatic ischemic infarcts are rare; often major vessel occlusion is recognized intraprocedurally and can be treated with thrombectomy by stent-retriever or administration of abciximab to dissolve the platelet aggregation

  Serial neurological exams must be performed after interventional procedures to identify both ischemic and hemorrhagic infarcts

  Of particular concern are posterior fossa infarcts, as these can cause progressive brainstem herniation and death

- **Catheter-associated vasospasm**

  Common in younger female patients;

  Nearly always asymptomatic and resolves in several minutes without treatment

  Seldom it may require administration of intra-arterial vasodilators such as verapamil or nitroglycerin if oligemia is suspected

INTRODUCTION TO THERMAL ABLATION METHODS

Background
- Thermal ablation methods include radiofrequency (RF) ablation, cryoablation, and microwave ablation. The definition of thermal ablation is applying direct thermal therapy to a tumor with the goal of complete or significant tumor destruction. Image-guided thermal ablation methods are commonly used to treat both benign and malignant tumors of the liver, kidneys, lungs, bone, and soft tissues. The next sections will specifically describe the most commonly used thermal ablation methods currently in use.

Radiofrequency Ablation (*J Vasc Inter Radiol* 2010;21:S179–86; *Radiographics* 2014;35:1344–62)
- Radiofrequency ablation (RFA) is a type of thermal ablation that uses electromagnetic radiation from the radiowave spectrum which consists of frequencies between 3 Hz and 300 GHz. The RFA system consists of a generator that produces electric current that is sent through an RF probe. The RF probe acts as a cathode. A large grounding pad which is placed on the patient acts as an anode. The grounding pad completes the electric circuit. The tip of the RF probe is very small and consists a significant amount of flux which causes tissue necrosis. The grounding pad disperses the flux and does not cause tissue necrosis when properly placed. As the electrical current is released from the tip of the RF probe, the dipole molecules which mostly consist of water will be agitated as they are flipped and realigned creating a significant rise in local tissue temperature. This process leads to coagulation necrosis. The tissue temperature exponentially decreases as the distance from the RF probe increases.
- The temperature of the tissue and duration of heating from the RF probe determines the success of the ablation. Tissue will necrose at approximately 2 s at 55°C and instantaneously at 100°C. However, if tissue is charred from heating too quickly or the temperature extends beyond 100°C, processes of vaporization, charring, and carbonization will result in increased tissue impedance of the electric current and act as an insulator. Therefore, the ideal temperature zone is from 55–100°C for a duration of approximately 4–6 min. To ensure that the entire tumor is ablated, 0.5–1 cm of normal tissue needs to be ablated around the margins of the tumor (*J Vasc Inter Radiol* 2010;21:S179–86)
- Another important concept to consider with RFA is the phenomenon of "heat sink." If there is a vessel >3 mm next to the tumor that is being ablated, the moving blood in the vessel will dissipate the heat. The tumor adjacent to the vessel will be harder to ablate and theoretically has a decreased risk of reaching complete necrosis
- The main disadvantages of RFA are the inability to reach large tumor margins, risks of vaporization/carbonization of tissue causing an insulating affect, and significant time to cause necrosis
- There have been many developments to overcome the limitations of RFA. To achieve a greater ablation zone margin, up to 3 RF probes can be placed parallel to 1 another but no more than 1 cm apart. If the distance of the probes are placed farther apart, there is an increased risk of incomplete tumor ablation
- The RF probes on the market have many variations. Some have traditional straight tipped electrodes while others have multi-tined, clustered, and expandable extensions with different shapes with the goal of increasing the ablation zone margin. Other devices use saline to cool the electrodes to increase the duration time of the ablation. There are also monopolar and bipolar electrodes. The more common are monopolar which consists of a single RF probe that is placed in the tumor that receives electrical current from a generator. The electrical circuit is then completed by a grounding pad. The bipolar electrodes consist of placing 2 RF probes in the tumor of interest with the electrical current received by the generator going back and forth through the 2 RF probes. There is minimal energy loss with the bipolar electrodes and they do not need a grounding pad (*Radiographics* 2014;35:1344–62)

Cryoablation (*Radiographics* 2014;35:1344–62; *Breast Cancer Res Treat* 1999;53(2):185–92; *Urology* 2002; 60 (suppl 1):S40–9; *Surgery* 2010;147(5):686–95; *Ann Surg* 2000;231(5):752–61)
- Cryoablation is a form a thermal ablation that freezes intratumoral tissue causing cell necrosis. Cryoablation uses the Joule–Thomson theory of expanding gases to freeze tissues. The cryogen that is typically used is Argon gas. Once the cryoprobe is

placed into the tumor of interest, the pressurized Argon gas is transferred to the tip which expands as the pressure decreases. The Argon gas is then returned through the tubing in the probe. The temperature at the probe tip can reach −160°C or lower. The cryoablation procedure persists for several freeze–thaw cycles. The average total time for freeze–thaw cycles is 25–30 min which is significantly longer than RFA or microwave ablation. An advantage over RFA or microwave ablation is the fact that the ablation zone can be visualized in real time under ultrasound, CT, or MRI guidance. The peripheral margin of tissue necrosis following cryoablation is 3–5 mm within the "iceball." Therefore, a 5–10 mm margin is typically recommended to achieve successful tumor ablation *(Radiographics 2014;35:1344–62)*

- Cell death can occur intra- or extracellularly depending on the method of the freeze and thaw cycle. The typical range of temperatures include −35 to −20°C. Faster freezing at lower temperatures will promote more intracellular ice crystals causing direct damage to cell membrane and organelles *(Breast Cancer Res Treat 1999;53(2):185–92)*. If slower rates of freezing occur, extracellular ice crystals form which lead to changes in osmolality and cell dehydration/death *(Urology 2002;60(suppl 1):S40–9)*

- Once the "iceball" melts within the ablation zone, the tumor is reperfused. During reperfusion, the cellular debris is rapidly released into the systemic circulation. Patients can have symptoms of a phenomenon called "Cryoshock" from these processes. Cyroshock phenomenon is a syndrome consisting of thrombocytopenia, disseminated intravascular coagulation, acute respiratory distress syndrome, hypotension, and multiorgan failure. The cause of cryoshock is thought to result from the release of cytokines from large volume freezing with multiple freeze–thaw cycles *(Surgery 2010;147(5):686–95; Ann Surg 2000;231(5):752–61)*

Microwave Ablation *(Radiographics 2014;35:1344–62; Radiographics 2005;25:S69–83; Am J Roentgenol 2009;192(2):511–4)*

- Microwave ablation is a form a thermal ablation which utilizes electromagnetic energy to cause tumor destruction. Microwave ablation technology offers similar benefits of RFA with the addition of several other advantages. Those advantages include: Faster ablation times, larger tumor ablation volumes, capability to use multiple applicators, ability to produce consistently higher intratumoral temperatures, lack of the need for a grounding pad, and potentially less procedural pain

- Located between the infrared and radiowaves on the electromagnetic spectrum, microwave radiation occurs between frequencies of 900–2450 MHz. Microwave radiation contains both positive and negative electrical charges as the waves oscillate back and forth. Microwave radiation takes advantage of the fact that water is a polar molecule that contains both a positive charge on the hydrogen atoms and negative charge on the oxygen atom. The microwave ablation frequency is designed to specifically interact with water molecules. When the oscillating microwaves interact with water, they cause the water molecules to flip causing tissue heating. The agitation of the water molecules produces friction and heat which leads to cellular death by coagulation necrosis. Compared to radiofrequency electric currents, microwaves can travel through all biological tissues including desiccated tissues.

- Different microwave systems can be separated by generation types. 1st-generation systems do not have antenna cooling. Because of this limitation, 1st-generation probes must use low power and short ablation time durations. The 2nd-generation systems do possess the ability for antenna cooling but are limited by generator power. 3rd-generation systems contain both antenna cooling and high-power generators. Within each system, they are then subdivided by applicator tip type, generator power, frequency control, phase control, number of antennae, and antenna diameter. All of the above factors should be considered and affect the volume of the microwave ablation zone. Frequency can also greatly affect the volume of the microwave ablation zone. The frequency of 915 MHz has been shown to create larger ablation zones compared to higher frequencies such as 2.45 GHz. The reason 915 MHz is more effective at creating larger ablation zones is due to the increase energy penetration *(Am J Roentgenol 2009;192(2):511–4)*. The highest heating of the ablation zone is greatest 1 cm from the antenna regardless of microwave ablation system. The average ablation time is approximately 2–8 min if using a high-powered system.

- In summary, microwave ablation is an effective thermal ablation method with similar benefits of RFA and additional potential benefits of faster ablation times, higher intratumoral temperatures, inhibition to electrical impedance, less sensitivity to heat sinks, and larger ablation zones

HEPATIC TUMOR ABLATION

Background
- When liver transplantation or surgical resection are not options for patients with early stage hepatocellular carcinoma (HCC), image-guided percutaneous local tumor ablation can be utilized to treat HCC. Also, patients who have limited metastatic disease of the liver and are not surgical candidates, could potentially benefit from percutaneous local tumor ablation to reduce disease burden. The ablation method that is most commonly used is Radiofrequency (RFA) ablation.

Patient Selection (*Handbook of Interventional Radiologic Procedures*. Philadelphia, PA: Wolters Kluwer; 537–48)

Indications
- **Hepatocellular carcinoma** → Unresectable liver tumors, single liver tumor <5 cm or up to 3 lesions <3 cm each, no vascular invasion, no extrahepatic spread, and Child A or B liver cirrhosis
- **Liver metastases** → Nonsurgical patients with limited metastatic disease to the liver (most commonly colorectal metastases) <3 cm in size. Total number of lesions is not an absolute contraindication; however, most will treat up to 5 lesions. Local tumor ablation of HCC and liver metastases can be used in conjunction with other endovascular treatments such as ^{90}Y radioembolization and TACE procedures

Contraindications
- **Absolute** → RFA is absolutely contraindicated for lesions <1 cm away from biliary ducts, intrahepatic bile duct dilation, exophytic location of tumor (seeding potential), and untreatable coagulopathy
- **Relative** → RFA is relatively contraindicated for prior bilioenteric anastomosis (risk of abscess), lesions close to the gastrointestinal tract, gallbladder, and pacemakers

Preprocedural Workup (*Handbook of Interventional Radiologic Procedures*. Philadelphia, PA: Wolters Kluwer; 537–48)
- History and physical
- Review imaging for extent of disease and planning for ablation. Specifically, identify size and location of the lesion and any adjacent vital structures such as blood vessels, bile ducts, gallbladder, and GI tract
- Labs: PT/INR (INR should be >1.5), baseline CBC, platelets (>50000/μL), complete metabolic panel (specifically check renal function [prefer GFR >60 or at least >30 if not in acute kidney injury if planning to give contrast]), tumor markers (α-fetoprotein for HCC and CEA for colorectal cancer)
- Hold antiplatelet medications for 10 d prior to the procedure (can be restarted 48–72 h after ablation)
- Warfarin should be held 5 d prior to the procedure (can be restarted 24 h after procedure)
- Heparin can be held 12–24 h prior to the procedure
- Patients should be NPO for at least 6 h prior to the procedure except for oral medications with a few sips of water
- Prophylactic antibiotics can be considered (Unasyn or Ciprofloxacin) if there is an allergy to those medications, Clindamycin can be used instead

Technical Procedure
- Consent the patient
- Liver ablation is usually performed with IV sedation (Fentanyl/Versed) or general anesthesia
- The access site is prepped and draped in the usual sterile fashion
- Using CT, MRI, US, or a combination of imaging modalities, the access site is anesthetized with 1 % lidocaine
- RFA probe, generator, and ground pad are connected according to manufacturer's protocol if RFA is chosen. If microwave ablation is chosen a grounding pad is not needed
- Using CT, MRI, or US guidance, the RFA or microwave probe(s) are inserted into the lesion(s) of interest
- Multiple probes can be used for 1 lesion to increase the thermal ablation zone (ideally the probes should be placed 1 cm apart from each other)
- Using RFA or microwave ablation, the probe tip is heated to 55–100°C for 4–6 min to cause irreversible tissue damage. The temperature should not exceed 100°C with RFA to prevent vaporization/carbonization of tissues that cause an insulating effect impeding the electrical charge
- The ablation margin should be 1–2 cm larger than the lesion to ensure complete margins

- The probes are then removed
- Sterile dressing is placed over the incision site
- Contrast CT or MRI can be performed after the procedure to verify the ablation zone

Postprocedural Care
- Patients can be discharged after 6–8 h or can be admitted for pain control
- If admitted, PCA or IV Dilaudid 2 mg every 2 h for pain and Zofran 4 mg every 4 h can be given for nausea
- Patients can be discharge when they are ambulating, eating, urinating, and pain and nausea are controlled with oral medications (Oxycodone 5–10 mg every 4–6 h as needed and Zofran 4 mg every 4 h as needed)
- Most patients resume full activity in 1 w

Complications (Handbook of Interventional Radiologic Procedures. Philadelphia, PA: Wolters Kluwer; 537–48)
- Cellulitis in incision site, liver abscess, tumor seeding, fever, malaise, abdominal pain, bleeding, skin burns, pleural effusions, and pneumothorax
- Procedural mortality is 0.1–0.5%

Surveillance
- CT or MRI with contrast examinations of the liver is obtained 4–8 w after the ablation. If there is concentric, symmetric, and uniform peripheral enhancement around an ablation zone, this is most commonly a transient effect of thermal ablation. However, eccentric, nodular, and scatter peripheral enhancement around an ablation zone is highly concerning for residual tumor

Results

Hepatocellular Carcinoma (Hepatology 2008;47:82–9; Radiology 2012;262:43–58; Radiology 2005;234:961–7; Radiology 2005;234:954–60)
- Thermal ablation is most optimal for very early HCC lesions <2 cm. Patients with very early HCC have had complete response rates as high as 97% and 5-y survival rates of 68% (Hepatology 2008;47:82–9)
- Early stage HCC (single tumor <5 cm or up to 3 tumors <3 cm) can be effectively treated with surgical resection, transplantation, or percutaneous ablation. Long-term survival rates have been reported as high as 75% (Radiology 2012;262:43–8)
- Important prognostic factors include severity of underlying cirrhosis and occurrence of new lesions. Early stage HCC in Child–Pugh class A patients had a 5-y survival rate of 51–77% and Child–Pugh class B patients had a 5-y survival rate of 31–38%. 5 y after treatment, the incidence of new HCC lesions is 80% (Radiology 2005;234:961–7)
- If there are vessels that are 3 mm or greater in size adjacent to the ablation zone, heat sink significantly affects local treatment (Radiology 2005;234:954–60)

Colorectal Hepatic Metastases (Ann Oncol 2012;23:2619–26; Radiology 2001;221(1):159–66; Radiology 2016;278(2):601–11)
- A phase II study by Ruers et al. compared efficacy of systemic chemotherapy with RFA and systemic chemotherapy alone for the treatment of metastatic colorectal cancer to the liver in 119 patients. The study demonstrated that the 30-mo overall survival rate was 61.7% for combined systemic chemotherapy and RFA and 57.6% for only systemic chemotherapy treatment. The median overall survival was 45.3 and 40.5 mo for combined systemic chemotherapy and RFA treatment and systemic treatment, respectively. The median progression-free survival was 16.8 mo and 9.9 mo, respectively. In conclusion, the 30-mo overall survival for the 2 groups were in a similar range. However, the systemic chemotherapy and RFA group had significantly longer progression-free survival (Ann Oncol 2012;23:2619–26)
- In a study by Sobiati, 179 metachronous colorectal carcinoma hepatic metastases were treated by RFA in 117 patients. The estimated medial survival was 36 mo. The 1-, 2-, and 3-y survival rates were 93%, 69%, and 46%, respectively (Radiology 2001;221(1):159–66)
- When treating metastatic colorectal carcinoma hepatic metastases with RFA, tumor size <3 cm and obtaining ablation margins >5 mm are critical to local tumor control with RFA. If the tumor size is >3 cm in size and there is presence of more than one site of extrahepatic disease, patients will have shorter overall survival (Radiology 2016; 278(2):601–11)

RENAL TUMOR ABLATION

Background (Handbook of Interventional Radiologic Procedures Philadelphia, PA: Wolters Kluwer; 548–54)
- Renal cancer is the 9th most commonly diagnosed cancer in the US. About 63990 new cases of kidney cancer will occur yearly in the US. Partial or complete

nephrectomy is still the standard of care for small renal cancers. However, thermal ablation is a growing treatment method for renal cancer with the potential addition benefit of preservation of normal renal tissue. The 2 most common thermal ablation methods used in common medical practice to treat primary renal malignancies are radiofrequency ablation (RFA) and cryoablation.

Patient Selection
- **Indications** → Patients who have T1 renal masses which are <7 cm without known contraindication to partial or complete nephrectomy, renal cell carcinoma in a patient with solitary kidney, prior partial nephrectomy, or prior contralateral radical nephrectomy. Patients with certain inherent diseases such as Von Hippel Landau, Birt Hogg Dubé syndrome, or multiple bilateral renal cell carcinomas
- **Contraindications**
  - **Absolute** → Uncorrectable coagulopathy
  - **Relative** → Anteromedial masses without safe access, hip prosthesis or pacemaker/defibrillators are relative contraindications in RFA because of possible increase risk of skin burn or interfering with pacemaker/defibrillator device, respectively. Cryoablation can be used in these patients.

Preprocedural Workup
- History and physical
- Labs: PT/INR (<1.5), Platelets (>50000/dL), creatinine, GFR (ideally >30 mL/min/1.73 m^2 if using IV contrast), baseline hemoglobin/hematocrit
- Hold antiplatelet medications for 10 d prior to the procedure (can be restarted 48–72 h after ablation)
- Warfarin should be held 5 d prior to the procedure (can be restarted 24 h after procedure)
- Heparin can be held 12–24 h prior to the procedure
- Patient should be NPO for at least 6 h prior to the procedure except for oral medications with a few sips of water
- Prophylactic antibiotics can be considered (Unasyn or ciprofloxacin) if there an allergy to those medications, Clindamycin can be used instead
- Review imaging: CT urogram with contrast or dynamic MRI of the kidneys can be performed for evaluation of renal mass(es) and their location to vital structures
- Important considerations when reviewing imaging include accessing the R.E.N.A.L nephrectomy score to assess complexity (4–6 low complexity, 7–9 medium complexity, and 10–12 high complexity), identifying any tumor extension into renal vein or IVC, and assessing surrounding structures bowel/pleura, and location of tumor to the hilum/ureters

R.E.N.A.L. Nephrectomy Score			
	1 point	2 points	3 points
(R)adius (maximal diameter of mass in cm)	≤4	>4 but <7	≥7
(E)xophytic/endophytic properties	≥50%	<50%	Entirely endophytic
(N)earness of the tumor to the collecting system or sinus (mm)	≥7	>4 but <7	≤4
(A)nterior/Posterior	No points given. Mass assigned a descriptor of a, p, or x		
(L)ocation relative to the polar lines	Entirely above the upper or below the lower polar line	Lesion crosses polar line	>50% mass is across the polar line (a) or mass crosses the axial renal midline (b) or mass is entirely between the polar lines (c)

- Choose ablation method: Cryoablation vs. RFA
- Discuss case with referring urologist

Technical Procedure
- Consent patient
- General anesthesia or deep conscious sedation
- Prep and drape in the usual sterile fashion
- Use CT with/without US guidance to confirm location of renal mass(es)
- 1% lidocaine anesthetic is used to anesthetize the access tract
- Before introducing the RFA or cryoablation probe consider performing hydrodissection by injecting sterile saline between bowel and the renal mass(es)

- Although not absolutely necessary, a biopsy of the renal mass can be performed before ablation under CT/US guidance
- Under CT/US guidance, the ablation probe(s) are advanced into the renal mass. If multiple probes are used, the probes should remain 1 cm apart from each other.
- Ablation is then started. See below for specific ablation methods.

Ablation Methods

Cryoablation
- If cryoablation is used, an appropriate size cryoprobe is chosen to appropriately account for desired ablation zone size. The probe(s) are then tested in a bowl of sterile saline to ensure that the probes are functioning properly. The tip of the probes should freeze the saline. Once the probes have been successfully tested, the probe(s) are inserted into the lesion of interest. Then at least 2 cycles of a 10-min freeze (argon gas) and 5-min thaw (nitrogen gas) are then performed. The ablation zone should extend >5 mm beyond the tumor surface. The probes are then removed. Hemostasis is then achieved with compression and sterile dressing that is placed over the incision site. An immediate post ablation CT scan is used to visualize the hypodense "iceball" ablation zone

RFA
- If RFA is used, the RFA probe should be appropriately connected to the device according to specific manufacturer's protocol. Under CT/US guidance, the probe(s) are advanced into the lesion of interest. The probe(s) are then heated between 60–100°C for a duration of time according to the manufacturer's protocol. The probes are then removed. Postablation CT with contrast is used to confirm the ablation zone. Peripheral hyperenhancement around ablation zone can be seen and is a transient affect. Hemostasis is then achieved with compression and sterile dressing is placed over the incision site

Postprocedural Care
- Patients should be on bedrest for 4–6 h
- Vitals are taken every 15 min for 1 h, every 30 min for the following 2 h, and every h thereafter
- Monitor hematuria (red tinge urine is expected up to 48 h, thick blood clots are concerning for more serious bleeding)
- Pain control: Percocet 5–10 mg/325 mg every 4–6 h as needed for 3–4 d following procedure
- NSAIDs should be avoided to prevent further renal dysfunction
- Nausea: Ondansetron 4 mg IV every 4 h as needed
- Hydration: 75–100 cc of normal saline while patient is NPO
- Monitor strict urine input and output
- Most patients can resume full activities in 7–10 d
- Patient may shower 1 d after the procedure (avoid soaking baths for 2–3 d)
- Patients are usually discharged same day but can be admitted for pain control or bleeding

Complications
- Pain at incision site, bleeding (20–40%), gross hematuria, hematoma (subcapsular/extracapsular), urine leak 1%, tumor track seeding, infection, nontarget ablation: rare but does occur including injury to nerves, bowel, or cause pneumothorax, skin burns from grounding pads used with RFA, renal/hepatic failure in cryoablation suspect cryoshock

Surveillance *(Handbook of Interventional Radiologic Procedures. Philadelphia, PA: Wolters Kluwer; 548–54)*
- Followup contrast enhanced renal mass protocol CT or MRI exams can be obtained in 1–3 mo. If no abnormal enhancement then imaging can be obtained every 3 mo for the 1st year, then every 1–2 y thereafter
- Thin peripheral enhancement is normal (up to 6 mo) and nodular enhancement is concerning for residual disease with RFA

Results *(J Urol 2008;179:1227–33; BJU Int 2012;110:1438–43; J Vasc Interv Radiol 2008;19:1311–20; Cancer 2008;113:2671–80; European Urolog 2015;67:252–9)*
- A meta-analysis of 99 studies involving 6471 renal tumors was performed by Kunckle et al. The study demonstrated that local recurrence of renal tumors occurred in 2.6% of patients after having nephron sparing surgery, 4.6 % after cyroablation, and 11.7% after RFA *(J Urol 2008;179:1227–33)*
- Whitson et al., conducted a retrospective cohort study using the Surveillance, Epidemiology, and End Results (SEER) database with 8818 patients with renal cell carcinoma <4 cm in size and no distant metastases who underwent either

nephron-sparing surgery or ablation. Patients who underwent ablation for T1a renal cell carcinoma had a twofold increase of renal cancer death. The 5-y survival rates for nephron-sparing surgery and ablation were 98% and 96%, respectively (*BJU Int 2012;110:1438–43*)
- A meta-analysis of 46 studies consisting of 1180 renal tumors in 1055 patients demonstrated that percutaneous ablation was safer than laparoscopic ablation with lower major complication rates. Further, percutaneous ablation was equally effective compared to laparoscopic ablation (*J Vasc Interv Radiol 2008;19:1311–20*)
- A meta-analysis of 47 studies consisting of 1375 renal lesions demonstrated that cryoablation had significantly lower rates of local tumor progression and fewer retreatments than RFA (*Cancer 2008;113:2671–80*)
- Within a cohort of 1424 patients with cT1a renal masses who underwent partial nephrectomy, cryoablation, or RFA, the local recurrence-free survival was similar among all three therapies. Metastases-free survival was significantly better with partial nephrectomy compared to cryoablation and RFA. Cryoablation had better metastases-free survival when compared to RFA (*European Urolog 2015;67:252–9*)

PULMONARY TUMOR ABLATION

Background (*Handbook of Interventional Radiologic Procedures. Philadelphia, PA: Wolters Kluwer; 530–7; Key Statistics for Lung Cancer.* Retrieved from https://www.cancer.org/cancer/non-small-cell-lung-cancer/about/key-statistics.html#written_by)
- Lung cancer is the 2nd most common cancer in men and women. Approximately, 14% of all new cancers are lung cancer. The American Cancer Society estimates that there will be approximately 222500 new lung cancers and 155000 lung cancer related deaths among men and women in the US every year. The majority of primary lung cancers are of the non-small cell lung cancer (NSCLC) subtype. Treatment options for NSCLC include surgical resection, local radiation, and ablation therapies. Another subtype of lung cancer, small cell lung cancer, is a more aggressive form of lung cancer with treatment options including systemic chemotherapy and radiation. Thermal ablation methods including radiofrequency ablation, microwave ablation, and cryoablation have been used to treat biopsy proven primary and metastatic pulmonary malignancies. Ablation therapy for salvage therapy can be used to treat aggressive small cell cancers for palliative measures to decrease patients' symptoms. The following sections will review thermal ablation therapy for primary and metastatic pulmonary malignancies.

Patient Selection (*Handbook of Interventional Radiologic Procedures. Philadelphia, PA: Wolters Kluwer; 530–7*)
- **Indications** → Nonsurgical candidates with primary non-small cell lung cancer without lymph node involvement, palliative treatment for metastatic disease, salvage therapy for recurrence status postradiation therapy, prior surgery, or for palliative symptoms
  - For lung lesions <3 cm in size cryoablation, RFA, and microwave are equally effective
  - For lung lesions >3 cm in size microwave is preferred over cryoablation and RFA
  - For lesions close to pleura (<1.5 cm), there is no difference in preference between the 3 ablation methods
  - For lesions next to airways or vessels with concern for heat sink, microwave ablation is preferred over cryoablation and RFA
  - If pacemakers/implantable medical devices are near lung lesions, cryoablation is preferred

Contraindications
- **Absolute contraindications** → Uncontrolled coagulopathy (INR >1.5, platelets <50,000 per uL, active infection/bacteremia
- **Relative contraindications** → Prior pneumonectomy, single functioning lung, pneumonia, life expectancy of <12 mo, pulmonary artery hypertension, poor lung function, and lesion close to vital structures (hilum, central airways, pulmonary artery, etc.)

Preprocedural Workup (*Radiology 2007;243:268–75; Ann Surg Oncol 2006;13:1529–37*)
- Important considerations while obtaining the complete history and physical include evaluating for any pacemakers/metallic implants that could be affected by ablation
- Assess cardiopulmonary status for sedation assessment
- All lesions should be biopsied before ablation procedure and typically need approximately 1 w for postbiopsy changes/hemorrhage to resolve prior to ablation
- PET/CT of chest, abdomen, and pelvis to access extent of disease and evaluate tumor size. Best results occur with tumor sizes <3 cm for both primary NSCLC and metastatic disease (*Radiology 2007;243:268–75; Ann Surg Oncol 2006;13:1529–37*)

Technical Procedure

- Consent patient
- Moderate sedation or general anesthesia is administered
- The patient is positioned, prone is preferred for a posterior approach
- Prep and drape in the usual sterile fashion
- If using RFA, grounding pads are applied to the opposite chest wall
- CT images are obtained and the trajectory to the lesion is chosen with the shortest path
- The access tract is anesthetized with 1% lidocaine extending to the parietal pleura
- The ablation probe (RFA, cryoablation, or microwave ablation probes) are advanced into the lesion of interest under CT guidance
- CT images are obtained to confirm the position of ablation probes (should allow ablation margin beyond 0.5–1 cm from the tumor)
- Ablation is performed based on the specific type of ablation and manufacturer's protocol
- Ablation probe(s) are then removed
- CT of the lesion is obtained to evaluate the ablation zone and rule out complications of pneumothorax or hemorrhage

Postprocedural Care (Handbook of Interventional Radiologic Procedures. Philadelphia, PA: Wolters Kluwer; 530–7)

- Immediately after ablation, an intraprocedural CT of the ablation zone should be obtained to evaluate the ablation zone, damage to adjacent structures, pulmonary hemorrhage, or pneumothorax
- The patient should be observed for at least 2–3 h and can be discharge on the same day of the procedure or can be admitted for observation depending on any complications that occurred or comorbidities
- A chest radiograph should be obtained at 2 h following the procedure to evaluate for new pneumothorax or assessment of existing pneumothorax
- If pneumothorax is enlarging or patient is symptomatic, a chest tube can be placed. The chest tube can usually be removed in 24 h
- Vitals should be monitor, oxygen should be administered. If hemorrhage is suspected an Hb/Hct can be ordered.
- Oral analgesics Percocet (5/325 mg) for moderate pain. PCA pumps or oral narcotics can be given if pain is severe or increasing
- NSAIDs (Ibuprofen 400–600 mg PO every 4 h PRN) for 3–5 d following discharge for pleural inflammation

Complications (Semin Intervent Radiol 2013;30:169–75)

- Pain at incision site, pneumothorax (11–49% of cases), pneumothroaces requiring chest tubes (6–29% of cases), pleural effusion (6–19% of cases), parenchymal hemorrhage (6%), hemoptysis (3–9%), postablation syndrome, infection, bronchopleural fistula (0.6%), tumor seeding, and air embolism (Semin Intervent Radiol 2013;30:169–75)

Surveillance (Handbook of Interventional Radiologic Procedures. Philadelphia, PA: Wolters Kluwer; 530–7)

- Baseline chest CT with IV contrast should be obtained at 1 mo- and at 3-mo intervals thereafter to evaluate for tumor recurrence. Normal CT findings include ground glass opacities around the ablation zone which can last up to 3 mo. Abnormal findings include irregular enhancement in or adjacent to the ablation zone. PET/CT can be obtained at 6 and 12 mo. A standard uptake value (SUV) >3.0 is suspicious for tumor recurrence

Results

Primary Lung Malignancies

Radiofrequency Ablation (Lancet Oncol 2008;9:621–8; Cancer 2015;121:3491–8)

- The Radiofrequency Ablation of Pulmonary Tumors Response Evaluation RAPTURE trial was a prospective, intention-to-treat, single-arm, multicenter clinical trial that showed that patients treated with RFA for non-small cell lung cancer 3.5 cm or less had overall survival rates of 70% at 1 y and 48% at 2 y and cancer-specific survival of 92% at 1 y and 73% at 2 y (Lancet Oncol 2008;9:621–8)
- A prospective multicenter study by Dupuy et al. showed that overall survival for patients treated with CT-guided RFA for medically inoperable Stage IA non-small cell lung cancer were 86.3% at 1 y and 69.8% at 2 y. Tumor size of <2 cm was associated with greater survival rate of 83% at 2 y (Cancer 2015;121:3491–8)

Cryoablation (J Vasc Interv Radiol 2015;26:312–9)

- A retrospective study to determine the long-term survival of 45 patients with T1N0M0 non-small cell lung cancer treated with cryoablation reported the 5-y overall survival, cancer-specific survival, and time to progression of disease were 67.8%, 56.6%, and 87.9%, respectively (*J Vasc Interv Radiol* 2015;26:312–9)

Microwave Ablation (*J Surg Onc* 2014;110:758–63)

- A retrospective study to evaluate the safety and effectiveness of CT-guided microwave ablation treatment of inoperable non-small cell lung cancer. The local control rates at 1, 3, and 5 y after microwave ablation were 96%, 64%, and 48%, respectively. The average cancer-specific and overall survivals were 47 mo and 33 mo. The overall survival rates at 1, 2, 3, and 5 y after microwave ablation were 89%, 63%, 43%, and 16%, respectively. Tumors ≤3.5 cm were associated with better survival (*J Surg Onc* 2014; 110:758–63)

Metastatic Lung Malignancies

Radiofrequency Ablation (*Lancet Oncol* 2008;9:621–28; *J Vasc Interv Radiol* 2007;18(10):1264–9; *Oncol Rep* 2009;22:885–91)

- RAPTURE showed an overall survival rate of 89% at 1 y and 66% at 2 y and the cancer-specific survival rate of 91% at 1 y and 68% at 2 y for patients treated with RFA of metastatic colorectal lesions smaller than 3.5 cm in the lungs (*Lancet Oncol* 2008;9:621–8)
- A retrospective study evaluated showed overall survival rates of 96%, 54%, and 48% at 1, 2, and 3 y, respectively. Pneumothorax occurred after 20 of the 41 sessions (49%), 3 of which necessitated chest tube placement. A small pleural effusion was found after 6 of the 41 sessions (15%) (*J Vasc Interv Radiol* 2007;18(10):1264–9)
- A study by Yamakado et al. evaluated long-term results of RFA in patients with colorectal lung metastases. The 1-, 3-, and 5-y local tumor progression rates were 10.1%, 20.6%, and 20.6%, respectively. The 1-, 3-, and 5-y survival rates were 83.9%, 56.1%, and 34.9%, respectively. The median survival time was 38.0 mo (*Oncol Rep* 2009;22:885–91).

Cryoablation (*J Thorac Oncol* 2015;10:1468–74)

- Multicenter prospective study of 40 patients with 60 lung metastases treated with cryoablation demonstrated local control rates of 96.6% and 94.2% at 6 and 12 mo, respectively. The overall survival at 1 y was 97.5% (*J Thorac Oncol* 2015;10:1468–74)

TRANSARTERIAL EMBOLIZATION AND CHEMOEMBOLIZATION FOR UNRESECTABLE HEPATOCELLULAR CARCINOMA AND METASTATIC LIVER DISEASE

Background (*Handbook of Interventional Radiologic Procedures*. Philadelphia, PA: Wolters Kluwer; 258–62; *Handbook of Interventional Radiologic Procedures*. Philadelphia, PA: Wolters Kluwer; 263–9)

- Transarterial embolization (TAE) and transarterial chemoembolization (TACE) are 2 methods that were developed to treat primary and metastatic hepatic neoplasms. Particles either bland (TAE) or combined with chemotherapeutic agent (Conventional TACE or DEB-TACE) are injected through the catheter to embolize the arteries supplying neoplastic lesions in the liver. The embolization process leads to tumor necrosis and has been proven to be an effective treatment of neoplastic lesions in the liver.

Patient Selection (*Handbook of Interventional Radiologic Procedures*. Philadelphia, PA: Wolters Kluwer; 258–62; *Handbook of Interventional Radiologic Procedures*. Philadelphia, PA: Wolters Kluwer; 263–9)

- **Indications** → Unresectable hepatocellular carcinoma, liver dominant hepatic metastases including hepatocellular carcinoma, cholangiocarcinoma, colorectal, ocular melanoma, carcinoids, and sarcomas, and downstaging to a resectable tumor or transplant criteria
- **Contraindications:**
  - **Absolute contraindications** → Hepatic encephalopathy, large tumor burden, poorly compensated liver failure, ECOG Score >2, and uncorrectable coagulopathy
  - **Relative contraindications** → Severe anaphylactic reactions to contrast agents or chemotherapy, bilirubin >3 mg/dL, portal vein occlusion, bilioenteric anastomosis, biliary stent, or prior sphincterotomy poses risk of cholangitis following hepatic artery embolization, biliary obstruction, cardiac failure, and renal insufficiency

Preprocedural Workup (*Handbook of Interventional Radiologic Procedures*. Philadelphia, PA: Wolters Kluwer; 258–62; *Handbook of Interventional Radiologic Procedures*. Philadelphia, PA: Wolters Kluwer; 263–9)

- Child-Pugh Scoring: A–C
- Laboratory Studies: PT/INR (<1.5), Platelets (>50000/dL), creatinine, GFR (ideally >30 mL/min/1.73 m^2), baseline hemoglobin/hematocrit
- Definite tissue sampling or equivocal imaging characteristics confident of diagnosis of the lesion(s) of interest

- CT/MRI imaging to exclude extrahepatic metastatic disease and review of relevant anatomy for the procedure
- NPO for at least 6 h
- IV hydration with normal saline solution
- Prophylactic antibiotic: IV Cephazolin 1 g
- Prophylactic antiemetic: IV Zofran 4 mg
- Foley catheter placement

Technical Procedure (*Handbook of Interventional Radiologic Procedures. Philadelphia, PA: Wolters Kluwer; 258–62; Handbook of Interventional Radiologic Procedures. Philadelphia, PA: Wolters Kluwer; 263–9*)

- Consent patient
- Patient is positioned supine
- Prep and drape the right groin in the usual sterile fashion
- Administer intravenous conscious sedation (Fentanyl/Versed)
- Gain access into the right common femoral artery
- Perform abdominal aortogram (15 cc/s for 30 cc)—allows evaluation of the celiac, renal, and superior mesenteric arteries
- Perform superior mesenteric arteriogram (3 cc/s for 30 cc) to evaluate accessory/ replaced hepatic arteries with/without patency of the portal vein on delayed
- Perform celiac arteriogram (3–4 cc/s for 12–15 cc)
- Perform common hepatic arteriogram (3 cc/s for 12–15 cc)
- Place a catheter as distal into the vessel that is supplying the tumor as possible to minimize collateral liver injury
- If TAE is desired, 100–300 micron particles can be administered with dilute contrast until hemostasis is achieved
- If TACE is desired, prepare 100 mg cisplatin, 50 mg doxorubicin, and/or 10 mg Mitomycin C in 10 cc contrast and 10 cc Ethiodol (Conventional TACE)
- Alternatively, DEB-TACE can be used which consists of delivery of drug-eluting beads: 75 mg doxorubicin on 100–300 micron beads; larger beads can be used if needed to produce hemostasis
- Administer the beads through the catheter until complete dose is given or hemostasis is achieved Perform common hepatic angiogram to confirm hemostasis of treated area and evaluate any other arteries supplying the tumor
- Removed catheter and sheath
- Achieve groin access hemostasis manually or with closure device

Postprocedural Care (*Handbook of Interventional Radiologic Procedures. Philadelphia, PA: Wolters Kluwer; 258–62; Handbook of Interventional Radiologic Procedures. Philadelphia, PA: Wolters Kluwer; 263–9*)

- Patients are occasionally admitted for observation
- IV hydration with normal saline (75–100 cc/h)
- Pain can be controlled with a PCA pump which is then transitioned to oral pain medications (5 mg oxycodone)
- Discontinue Foley Catheter
- Antiemetics: 4 mg IV zofran
- Some IR physicians will send patients home with 5–10 d of antibiotics

Complications (*Handbook of Interventional Radiologic Procedures. Philadelphia, PA: Wolters Kluwer; 258–62; Handbook of Interventional Radiologic Procedures. Philadelphia, PA: Wolters Kluwer; 263–9*)

- Postembolization syndrome (patient experiences pain, nausea, and fever)—Treated with hydration, NSAIDs, and Zofran 4 mg PO Q4h
- Liver failure/encephalopathy which are related to poor liver function reserve prior to TACE. Treatment is IV hydration, blood pressure support, lactulose, rifaximin, and Flagyl until liver function improves
- Liver abscess. Treatment is percutaneous drainage with antibiotics
- Nontarget embolization leading to gastritis/enteritis. Treatment consists of omeprazole 20 mg PO twice a day, NPO, and IV hydration

Surveillance (*Handbook of Interventional Radiologic Procedures. Philadelphia, PA: Wolters Kluwer; 258–62; Handbook of Interventional Radiologic Procedures. Philadelphia, PA: Wolters Kluwer; 263–9*)

- An MRI of the liver should be performed at ~4–8 w after the procedure, depending on individual practice patterns
- Repeat BMP, CBC, PT/INR, and specific tumor markers at 4–6 w after procedure

Results

Transarterial Embolization (TAE) (*Cardiovasc Intervent Radiol 2007;30:6–25; J Vasc Interv Radiol 2008;19:862–9; J Clin Oncol 2016;35:2046–53*)

- The meta-analysis performed by Marelli et al. of 3 randomized controlled trials confirmed that when TACE is compared to TAE alone there is no demonstrated survival difference (*Cardiovasc Intervent Radiol 2007;30:6–25*)

- A retrospective study by Maluccio et al. involing 322 patients with unresectable HCC who underwent TAE with polyvinyl alcohol or spherical embolic particles demonstrated median survival time of 21 mo and 1-, 2-, and 3-y overall survival rates of 66%, 46%, and 33% (*J Vasc Interv Radiol* 2008;19:862–9)
- A randomized prospective study was conducted to evaluate outcomes of treating HCC with microspheres alone vs. chemoembolization with Doxorubicin drug eluting microspheres. In the study, 51 patients were assigned to the Beadblock (microspheres alone group) and 50 patients to the Doxorubicin drug eluting microscpheres group. There was no difference in RECIST tumor response between the groups: Beadblock, 5.9% versus Doxorubicin drug eluting microspheres 6.0%. The median progression-free survival was 6.2 vs. 2.8 mo and overall survival 19.6 vs. 20.8 mo for Beadblock and Doxorubicin drug-eluting microspheres, respectively. The study concluded that there is no apparent difference between the 2 groups (*J Clin Oncol* 2016;35:2046–53)

Conventional TACE (Lancet 2002;359:1734–9; Am J Roentgenol 2010;194(3):830–7)

- Llovet et al. conducted a randomized controlled trial which was terminated early because conventional TACE showed significant survival benefit for treatment of unresectable hepatocellular carcinoma compared to supportive care. The 1- and 2-y survival was 82% and 63% for conventional TACE, 75% and 50% for embolization only, and 63% and 27% for supportive care (*Lancet* 2002;359:1734–9)
- A prospective nonrandomized observational cohort study involving 11030 patients who either received TACE or transarterial infusion therapy without embolization to identify if one method is superior to treat unresectable HCC. The study showed that TACE was associated with significantly better overall survival rates than transarterial infusion therapy without embolization. The 1-, 3-, and 5-y survival rates were 81%, 46%, and 25% and 71%, 33%, and 16% for the TACE and transarterial infusion therapy without embolization groups, respectively (*Am J Roentgenol* 2010;194(3):830–7)

DEB-TACE (Cardiovasc Intervent Radiol 2010;33:541–51; Cardiovasc Intervent Radiol 2010;33(1):41–52; Cardiovasc Intervent Radiol 2012;35(5):1119–28)

- In a prospective randomized study comparing DEB-TACE and bland embolization treatment of immediate stage hepatocellular carcinoma, DEB-TACE demonstrated a better local response, fewer recurrences, and a longer time to progression than bland embolization with BeadBlock (*Cardiovasc Intervent Radiol* 2010;33:541–51)
- In a randomized control trial that was conducted to compare the effectiveness of conventional TACE vs. drug-eluting beads-TACE (DC Beads) concluded that the DEB-TACE group showed higher rates of complete response, objective response, and disease control compared with the conventional TACE group. DEB-TACE had more of an objective tumor response in patients with more severe liver disease and limited side effects. DEB-TACE with DC Beads/Doxorubicin is an effective and safe treatment for HCC with additional benefit for patients with more advanced liver disease (*Cardiovasc Intervent Radiol* 2010;33(1):41–52)
- In a study by Malagari et al., 5-y survival of 173 patients who were treated with DC Bead loaded doxorubicin (DEB-DOX) for hepatocellular carcinoma that was not suitable for curable treatments. The overall survival at 1, 2, 3, 4, and 5 y was 93.6%, 83.6%, 62%, 41%, and 22.5%, respectively. Higher rates were achieved in Child–Pugh A patients compared to Child–Pugh B patients (*Cardiovasc Intervent Radiol* 2012;35(5):1119–28).

RADIOEMBOLIZATION TREATMENT OF UNRESECTABLE HEPATOCELLULAR CARCINOMA AND METASTATIC LIVER DISEASE

Background (Handbook of Interventional Radiologic Procedures. Philadelphia, PA: Wolters Kluwer; 269–75)

- Radioembolization therapy involves an isotope of Yttrium-90 (^{90}Y) that is impregnated to glass or resin microspheres. The impregnated microspheres are injected through a catheter into the hepatic arteries that are supplying either hepatocellular carcinoma or metastases. The intrinsic characteristics of ^{90}Y make it ideal intra-arterial brachytherapy. ^{90}Y has a physical half-life of 64.1 h. During decay, ^{90}Y releases beta particles with an average energy of 0.9368 MeV. The mean tissue penetration of the beta particles is 2.5 mm and maximum tissue penetration is 10 mm. There are 2 commercially available microspheres for the treatment of hepatocellular carcinoma or metastatic liver disease, SIR-Spheres (Sirtex Medical, Lane Cove, Australia) and Theraspheres (MDS Nordion, Kanata, Canada). Comparison of the two microspheres is listed below.

Differences between SIR-Spheres and Theraspheres

Brand	SIR-Spheres	Theraspheres
Company	Sirtex Medical, Lane Cove, Australia	MDS Nordion, Kanata, Canada
Approved Indication	Approved by FDA (2002) for treatment of metastatic colorectal cancer to the liver with concomitant use of floxuridine	Approved by FDA (1999) under Humanitarian Device exemption for treatment of unresectable hepatocellular carcinoma with or without portal vein thrombosis or bridged to liver transplantation
Particle Type	Resin with bound Yttrium-90	Glass with Yttrium-90 in matrix
Mean Spherical Diameter	20–60 μm	20–30 μm
Activity per Microsphere	50 Bq	2500 Bq
Number of Particles	40–80 million	1.2 million

Patient Selection (Handbook of Interventional Radiologic Procedures. Philadelphia, PA: Wolters Kluwer; 269–75)

- **Indications** → Unresectable hepatic primary or metastatic cancer, liver-dominant tumor burden, and life expectancy of at least 3 mo
- **Absolute contraindications** → Hepatopulmonary lung shunting; Therasphere (30 Gy per infusion or 50 Gy cumulative limit) SIR-Spheres (Lung Shunt Fraction limit of 20%), uncorrectable coagulopathy, inability to gain arterial access due to underlying severe peripheral vascular disease, anaphylaxis to iodinated contrast, severe decrease renal function, and life-threatening extrahepatic disease
- **Relative contraindications** → poor performance status equating to the Eastern Cooperative Oncology Group (ECOG) performance status score of <2 (see ECOG Description below), total bilirubin >2 times normal, biliary obstruction, and portal vein thrombosis

ECOG Score	ECOG Description
0	Fully active, able to carry on all predisease performance without restriction
1	Restricted in physically strenuous activity but ambulatory and able to carry out work of a light or sedentary nature, eg, light house work, office work
2	Ambulatory and capable of all self-care but unable to carry out any work activities; up and about more than 50% of waking hours
3	Capable of only limited self-care; confined to bed or chair more than 50% of waking hours
4	Completely disabled; cannot carry on any self-care; totally confined to bed or chair

Pre-Procedural Workup (Handbook of Interventional Radiologic Procedures. Philadelphia, PA: Wolters Kluwer; 269–75)

- History and physical (Mallampati score for conscious sedation)
- Labs: PT/INR (<1.5), Platelets (>50000 /dL), creatinine, GFR (ideally >30 mL/min/1.73 m^2), baseline hemoglobin/hematocrit
- CT of chest, abdomen, and pelvis to evaluate for metastasis and patency of portal vein
- Arteriography and MAA lung shunt study
- Patients should be NPO for at least 6 h before the procedure
- Patients will require IV access for conscious sedation

Technical Procedure

Part 1: Pretreatment Angiography and MAA administration for defining vascular anatomy, embolization of vessels at risk for nontarget embolization, and evaluation of vascular shunts that would be contraindications to ^{90}Y therapy based on the MAA administration

- Consent patient
- Prep and draped the right groin in the usual sterile fashion
- Administer moderate conscious sedation (Fentanyl/Versed)
- Obtain right common femoral artery access
- Perform abdominal aortogram (15 cc/s for 30 cc)—allows evaluation of the celiac, renal, and superior mesenteric arteries
- Perform superior mesenteric arteriogram (3 cc/s for 30 cc) to evaluate accessory/ replaced hepatic arteries with/without patency of the portal vein on delayed

- Perform celiac arteriogram (3–4 cc/s for 12–15 cc)
- Perform common hepatic arteriogram (3 cc/s for 12–15 cc)
- If tumor is near the dome of the liver, consider phrenic arteriogram (1–2 cc/s for 10–12 cc)
- The IR physician can embolize any nonvital artery with coils that may be an increased risk of nontarget embolization
- Identify arteries that directly supply the tumor(s) of interest and advance a microcatheter as selective and distal as possible
- Through the microcatheter the 4–5 mCi of Tc-99m MAA particles are administered to evaluate the Lung Shunt function
- After Tc-99m MAA particles are administered, the catheters and sheaths are removed and hemostasis is achieved at the access site either from manual compression or closure device
- The patient is brought to nuclear medicine to have SPECT imaging and evaluate lung and GI shunts. If there are no clinically significant shunts that would prevent ^{90}Y radioembolization. The patient is brought back another day to have the ^{90}Y radioembolization therapy.

Part 2: Administration of ^{90}Y
- Consent patient
- Prep and draped the right groin in the usual sterile fashion
- Administer moderate conscious sedation (Fentanyl/Versed)
- Obtain right common femoral artery access
- Access to the arteries supplying the hepatic tumors of interest is obtained the exact way that was done on the mapping portion of the procedure
- Once the microcatheter is in place, the ^{90}Y microspheres are infused through the catheter with dilute contrast slowly until dose is completely administered or hemostasis is achieved
- Perform selective post-embolization arteriogram
- Achieve right common femoral artery access hemostasis manually or with closure device
- SPECT is performed for evaluation of treatment

Postprocedural Care
- Prior to discharge the arteriotomy site should be inspected for hematoma
- With femoral arteriotomies, patients should be observed for 2 h if a closure device is used or 6 h if manual compression was used to achieve hemostasis
- Patients should be discharged home on proton pump inhibitor (Omeprazole 20 mg orally once a day) to prevent gastritis Followup labs (tumor markers AFP, CEA, CA-19-9, or chromogranin A, liver function tests, CBC, and CMP) and CT/MRI imaging in 4–6 mo is obtained to access treatment response

Complications and Management
- Postembolization syndrome (patient experiences pain, nausea, and fever)—Treated with hydration, NSAIDs, and Zofran 4 mg PO Q4h
- Nontarget embolization leading to gastritis/enteritis. Treatment consists of omeprazole 20 mg PO twice a day, NPO, and IV hydration
- Biloma—Treated with percutaneous drainage
- Radiation cholecystitis—Treated with cholecystectomy
- Abscess—Antibiotics with/without percutaneous drainage

Results

^{90}Y Radioembolization Treatment of Hepatocellular Carcinoma (J Surg Oncol 2006;94:572–86; Int J Radiat Oncol Biol Phys 1998;40:583–92; Hepatology 2008;47:71–81; J Clin Oncol 2017;35(15):4083–183; Gastroenterology 2010;138(1):52–64; Hepatology 2014;60:192–201; J Vasc Interv Radiol 2017;28:1371–7)
- Intra-arterial administration of ^{90}Y for T3 unresectable hepatocellular carcinoma is an effective therapy to use as a bridge to liver transplantation, surgical resection, or ablation. The 1-, 2-, and 3-y overall survival rates were 84%, 54%, and 27%, respectively (J Surg Oncol 2006;94:572–86)
- In a study by Lau et al., 71 patients with unresectable hepatocellular carcinoma were treated with ^{90}Y microspheres. The treatment proved to be effective with the median survival of 9.4 mo (range 1.8–46.4 mo). The treatment was well tolerated without bone-marrow toxicity, radiation hepatitis, or pneumonitis (Int J Radiat Oncol Biol Phys 1998; 40:583–92)
- ^{90}Y therapy for hepatocellular carcinoma with known portal vein thrombosis has be proven safe with limited toxicities (Hepatology 2008;47:71–81)

- Treatment with Sorafenib and ^{90}Y radioembolization in patients with metastatic HCC is tolerable and was associated with longer overall survival and progression-free survival compared to previous studies which evaluated Sorafenib alone (*J Clin Oncol* 2017:35:(15):4083–183)
- In a single center, prospective, longitudinal cohort study involving 526 patients who underwent ^{90}Y radioembolization treatment of unresectable HCC, the response rates were 42% and 57% based on WHO and EASL criteria. Overall time to progression was 7.9 mo. Survival times were significantly longer in Child–Pugh A patients vs. Child–Pugh B patients (17.2 mo vs. 7.7 mo) (*Gastroenterology* 2010;138(1):52–64)
- A study by Vouche et al. demonstrated the efficacy of radiation segmentectomy with ^{90}Y radioembolization of solitary HCC ≤5 cm not amenable to RFA or resection. mRECIST complete response, partial response, and stable disease were 47%, 39%, and 12%, respectively. Median time-to-disease-progression was 33.1 mo. Median overall survival was 53.4 mo (*Hepatology* 2014;60:192–201)
- ^{90}Y radioembolization and drug-eluting embolization have similar overall survival for infiltrative HCC without portal vein invasion. However, abdominal pain and fever were more common with patients receiving drug-eluting embolization (*J Vasc Interv Radiol* 2017:28:1371–7)

^{90}Y Radioembolization Treatment of Colorectal Metastasis (*Int J Radiat Oncol Biol Phys* 2006;65:412–25; Cancer 2009;115(9):1849–58; J Clin Oncol 2016;34:1723–31; Ann Oncol 2001;12:1711–20; Ann Surg Oncol 2015;22:794–802)

- In a study by Kennedy et al., a total of 208 patients with unresectable colorectal liver metastases that were refractory to oxaliplatin and irinotecan underwent salvage ^{90}Y radioembolization at 7 institutions. The median survival was 10.5 mo for responders (*Int J Radiat Oncol Biol Phys* 2006;65:412–25)
- In a study by Mulchay et al., 72 patients with unresectable hepatic colorectal metastases were treated with ^{90}Y therapy and showed overall survival from the 1st ^{90}Y treatment up to 14.5 mo (*Cancer* 2009;115(9):1849–58)
- SIRFLOX Trial: Addition of SIRT with FOLFOX-based 1st-line chemotherapy in patients with liver dominant or only colorectal liver metastases showed no significant difference in progression free survival but significantly delayed disease progression in the liver (*J Clin Oncol* 2016;34:1723–31)
- A phase III randomized trial by Gray et al. showed that a combination of a single injection of SIR-Spheres plus hepatic artery chemotherapy is substantially more effective in increasing tumor responses and progression-free survival than the same regimen of hepatic artery chemotherapy in patients with bilobar nonresectable liver metastases from primary adenocarcinoma of the larger bowel. The 1-, 2-, 3-, and 5-year survival for patients receiving SIR-Spheres and hepatic artery chemotherapy was 72%, 39%, 17%, and 3.5%, compared to 68%, 29%, 6.5%, and 0% for hepatic artery chemotherapy alone (*Ann Oncol* 2001;12:1711–20)
- A study by Saxena et al. showed that resin-based ^{90}Y radioembolization for nonresectable chemorefractory colorectal liver metastases in 302 patients is a safe and effective treatment. The median survival was 10.5 mo and a 24-mo survival of 21% (*Ann Surg Oncol* 2015;22:794–802)

Alternative Treatments for Advanced Hepatocellular Carcinoma (*Cancer Res* 2004:64:7099–109; Cancer Chemother Pharmacol 2007;59:561–74; N Engl J Med 2008;359:378–90)

- Sorafenib (Nexavar, Bayer Healthcare Pharmaceuticals—Onyx Pharmaceuticals) is a promising systemic therapy for treatment of unresectable advanced hepatocellular carcinoma. Sorafenib is an inhibitor of tumor angiogenesis and cell proliferation by inhibiting a series of cell signaling pathways including: The serine-threonine kinase Raf1 and Raf2, receptor tyrosine kinase activity of endothelial growth factor receptors of VEGFR 1,2, and 3, and platelet-derived growth factor receptor β (PDGFR-β) (*Cancer Res* 2004:64:7099–109, Cancer Chemother Pharmacol 2007;59:561–74). The standard treatment dose is 400 mg PO twice daily. A multicenter, double-blinded randomized placebo controlled trial was conducted with 602 patients with advanced hepatocellular carcinoma who have not yet received treatment with Sorafenib or placebo. Patients who received Sorafenib (400 mg twice daily) had significant increase in overall survival compared to placebo group (10.7 mo Sorafenib group vs. 7.9 mo placebo group). However, there was no significant difference in time to progression of disease (*N Engl J Med* 2008;359:378–90)

CHRONIC PAIN

Background (Clin J Pain 1993;9:174–82; Classification of Chronic Pain: Descriptions of Chronic Pain Syndromes and Definition of Pain Terms. 2nd ed. Seattle, WA: IASP Press; 1994; Spine 1995;20:11–9; Pain Physician 2013;16:S1–48; Pain Physician 2013;16:549–283)

- Pain which persists beyond the timeframe expected for normal healing of a comparable pathologic process
- Unlike acute pain, which may have a purpose in signaling injury or pathology, chronic pain serves no useful purpose and leads to long-term functional disability
- Associated with higher rates of cardiovascular disease and obesity
- Very common, with incidence of persistent pain for 6 mo reported in up to 49% of the adult population
- The division between acute and chronic pain is generally defined as 3 mo, though may be shortened in instances when healing of the cause of pain may never occur, such as with cancer-related pain
- Often multifactorial, may be associated with chronic nervous system remodeling and sensitization reinforcing pain signaling, and may not be amenable to routine pain control methods

Etiologies and Presentation (Clin J Pain 1993;9:174–82; Classification of Chronic Pain Syndromes and Definition of Pain Terms. 2nd ed. Seattle, WA: IASP Press; 1994; N Eng J Med 2001;344:262–70; Radiology 2016;281(3):669–88; Spine 2004;29:17–25; N Eng J Med 2008;358:818–25; Joint Bone Spine 2006;73:151–8; Spine 2008;33(23):2560–5)

- **Numerous etiologies:** Chronic noncancer-related pain disorders include: Neck and back pain, complex regional pain syndrome, temporomandibular disorders, osteoarthritis, rheumatoid arthritis, inflammatory bowel syndrome, fibromyalgia, headache, and lateral epicondylalgia
- **Chronic back pain** accounts for most chronic pain problems. It is the 2nd most common complaint in primary care and the most likely cause of chronic pain to present to the interventional pain clinic
- Includes pain involving the cervical, thoracic, lumbar, and sacral spine for >3 mo
- Symptoms may wax and wane
- Often related to nonemergent muscular or ligamentous injury, degenerative joint disease, spinal stenosis, or disc herniation
- In most cases (up to 80%) the origin of pain cannot be definitively diagnosed
- Axial vs. radicular pain suggests different pain generators
- **Radicular pain** radiates along dermatomal distributions to the extremities and suggests irritation of a spinal nerve root or dorsal root ganglion due to:

  Mechanical causes
  - Spinal canal or foraminal narrowing resulting in symptoms and signs of intraspinal nervous and vascular structure entrapment
  - Narrowing due to degenerative stenosis (osteophytes, facet joint arthropathy, spondylolisthesis, or ligamentum flavum thickening), disc herniation, or synovial facet cysts
  - Disc herniation most common at L4–S1
  - Two-third of disc herniation cases demonstrate spontaneous partial or complete resolution after 6 mo

  Nonmechanical causes
  - Chemical mediated inflammation without obvious entrapment from adjacent inflammatory process, local trauma, or nerve root exposure to nucleus pulposus material leakage from annular fissures
- Spinal canal narrowing often with bilateral polyradicular symptoms
- Isolated neural foraminal narrowing or radiculitis is unilateral
- **Axial pain** without radiculopathy typically related to degenerative joint disease of involving the facet or sacroiliac joints, lumbosacral pseudarthrosis, or internal disc derangement
- Facet arthropathy present in up to 89% of the population aged 60–69 y old (Spine 2008;33(23):2560)
- **Other differential considerations of chronic back pain:** Cauda equina syndrome, metastatic disease, vascular claudication, infection (osteomyelitis/discitis/epidural abscess), spondyloarthropathies, psychiatric illness, malingering

Axial vs. Radicular Pain

		Axial Pain	Radicular Pain
Symptoms			
	No radicular pattern, but may refer to buttocks and posterior thigh		Dermatomal distribution
	Dull, aching, deep		Shooting, burning electric
	Ill defined		Well defined
	Midline back pain		Extremity pain often worse than back pain
	Worsens with extension		Worsens with flexion
	No paresthesia		Associated paresthesia
Signs			
	Negative straight leg test		Positive straight leg test
	Atrophy uncommon		Associated muscular atrophy
	Subjective weakness		Objective weakness

Evaluation (N Eng J Med 2001;344:262–70, Radiology 2016;281(3):669–88, Spine 1995;20:2613–23, Radiology 2005;237:597–04; J Bone Joint Surg Am 1990;72(3):403–8)

- **History:** Focused clinical history to determine: Location of pain allowing targeted inspection of imaging, axial or radicular symptoms (Table 22-1), functional limitation, and history of trauma. Associated symptoms to suggest alternative diagnosis: Fever, infection, IVDU, weight loss, saddle anesthesia, incontinence, history of malignancy, depression
- Progressive neurologic deficit, saddle anesthesia, or incontinence should prompt early surgical evaluation
- **Physical:** Observation of gait (wide gait can be seen with spinal stenosis), palpation of spine for focal tenderness, neurologic exam (sensation, strength, reflexes), provocative maneuvers (flexion, extension, straight leg raise)
- **Imaging:** False-positive abnormal imaging is common in asymptomatic population but useful for symptom-imaging correlation to identify the potential origin of pain generator
- CT best for evaluation of osseous structures
- MRI best to evaluate marrow signal intensity and soft tissues: Signal characteristics of the spinal cord, thecal effacement, fluid collections, intraspinal masses, etc.

Management (Pain Physician 2013;16:S49–283; N Eng J Med 2001;344:262–70; N Eng J Med 2008;358:818–25; Spine 2013;13(11):1438–48; Spine 2017;17(10):1480–8; Spine 2009;34(10):1094–109; Spine 2009;34(10):1066–77)

- Initial nonoperative management in absence of progressive neurologic symptoms
- Multidisciplinary approach utilizing cognitive–behavioral therapy, patient education, intensive physical rehabilitation
- **Medications:** NSAIDs, SSRIs, TCAs. No role for chronic opioid therapy in noncancer-related chronic back pain
  Spinal injections: Both diagnostic and therapeutic benefit, best indication in the setting of chronic radicular pain
- **Surgery:** Discectomy/microdiscectomy for disk herniation causing radicular pain and laminectomy or intraspinous spacer placement for symptomatic spinal stenosis associated with short-term benefits which diminish over time compared to conservative management
- Vertebral fusion may be considered for patients with >1 y disabling back pain refractory to behavioral modification/intensive interdisciplinary rehabilitation

SPINAL INJECTIONS

Background

- Procedures performed on an outpatient basis, are minimally invasive, and serve as an adjunct to conservative management or for presurgical planning
- See **Fig. 20-1** for needle trajectory of the following procedures
  Selective Nerve Root Blocks (**SNRBs**) and Epidural Steroid Injections (**ESI**) are useful for the diagnosis and/or treatment of single or multilevel radicular pain
- Facet and sacroiliac (SI) joint injections are useful for treatment of axial nonradicular pain
- Imaging guidance demonstrates improved localization of needle and outcomes
- Radicular pain symptoms from irritation of the nerve root is the presumed cause of the pain whether due to inflammation or compression

Figure 20-1

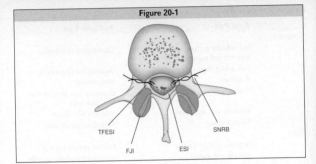

TFESI   SNRB   FJI   ESI

- Axial pain symptoms from nociceptor nerve fibers innervating the joint capsule
- With all spinal injections, local anesthetic, with or without corticosteroids, is injected into or around the suspected pain generator
- **ESI**—Needle placement is targeted at the posterior epidural space. Approach may be interlaminar (more common) or transforaminal.
- **SNRB**—Needle placement is targeted at the foraminal epiradicular space (around the nerve root and dorsal root ganglion). Approach may be transforaminal (most common) or interlaminar.
- **Facet and SI Joint Injections**—Periarticular or intraarticular needle placement is directed at the suspected painful joint space
- Local anesthetic useful for temporary pain relief and to test if treated target/level is the pain generator. Relief with local anesthetic may correspond to favorable surgical outcomes.
- Diagnostic SNRB or joint injections with a comparative block useful prior to therapeutic procedure or surgery to confirm pain generator if diagnosis unclear
  - Comparative blocks performed at 2 separate time points with a long- and short-acting local anesthetic. Symptomatic relief correlating with expected anesthetic duration confirms pain generator.
- Steroids useful to reduce nerve root inflammation
- SNRB is more focused and has been reported to have improved short-term pain outcomes when compared with interlaminar ESI (N Eng J Med 2001;344:262–70)
- Image guidance allows identification of the needle tip and more accurate placement

Patient Selection (Radiology 2016;281(3):669)

- May require one or a combination several types of injection if back and neck pain is multilevel or complex
- Spine injections are a useful adjunct to conservative therapy for patients who are not surgical candidates or if they are unable to tolerate systemic therapy or oral medications
- **Symptom-Imaging correlation** important to determine if intervention is appropriate and guide selection of the appropriate procedure. Abnormal imaging is common in asymptomatic patients. Therefore, symptoms must direct a targeted review of available imaging.
- Point tenderness or dermatomal distribution of radicular pain helpful to direct review of imaging at a specific level. Imaging may not be abnormal, especially in the setting of axial pain generators (facet joint or SI pain) where there is low correlation between imaging and symptoms.
- If pain is unilateral, radicular, and associated with disc herniation or foraminal stenosis → **SNRB**
- If pain is bilateral, radicular, and associated with spinal canal stenosis, spondylolisthesis, or bilateral foraminal stenosis → **ESI, or bilateral SNRB**
- SNRB and ESI also useful for post spinal surgery radicular pain
- If pain is axial, paraspinal, and associated with facet arthropathy, spondylolysis, facet marrow signal changes → **Facet injection or ESI**
- Also consider **facet injections** if the patient has failed to have pain relief after other spine-targeted interventions
- If axial pain originates from the buttocks, unilateral or bilateral SI joints, and is associated with sitting intolerance, groin pain, and history of noninfectious sacroiliitis → **SI joint injection**

- Coagulopathy (INR >1.5, platelets <50000/μL)
- Systemic or local infection at site of needle placement
- Progressive neurologic disorder which may be masked by the intervention
- Pilonidal cysts (for lumbar or SI injections)
- Allergy to local anesthetic
- Pregnancy (for lumbar or SI injections)
- If the dura is punctured at any point during an epidural injection the procedure should be terminated to avoid intrathecal administration of corticosteroid or anesthetic and the procedure can be reattempted on another day

Preprocedural Workup

- **History:** Note pain quality, severity, and location for symptom-imaging correlation, above
- Frequency and use of pain medication useful for postintervention comparison
- Review surgical history, infectious history, history of trauma, pertinent allergies
- **Physical:** Evaluate for signs of infection: Fever or cellulitis overlying injection site
- Provocative maneuvers: Flexion, extension, straight leg test, observe gait
- **Imaging:** Helpful for symptom imaging correlation, but low correlation between imaging findings and symptoms
- MRI useful to evaluate marrow signal intensity and soft tissues. Signal characteristics of the spinal cord, thecal effacement, fluid collections, intraspinal masses, etc. Most sensitive for identifying disc degeneration, but severity may not have a linear correlation with pain symptoms
- CT also useful for preprocedural planning and to evaluate osseous structures which may obstruct percutaneous approach
- Review of existing plain films useful to evaluate whether fluoroscopic approach likely to be successful, or if CT guidance needed
- Nuclear SPECT imaging specific, but not sensitive for painful facet arthropathy
- **Labs:** PT/INR (<1.5), Platelets (>50000/dL), baseline hemoglobin/hematocrit
- Contrast used to confirm location is such a small volume that renal function testing is generally not required
- **Medications**
- Hold antiplatelet medications for 10 d prior to SNRB or ESI (Can be restarted 24 h after injection). Hold of antiplatelet medications not needed for facet or SI injections.
- Warfarin should be held 5 d prior to the procedure (Can be restarted 24 h after procedure)
- Unfractionated heparin may be held 6–12 h prior to the procedure

ESI/SNRB

Procedural Preparation

- **Imaging Guidance**
- Fluoroscopy is fast and most cost-effective. Biplane fluoroscopy useful when available to reduce procedure time
- CT useful when fluoroscopic access failed, extensive productive osseous disease which may hinder access, and improved accuracy of needle placement to avoid treatment of adjacent pain generators during diagnostic SNRB, especially if an interlaminar approach is utilized
- MR guidance has also been reported and minimizes radiation exposure, but is much less common

Anesthesia/Sedation

- Withhold pain medications the day of a diagnostic procedure, so the effect of the intervention is not masked
- Cutaneous and tract anesthesia with 1% lidocaine is generally sufficient
- Intravenous conscious sedation may be administered if the patient is excessively anxious or in pain. Example conscious sedation schedule:
  - Anxiolysis: Midazolam 1 mg, initially, and 0.5–1.0 mg (0.5 mg if elderly or debilitated) as needed up to 4 mg with 3–5-min intervals between doses
  - Pain control: Fentanyl 50 μg, initially, and 25–50 μg as needed up to 200 μg with 3–5-min intervals between doses
- **Monitoring:** Baseline vital signs prior to procedure. Continuous physiologic monitoring only required with conscious sedation, to include pulse oximetry and intermittent blood pressure measurements
- **Pharmacologic Agents** (*Radiology* 2016;281(3):669–88; FDA Drug Safety Communication: FDA requires label changes to warn of rare but serious neurologic problems after epidural corticosteroid injections for pain. http://www.fda.gov/downloads/Drugs/DrugSafety/ UCM394286.pdf. Published April 23, 2014. Accessed

November 2017; Clin J Pain 2011;27(6):518–22 (ISSN: 1536–5409); Reg Anesth Pain Med 2011;36(6):572–8; Skeletal Radiology 2015;44(2):149–55; Pain Physician 2016;19:E365–10)

- 1–2 mL of a low osmolal nonionic contrast agent may be used to confirm needle positioning
- Injectate mixture and dose varies greatly in the literature, no standard has been established and may vary by institution
- Local anesthetic: lower volume, and concentration of anesthetic demonstrate preferential sensory block vs. motor block
  - Short-acting local anesthetic, such as lidocaine 1%
  - Long-acting local anesthetic, such as bupivacaine 0.25–0.5%
- Corticosteroid choice is controversial and not standardized. Epidural administration is considered off-label use in US by the FDA.
  - Dexamethasone 4 mg/mL, a water-soluble nonparticulate corticosteroid, demonstrates equivalent efficacy and the least theoretical and reported risk of, potentially catastrophic, vascular embolization
  - Other commonly used corticosteroids include particulate steroids: Triamcinolone, betamethasone, and methylprednisolone
- **Consent:** Risk of bleeding, infection, transient sensory and motor block, allergic reaction, potential for no relief or possible worsening of pain

Technical Procedures

Fluoroscopic Lumbar Interlaminar ESI

- Patient positioned prone over a bolster to open interlaminar space
- Obtain AP view centered on spinous processes with slight craniocaudal angulation of the C-arm to visualize the interlaminar space
- Mark skin surface at planned insertion site in midline, or for a paramedian approach if significant interspinous ligament calcification
- Prep and drape in the usual sterile fashion
- Infiltrate skin and tract with lidocaine 1%
- Insert 22G spinal needle with slight craniocaudal angulation, to match C-arm angulation
- Advance needle under lateral fluoroscopy
- As the needle tip nears the posterior margin of the spinal canal, remove stylet, and attach tubing and glass syringe or specialized low resistance plastic syringe for "loss-of-resistance" technique detection of the epidural space
- Apply firm pressure on the syringe plunger with further needle advancement
- Immediate loss of resistance to plunger pressure once the posterior epidural space is entered
- Remove syringe and observe for CSF return or blood. If there is return of CSF, the thecal sac has been entered and the procedure should be terminated and rescheduled for a later date to avoid intrathecal administration of anesthesia or corticosteroid. If there is blood return, the needle is intravascular and should be repositioned.
- Under lateral fluoroscopy, 2–3 mL of nonionic myelography-approved contrast is then administered under low pressure. Contrast should collect in the epidural space posterior to the thecal sac. If intrathecal, the contrast will layer dependently in the thecal sac, and the procedure should be terminated, as above. Needle may need to be readjusted if contrast is intravascular or pools on contralateral side of symptoms. If met with resistance, may indicate intraligamentous placement or dural adhesions and repositioning may be required.
  - The plica medians is a midline dural reflection which may confine injected material to 1 side
- After confirmation of epidural placement, direct bevel toward symptomatic side and inject 3–5 mL mixture of 1 mL dexamethasone 4 mg/mL and lidocaine 1%, under low pressure
  - Epidural steroids alone or with bupivacaine are not effective for pain due to spinal stenosis or radiculopathy (Pain Physician 2016;19(3):E365)
- The needle is then removed
- Clean insertion site and apply bandage
- Instruct patient to lay on symptomatic side for 10 min following procedure

Fluoroscopic Caudal/Sacral ESI

- Patient positioned prone
- Obtain AP view including the median sacral ridge and sacral cornua (bony border of the sacral hiatus)
- Mark skin in the midline 2–3 cm below the sacral hiatus
- Place gauze between the buttocks to prevent irritation of the perineum from povidone–iodine

- Prep and drape in the usual sterile fashion
- Infiltrate skin and tract with lidocaine 1%
- Advance a 5-in 22G spinal needle cranially into the sacral hiatus
- Lateral fluoroscopy useful for advancement
- Keeping the spinal needle as horizontal as possible, advance the needle to the S2/S3 level
- Remove stylet and connect tubing
- Under intermittent fluoroscopy, inject 2–3 mL of nonionic myelography-approved contrast to confirm epidural placement. If intrathecal, terminate and reschedule procedure, as above.
- Injection of anesthetic and corticosteroid, such as 8 mg dexamethasone or 6 mg betamethasone mixed with 10–12 mL bupivacaine, maybe diluted with ~15 normal saline

Fluoroscopic Transforaminal Lumbar SNRB
- Patient positioned prone.
- C-arm is obliqued 25–30° toward the side to be injected and craniocaudally to parallel the vertebral body endplates at the level to be treated
- Mark skin surface at planned insertion site for a posterolateral approach to target just above the nerve root to be treated, the supraneural space or "safe triangle," bounded superiorly by the pedicle, inferomedially by the nerve root and laterally be the lateral margin of the vertebral body. The exiting nerve root typically passes just below the pedicle.
- If treating L5, the needle will need exaggerated craniocaudal angulation to avoid the ipsilateral iliac wing
- If treating S1, less lateral obliquity of the C-arm is needed, and the needle is targeted at the center of the sacral foramen
- The patient is prepped and draped in the usual sterile fashion
- Infiltrate skin and tract with lidocaine 1%
- A 22G spinal needle is advanced slightly cranially toward the inferolateral aspect of the pedicle
- As the needle approaches the nerve root, the patient may complain of provocation of pain symptoms
- Lateral and AP fluoroscopy useful to confirm location
- Connect tubing and inject 2–3 mL of nonionic myelography-approved contrast under low pressure. Contrast should course freely along the nerve root. If contrast is intravascular or there is resistance, possibly indicating intraneural injection, repositioning is required.
- If repositioning is required, target the "Kambin triangle." It is the inferoposterior aspect of the foramen over the lateral aspect of the intervertebral disc and is bounded superiorly by the exiting nerve root, laterally by the lateral margin of the disc, inferiorly by the lower vertebral body pedicle, and medially by the facet joint. Targeting the Kambin triangle also avoids the artery of Adamkiewicz which may course across the safe triangle within the upper lumbar spine. This artery is important for supplying the anterior spinal artery, and a potential embolization risk.
- After confirming positioning, diagnostic SNRB performed by injection 1–2 mL of lidocaine 1% or bupivacaine 0.25%. Therapeutic SNRB achieved with injection of 3 mL mixture of local anesthetic and corticosteroid, such as 2 mL lidocaine 1% or bupivacaine 0.25% and 1 mL dexamethasone 4 mg/mL. Injectant administered over 1–2 min.
- The needle is then removed
- Clean insertion site and apply bandage

Lumbosacral Transforaminal ESI
- Variant of the transforaminal SNRB procedure, above, however the target of the injectant is the intraspinal epidural space rather than the foraminal epiradicular space
- Useful when interlaminar approach is obstructed by postsurgical bony fusion bodies or hardware
- Similar identical, however the inferomedial aspect of the pedicle is targeted instead of the inferolateral aspect
- Addition of 2–3 mL normal saline to the anesthetic–corticosteroid mixture increases dispersal of injectant into intraspinal epidural space

Postprocedural Care
- Patient observed for 15–30 min unless conscious sedation administered, then observe for an hour
- Patient should have someone else drive them home

- May resume normal activities
- Pain relief, if present, may occur within minutes of injection due to the local anesthetic and last up to a few hours
- Important to document pain relief, if present, as evidence of correct location
- Effects of corticosteroids onset in 2–3 d, with peak effect in 2–3 w. Anti-inflammatory effects will return to baseline within 6–8 w and pain may return.
- If performed for disc herniation, pain relief may last longer as herniated fragment is resorbed

Complications (Curr Rev Musculoskelet Med 2008;1(3–4):212)
- Bleeding along the needle trajectory, with rare but potentially serious epidural hematomas occurring in <1 in 150000 procedures
- Infection occurs in up to 1–2% of procedures, with severe infection including meningitis, epidural abscess, or osteomyelitis occurring in 0.01–0.1%
- Temporary and permanent nerve root injuries have been reported due to direct trauma from the needle
- Intravascular penetration as frequent as 11.2% with transforaminal injections and 1.8% with interlaminar injections. Intravenous injection is most common with minimal sequelae, however, there are case reports of spinal infarct and paraplegia due to intraarterial injection of particulate steroids (artery of Adamkiewicz). Risk reduced with soluble steroids and use of contrast to confirm needle placement.
- Dural puncture can result in spinal anesthesia if anesthetic administered intrathecally
- Rarely epidural corticosteroid administration has resulted in transient suppression of the hypothalamus–pituitary–adrenal axis and Cushingoid syndrome

FACET AND SI JOINT INJECTIONS

Procedural Preparation

Imaging Guidance
- Usually performed under fluoroscopy, however, CT guidance may be useful in the setting of difficult access due to advanced productive osseous degenerative disease
- MRI guidance may also be a consideration, if available, for SI joint injections in the setting pain from sacroiliitis due spondyloarthropathy since this modality carries no radiation dose and these patients are often between the ages of 20–30 y

Anesthesia/Sedation
- Withhold pain medication the day of a diagnostic procedure, so the effect of the intervention is not masked
- Cutaneous and tract anesthesia with 1% lidocaine is generally sufficient. Conscious sedation rarely required, but may be administered, as with *ESI/SNRBs* above.
- **Monitoring:** Baseline vital signs prior to procedure. Continuous physiologic monitoring only required with conscious sedation, to include pulse oximetry and intermittent blood pressure measurements

Pharmacologic Agents
- Intraarticular spaces are smaller than the epidural space, therefore volume of injectant should be less than that used for ESI and SNRBs
- Injectate mixture and/or doses may vary by institution
- 0.25–0.5 mL of a low osmolal nonionic contrast agent may be used to confirm location
- For comparative diagnostic facet joint injections, 1 mL of local anesthetic, lidocaine 1–2% for short-acting block and bupivacaine 0.25–0.5% for a longer-acting comparison block can be used
- For therapeutic facet injections, a corticosteroid, such as 40 mg triamcinolone acetonide (1 mL), is added to 1 mL of lidocaine 1–2% for a longer therapeutic effect
- **Consent:** Risk of bleeding, infection, transient sensory and motor block, allergic reaction, potential for no relief or possible worsening of pain

Technical Procedures

Fluoroscopic lumbar Facet Joint Injection
- Patient placed in the prone position over a bolster to open the articular recesses
- Patient and/or C-arm is rotated laterally until the projection is parallel to and centered on the joint space to be injected, so that it is seen in profile
- Skin insertion site is marked over the joint for a vertical approach to the joint
- Prep and drape in the usual sterile fashion
- Infiltrate skin and tract with lidocaine 1%
- Advance a 22G spinal needle toward the cartilage interface or capsular recesses of joint under lateral and AP fluoroscopy

- A pop may be felt upon entering the joint space, and the patient may complain of reproduction of their pain symptoms
- Remove stylet and connect catheter tubing
- Inject contrast to confirm intraarticular placement
- Inject local anesthetic if diagnostic injection, or local anesthetic–corticosteroid mixture if a therapeutic injection
- Even extra-articular injection around joint capsule has been shown to provide partial pain relief in approximately 50% of patients, if intra-articular placement is not obtainable (*J Bone Joint Surg Br* 1986;68(1):138–41)
- The needle is then removed and the insertion site is cleaned and dressed

Fluoroscopic Sacroiliac Joint Injection
- Patient is placed in the prone oblique position, with the side to be injected facing down
- C-arm is centered on the SI joint and oblique laterally 0–20° to profile the posterior recess of the sacroiliac joint. The sacroiliac joints are oriented obliquely, so the posterior aspect of the joint will be medial to the anterior aspect of the joint on an AP projection.
- Skin insertion site is marked for a vertical approach targeting the synovial portion of joint, the caudal most one-third. Slight medial or lateral angulation of the spinal needle may be useful if osteophytic disease is present
- Prep and drape in the usual sterile fashion
- Infiltrate skin and tract with lidocaine 1%
- Advance a 22G spinal needle into the posterior-inferior one-third of the joint. Gentle pressure may be required to advance the needle through the fibrous joint capsule and overlying ligamentous assembly.
- Once the joint is entered, place the patient prone
- Remove the stylet and connect catheter tubing to the needle
- Inject 0.25–5 mL of contrast under AP fluoroscopy to confirm needle location in the joint. Contrast should outline the joint, including the more laterally oriented anterior joint space.
- Following confirmation of intraarticular placement, inject 1 mL of local anesthetic for a diagnostic injection, or 2–3 mL of anesthetic–corticosteroid mixture for a therapeutic injection
- The needle is then removed and the insertion site is cleaned and dressed

Postprocedural Care
- Patient is observed for 15–30 min unless conscious sedation administered, then observe for an hour
- Patient should have someone else drive them home
- May resume normal activities
- Pain relief, if present, may occur within minutes of injection due to the local anesthetic, and last up to a few hours
- Important to document relief of pain, if present, as evidence of correct location
- Effects of corticosteroids may be present for 2–3 d, with peak effect in 2–3 w. Anti-inflammatory effects will return to baseline within 6–8 w and pain may return

Complications (*Pain Physician* 2012;15(2):E143–50; *PMR* 2012;4(7):473–8)
- Mild local bleeding most common, serious sequelae are less common than with intraspinal procedures
- Vasovagal reaction
- Injection site soreness
- Nerve root irritation
- Intravascular penetration

INTERVENTIONAL
20-8

STELLATE GANGLION BLOCKS

Background (*Brit J Anesth* 1955;27:616–21; *AJR* 1992;158:655–9; *Pain Physician* 2000;3(3):294–304)
- The stellate ganglia are bilateral sympathetic ganglia formed by the fusion of the inferior cervical ganglia and the upper thoracic sympathetic chain, with involvement of the 1st and 2nd thoracic ganglia in 80% of patients
- They are star-shaped structures measuring up to 3 cm in craniocaudal length and 1 cm in width, located along the anterior surface of the prevertebral fascia anterior to the transverse processes of C7 and T1 vertebral bodies and just lateral to the longus colli muscles. Important adjacent structures include the ipsilateral vertebral artery which is typically closely apposed to the ganglion anteriorly and may be circumscribed by sympathetic fiber as it passes posteriorly into the transverse foramen at C7. The ipsilateral subclavian artery and apical pleural space are anteroinferior and the carotid artery anterolateral to the ganglia.

- Each ganglion relay sympathetic nerve fibers supplying the ipsilateral head, neck, cardiac visceral afferent fibers, and most or all the sympathetic fibers of each ipsilateral upper extremity
- The ganglia have been implicated in multiple chronic pain and vascular syndromes and anesthetic blocks of the ganglia have shown benefit in the treatment and diagnosis of these disorders, and may predict therapeutic response to surgical sympathectomy
- Historically, the procedure was performed with only palpation, however, fluoroscopy or ultrasound are now typically utilized for guidance

Patient Selection

- Stellate ganglion blocks have been used for the treatment of multiple pain and vascular syndromes affecting the upper extremities, head, and neck
- Prior to considering treatment with anesthetic block, management with conservative therapy; including anti-inflammatory medication and physical therapy is advised
- **Pain Syndromes** (Pain Physician 2000;3(3):294–304; Pain Medicine 2007;6(4):326–31; Clin J Pain 2002;18(4):216–33; BMJ 1998;316(7134):792–3; Reg Anesth 1997;22(3):287–90; Pain 2000;87(1):103–05)
- Historically, the most common pain syndrome treated with a stellate ganglion block is Complex Regional Pain Syndrome (CRPS) involving an upper extremity, a syndrome once thought to entirely mediated by sympathetic nerve dysfunction
  - CRPS is a chronic pain syndrome which often affects the extremities and which also often has an important, but controversial, sympathetic-mediated component
  - Characterized by persistent pain out of proportion to the inciting event, allodynia, motor weakness, edema, asymmetric color or temperature changes from the contralateral extremity, increased sweating, and atrophy of skin, hair, or nails
  - Repeated injury or noxious stimuli leads to sensitization of peripheral and central nociception pathways lowering the threshold for excitation of nerve fibers leading to increased synaptic activity in response to previously nonpainful stimuli
  - Subtypes of CRPS is based on the inciting cause rather than differences in clinical features or management
    - Type 1, formerly known as reflex sympathetic dystrophy syndrome, caused by an injury which did not directly damage the nerves of the affected extremity such as fracture, soft tissue injury, stroke, or prolonged immobilization
    - Type 2, formerly known as causalgia, caused by direct damage to the nerves of the affected extremity
  - Sympathetic-mediated pain is not present in all patients with CRPS, but can be an important component in many patients
  - The role of the sympathetic nervous system in CRPS is not entirely understood but likely related to pathologic interaction of sensitized dysfunctional afferent nociception fibers with efferent sympathetic fibers within the dorsal root ganglion or affected limb
  - Many patients with a sympathetic-mediated component that will respond to sympathetic block, however, many patients will not receive significant relief from sympatheticolysis
  - Evidence for the long-term benefit of stellate ganglion blocks for CRPS is limited. Benefits may be related to sympathetic blockade or possibly due to local infiltration of the anesthetic agent around the site of injection and effect on the peripheral nociceptive fibers themselves
- Evidence is limited, but other pain syndromes which have been treated with stellate ganglion blocks include: Herpes zoster (shingles), postherpetic neuralgia, recalcitrant angina, phantom limb pain, frostbite or burn wounds

Vascular Syndromes (Pain Physician 2000;3(3):294–304)
- Anesthetic blockade of the stellate ganglion can inhibit sympathetic mediated vasoconstriction within the ipsilateral upper extremity, thus improving blood flow in the affected extremity and treat syndromes characterized by reduced peripheral blood flow
- Such syndromes include: Raynaud's syndrome, scleroderma, arterial vascular insufficiency, vasospasm, and postembolic syndromes

Miscellaneous Syndromes (Pain Physician 2000;3(3):294–304; Lancet Oncol 2008;9(6):523–32; Clin Cardiol 1985;8:111–3; Circulation 2000;102:742–7; Circulation 2010;121:2255–62; Circulation 2004;109:1826–33; N Engl J Med 2008;358:2024–9)
- Palmar hyperhidrosis
- Hot flashes in women with history of breast cancer, and who are therefore unable to be treated with hormonal therapy
- Recurrent ventricular arrhythmias following myocardial infarction (electrical storm)
- Long QT syndrome

Contraindications
- Coagulopathy (INR >1.5, platelets <50000/μL)
- Systemic or local infection at site of needle placement
- Progressive neurologic disorder which may be masked by the intervention
- Allergy to local anesthetic
- Glaucoma
- Pathologic bradycardia or severe cardiac conduction block

Preprocedural Workup
- **History:** Varies with indication, useful to exclude important differential diagnoses
- Evaluate for soft tissue infection or arterial/venous occlusion, as these may also cause unilateral upper-extremity pain, edema, and erythema which may be seen in CRPS
- Frequency and use of pain medication useful for postintervention comparison
- Review surgical history, infectious history, history of trauma, and pertinent allergies
- **Physical:** Evaluate for signs of infection: Fever or cellulitis within affected limb or overlying injection site

Imaging
- Nuclear medicine triple phase bone scintigraphy may be useful in CRPS. The affected limb demonstrates decreased radiotracer uptake in the perfusion and blood pool phases and increased asymmetric periarticular uptake in the delayed mineralization phase, when compared to the unaffected limb
- Doppler ultrasound useful to exclude arterial or venous occlusive disease in the affected extremity
- Targeted ultrasound may be useful to identify the stellate ganglion and surrounding soft tissue structures

Labs
- PT/INR (<1.5), Platelets (>50000/dL), baseline hemoglobin/hematocrit
- Procedural contrast used to confirm location is such a small volume that renal function testing is generally not required

Medications
- Hold antiplatelet medications for 10 d prior to procedure (can be restarted 24 h after injection)
- Warfarin should be held 5 d prior to the procedure (Can be restarted 24 h after procedure)
- Unfractionated heparin may be held 6–12 h prior to the procedure

Technical Procedure (Pain Physician 2000;3(3):294–304; Clin J Pain 2002;18(4):216–33; BMJ 1998;316(7134): 792–3; Reg Anesth 1997;22(3):287–90; Pain 2000;87(1):103–5; Lancet Oncol 2008;9(6):523–32; Clin Cardiol 1985;8: 111–3; Circulation 2000;102:742–7; Circulation 2010;121:2255–62; Circulation 2004;109:1826–33; N Engl J Med 2008;358:2034–9; Pain Physician 2004;7:327––31; J Anaesthesia 2011;55:52–6; Acta Anaesth Belg 2016;67:1–5)

Imaging Guidance
- Commonly performed under fluoroscopic guidance allowing visualization of osseous targets. The target endpoint for injection under fluoroscopic guidance is contact with the bony surface of the vertebral body
- Ultrasound guidance may also be used, and has the benefit of visualizing the soft tissue and vascular structures surrounding the stellate ganglion. With ultrasound, the target endpoint is the prevertebral fascia covering the anterior surface of the adjacent longus colli muscle
- CT may also be used but increases radiation dose, as well as procedure time
- If utilizing fluoroscopic or CT guidance, a small amount of iodinated contrasted may be used to confirm needle placement

Anesthesia/Sedation
- Often performed under sedation
- Example conscious sedation schedule:
  - Anxiolysis: Midazolam 1 mg, initially, and 0.5–1.0 mg (0.5 mg if elderly or debilitated) as needed up to 4 mg with 3–5-min intervals between doses
  - Pain control: Fentanyl 50 μg, initially, and 25–50 μg as needed up to 200 μg with 3–5-min intervals between doses
- Cutaneous anesthesia with 1% lidocaine
- **Monitoring:** Baseline vital signs prior to procedure. Continuous physiologic monitoring is required, to include pulse oximetry, electrocardiography, and intermittent blood pressure measurements
- Upper-extremity skin temperature changes can indicate a successful block, and can be monitored over the distal bilateral arms, with monitoring devices placed in mirrored positions for useful comparison

Pharmacologic Agents
- 1–2 mL of a low osmolal nonionic contrast agent may be used to confirm needle positioning
- Local anesthetic with bupivacaine 0.25% or lidocaine 1%

Procedure

Fluoroscopic Guided Stellate Ganglion Block
- The patient is positioned supine with the neck slightly extended over a pillow under the shoulders. The head should be slightly rotated away from the side to be treated.
- In AP direction, the fluoroscopy tube is centered on the C6/C7 intervertebral space. Craniocaudal angulation can be used to orient the projection parallel to the endplates at the C6/C7 disc space.
- The fluoroscope is then obliqued laterally toward the side to be treated to open the view of the ipsilateral neuroforamen
- The planned insertion site on the skin is then marked over the junction of the uncinate process of the C7 with the vertebral body proper
- The patient is prepped and draped in the usual sterile fashion
- The skin is infiltrated with lidocaine 1% at the planned insertion site
- A 25G spinal needle is then advanced to the junction of the uncinate process and vertebral body of C7, until bone is contacted with the needle tip. The needle is then retracted 1–2 mm
- The stylet is removed, and catheter tube attached
- Gentle aspiration performed, if blood or CSF is aspirated the needle is in the wrong position
- 1–2 mL of contrast is then injected to confirm placement and exclude intravascular or intrathecal placement, the contrast should track along the longissimus coli
- A test dose of 0.5 mL of the local anesthetic may be administered. If there is intra-arterial placement of the needle, even this low dose may be enough to cause almost immediate seizures
- An additional 3–4 mL of local anesthetic may then be injected
- If successful block of the stellate ganglion is achieved, the ipsilateral arm skin temperature may increase by 1–3°C. The patient may also demonstrate signs of ipsilateral Horner's syndrome (ptosis and miosis) within minutes of injection.
- The catheter is then disconnected and the stylet replaced
- The needle is then removed and the insertion site is cleaned and dressed
- **Other fluoroscopic approaches have been described.** The most common alternative approach directs the needle at the anterior tubercle (Chassaignac tubercle) of the transverse process of C6, and enough anesthetic is injected to track caudally to the level of the stellate ganglion. This approach is a carryover from when the procedure was performed without image guidance, in an effort to avoid the vertebral artery and pleural space. However, it requires more injectant and has been shown to be less effective at actually achieving anesthetic block of the stellate ganglion, successful less than 50% of the time (*Anesthesiology* 1998;15:871–7)

Postprocedural Care
- Patient observed for 60 min following the procedure, and should be able to swallow liquids without aspiration
- Patient should have someone else drive them home
- May resume normal activities
- The anesthetic effects last for several hours following injection and expected side effects, such as Horner's syndrome, will subside along with the duration of the anesthetic
- Pain relief is unpredictable. The patient may have none, partial, or full relief of pain. If relief is achieved, it may last longer than the duration of anesthetic, sometimes days or weeks. This is likely to occur after repeated injections, so if the patient has any relief, additional treatment is recommended.

Complications (*Pain Physician* 2000;3(3):294–304)
- Injury to adjacent soft tissue structures and nerves: Tracheal or esophageal perforation, pneumothorax or hemothorax, bleeding from vascular injury. These are reduced with image guidance.
- Infection such as cellulitis or osteomyelitis
- Voice hoarseness due to recurrent laryngeal nerve anesthetic block or injury and associated paralysis
- Arm weakness or numbness if there is anesthetic block or the nerve roots or brachial plexus
- High spinal blockade with intrathecal injection
- Seizures due to intravascular injection
- Bradycardia and hypotension due to blockade of afferent cardiac sympathetic fibers

PRIAPISM

Definition
- Persistent and often painful penile erection lasting hours after, or in the absence of, sexual arousal

Physiology
- Normal tumescence occurs largely from parasympathetic neurotransmitter (nitric oxide) mediated smooth muscle relaxation of the corpora cavernosa and increased arterial inflow. Engorgement of the cavernosa compress venous outflow causing penile tumescence and rigidity.
- Sympathetic-mediated signaling stimulates cavernosa smooth muscle contraction, reducing arterial inflow and promoting venous outflow
- Priapism primarily involves the corpora cavernosa, not the corpus spongiosum or glans

Etiology (J Urol 2003;170:1318–24)

Ischemic/Low Flow
- Most common cause
- Venous outflow obstruction leads to ischemia and thrombosis with eventual fibrosis and erectile dysfunction
- Medical emergency—A compartment syndrome
- Delayed treatment can lead to fibrosis and erectile dysfunction
- Causes include:
  - **Mechanical occlusion** (thromboembolic/hypercoagulable state)
    - Sickle cell crisis (most common cause in children) (J Pediatr Urol 2014;10(1):11–24)
    - Hematologic dyscrasia or malignancy
    - Metastatic disease
    - Dialysis
    - Rebound hypercoagulable states with anticoagulant medications
  - **Prolonged smooth muscle relaxation**
    - Intracavernosal injection of vasodilator therapy for erectile dysfunction: Alprostadil, papaverine, prostaglandin E1, phentolamine
      - Most cause common in adults (Urology 2001;57(5):970–2)
    - Antihypertensives: CCBs, alpha antagonists(prazosin), hydralazine
    - Psychotropics: Trazodone, haloperidol, SSRIs, phenothiazine
    - Chronic cocaine use (depletes sympathetic neurotransmitters) (Urology 2003;62(1):187–92)
    - Spinal cord injury (Urology 2005;65(6):1195–7)

Nonischemic/High Flow
- Less common
- Unregulated arterial inflow. Maybe idiopathic, but often due to fistula from prior penile or pelvic trauma.
  - May also result from intracavernosal injections if cavernosal artery is lacerated by needle
- Does not cause ischemia and consequent fibrotic changes, relatively benign (J Urol 1986;135(1):142–7)
- Urgent treatment not necessary

Stuttering/Intermittent
- Recurrent episodes of ischemic priapism with an interval period of detumescence
- Often idiopathic but associated with the systemic causes of ischemic priapism (ie, sickle cell disease)

Clinical Manifestations
- Must differentiate ischemic vs. nonischemia (ischemic requires urgent intervention)
- Ischemic/Low Flow: Severe pain, rigid penis, history of intracavernosal injection therapy, hematologic abnormality or thromboembolic state
- Nonischemic/High Flow: Generally not painful, history of trauma, tumescent but not fully rigid penis, may be chronic

Diagnostic Studies
- Often the diagnosis is readily apparent
- Corpus cavernosa blood gas testing
  - Ischemic: Dark aspirated blood, pH <7.25, pO_2 <30 mmHg, pCO_2 >60 mmHg
    (Int J Impot Res 1994;6(1):9–16)

- Nonischemic: Normal arterial blood, bright red, pH 7.4, PO_2 >90 mmHg, pCO_2 <40 mmHg
- Doppler ultrasound of the penis (*Radiographics* 2013;33(3):721–40)
  - Ischemic: Coarsened cavernosal echotexture related to edema, absence of normal blood flow within the substance of the corpora cavernosa
  - Nonischemic: High blood flow in the cavernosal artery, a pseudoaneurysm, or an arterial-lacunar (arterial cavernous) fistula may be visualized
- Workup of etiology may include CBC, Hemoglobin electrophoresis, drug screening

Treatment

Ischemic (*J Urol* 2003;170:1318–24)
- Immediate intracavernous treatment required. Often performed in emergency department or by urology.
  - Less successful if treatment delayed >48 h from onset
- Cavernosal aspiration and sympathomimetic administration is successful in 77%, opposed to aspiration or sympathomimetic therapy alone, 36% and 58%, respectively
- Clean and prep skin, administer local anesthetic at planned puncture site
- Aspirate either corpora cavernosa at base or shaft of penis with 16G–21G needle in the 3 or 9 o'clock position, avoiding the dorsal vessels and nerves
  - Avoid deep insertion of needle to minimize risk of cavernosal artery injury
- Aspirate until outflow of dark hypoxic blood ceases and bright arterial blood is obtained
  - If aspiration is difficult due to thrombus, consider irrigating with 10 mL
- Intracavernosal injection of a sympathomimetic
  - In patients with high cardiovascular risk continuous blood pressure and ECG monitoring recommended
  - Phenylephrine (selective alpha-1 agonist) is agent of choice due to less associated adverse effects
    - Administer 1 mL of 100–500 µg/mL every 3–5 min for up to 1 h
      - Lower dose for children and patients with severe heart disease
- Treatment of systemic cause, if identified, should be performed concurrently (hydration, oxygenation, transfusion, alkalinization, pheresis)
- If unsuccessful, surgical cavernoglanular shunt placement is next step

Nonischemic (*J Urol* 2003;170:1318–24; *JVIR* 2007;18(10):1222–6)
- Treatment not urgent, initial management is observation
  - May resolve spontaneously
  - Time from onset to presentation does not impact outcomes
  - Goal is to close arteriocavernous fistula while maintaining erectile function
- Selective arterial embolization, if intervention desired
  - Access right or left femoral artery
  - Selective angiography of bilateral internal iliac arteries and subselective angiography of the internal pudendal arteries
    - See *Arterial Interventions*
  - Look for abnormal cavernosal blush or arteriovenous fistula
  - Subselectively catheterize the internal pudendal artery with a microcatheter and advance the microcatheter as close as possible to the fistula
  - Embolization is often first performed using a temporary embolic agent (gelatin sponges, autologous blood clot)
  - If there is recurrence of high flow priapism, repeat embolization using a permanent embolic agent can be considered
    - Limited evidence suggests equivalent rates of success (74–78%) but higher rate of erectile dysfunction (up to 30%) with use of permanent agents (microcoils, PVA particles, ethanol, acrylic glue)
  - Generally well tolerated without need for postoperative narcotics or hospitalization
  - Complications include erectile dysfunction (5–20%) and recurrence
- If embolization fails, surgical ligation of the vascular lesion can be performed
  - Associated with higher rates of erectile dysfunction

Stuttering (*J Urol* 2003;170:1318–24)
- Treatment based on prevention of recurrent ischemic episodes by treating the underlying systemic causes and avoidance of provoking stimuli
- Ischemic episodes should be treated emergently, as above

ADDITIONAL RESOURCES

1. Goodman, Bradly S, Mallempati S, et al. Complications and pitfalls of lumbar inter-laminar and transforaminal epidural injections. *Curr Rev Musculoskelet Med* 2008; 1(3–4): 212–22.
2. Lilius G, Laasonen EM, Myllynen P, et al. Lumbar facet joint syndrome: A randomised clinical trial. *J Bone Joint Surg Br* 1989;71(4):681–4.
3. Riew KD, Park JB, Cho YS, et al. Nerve root blocks in the treatment of lumbar radicular pain: A minimum 5-year follow-up. *J Bone Joint Surg Am* 2006;88:1722–5.
4. Sarazin L, Chevrot A, Pessis E, et al. Lumbar facet joint arthrography with the posterior approach. *RadioGraphics* 1999;19:93–104.
5. Schaufele MK, Hatch L, Jones W. Interlaminar versus transforaminal epidural injections for the treatment of symptomatic lumbar intervertebral disc herniations. *Pain Physician* 2006;9(4):361–66.

Background (CDC 2011)
- Overall prevalence of 5.8–12.9% of adults in the US

Etiology and Presentation (ADA 2011)
- Type 1 accounts for 5–10% of cases
  - Deficiency in insulin production
  - Autoimmune disease with destruction of pancreatic β-islet cells
  - Present with acute symptoms, often in acute DKA
- Type 2 accounts for >90% of cases
  - Insulin resistance secondary to obesity
  - Obesity generates increased free fatty acid plasma levels increasing muscle insulin resistance and decreasing glucose uptake
  - Often diagnosed with screening UA or serum analysis, as well as in association with other chronic conditions
- Common symptoms for both types include polyuria, polydipsia, polyphagia, fatigue, blurred vision, neuropathy, weight loss
- Wide variety of microvascular and macrovascular complications

Evaluation
- Mostly diagnosed on screening studies as outpatient (except for Type 1 initially presenting in acute DKA)
- Testing diagnostic criteria
  - Fasting plasma glucose >126 mg/dL on 2 occasions
  - Random plasma glucose >200 mg/dL with symptoms
  - Hemoglobin A1c >6.5%
  - 2-h postprandial >200 mg/dL

Treatment
- Type 1 requires insulin replacement
- Type 2
  - Diet and exercise are first line conservative treatment
  - Oral hypoglycemic agents may be added if diet and exercise alone do not control glucose levels
  - May ultimately require insulin therapy if conservative and oral agent treatments fail
- Oral hypoglycemic
  - Metformin
  - Sulfonylureas (Glipizide, Glyburide)
  - Thiazolidinedione's (Pioglitazone, Rosiglitazone)
  - Alpha-glucosidase inhibitors (Acarbose, Miglitol)
  - Nonsulfonylurea insulin secretagogues (Repaglinide, Nateglinide)
  - Dipeptidyl peptidase-IV inhibitors (Sitagliptin, Saxagliptin, Linagliptin, Alogliptin)
  - Sodium glucose–linked transporter-2 inhibitors (Canagliflozin, Empagliflozin, Dapagliflozin)
  - Glucagon-like peptide-1 agonists (Exenatide, Liraglutide, Albiglutide, Dulaglutide)

Insulin Types

Type	Onset	Duration (hours)
Human insulin lispro	15 min	4 h
Regular insulin	30–60 min	4–6 h
NPH insulin	2–4 h	10–18 h
Ultralente insulin	6–10 h	18–24 h
NPH 70/Regular 30	30 min	10–16 h
Glargine (Lantus)	3–4 h	24 h

(Adapted from Agabegi SS, Agabegi ED. Step-Up to Medicine. Lippincott Williams & Wilkins; 2012.)

Chronic Complications
- Macrovascular complications
  - Increased risk of stroke, MI, CHF, CAD, and peripheral vascular disease
  - Etiology is accreted atherosclerosis
- Microvascular complications
  - Diabetic neuropathy
    - Sensory nerves in common stocking/glove pattern
    - Presents as numbness and paresthesia
    - Leads to ulceration and ischemia

*This is the dedicated Diabetes chapter.

- Diabetic nephropathy
  - Nephrotic disease with glomerulus basement membrane thickening
- Diabetic retinopathy
  - Hemorrhage, exudates, microaneurysms, and venous dilatation on funduscopic exam
  - Macular edema that leads to vision loss

Acute Complications
- Diabetic ketoacidosis (DKA)
  - Severe hyperglycemia with increased ketogenesis
  - Most common in Type 1, may be initial presentation
  - Symptoms include nausea, vomiting, acetone (fruity) breath, dehydration, tachycardia, polydipsia, polyuria, fatigue, altered mental status, Kussmaul's respirations (rapid deep breathing)
  - Clinical features
    - Hyperglycemia >450 mg/dL
    - Metabolic acidosis with anion gap
    - Serum and urine positive ketones
    - Hyponatremia
    - Potassium may be elevated on serum studies but total body potassium is low due to intracellular shift of potassium into the cells
  - Treatment
    1. Fluid replacement: Isotonic (normal) saline
       - May add 5% glucose to IV fluid once blood glue reaches <250 mg/dL to limit hypoglycemia
    2. Potassium replacement if <5.3 me/L
       - If <3.3 mEq/L, use 40 mEq/h IV potassium
       - If 3.3–5.3 mEq/L, use 20–30 mEq/L IV potassium
       - Goal potassium 4.0–5.0 mEq/L
    3. Insulin
       - Potassium replacement **before** insulin therapy since insulin drives potassium into cells worsening hypokalemia
       - Use IV regular insulin: Initial bolus of 0.1 μ/kg then 0.1 μ/kg/h maintenance
       - Monitor blood glucose levels closely
       - Continue IV insulin until anion gap is closed
       - Transition to subcutaneous insulin once patient is tolerating PO diet
- Hyperosmolar hyperglycemic state (HHS)
  - Severe hyperglycemia in Type 2 diabetics
  - Similar symptoms to DKA with dehydration, polyuria, fatigue, altered mental status
  - Hyperglycemia >900 mg/dL, serum osmolarity >320 mOsm/L
  - No acidosis or anion gap, minimal to no ketosis
  - Same treatment as DKA

Floor Management Tips
- For diabetic patients on the floor, utilize a sliding insulin scale dosing schedule with finger stick glucose checks with 3 meals and at bedtime
- Utilize ½ to ⅔ of patient's home dose insulin plus sliding scale
- Hold meal time insulin dosing when patient is NPO and prior to procedure
- Be aware of peak activity times for medium and long acting insulin schedules to avoid hypoglycemia on procedure day when patient will be NPO
- Example regular insulin sliding scale: 2 units per 50 mg/dL blood glucose >150
  - BG 150–200 = 2 units regular insulin
  - BG 201–250 = 4 units regular insulin
  - BG 251–300 = 6 units regular insulin
  - BG 301–350 = 8 units regular insulin
  - BG 351–400 = 10 units regular insulin
  - BG >400 = Call covering physician (may require adjustment to scheduled insulin dosing)

Source: American Diabetes Association Standards of Medical Care in Diabetes 2017, http://care. diabetesjournals.org/content/diacare/suppl/2016/12/15/40.Supplement_1.DC1/DC_40_S1_final.pdf

HYPERTENSION

Background
- Hypertension (HTN) affects ~50% patients > 60 y and is responsible for 7.6 million deaths worldwide each year (*NEJM* 2010:362:2102)

Definition	Treatment
Normal SBP <120 and DBP <80	Encourage healthy lifestyle
Elevated Systolic between 120–129 and diastolic less than 80	Lifestyle modification for 3 mo (*JACC* 2017;11:6): • Weight loss (↓ 0.5–2 mmHg/kg lost) • DASH diet rich in fruits, vegetables, low fat (↓ 8–14 mmHg) (http://www.nhlbi.nih.gov/health/public/heart/hbp/dash/new_dash.pdf) • Sodium reduction <2.4 g/d (↓ 2–8 mmHg) • Aerobic exercise >30 min/d, intensity more effective than frequency (↓ 4–9 mmHg) • Moderate ETOH consumption <2 drinks/d men, <1 drink/d women (↓ 2–4 mmHg)
Stage 1: Systolic between 130–139 or diastolic between 80–89	Lifestyle modification *and* Patients without compelling indication: Hydrochlorothiazide 12.5 mg PO QD Patients with compelling indication see below
Stage 2: Systolic at least 140 *or* diastolic at least 90 mmHg	Lifestyle modification *and* Patients without compelling indication: ACEI + CCB (**Accomplish** *NEJM* 2008:2417) Patients with compelling indication see below
Hypertensive urgency SBP >180 or DBP >120	Treatment for stage II plus close followup (1–3 d), home BP monitoring
Hypertensive emergency (evidence of end organ damage)	Headache, chest pain, visual changes, altered mental status, CVA, neurologic symptoms, pulmonary edema, bleeding, aortic dissection, renal failure, CHF, pre-eclampsia/eclampsia. Requires emergency referral for IV agents.

Compelling Indications (*NEJM* 2006;355:385)
• **Afib:** BB or CCB (ie, diltiazem) for rate control
• **DM2:** ACEI (renoprotective). ACEI + CCB for combined therapy (ACCOMPLISH *NEJM* 2008;359:2417). Goal BP <140/90 in absence of nephropathy/CKD (ACCORD *NEJM* 2010;362:1575)
• **High CAD risk:** ACEI, BB, CCB, thiazide
• **CKD:** ACEI/ARB plus a loop diuretic
• **CHF:** ACEI, ARB, BB, diuretics, aldosterone antagonist
• **H/o CVA:** Thiazide, ACEI
• **H/o MI:** ACEI, BB, aldosterone antagonist

Special Populations
• **African-ancestry:** Thiazide or CCB
• **Angina:** BB or CCB
• **BPH:** α-Blocker
• **Elderly:** Thiazide or CCB. SBP <140 (*NEJM* 2007;357:789)
• **Nephrolithiasis:** Thiazide (decreases renal calcium clearance)
• **Osteoporosis:** Thiazide
• **Pregnancy:** Methyldopa (Pregnancy risk factor B), hydralazine, or nifedipine sustained release (Pregnancy risk factor C)
• **Younger patients (<50 y):** ACEI or ARB

Second-Line Agents
• Loop diuretics (ie, furosemide) useful in refractory HTN with renal insufficiency (Cr >1.5)
• Combined α- and β-blockers (ie, labetalol)
• Combined calcium channel blockers (ie, diltiazem/verapamil + amlodipine) or ARB and ACEI with careful K/Cr monitoring
• Clonidine available in transdermal dosing
• Hydralazine
• Aliskiren (oral renin inhibitor)

Medication Side-Effects
• **α-Blockers:** Increased risk of CHF (doxazosin), postural hypotension
• **ACEI:** Cough (~15% pts). Hyperkalemia in renal insufficiency. Angioedema. Contraindicated in pregnancy.
• **Aldosterone antagonists:** Hyperkalemia, especially w/ ACEI, DM, renal insufficiency. Gynecomastia and breast pain (less so with eplerenone).

- **ARB:** Contraindicated in pregnancy
- **BB:** Angina/rebound HTN on abrupt discontinuation. May mask hypoglycemic symptoms in DM. May exacerbate asthma/COPD, impotence. Contraindicated in heart block. Nightmares, fatigue, decreased exercise tolerance. Use in patients w/ pheochromocytoma may exacerbate HTN by unopposed α-stimulation.
- **CCB:** Verapamil is a negative inotrope and is contraindicated in heart block. Peripheral edema.
- **Clonidine:** Rebound HTN on discontinuation
- **Thiazides:** Hypokalemia, most common in 1st weeks of treatment, prevent by dietary salt restriction. Hyperglycemia, especially in diabetics. Hyponatremia. May exacerbate gout.

COMMON COMORBIDITIES

Congestive Heart Failure (CHF)
- **Background**
  - Decreased cardiac output secondary to wide variety of etiologies
    - Ischemic heart disease, hypertension to myocardial hypertrophy, aortic stenosis, aortic regurgitation, mitral stenosis, restrictive cardiomyopathy (amyloidosis, sarcoidosis)
- **Symptoms**
  - Dyspnea, orthopnea, paroxysmal nocturnal dyspnea, nocturnal cough
- **Physical exam**
  - Left-sided heart failure
    - Leftward displaced point of maximal impulse
    - Pathologic S_3
    - S_4 Gallop
    - Lung base rales or crackles
  - Right-sided heart failure
    - Peripheral pitting edema
    - Nocturnal
    - Jugular venous distention
    - Hepatojugular reflex
    - Ascites
- **Diagnosis**
  - Echocardiogram to look for cardiomegaly and determine EF
  - Stress testing
  - Cardiac catheterization
- **Treatment**
  - Initially with lifestyle modification including sodium diet restriction, weight loss, stop smoking and alcohol, and exercise
  - Utilize New York Heart Association classifications
    - Mild CHF (NYHA Class I–II)
      - Restrict sodium and encourage physical activity
      - Start loop diuretic (Furosemide)
    - Mild to Moderate (NYHA Class II–III)
      - Loop diuretic and ACE inhibitor
      - Add β-Blocker if symptoms are not controlled
    - Moderate to Severe (NYHA Class III–IV)
      - Add digoxin along with continued loop diuretic and ACE Inhibitor
      - If symptoms still not controlled, consider adding spironolactone
  - ICD lower mortality in patients with EF <35% with class II or III symptoms not controlled with optimal medical management
- **Acute decompensated heart failure exacerbation**
  - Acute dyspnea with increased left heart pressures and pulmonary edema
  - Add supplemental oxygen with nasal cannula, non-rebreather, or intubation as needed
  - IV diuretics to remove excess fluid overload

Coronary Heart Disease (CAD)
- **Background**
  - Increased calcification of coronary arteries resulting in decreased cardiac perfusion
- **Symptoms**
  - Varies from asymptomatic, stable angina, unstable angina, to myocardial infarction

- **Physical exam and diagnosis**
  - Physical exam is typically normal and unrevealing
  - ECG during chest pain symptoms to look for T wave or ST segment abnormalities
  - Cardiac stress test to look for exercise-induced ischemia
    - ECG, echocardiogram, and pharmacologic stress tests are all modality options depending on patient's tolerance
  - Cardiac catheterization
    - Most sensitive and specific test for CAD
    - Angiography allows for visualization of coronary vessels
    - Can measure degree of stenosis and provide intervention/treatment concurrently
- **Treatment**
  - Initially with lifestyle and risk factor modification similar to CHF
    - Restrict fat and cholesterol in diet, smoking cessation, weight control, hypertension and hyperlipidemia management, and regular exercise
  - Medical treatments
    - Aspirin decreases morbidity and reduces myocardial infarction risk
    - β-blockers reduce frequency of acute coronary events
    - Nitrates relieve acute angina/chest pain symptoms
    - Calcium channel blockers may be added on top of β-blockers for further management
  - Cardiac catheterization
    - May include balloon and stenting options based on degree of disease
    - Can be done prophylactically
  - Coronary artery bypass grafting (CABG) in severe multivessel disease

Source: 2013 ACCF/AHA Guideline for the Management of Heart Failure: Executive Summary, https://doi.org/10.1161/CIR.0b013e31829e8807

Chronic Obstructive Pulmonary Disease (COPD)
- **Background**
  - Defined as two subtypes that regularly coexist
    - Chronic bronchitis: Chronic cough with productive sputum for >3 mo of year for >2 y
    - Emphysema: Enlargement of airspaces secondary to destruction of alveolar walls
- **Symptoms**
  - Cough, dyspnea, sputum production, wheezing, crackles, cyanosis, tachypnea, increased work of breathing, use of accessory respiratory muscles
- **Diagnosis**
  - Clinical diagnosis based on symptoms
  - Pulmonary function testing
    - Significantly decreased FEV_1
    - Decreased FEV_1/FVC ratio
    - Total lung capacity (TLO) and residual volume (RV) increased
  - Chest radiography may demonstrate hyperinflated lungs and flattened diaphragm, prominent hilar vessels, and decreased peripheral bronchovascular markings
- **Treatment**
  - Stop smoking
  - Oxygen therapy
    - Only option to improve mortality
    - Qualify if walking pulse oximetry is <90%
  - Medicine
    - Inhaled β_2-agonist (albuterol)
    - Inhaled anticholinergic (ipratropium)
    - Inhaled corticosteroids (fluticasone)
    - Antibiotics in acute exacerbation
  - Start with lifestyle modification, add home medicine inhalers for mild to moderate symptom control, and home oxygen therapy for severe disease with associated hypoxia
- **Acute COPD exacerbation**
  - Acute persistent dyspnea and respiratory failure not relieved by bronchodilators
  - Treatment steps
    - Supplemental oxygen via nasal cannula, face mask, noninvasive positive-pressure ventilation (BiPAP or CPAP), or intubation with mechanical ventilation depending on respiratory stability
    - Systemic corticosteroids, IV then oral taper (do not use inhaled delivery)

- Antibiotics only if there are 2 of 3 symptoms: Increased dyspnea, increased sputum volume, or increased sputum purulence
  - Goal is to limit antibiotic use to exacerbation that truly include infectious etiology

Source: Global Strategy for the Diagnosis, Management and Prevention of COPD, Global Initiative for Chronic Obstructive Lung Disease (GOLD) 2017. http://www.goldcopd.org

Acute Kidney Injury (AKI)
- **Background**
  - Acute decrease in kidney function measured by glomerular filtration rate
  - Risk, Injury, Failure, Loss and End-Stage Kidney (RIFLE) multi-level classification system established in 2004 based upon increasing severity of disease (Fig. 21-1)

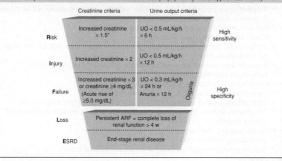

Figure 21-1 RIFLE classification scheme for Acute Kidney Injury. Adapted from Bellomo, Crit Care 2004. (Source: Kidney Disease: Improving Global Outcomes (KDIGO) Acute Kidney Injury Work Group. KDIGO Clinical Practice Guideline for Acute Kidney Injury. Kidney inter., Suppl. 2012;2:1–138.)

- **Symptoms and diagnosis**
  - Measured as increase in creatinine
  - Various symptoms based on etiology and risk factors for underlying AKI cause
- **Classification**
  - Prerenal causes
    - Volume depletion (hemorrhage)
    - Hypotension
    - Sepsis
    - Heart failure (decreased cardiac output)
    - Liver failure
  - Intrinsic renal
    - Medication induced acute interstitial nephritis (NSAIDs)
    - Acute tubular necrosis (ATN) from nephrotoxic agents such as iodinated contrast
    - Direct glomerular damage (autoimmune diseases, nephrotic/nephritic syndromes)
    - Renal vascular damage (thrombosis of renal artery/vein)
  - Postrenal causes
    - Urinary obstruction
    - Bladder outlet obstruction
    - Renal pelvis obstruction
- **Treatment**
  - Management priorities are mainly supportive and include:
    - Preventing further insult (renal toxic agent)
    - Treating life threatening complications (hyperkalemia, metabolic acidosis)
    - Providing support by renal replacement (dialysis) with the anticipated goal of renal recovery
  - Dialysis in the form of continuous verses intermittent have similar outcomes

Background
- Used to treat respiratory failure that has not resolved with other oxygen delivery systems (nasal cannula, venture mask, no rebreathing mask, etc.)
- Main goals for mechanical ventilator is to correct hypoxemia and preserve alveolar ventilation
- Other indications include impaired consciousness, inability to protect airway, respiratory muscle disability

Modes
- Assisted control (AC)
  - Typically, the initial mode during respiratory failure
  - Ventilator delivers all breaths
  - Machine always provides same preset tidal volume with every breath
  - Patient can initiate own breath and ventilator will provide set tidal volume and rate
  - If patient doesn't breathe, a backup breath with the same tidal volume will be initiated
  - Patient can breathe "over" the ventilator
- Synchronous intermittent mandatory ventilation (SIMV)
  - Used for maintenance and weaning
  - Similar to AC but ventilator does not provide predetermined tidal volume when patient initiates breath
  - If patient does not initiate breath, ventilator will provide tidal volume
  - Follows set respiratory rate
- Continuous positive airway pressure (CPAP)
  - Used in weaning trial and some maintenance scenarios
  - Only utilizes positive end-expiratory pressure (PEEP) and pressure support
  - Continuous delivery of positive pressure, patient breaths on their own, no tidal volume breaths are provided
- Pressure-support ventilation (PSV)
  - Used during weaning trials
  - Positive pressure is provided only when patient initiates breath

Parameters
- Minute ventilation
  - Respiratory Rate X Tidal volume
  - Normal tidal volume is 8–10 mL/kg
  - Normal respiratory rate is 10–12 breaths/min
  - Goal is to maintain baseline $PaCO_2$
- Fraction of inspired oxygen (FiO_2)
  - Start at 100%
  - Titrate down and use lowest setting to maintain saturation >90%
  - May add PEEP or CPAP to help further decrease FiO_2
- Inspiratory–expiratory ratio (I:E)
  - Time of inspiration versus time in expiratory during one complete breath
  - Typical 1:2, minimal adjustments
- Positive end-expiratory pressure
  - Positive pressure delivered at the end of exhalation
  - Can be added with any ventilation modes
  - Increases lung compliance and prevents alveolar collapse
  - Prolonged PEEP increases risk of barotrauma and pneumothorax

Complications
- Regular maintenance and monitoring of settings required
- Suctioning of secretions, ICU level of care
- Pneumonia/infection, increased risk of nosocomial microbes
- Self or accidental extubating
- Pain and agitation
  - Balance sedation with benzodiazepines, opioids, and induction agents
- Extended intubation causes softening of trachea supportive cartilage; tracheostomy is done when >2 w of continuous mechanical ventilation anticipated

Other Types of Oxygen Delivery
- Nasal cannula: Easy access
- Face mask: Increased flow rate compared to nasal cannula
- Ventura mask: Better control of oxygenation, ideal for CO_2 retention
- Nonrebreather mask: Even greater control of oxygenation compared to Venturi

Source: Agabegi SS, Agabegi ED. Step-Up to Medicine. Lippincott Williams & Wilkins; 2012.

Acute Respiratory Distress Syndrome (ARDS)

- ARDS initially defined as an acute condition characterized by bilateral pulmonary infiltrates and severe hypoxemia in the absence of evidence for cardiogenic pulmonary edema

Figure 21-2 Acute Respiratory Distress Syndrome redefined in 2012 using the Berlin criteria. (Reprinted from Ashbaugh DG, Bigelow DB, Petty TL, et al. Acute respiratory distress in adults. *Lancet* 1967;2(7511):319–23. Copyright ©1967 Elsevier, with permission.)

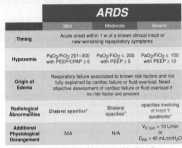

ARDS			
	Mild	Moderate	Severe
Timing	Acute onset within 1 w of a known clinical insult or new worsening respiratory symptoms		
Hypoxemia	PaO_2/FiO_2 201–300 with $PEEP/CPAP \geq 5$	$PaO_2/FiO_2 \leq 200$ with $PEEP \geq 5$	$PaO_2/FiO_2 \leq 100$ with $PEEP \geq 5$
Origin of Edema	Respiratory failure associated to known risk factors and not fully explained by cardiac failure or fluid overload. Need objective assessment of cardiac failure or fluid overload if no risk factor are present		
Radiological Abnormalities	Bilateral opacities*	Bilateral opacities*	opacities involving at least 2 quadrants*
Additional Physiological Derangement	N/A	N/A	$V_{E\,Corr} > 10$ L/min or $C_{RS} < 40$ mL/cmH₂O

*Not fully explained by effusion, nodules, masses, or lobar/ lung collapse; use training set of CXRs; $V_{E\,Corr} = V_E \times PaCO_2/40$ (corrected for Body Surface Area)

- Risk factors:

Direct Risk Factors	Indirect Risk Factors
Pneumonia	Nonpulmonary sepsis
Aspiration of gastric contents	Major trauma
Inhalation injury	Multiple transfusions
Pulmonary contusion	Major burns
Near drowning	Pancreatitis
	Noncardiogenic Shock

- Management includes source control, oxygen supplementation, fluid restriction, nutritional support, ventilator support
- Low tidal volume (6 cc/kg predicted body weight) shown to have a survival benefit (Reference-Acute Respiratory Distress Syndrome Network: Ventilation with lower tidal volumes as compared with traditional tidal volumes for acute lung injury and acute respiratory distress syndrome. *N Engl J Med* 2000;342:1301–8)
- With increasing severity, various therapeutic management options have been proposed (Fig. 21-3)

Figure 21-3 Therapeutic options in Acute Respiratory Distress Syndrome based upon disease severity. (Reprinted from Ashbaugh DG, Bigelow DB, Petty TL, et al. Acute respiratory distress in adults. *Lancet* 1967;2(7511):319–23. Copyright ©1967 Elsevier, with permission.)

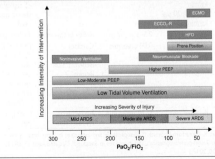

INTRODUCTION TO VASOPRESSORS

Shock

- Inadequate tissue perfusion with impaired oxygen and nutrient delivery
- Multiple types of shock including hemorrhagic, septic, neurogenic, cardiogenic, and adrenal insufficiency (endocrine shock)
- For all types of shock, vasopressors should only be initiated with/after adequate resuscitation is provided with crystalloids, colloids, and/or blood products
- Hemorrhagic shock
  - Vasopressors are not recommended in initial stabilization of hemorrhagic shock
  - May utilize permissive hypotension until bleeding source is controlled
  - If hypotension persists after despite blood/fluid resuscitation and surgical intervention, consider alternative shock etiology and appropriate vasopressor
- Septic shock
  - Maintain mean arterial pressure (MAP) ≥65 mmHg for goal of adequate end-organ perfusion
  - Norepinephrine is 1st-line agent
  - Epinephrine may be added to norepinephrine if hypotension persists
  - Vasopressin optimizes therapeutic efficacy of norepinephrine
  - Dobutamine may be initiated in combination with norepinephrine when patient has myocardial dysfunction
  - Dopamine should not be used for renal protective effects
- Neurogenic shock
  - Vasopressors may be initiated early to avoid volume overload
  - Norepinephrine is first line agent
  - Phenylephrine should be avoided due to unopposed alpha activity resulting in reflex bradycardia
- Cardiogenic shock
  - Vasopressors and/or inotropes may be initiated early when there is clinical evidence of volume overload
  - Dobutamine may be initiated in combination with norepinephrine in low output cardiac state
- Adrenal insufficiency/endocrine shock
  - Random serum cortisol <20 µg/dL
  - Give steroid replacement (hydrocortisone 50 mg IV q6 or 100 mg IV q8)
  - Home oral steroid taper recommended if on steroid therapy for >7 d

Drug	Receptor Affinity	Dose	Adverse Events	Notes
Norepinephrine	$\alpha_1 > \beta_1$	0/05–1 µg/kg/min	Tachycardia, Peripheral/GI ischemia	
Epinephrine	$\beta_1 > \alpha_1$ Low doses = β High doses = α	0/05–0/5 µg/kg/min	Tachycardia, Peripheral/GI ischemia	
Dopamine	DA = <5 µg/kg/min β_1 = 5–10 µg/kg/min α_1 = 10–20 µg/kg/min	5–20 µg/kg/min	Tachycardia, Arrhythmias	Renal protective doses of <5 µg/kg/min should not be used
Phenylephrine	α_1	0.5–5 µg/kg/min	Reflex bradycardia	Tachyphylaxis
Vasopressin	V_1	0.04 units/min	Cardiac/mesenteric ischemia, Skin lesions	DO NOT TITRATE (doses >0.04 units/min can result in cardiac ischemia
Dobutamine	β_1, β_2	5–20 µg/kg/min	Arrhythmias, Hypotension	Inotropic agent

(Source: Rojas K, Birrer K, Cheatham M, Smith C. Vasopressors and Inotropes in Shock. http://www.surgicalcriticalcare.net/Guidelines/Vasopressors and Inotropes in Shock.pdf. Updated April 19, 2011. Accessed December 20, 2017.)

Definition
- **Guidelines for the diagnosis and management of sepsis first authored in 2004**
- **Most recent update** (*JAMA* 2016;315(8):801–10) **defines three definitions of sepsis:**
  - Sepsis—Life-threatening organ dysfunction caused by dysregulated host response to infection
  - Septic Shock—Subset of sepsis with circulatory and cellular/metabolic dysfunction associated with higher risk of mortality
  - "Sepsis" in place of "Severe Sepsis"
- **2016 update provide 93 Recommendations:**
  - 32 Strong recommendations: "We recommend"
  - 39 Weak recommendations: "We suggest"
  - 18 Best Practice Statements
- **Acute resuscitation**
  - Begin goal-directed resuscitation during 1st 6 h after recognition
  - Begin initial fluid resuscitation with crystalloid (strong recommendation) and consider the addition of albumin (weak recommendation)
  - Begin initial fluid challenge in patients with tissue hypoperfusion and suspected hypovolemia, to achieve ≥30 mL of crystalloids per kilogram of body weight within the 1st 3 h (strong recommendation)
  - Use norepinephrine as the 1st-choice vasopressor to maintain a mean arterial pressure of ≥65 mmHg (strong recommendation)
  - Use epinephrine when an additional agent is needed to maintain mean arterial pressure of ≥65 mmHg (weak recommendation)
  - Add vasopressin (at a dose of 0.03 µ/min) with weaning of norepinephrine (weak recommendation)
  - Avoid the use of dopamine except in carefully selected patients (eg, patients with a low risk of arrhythmias and either known marked ventricular systolic dysfunction or low heart rate)
  - Infuse dobutamine or add it to vasopressor therapy in the presence of myocardial dysfunction (eg, elevated cardiac filling pressures or low cardiac output) or ongoing hypoperfusion despite adequate intravascular volume and mean arterial pressure
  - Avoid the use of intravenous hydrocortisone if adequate fluid resuscitation and vasopressor therapy restore hemodynamic stability; if hydrocortisone is used, administer at a dose of 200 mg/d (weak recommendation)
  - Target a hemoglobin level of 7–9 g/dL in patients without hypoperfusion, critical coronary artery disease or myocardial ischemia, or acute hemorrhage
- **Infection control**
  - Obtain blood cultures before antibiotic therapy is administered
  - Perform imaging studies promptly to confirm source of infection
  - Administer IV antibiotic therapy within 1 h after diagnosis of either sepsis or septic shock (strong recommendation)
  - Administer empiric broad-spectrum therapy with one or more antimicrobials to cover most likely pathogen (strong recommendation)
  - Reassess antibiotic therapy daily for de-escalation when appropriate
  - Perform source control with attention to risks and benefits of the chosen method as soon as medically and logistically practical after diagnosis made (best practice statement)
- **Respiratory support**
  - Use a low tidal volume and limitation of inspiratory-plateau-pressure strategy for adult patients with sepsis induced respiratory failure without ARDS (strong recommendation)
  - Administer higher rather than lower positive end-expiratory pressure for patients with sepsis-induced moderate to severe ARDS (weak recommendation)
  - Use prone positioning in patients with sepsis-induced ARDS and a ratio of the partial pressure of arterial oxygen (mmHg) to the fraction of inspired oxygen of <150, In facilities that have experience with such practice (strong recommendation)
  - Elevate the head of the bed in patients undergoing mechanical ventilation, unless contraindicated
  - Use a conservative fluid strategy for established acute lung injury or ARDS with no evidence of tissue hypoperfusion

- Use of HFOV in adult patients with sepsis induced ARDS is not recommended (strong recommendation)
- **General Support**
  - Use a protocol-specified approach to blood glucose management, with the initiation of insulin after 2 consecutive blood glucose levels of >180 mg/dL (10 mmol/L) targeting a blood glucose level <180 mg/dL (strong recommendation)
  - We suggest against the use of renal replacement therapy in patients with sepsis and acute kidney injury for increase in creatinine or oliguria without other definitive indication for dialysis (weak recommendation)
  - Use the equivalent of continuous venovenous hemofiltration or intermittent hemodialysis as needed for renal failure or fluid overload
  - Administer prophylaxis for deep-vein thrombosis
  - Administer stress-ulcer prophylaxis to prevent upper gastrointestinal bleeding
  - Administer oral or enteral feedings, as tolerated, rather than either complete fasting or provision of only intravenous glucose within the 1st 48 h after a diagnosis of severe sepsis or septic shock (weak recommendation)
  - Address goals of care, including treatment plans and end-of-life planning as appropriate (strong recommendation)
  - Goals of care should be addressed as early as feasible, but no later than within 72 h of ICU admission (weak recommendation)

INTRODUCTION TO CARDIAC INTENSIVE CARE

- **Common Dysrhythmias**
  - Sinus bradycardia (Heart rate <60 bpm)
    - Causes: MI, ↓ Thyroid, ↓ Temp, ↓ Glucose, Medications (Beta blockers)
    - Management: Atropine, Pacing if associated with hypotension
  - Sinus Tachycardia (Heart rate 101–160 bpm)
    - Causes: HTN, Fever, Stress, Stimulants, Pain, ↑ Thyroid, Hypoxia
    - Management: Address underlying etiology, Manage sepsis for patient with SIRS
      - Narrow QRS → Vagal stimulation, Adenosine, Beta blockers, Cardioversion
      - Wide QRS → Procainamide, Amiodarone, Sotalol
  - Atrial Fibrillation (Irregular Heart Rate 350–400 bpm)
    - Causes: Hypoxia, CHF, CAD, ↑ Thyroid, SA node dysfunction
    - Management: Beta blockers, Calcium channel blockers, Amiodarone, Digoxin
  - Atrial Flutter (Heart Rate 250–400 bpm)
    - Causes: Ischemia, COPD, Thickened heart muscle
    - Management: Cardioversion (Tx of choice), Procainamide, beta blocker, Diltiazem, Heparin for thrombus prevention
  - Sinus Ventricular Tachycardia (Heart Rate 150–250 bpm)
    - Causes: Hypoxia, Stimulants, Hypokalemia, CAD
    - Management: Cardioversion if hypotensive, Vagal stimulation, Adenosine
  - Ventricular Tachycardia (Heart Rate 101–250 bpm)
    - Causes: CAD, MI, QT prolongation, Digoxin toxicity
    - Management: ACLS protocol (see figure), Recurrent → may require ICD placement
  - Ventricular Fibrillation (Heart Rate not discernable)
    - Causes: MI, Electrolyte imbalances, ↓ Temp, Trauma, Drug toxicity/overdose
    - Management: ACLS (see figure)
  - Torsades de Pointes (Heart Rate 150–250)
    - Causes: Prolonged QT interval, Hypokalemia, Hypomagnesemia, TCA overdose
    - Management: Replace electrolytes, Cardioversion if hypotensive, Correct causing factors
- **Acute Coronary Syndrome**
  - Defined as a spectrum of conditions caused by sudden blockage of the blood supply to the heart. Three types include potentially reversible **unstable angina (UA)**, irreversible cell death by either an **ST-segment elevation MI (STEMI)** or a **non-ST-segment elevation MI (NSTEMI)**
  - Risk factors:
    - **HTN**
    - **High cholesterol**
    - **Obesity**
    - **Smoking**
    - **Diabetes**

- **Family history**
- **Older age**
- **Initial management:**
  - Assess ABC's: Airway (need for intubation), Breathing (O_2 supplementation, Sats > 90%), Circulation (vitals and IV access)
  - Obtain 12-lead ECG as soon as possible
  - Performed focused history physical
  - Obtain blood: Troponin, electrolytes, H/H, coags
  - ASA 325 mg PO if no contraindication; Give rectally if PO contraindicated
  - Sublingual nitroglycerine for persistent chest pain
  - Beta blockers if no contraindications (signs of HF, hemodynamically unstable)
  - Morphine sulfate for discomfort/anxiety related myocardial ischemia
  - Initiate statin therapy
  - Early Cardiology consult

Consults

Background
- A focused yet thorough evaluation of appropriateness and pt candidacy for a procedure
- Important to remember your role as a consultant/specialist; many medical mgmt issues are better addressed by other specialists

Evaluation
- History: Chart review, onset of sx, location, exacerbating/ relieving factors, pt ability undergo procedure, ability to consent, NPO status
- Assoc. sx: Fevers/chills, N/V, Δ in bowel habits (diarrhea/ constipation, stool quality, or color hematochezia, melena), jaundice, menstrual hx
- PMHx: previous procedures/surgeries, prior vascular access or endovascular intervention, contrast reactions, renal function or dz likely to impair renal function (eg, DM, HTN, PVD, receiving nephrotoxic drugs), coagulopathy or dz likely to impair clotting (eg, cirrhosis, uremia), drug allergies, contrast rxns
- Exam: VS; general appearance and posture, lines and tubes, mobility, neck ROM, CV/ pulses, respirations, abd exam, ASA score, Mallampati score
- Labs: CBC, coags, lytes, pregnancy test, ± LFT, ± EKG
- Imaging: Review all imaging and determine if any additional pre-op imaging is req
- Assessment: Is the pt hemodynamically stable? Is urgent intervention req.? Can the pt. be medically optimized prior to intervention? (eg, hydration, correct electrolyte imbalance, hold potentially high-risk meds—anti-coagulants, NSAIDs etc.)

ASA Classification		
ASA PS Classification	**Definition**	**Examples, including but not limited to:**
ASA I	Normal, healthy pt	Healthy, nonsmoking, no or min EtOH use
ASA II	Pt w/ mild systemic dz	Mild dz w/o substantive functional limitations; current smoker, social EtOH use, BMI 30–40, controlled DM or HTN, mild lung dz, pregnancy
ASA III	Pt w/ severe systemic dz	Substantive functional limitation, ≥1 moderate to severe dz, uncontrolled DM or HTN, COPD, BMI ≥40, alcoholic hepatitis, EtOH dependence, ESRD on HD, MI >3 mo ago, TIA, CAD/stents
ASA IV	Pt with severe systemic dz that is a constant threat to life	MI <3 mo ago, ongoing cardiac ischemia, severe valvular dysfxn, sepsis, DIC, ARDS
ASA V	Moribund pt not expected to survive w/o the procedure	Ruptured AAA, massive trauma, intracranial bleed w/ mass effect, ischemic bowel in the face of sig. cardiac dz or multiorgan failure
ASA VI	Pt declared brain-dead, organs are being removed for donor purposes	

(Adapted from Hurwitz EE, Simon M, Vinta SR, et al. Adding examples to the ASA-Physical Status Classification improves correct assignment to patients. *Anesthesiology* 2017;126(4):614–22. DOI: 10.1097/ALN.0000000000001541, with permission.)

*The addition of "E" denotes emergency surgery, ie, any delay in Tx would lead to sig. incr. in the threat to life or body part.

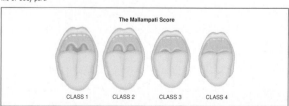

The Mallampati Score

CLASS 1 CLASS 2 CLASS 3 CLASS 4

(Adapted from Brunicardi F, Andersen DK, Billiar TR, et al. *Schwartz's Principles of Surgery.* 10th ed.; 2014.)

POSTPROCEDURE PAIN MANAGEMENT

Background (*JVIR* 2003;14:1373–85)
- IR procedures may not require any analgesia; however, some are intrinsically painful (eg, uterine artery or hepatic embolizations) and often require post-op analgesia
- High-intensity or refractory pain should be assessed to reveal any new medical or surgical complication

Evaluation
- History: Type of procedure, nature of pain (onset, location, quality, intensity, aggravating and relieving factors, prev. Rx, barriers to assessment), Numeric Pain Scale (0 = "no pain" → 10 = "worst pain ever"), pain w/in the expectation of the procedure?
- Exam: VS, RS, inspect incision for signs of infxn (eg, rubor, calor, tumor, dolor)

Treatment (*Anesthesiology* 2013;118:251–70; *JPAIN* 2016;17(2):131–57)
- Multimodal analgesia (ie, Rx w/ a combination of analgesic meds with diff. MOA and nonpharm interv.) is the gold standard of pain mgmt
- PO preferred over IV admin of opioids for postop analgesia
- Certain procedures respond better to particular types of analgesia (eg Tumor lysis syndrome and postfibroid embolization syndrome are best treated with NSAIDS and meperidine (for shaking); opioids are a 2nd line)

Select Analgesics		
Drug	**Typical Clinical Dose**	**Comments**
Acetaminophen	PO or IV 500–1000 mg q4h (max dose = 4 g/24 h)	NSAID, COX inhibitor, C/I: Hepatotoxic
Ibuprofen	PO 400–600 mg q4–6h (max dose = 3.2 g/24 h)	NSAID, COX inhibitor C/I: Active bleeding, peptic ulceration, CV events, renal dysfxn
Ketorolac	IV 15 mg q6h (max dose = 120 mg)	
Oxycodone	PO 5–10 mg q4–6h	Opioid, 1° effect is on CNS S/E: Constipation, sedation and decreased respiratory drive
Hydromorphone	PO 2–6 mg q4–6h IV 0.2–0.5 mg q4–6h	

POSTOPERATIVE FEVER

Background (Weed H & Baddour L, *Postoperative Fever.* In: UpToDate, Post TW (Ed), UpToDate, Waltham, MA, Accessed October 31, 2017)
- Fever is common in the early postop period, etiology is typically noninfectious and is caused by inflammatory cytokines and pyrogens
- SIRS response can occur after abscess drainage or drain manipulation due to transient bacteremia
- Five W's: Wind (atelectasis/PNA), Water (UTI), Wound (incision, access site), Walking (DVT/PE), What did we do? (Type of intervention, infusions, transfusion rxn, drug rxn, newly placed lines or indwelling drains)

Evaluation
- History: S/sx, onset of sx, time since procedure, type of procedure, any complications, medications, or blood transfusion
- Exam: Evaluate incision, site of lines/tubes placed, signs of DVT or PE
- Workup: Consider CBC w/ diff., CXR, blood cx, UA/ UCx, CT
(Note: Embolization of large benign soft tissue masses (eg, fibroids) or any malignant mass can induce a "postembolization syndrome"—this causes fevers w/in the 1st few days that responds well to acetaminophen and/or ibuprofen. This should not be confused with postoperative infxn which usually presents several days later. A workup for infxn may not be needed if fever is w/in the 1st 2–3 d if postembolization syndrome is anticipated.)

BLEEDING FROM PUNCTURE SITE

Evaluation
- History: Type of procedure, ΔVS, what intervention has been attempted? How the procedure was performed? (eg, site of vascular or percutaneous punctures), what was used for closure, etc
- PMHx: Bleeding d/o, liver dz, recent anticoag or antiplt admin
- Exam: VS, type of bleed (eg, superficial bleeding from skin, venous ooze, brisk arterial), skin discoloration, palpate for hematoma

Treatment

- Superficial bleeding or venous ooze: Hold firm pressure at puncture site, consider applying pressure dressing, elevate the extremity or the pt to decrease bleeding, if pt is not taking any anticoag/ antiplt meds approximate skin with a simple buried interrupted suture w/ absorbable (eg, monocryl or vicryl) 3-0 or 4-0 suture. *(Note: Do not close incision if pt is currently on anticoag/antiplt meds as this can lead to hematoma formation.)*
- Arterial bleeding: Try to palpate the vessel and hold firm pressure at or slightly above puncture site. Pulse in the underlying vessel should be palpable, do not occlude the vessel. Hold pressure 3 min for every 1F sheath used (eg, 7F sheath hold pressure for 21 min). If bleeding persists consider vasc surg consult. FFP or plt transfusion may be needed.
- Consider evaluation of the puncture sites with ultrasound if there is persistent bleeding or physical exam findings to suggest a pseudoaneurysm
- Have a low threshold to evaluate w/ CT for high arterial sticks—retroperitoneal bleeding is difficult to detect clinically, can lead to rapid clinical decompensation. If concern for RP hemorrhage with clinical decompensation, consider empiric RBC transfusion.

SECURING A CATHETER

Background

- A suture should always be placed to secure a catheter to the pt; technique is provider specific
- Discussion w/ the pt and careful consideration should be made to maximize pt comfort while preventing catheter movement

Technique *(NEJM 2007;357;e15)*

- Instruments: Needle driver, nonabsorbable monofilament suture (eg, Nylon or Prolene) on a cutting needle. *(Note: Monofilament is preferred over silk or other braided suture; lower potential for infxn and skin irritation.)*
- Take a large bite of tissue using the curve of the needle on the obtuse side of the catheter—taking care to avoid puncturing the catheter. Once through the tissue cut off the needle and dispose.
- Tie an air knot on the clamp. *(Note: If there is a size mismatch of the catheter and the skin incision, tie down to the skin to gently approximate the tissue.)*
- Wrap suture around the catheter once and tie down on the catheter, repeat this action once more. *(Note: A slight crimp in the catheter is ok, but avoid excessively tight sutures on the catheter itself.)*
- We do not recommend using the "Roman-sandal" technique as this has been shown to be associated w/ catheter dislodgement *(J R Nav Med Serv 2015;101(1):42–6)*

REMOVING A TUNNELED CENTRAL VENOUS CATHETER

Background *(JVIR 2007;18:1232–40)*

- Typically indicated when pt no longer has need for central venous access or there is suspected catheter associated line infxn

Technique

- Instruments: Sterile drape, chlorhexidine scrub, local anesthetic (eg, buffered 1% lidocaine solution), curved forceps, suture scissor
- Place pt in a semirecumbent position and use a scissor to remove any retention sutures
- Prep and drape the catheter exit site in a sterile fashion
- Administer the local anesthetic into the subq tissue, infiltrating around the polyester cuff
- Using the curved forceps—gently dissect through the tunnel exit site to loosen the cuff. *(Note: A polyester cuff located deep to the catheter exit site may be very difficult to dissect, in such cases consider making a small skin incision at the site of the cuff to improve exposure.)* Keep backtension on the catheter with one hand while dissecting with the other to help free the cuff
- Never use a sharp instrument to dissect the cuff unless you can clearly visualize the dissection plane—cutting the catheter can result in retraction of the catheter inside the subq tunnel and could require a cutdown and/or operative intervention
- Remove the catheter and apply manual pressure above the exit site/at the venotomy for at least 5 min
- Confirm hemostasis and apply a sterile dressing. Inspect catheter to make sure it is intact

DRAINAGE CATHETER-RELATED COMPLICATIONS

Background (*Semin Intervent Radiol 2006;23:194–204*)
- Percutaneous fluid drainage is common, and once successfully placed, the next priority is maintaining optimal position
- Self-locking pigtail catheters are most commonly used and have resulted in reduced frequency of catheter dislodgment
- Functional parameters for catheters incl: output, access site leakage or infxn, lab and clinical findings of complication or failure of drainage

Catheter has Come Out (*RadioGraphics 2002;22:305–22*)
- Catheter falls out or is inadvertently removed
- Replacement can often be achieved w/o repuncture, depending on the maturity of the tract and time since catheter fell out
- Pt should return to the IR suite w/ in 24 h and the tract assessed under fluoroscopic guidance
- If catheter was placed w/in the last few hours or days, the tract will likely have closed and a new puncture must be performed
- Catheters dislodged later (see section below)—tract is formed, new catheter may be repositioned through existing tract under fluoroscopic guidance
- If immediate repositioning/replacement cannot be performed and catheter is dislodged but not entirely out, tightly secure the catheter to the pt wherever it is at that point—salvage may be possible

Should the Catheter Come Out?
- Most important factor is the clinical status of the pt:
  (-) Fever, (-) Leukocytosis, Drain output <10–20 cc for 2 consecutive d, no catheter-related issue to explain low output (eg, malposition, occlusion, or kinking)
  Imaging features: Small, well-drained cavity, w/o any undrained or loculated collections
  (*Note: Catheter injection should always be performed prior to removal if fistulous communication with intestine, biliary tract, urinary tract, or pancreatic duct is suspected to avoid reaccumulation of the collection*)

Catheter Site Infection
- Local infxn at access site typically results from prolonged catheterization
- If refractory to cx sp. or broad spec. abx, removal and placement at a different site may be required
- Large, indurated, painful or crepitant skin may indicate underlying abscess or necrotizing fasciitis → obtain CT or ultrasound

Bleeding
- Drainage procedures carry inherent risk of bleeding; fluid collections may be adjacent to, surrounding or w/in vascular structures (eg, liver or spleen), or encased by hypervascular or inflamed tissue
- If bleeding occurs → obtain imaging before manipulating or removing the catheter; premature removal can result in catastrophic escalation of bleeding
  (*Note: Catheters can produce a tamponade effect on venous structures—removing them can cause significant bleeding in cases where the catheter traverses larger vessels*)
- Most bleeds are typically self-limited and result from small surrounding vessels → manage conservatively with IVF, or transfusion if necessary
- **Pericatheter bleeding** is often the result of superficial vessels at the exit site or w/in a subq. tunnel (eg, tunneled CVC)
  Rx → manual compression at the exit site or along the subq. tunnel, consider correcting coagulopathy/stopping anticoag/antiplt meds. Uremia inhibiting platelet function can also contribute to tunneled HD catheter-related bleeding.
  If pt is not currently receiving any anticoag/antiplt meds a simple buried interrupted suture, using absorbable (eg, monocryl or vicryl) 3-0 or 4-0 suture, may be placed at the exit site to approximate the skin edges

Pericatheter Leakage (*Semin Intervent Radiol 2015;32:67–77*)
- **Gastrostomy tubes**—Most common cause is poor seal around the tube due to inadequate tract formation
  ↑ Risk a/w malnutrition, malignancy, or poor inflammatory response
  Buried Bumper Syndrome—Erosion of the internal retention bumper or balloon into the stomach or bowel wall. Clinical findings incl: skin ulceration, enlarging incision around the tube, to complete erosion of the retention bumper or balloon
- **Percutaneous Transhepatic Biliary Drainage Catheters (PTBD) and Percutaneous Nephrostomy (PCN)**—Most common cause is catheter obstruction

Obstructed or malpositioned catheter → ↑ Intrabiliary or intrarenal pressure → leak occurs from path of least resistance; around the catheter

(Note: Pt w/ ascites, pericatheter leakage of ascitic fluid may be mistaken for bile; in this case, ongoing drainage of ascites is recommended to allow for adequate tract formation)

- **Abscess Drainage Catheters**—Most common cause is obstruction or malposition, typically requiring fluoroscopic eval and catheter exchange

  Viscous fluid leakage—Consider catheter upsizing

  High-output intra-abdominal drain—Suspect bowel leak/fistula

  High-output pseudocyst drain—Suspect communication with pancreatic duct

Catheter Dislodgement

- **Gastrostomy tubes**—mgmt is determined by tract maturity

  <4 w after placement—Tract may not be fully matured; reinsertion should be performed under image guidance. If tube was placed endoscopically, stomach or jejunum may not be fixed to the anterior abdominal wall and enteric contents may leak into the peritoneal cavity.

  >4 w after placement—Mature tract, G-tube can usually be replaced at the bedside. If any concern exists of tract immaturity fluoroscopic eval should be performed.

  For all GJ- and J- tubes, reinsertion should be performed over a guidewire under fluoroscopic guidance

- **Percutaneous Transhepatic Biliary Drainage Catheters (PTBD)**

  Internal–external PTBD catheters are typically secured via a suture anchor at the skin and an internal retention loop in the duodenum

  External PTBDs, used when biliary obstruction cannot be traversed, are more frequently displaced or retracted. If retraction occurs, tape the catheter in place, and take the pt for fluoroscopic eval. as soon as possible.

  PTBD catheter dislodgement/obstruction is a/w new pericatheter leakage, persistent pain, and abrupt Δ in output

  Initial eval. w/ KUB, followed by fluoroscopic eval. and tractogram if position is uncertain, if tract is mature catheter reinsertion should be attempted w/in 2 d of dislodgement

- **Percutaneous Nephrostomy (PCN)**

  If PCN is completely dislodged, limited window to successfully reinsert catheter into the existing tract. Continuous leakage of urine from the exit site is a sign of a mature tract.

  Similar to PTBD reinsertions, a fluoroscopic eval. and tractogram for reinsertion can be attempted

Catheter Obstruction

- **Gastrostomy tubes**—Initial conservative mgmt. with saline or water flushes should be attempted. If failure of conservative measures; manage same as catheter dislodgement (see above).

- **Percutaneous Transhepatic Biliary Drainage Catheters (PTBD)**

  Obstruction typically results from bile stones, biliary sludge, or blood clots. Daily flushes help prevent obstructive episodes. Thicker output will need more frequent flushes.

  S/Sx: ↑ Bili, RUQ pain, fever, ↑ WBC, jaundice, pruritus, N/V, abrupt Δ in output, resistance to flushing, pericatheter leakage

  Catheter colonization + obstruction → Ascending cholangitis and sepsis; therefore empiric catheter exchange is advised if pt is symptomatic

- **Percutaneous Nephrostomy (PCN)**

  Obstruction typically results from mineral encrustation w/in the catheter lumen, or blood clots

  S/Sx: Pericatheter leakage, flank pain, fever and/or sepsis

  Similar to PTBD obstruction, catheter exchange (and possible upsizing) should be performed as soon as possible to mitigate risk of sepsis

- **Vascular Catheters (Venous, Arterial)**

  Arterial catheters may become obstructed if they are in small vessels, usually due to clotting, or when the catheter is abutting the vessel wall or plaque

  Repositioning the catheter will typically relieve the obstruction

  Venous catheters become obstructed due to blood clots or side-holes that become blocked by the vessel wall

  Instill 2–4 mg tPA, dwell and let it sit for 20 min—attempt to flush and aspirate NS

  If still obstructed, may attempt a second round of tPA

  If still obstructed, the catheter may need to be exchanged or repositioned over a wire

  (Note: Fibrin sheaths along the tip of a longer-term indwelling venous catheter may form and may lead to obstruction—management can include slow TPA infusion, catheter exchange, fluoroscopic removal/stripping)

CONTRAST REACTIONS

The following tables describe a classification system for acute reactions to contrast media—which can be either allergic-type or physiologic

Severity	Allergic-type	Physiologic
Mild *Self-limited without evidence of progression*	Limited urticaria/pruritus or cutaneous edema "Itchy"/"scratchy" throat Nasal congestion, sneezing/conjunctivitis/rhinorrhea	Limited nausea/vomiting Transient flushing/warmth/chills HA, dizziness, anxiety Mild HTN Vasovagal rxn w/ spon. resolution
Moderate *More pronounced and may req. mgmt* *May progress to severe*	Diffuse urticaria/pruritis, erythema w/ stable VS Facial edema w/o dyspnea Throat tightness or hoarseness w/o dyspnea Mild wheeze or bronchospasm w/o hypoxia	Protracted nausea/vomiting HTN urgency Isolated chest pain Vasovagal rxn responsive to Rx
Severe *Life-threatening, may result in CP arrest.* *Act quickly!*	Diffuse or facial edema w/ dyspnea, erythema w/ HoTN Laryngeal edema w/ stridor ± hypoxia Severe wheeze or bronchospasm w/ hypoxia Anaphylactic shock (HoTN + tachy)	Vasovagal rxn nonresponsive to Rx Arrhythmias Convulsions, seizures HTN emergency

Treatment of Acute Reactions to Contrast Media

Urticaria	Treatment	Dosing
Mild *scattered/transient*	No treatment often needed If symptomatic, consider Diphenhydramine (Benadryl) or Fexofenadine (Allegra) [Adults]	Adult: Diphenhydramine: 25–50 mg PO or IV, Fexofenadine: 180 mg PO Peds: Diphenhydramine: 1 mg/kg (max = 50 mg) PO, IM or IV; admin IV dose slowly over 1–2 min
Moderate *More numerous/bothersome*	Monitor VS, IV access, consider Diphenhydramine (Benadryl) (PO or IV) Fexofenadine (Allegra)	
Severe *Widespread/progressive*	Monitor VS, IV access, Diphenhydramine (Benadryl) (IV)	

Diffuse Erythema	Treatment	Dosing
All forms	IV access, monitor VS, suppl. O_2	6–10 L/min
Normotensive	No other Rx req.	
Hypotensive *Widespread/progressive*	IV fluids: NS or LR	Adult: 1000 mL rapidly Peds: 10–20 mL/kg (max = 500–1000 mL)
	Epinephrine*	Adult: IV 0.1 mg (max = 1 mg) IM 0.3 mg, q5–15 min (max = 1 mg) Peds: IV 0.01 mg/kg; (max single dose = 0.1 mg), q5–15 min (max total = 1 mg) IM 0.01 mg/kg (max single dose = 0.3 mg); q5–15 min (max total = 1 mg)

Bronchospasm	Treatment	Dosing
All forms	IV access, monitor VS, suppl. O_2, consider calling rapid response team	6–10 L/min
Mild	*Short-acting* inh β_2-agonist (SABA): Albuterol Rx of choice	2 puffs (90 µg/puff) for a total of 180 µg can repeat × 3
Moderate	SABA ± Epinephrine* (IM or IV)	Adult: IV 0.1 mg (max = 1 mg) IM 0.3 mg, q5–15 min (max = 1 mg) Peds: IV 0.01 mg/kg;(max single dose = 0.1 mg), q5–15min (max total = 1 mg) IM 0.01 mg/kg (max single dose = 0.3 mg); q5–15 min (max total = 1 mg)
Severe	SABA + Epinephrine* (IM or IV)	

Laryngeal Edema	Treatment	Dosing
All forms	IV access, monitor VS, O_2, call rapid response team	6–10 L/min
	Epinephrine* (IM or IV)	Adult: IV 0.1 mg (max = 1 mg) IM 0.3 mg, q5–15 min (max = 1 mg) Peds: IV 0.01 mg/kg (max single dose = 0.1 mg), q5–15 min (max total = 1 mg) IM 0.01 mg/kg (max single dose = 0.3 mg); q5–15 min (max total = 1 mg)

HoTN	Treatment	Dosing
All forms *Adults: SBP <90* *Peds: variable*	IV access, monitor VS, elevate legs >60°	
	O_2	6–10 L/min
	IV fluids (NS or LR)	Adult: 1000 mL rapidly Peds: 10–20 mL/kg (max = 500–1000 mL)
HoTN w/ persistent bradycardia *(Vasovagal rxn)*	Add Atropine (IV)	Adult: 0.6–1 mg (max = 3 mg) Peds: IV 0.02 mg/kg; Min single dose = 0.1 mg Max single dose = 0.6–1 mg Max total dose = 1 mg for infants and children 2 mg for adolescents
HoTN w/ persistent tachycardia *(Anaphylactoid rxn)*	Epinephrine* (IV or IM)	Adult: IV 0.1 mg (max = 1 mg) IM 0.3 mg, q5–15min (max = 1 mg) Peds: IV 0.01 mg/kg;(max single dose = 0.1 mg), q5–15 min (max total = 1 mg) IM 0.01 mg/kg (max single dose = 0.3 mg); q5–15 min (max total = 1 mg)

Unresponsive and Pulseless	Treatment	Dosing
All forms	Activate emergency response team, initiate BLS/ACLS/PALS	
	Start CPR	
	Get defibrillator, apply pads, shock as indicated	
	Epinephrine* (IV or IM)—given per ACLS algorithm (see below)	IM 0.01 mg/kg (max single dose = 0.3 mg); can repeat q5–15 min, PRN (max total = 1 mg) IV 0.01 mg/kg (max single dose (0.1 mg) can repeat q5–15 min, PRN (max total = 1 mg)

Reaction Rebound Prevention	Treatment	Dosing
Note: IV steroids may prevent a recurrence of an allergic-like rxn, not for acute Rx	Hydrocortisone (Solu-Cortef) (IV)	IV 5 mg/kg; admin over 1–2 min; (max = 200 mg)
	Methylprednisolone (Solu-Medrol) (IV)	IV 1 mg/kg; admin over 1–2 min; (max = 40 mg)

Pulmonary Edema	Treatment	Dosing
All forms	IV access, monitor VS, elevate HOB	
	O₂	6–10 L/min
	Furosemide (Lasix) (IV)	Adult: 20–40 mg IV Peds: IV 0.5–1 mg/kg (max = 40 mg)

Seizures	Treatment	Dosing
All forms	Observe and protect the pt Turn patient on side to avoid aspiration Suction airway PRN IV access Monitor VS	
	O₂	6–10 L/min
	Lorazepam (IV) [Adult]	IV 2–4 mg IV (max = 4 mg)

Hypoglycemia	Treatment	Dosing
All forms	IV access	
	O₂	6–10 L/min
Tolerating PO	Observe	
	Admin PO glc	2 sugar packets or 15 g glc tab or ½ cup (4 oz) fruit juice
Cannot tolerate PO	Dextrose (IV)	Adult: IV D50W 1 amp + D5W or D5WNS @100 mL/h Peds: IV D25 2 mL/kg; over 2 min
	Glucagon (IM/SQ)	Adult: IM 1 mg Peds: IM/SQ 0.5 mg if <20 kg IM/SW 1 mg if >20 kg

Hypertensive Crisis	Treatment	Dosing
Adults: *SBP >200* *DBP >120*	IV access, monitor VS, pulse ox	
	O₂	6–10 L/min
	Labetalol (IV)	20 mg IV, may incr dose × 2 q10 min
	Nitroglycerine tab (SL) + Furosemide (Lasix) (IV)	0.4 mg tab, q5–10 min 20–40 mg IV

Anxiety	Treatment	Dosing
All forms	Dx of exclusion	
	Assess pt for s/s of other rxns	
	IV access	
	Monitor VS	
	Pulse oximeter	
	Reassure	

(Adapted from ACR Manual on Contrast Media. 2017. 978-1-55903-012-0.)
*Epinephrine IV 0.1 mL/kg 1:10,000 dilution, IM 0.01 mL/kg of 1:1000 dilution, or Epinephrine auto-injector (<30 kg: Pediatric [EpiPen Jr or equivalent], >30 kg: Adult [EpiPen or equivalent])

ACLS

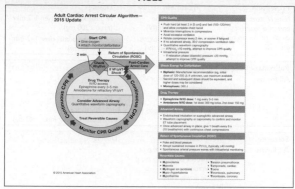

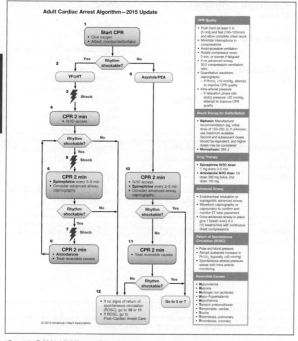

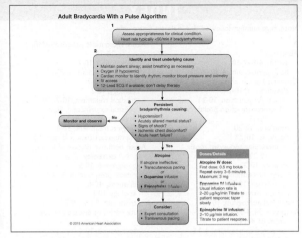

(Copyright © 2016 ACLS Training Center, https://www.acls.net. This document is current with respect to 2015 American Heart Association Guidelines for CPR and ECC. These guidelines are current until they are replaced on October 2020. If you are reading this page after October 2020, please contact ACLS Training Center at support@acls.net for an updated document.)

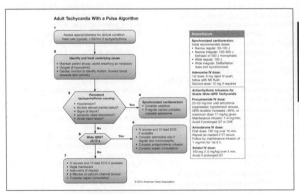

(Copyright © 2016 ACLS Training Center, https://www.acls.net. This document is current with respect to 2015 American Heart Association Guidelines for CPR and ECC. These guidelines are current until they are replaced on October 2020. If you are reading this page after October 2020, please contact ACLS Training Center at support@acls.net for an updated document.)